Understanding Diabetes Mellitus

Understanding Diabetes Mellitus

Edited by Carlos Rickman

hayle medical
New York

Hayle Medical,
750 Third Avenue, 9th Floor,
New York, NY 10017, USA

Visit us on the World Wide Web at:
www.haylemedical.com

ISBN: 978-1-63241-523-3

The publisher's policy is to use permanent paper from mills that operate a sustainable forestry policy. Furthermore, the publisher ensures that the text paper and cover boards used have met acceptable environmental accreditation standards.

Printed in China.

Cataloging-in-Publication Data

Understanding diabetes mellitus / edited by Carlos Rickman.
p. cm.
Includes bibliographical references and index.
ISBN 978-1-63241-523-3
1. Diabetes. I. Rickman, Carlos.

RC660 .U53 2018
616.462--dc23

Table of Contents

Preface IX

Chapter 1 **The Gut Microbiota Modulates Glycaemic Control and Serum Metabolite Profiles in Non-Obese Diabetic Mice** 1
Thomas U. Greiner, Tuulia Hyötyläinen, Mikael Knip, Fredrik Bäckhed, Matej Orešič

Chapter 2 **Modeling of Hypo/Hyperglycemia and their Impact on Breast Cancer Progression Related Molecules** 11
Sirin A. I. Adham, Hasina Al Rawahi, Sumaya Habib, Mansour S. Al Moundhri, Alicia Viloria-Petit, Brenda L. Coomber

Chapter 3 **High Variability in Oral Glucose Tolerance among 1,128 Patients with Cystic Fibrosis: A Multicenter Screening Study** 22
Nicole Scheuing, Reinhard W. Holl, Gerd Dockter, Julia M. Hermann, Sibylle Junge, Cordula Koerner-Rettberg, Lutz Naehrlich, Christina Smaczny, Doris Staab, Gabriela Thalhammer, Silke van Koningsbruggen-Rietschel, Manfred Ballmann

Chapter 4 **Access to Diagnostic Tests and Essential Medicines for Cardiovascular Diseases and Diabetes Care: Cost, Availability and Affordability in the West Region of Cameroon** 28
Ahmadou M. Jingi, Jean Jacques N. Noubiap, Arnold Ewane Onana, Jobert Richie N. Nansseu, Binhuan Wang, Samuel Kingue, André Pascal Kengne

Chapter 5 **Decrease in Urinary Creatinine Excretion in Early Stage Chronic Kidney Disease** 36
Elena Tynkevich, Martin Flamant, Jean-Philippe Haymann, Marie Metzger, Eric Thervet, Jean-Jacques Boffa, François Vrtovsnik, Pascal Houillier, Marc Froissart, Bénédicte Stengel

Chapter 6 **HLA Class I and Class II Associations with ESRD in Saudi Arabian Population** 47
Nuha Mahmoud Hamdi, Fadel Hassan Al-Hababi, Amr Ekhlas Eid

Chapter 7 **Regional Differences of Undiagnosed Type 2 Diabetes and Prediabetes Prevalence are not Explained by known Risk Factors** 60
Teresa Tamayo, Sabine Schipf, Christine Meisinger, Michaela Schunk, Werner Maier, Christian Herder, Michael Roden, Matthias Nauck, Annette Peters, Henry Völzke, Wolfgang Rathmann

Chapter 8 **Lifestyle Factors Associated with Type 2 Diabetes and use of Different Glucose-Lowering Drugs** 69
Sinna P. Ulrichsen, Anil Mor, Elisabeth Svensson, Finn B. Larsen, Reimar W. Thomsen

Chapter 9 **Impaired Glucose Metabolism in Response to High Fat Diet in Female Mice Conceived by *In Vitro* Fertilization (IVF) or Ovarian Stimulation Alone** 79
Miaoxin Chen, Linda Wu, Fang Wu, Gary A. Wittert, Robert J. Norman, Rebecca L. Robker, Leonie K. Heilbronn

Chapter 10 **Assessment of CD4+ T Cell Responses to Glutamic Acid Decarboxylase 65 using DQ8 Tetramers Reveals a Pathogenic Role of GAD65 121-140 and GAD65 250-266 in T1D Development** 88
I-Ting Chow, Junbao Yang, Theresa J. Gates, Eddie A. James, Duy T. Mai, Carla Greenbaum, William W. Kwok

Chapter 11 **Foreign Body Response to Subcutaneous Implants in Diabetic Rats** 97
Teresa Oviedo Socarrás, Anilton C. Vasconcelos, Paula P. Campos, Nubia B. Pereira, Jessica P. C. Souza, Silvia P. Andrade

Chapter 12 **Hypoxia in Vascular Networks: A Complex System Approach to Unravel the Diabetic Paradox** 107
Yérali Gandica, Tobias Schwarz, Orlando Oliveira, Rui D. M. Travasso

Chapter 13 **Generation of Insulin-Producing Cells from the Mouse Liver using β Cell-Related Gene Transfer Including *Mafa* and *Mafb*** 115
Haruka Nagasaki, Tokio Katsumata, Hisashi Oishi, Pei-Han Tai, Yukari Sekiguchi, Ryusuke Koshida, Yunshin Jung, Takashi Kudo, Satoru Takahashi

Chapter 14 **Relationship of Dickkopf1 (DKK1) with Cardiovascular Disease and Bone Metabolism in Caucasian Type 2 Diabetes Mellitus** 124
Antonia Garcia-Martín, Rebeca Reyes-Garcia, Beatriz García-Fontana, Sonia Morales-Santana, Ana Coto-Montes, Manuel Muñoz-Garach, Pedro Rozas-Moreno, Manuel Muñoz-Torres

Chapter 15 **Health Behaviour in Children and Adolescents with Type 1 Diabetes Compared to a Representative Reference Population** 131
Sebastian Kummer, Anna Stahl-Pehe, Katty Castillo, Christina Bächle, Christine Graf, Klaus Straßburger, Burak Salgin, Ertan Mayatepek, Guido Giani, Reinhard W. Holl, Thomas Meissner, Joachim Rosenbauer

Chapter 16 **Proximal Tubule Dysfunction is Associated with Podocyte Damage Biomarkers Nephrin and Vascular Endothelial Growth Factor in Type 2 Diabetes Mellitus Patients** 142
Ligia Petrica, Adrian Vlad, Gheorghe Gluhovschi, Florica Gadalean, Victor Dumitrascu, Cristina Gluhovschi, Silvia Velciov, Flaviu Bob, Daliborca Vlad, Roxana Popescu, Oana Milas, Sorin Ursoniu

Chapter 17 **Protective Effects of Astragaloside IV on db/db Mice with Diabetic Retinopathy** 150
Yuzhi Ding, Songtao Yuan, Xiaoyi Liu, Pingan Mao, Chen Zhao, Qiong Huang, Rihua Zhang, Yuan Fang, Qinglu Song, Dongqing Yuan, Ping Xie, Yun Liu, Qinghuai Liu

Chapter 18 **Glycemic Effects and Safety of L-Glutamine Supplementation with or without Sitagliptin in Type 2 Diabetes Patients** 158
Dorit Samocha-Bonet, Donald J. Chisholm, Fiona M. Gribble, Adelle C. F. Coster, Kevin H. Carpenter, Graham R. D. Jones, Jens J. Holst, Jerry R. Greenfield

Chapter 19 **The Sodium-Glucose Co-Transporter 2 Inhibitor Empagliflozin Improves Diabetes-Induced Vascular Dysfunction in the Streptozotocin Diabetes Rat Model by Interfering with Oxidative Stress and Glucotoxicity** 165
Matthias Oelze, Swenja Kröller-Schön, Philipp Welschof, Thomas Jansen, Michael Hausding, Yuliya Mikhed, Paul Stamm, Michael Mader, Elena Zinßius, Saule Agdauletova, Anna Gottschlich, Sebastian Steven, Eberhard Schulz, Serge P. Bottari, Eric Mayoux, Thomas Münzel, Andreas Daiber

Chapter 20 **Influence of the Time of Day and Fasting Duration on Glucose Level following a 1-Hour, 50-Gram Glucose Challenge Test in Pregnant Women** 178
Panchalli Wang, Mei-Chun Lu, Cheng-Wei Yu, Yuan-Horng Yan

Chapter 21 **The 5-Year Onset and Regression of Diabetic Retinopathy in Chinese Type 2 Diabetes Patients** 185
Peiyao Jin, Jinjuan Peng, Haidong Zou, Weiwei Wang, Jiong Fu, Binjie Shen, Xuelin Bai, Xun Xu, Xi Zhang

Chapter 22 **Measurement of Visceral Fat: Should we Include Retroperitoneal Fat?** 192
Chi-Sheng Hung, Jen-Kuang Lee, Chung-Yi Yang, Hung-Ren Hsieh, Wen-Ya Ma, Mao-Shin Lin, Pi-Hua Liu, Shyang-Rong Shih, Jyh-Ming Liou, Lee-Ming Chuang, Ming-Fong Chen, Jou-Wei Lin, Jung-Nan Wei, Hung-Yuan Li

Chapter 23 **Differential Regulation of Human Aortic Smooth Muscle Cell Proliferation by Monocyte-Derived Macrophages from Diabetic Patients** 200
Te-Chuan Chen, Mao-Ling Sung, Hsing-Chun Kuo, Shao-Ju Chien, Chia-Kuang Yen, Cheng-Nan Chen

Chapter 24 **Possible Contribution of Taurine to Distorted Glucagon Secretion in Intra-Islet Insulin Deficiency: A Metabolome Analysis using a Novel α-Cell Model of Insulin-Deficient Diabetes** 208
Megumi Bessho, Yuko Murase-Mishiba, Akihisa Imagawa, Jungo Terasaki, Toshiaki Hanafusa

Permissions

List of Contributors

Index

Preface

This book has been an outcome of determined endeavour from a group of educationists in the field. The primary objective was to involve a broad spectrum of professionals from diverse cultural background involved in the field for developing new researches. The book not only targets students but also scholars pursuing higher research for further enhancement of the theoretical and practical applications of the subject.

Diabetes is a disorder which is caused by high sugar levels for a long period of time. Some of the symptoms of this illness are increased thirst and hunger, fatigue, weight loss and blurred vision. If not treated initially it can cause heart diseases, chronic kidney failure, foot ulcers and problems in the eye. Maintaining a healthy lifestyle with a proper diet and exercise can help in management of diabetes. This book provides comprehensive insights into the topic of diabetes mellitus. For all those who are interested in studying diabetes, this book can prove to be an essential guide.

It was an honour to edit such a profound book and also a challenging task to compile and examine all the relevant data for accuracy and originality. I wish to acknowledge the efforts of the contributors for submitting such brilliant and diverse chapters in the field and for endlessly working for the completion of the book. Last, but not the least; I thank my family for being a constant source of support in all my research endeavours.

Editor

1

The Gut Microbiota Modulates Glycaemic Control and Serum Metabolite Profiles in Non-Obese Diabetic Mice

Thomas U. Greiner[1], Tuulia Hyötyläinen[2,3], Mikael Knip[4,5,6,7], Fredrik Bäckhed[1,8]*, Matej Orešič[2,3]*

1 The Wallenberg Laboratory and Sahlgrenska Center for Cardiovascular and Metabolic Research, Department of Molecular and Clinical Medicine, Institute of Medicine, University of Gothenburg, Gothenburg, Sweden, **2** VTT Technical Research Centre of Finland, Espoo, Finland, **3** Steno Diabetes Center, Gentofte, Denmark, **4** Children's Hospital, University of Helsinki and Helsinki University Central Hospital, Helsinki, Finland, **5** Diabetes and Obesity Research Program, University of Helsinki, Helsinki, Finland, **6** Folkhälsan Research Center, Helsinki, Finland, **7** Department of Pediatrics, Tampere University Hospital, Tampere, Finland, **8** Novo Nordisk Foundation Center for Basic Metabolic Research, Section for Metabolic Receptology and Enteroendocrinology, Faculty of Health Sciences, University of Copenhagen, Copenhagen, Denmark

Abstract

Islet autoimmunity in children who later progress to type 1 diabetes is preceded by dysregulated serum metabolite profiles, but the origin of these metabolic changes is unknown. The gut microbiota affects host metabolism and changes in its composition contribute to several immune-mediated diseases; however, it is not known whether the gut microbiota is involved in the early metabolic disturbances in progression to type 1 diabetes. We rederived non-obese diabetic (NOD) mice as germ free to explore the potential role of the gut microbiota in the development of diabetic autoimmunity and to directly investigate whether the metabolic profiles associated with the development of type 1 diabetes can be modulated by the gut microbiota. The absence of a gut microbiota in NOD mice did not affect the overall diabetes incidence but resulted in increased insulitis and levels of interferon gamma and interleukin 12; these changes were counterbalanced by improved peripheral glucose metabolism. Furthermore, we observed a markedly increased variation in blood glucose levels in the absence of a microbiota in NOD mice that did not progress to diabetes. Additionally, germ-free NOD mice had a metabolite profile similar to that of pre-diabetic children. Our data suggest that germ-free NOD mice have reduced glycaemic control and dysregulated immunologic and metabolic responses.

Editor: Paolo Fiorina, Children's Hospital Boston/Harvard Medical School, United States of America

Funding: This work was supported by the Human Frontier of Science Program (RGY64/2008 to FB and MO), Juvenile Diabetes Research Foundation (36-2008-919 to MO and FB), DIAPREPP and BETABAT projects of the Seventh Framework Program of the European Community (HEALTH- 2008-202013 and HEALTH-2011-277713, respectively, to MO), Academy of Finland Centre of Excellence in Molecular Systems Immunology and Physiology Research (SyMMyS, 2012-2017, Decision No. 250114 to MO and MK), The Swedish Research Council, The Swedish Child Diabetes Foundation, Swedish Foundation for Strategic Research and a LUA-ALF grant from Västra Götalandsregionen. The funders had no role in study design, data collection and analysis, decision to publish, or preparation of the manuscript.

* Email: fredrik.backhed@wlab.gu.se (FB); mtjo@steno.dk (MO)

Introduction

Type 1 diabetes is an autoimmune disorder characterized by the specific destruction of insulin-producing beta cells in the pancreas [1]. The incidence of type 1 diabetes among children and adolescents has increased markedly in western countries in recent decades [2]. In contrast to other autoimmune diseases with a clear female bias, type 1 diabetes has no clear gender separation in children and has a male bias in young adults [3]. Genetic risk factors affect disease incidence; however, less than 10% of the individuals carrying human leukocyte antigen (HLA) risk alleles develop diabetes and the concordance between monozygotic twins is less than 40%, suggesting that environmental factors are important for disease development [4,5]. Infections as well as dietary factors have been implicated as triggers of autoimmunity and disease progression [6] and, according to the hygiene hypothesis, infections early in life could prevent allergic diseases [7]. Despite promising results in rodent models, clinical trials to treat type 1 diabetes using immunotherapy such as anti-CD3 monoclonal antibodies or cytotoxic T lymphocyte antigen-immunoglobulin (CTLA4-Ig) have only shown a partial improvement of the disease [8–10]. Recent trials using haematopoietic stem cell transplantation as a treatment of type 1 diabetes have shown promising results but it is still unclear whether it can safely be used to treat all patients [8]. Thus, there is still a need to identify new factors that trigger type 1 diabetes that may be targeted in treatment of the disease.

The gut microbiota is a complex microbial ecosystem that is considered to be a major driving force in immunological maturation [11]. Its profound role in regulating host metabolism has become evident in recent years [12] and emerging evidence indicates that it is a possible modulator of diabetes. Several reports have demonstrated that an altered microbiota is associated with risk of developing type 2 diabetes [13,14] and both preclinical and clinical type 1 diabetes [15,16]. Furthermore, maternal use of phenoxymethyl or quinolone antimicrobials before pregnancy is associated with an increased risk of type 1 diabetes in the offspring [17,18]. Studies in non-obese diabetic (NOD) mice suggest a direct involvement of the gut microbiota in the development of autoimmune diabetes [19,20]. However, the mechanisms that link the microbiota with autoimmune disease remain to be determined.

A recent report suggested that microbially driven increases in testosterone levels can explain the relative protection against diabetes observed in male NOD mice [21]. However, because puberty does not confer protection against type 1 diabetes in men [3], it is unclear whether this microbially derived effect is present in humans and suggests that there are additional effects of the microbiota on type 1 diabetes development that are not gender dependent.

Changes in the microbiota have been shown to affect the metabolome of the host and our previous metabolomics study revealed that metabolic abnormalities precede islet autoimmunity in children who later progress to type 1 diabetes independent of HLA-associated genetic risk [22]. We also showed that lipidomic profiles of children who progress to type 1 diabetes are similar to those of female NOD mice [23]. Here we rederived NOD mice as germ free (GF) to investigate the microbial influence on diabetic autoimmunity and to directly investigate whether the metabolic profiles associated with the development of type 1 diabetes can be modulated by the gut microbiota.

Materials and Methods

Mice

GF NOD mice were rederived at Taconic farms and were thereafter maintained in flexible plastic film isolators under a strict 12-h light cycle (lights on at 06:00 h) at the University of Gothenburg. GF status was verified regularly by anaerobic culturing in addition to PCR for bacterial 16S rDNA. Both GF and conventionally raised (CONV-R) NOD mice were fed autoclaved chow diet (Labdiet) *ad libitum*. Diabetes incidence was determined by monitoring blood glucose levels weekly by sampling of a small volume of blood from the tail vein. Mice were considered diabetic when values exceeded 18 mM for two consecutive weeks or 25 mM for one week. Blood for metabolomics and cytokine analyses was collected from the *vena cava* at the termination of the experiment under deep isoflurane anesthesia after a 4 h fast, unless otherwise stated. This study was carried out in accordance with the recommendations for Laboratory Animals in Sweden. The protocol was approved by the Committee on the Ethics of Animal Experiments at the University of Gothenburg (Permit Number: 338–2012). All efforts were made to minimize animal suffering.

Insulitis and beta cell area

Sections 200–300 μm apart from the pancreas of 4-, 9- and 23-week-old mice were stained with haematoxylin and eosin and scored according to the following criteria: no infiltration (0); peri-insulitis (1); ≤50% destruction of islet (2); ≥50% destruction of islet (3). We scored 100 (at 4 and 9 weeks) and 50 (at 23 weeks) islets per mouse. For beta cell area, sections 300 μm apart through the whole pancreas were stained with guinea pig anti-insulin (Dako), visualized using VECTASTAIN ABC and Vulcan Fast Red Chromogen Kit 2 (Histolab), and counterstained with haematoxylin. The area stained for insulin was compared with the total area of the tissue using Biopix software.

Insulin autoantibodies

Serum insulin autoantibodies (IAA) were analysed using a competitive radiobinding assay as previously described [15]. The results were expressed in relative units (RU) based on standard curves run on each plate. The cut-off value for mouse IAA positivity was set at the mean+3SDS in 29 BALB-mice, i.e. 0.88 RU.

Cytokine measurements

Serum from mice at 15 and 23 weeks was analysed with Mesoscale 9-plex cytokine assay according to the manufacturer's instructions.

Oral glucose tolerance test (OGTT) and insulin measurements

Mice aged 17–18 weeks were fasted for 4 h and orally gavaged with 20% D-glucose (2 g/kg). Blood was drawn from the tail vein at 0, 15, 30, 60, 90 and 120 min and blood glucose levels were measured using a HemoCue glucometer. Insulin levels were measured at 0, 15 and 30 min after gavage. In mice that did not progress to diabetes by 30 weeks of age, insulin levels were measured after a 4 h fast. Insulin was measured using insulin ELISA-kit (Crystal Chem).

Analysis of polar metabolites by GC×GC-TOFMS

An established metabolomics platform using two dimensional gas chromatography coupled to time-of-flight mass spectrometry (GC×GC-TOFMS) was used to analyse polar metabolites in serum [24]. Serum samples (30 μl) were combined with 10 μl of an internal standard, labelled palmitic acid (16:0–16,16,16d3; 500 mg/l), and 400 μl of methanol, vortexed for 2 min and incubated for 30 min at room temperature. The supernatant was separated by centrifugation at 5590 *g* for 5 min at room temperature. The sample was dried under a constant flow of nitrogen. Twenty-five μl of 2% methoxyamine hydrochloride in pyridine was added to the dried sample and incubated at 45°C for 1 h and then derivatized with 25 μl of N-methyl-N-(trimethylsilyl)-trifluoroacetamide by incubating at 45°C for 1 h. Five μl of retention index standard mixture with five alkanes (400 mg/l) was added to the metabolite mixture. Sample order for analysis was established by randomization. The samples were analysed on a Leco Pegasus 4D GC×GC-TOF mass spectrometer with Agilent technologies 6890N GC and Combi PAL autosampler. Data were processed using the Guineu software [24].

Analysis of molecular lipids by UPLC-MS

An established platform based on Acquity Ultra Performance LC coupled to time-of-flight mass spectrometry (UPLC-MS) was used to analyse the molecular lipids in aliquots (10 μl) of serum samples [25]. The data were processed using MZmine 2 software [26] and the lipid identification was based on an internal spectral library or on *de novo* identification using tandem MS [25].

Statistical analysis

Data were analysed by Student's t test and presented as mean ± SEM or SD. Survival curves were analysed with log-rank (Mantel-Cox) test. IAA positivity was analysed by Fisher's exact test. Univariate statistical analysis of metabolomics data used MATLAB r2012a. Clustering was performed and visualized using the MeV software [27].

Results

Colonization status affects insulitis and the presence of IAA in NOD mice

To investigate the potential role of the gut microbiota in the development of type 1 diabetes, we rederived NOD mice as GF. Female NOD mice developed diabetes at a higher rate and at an earlier time point than male NOD mice (Fig. 1A), in agreement with a previous report [28]. Disease onset was earlier in GF compared with CONV-R male NOD mice but no difference was observed between female GF and CONV-R NOD mice (Fig. 1A). There was no significant difference between diabetes progression of GF and CONV-R NOD mice (both male and female) by 30 weeks (Fig. 1A).

To further investigate autoimmunity in the NOD mice, we investigated the rate of islet infiltration (Fig. 1B). At 9 weeks, there was a tendency towards enhanced insulitis in male GF NOD mice and a significant increase in insulitis in female GF NOD mice compared with their CONV-R NOD counterparts (Fig. 1C, D). The difference in rate of infiltration was only transient since there was no difference in insulitis score between GF and CONV-R NOD mice that had not yet progressed to diabetes at 23 weeks

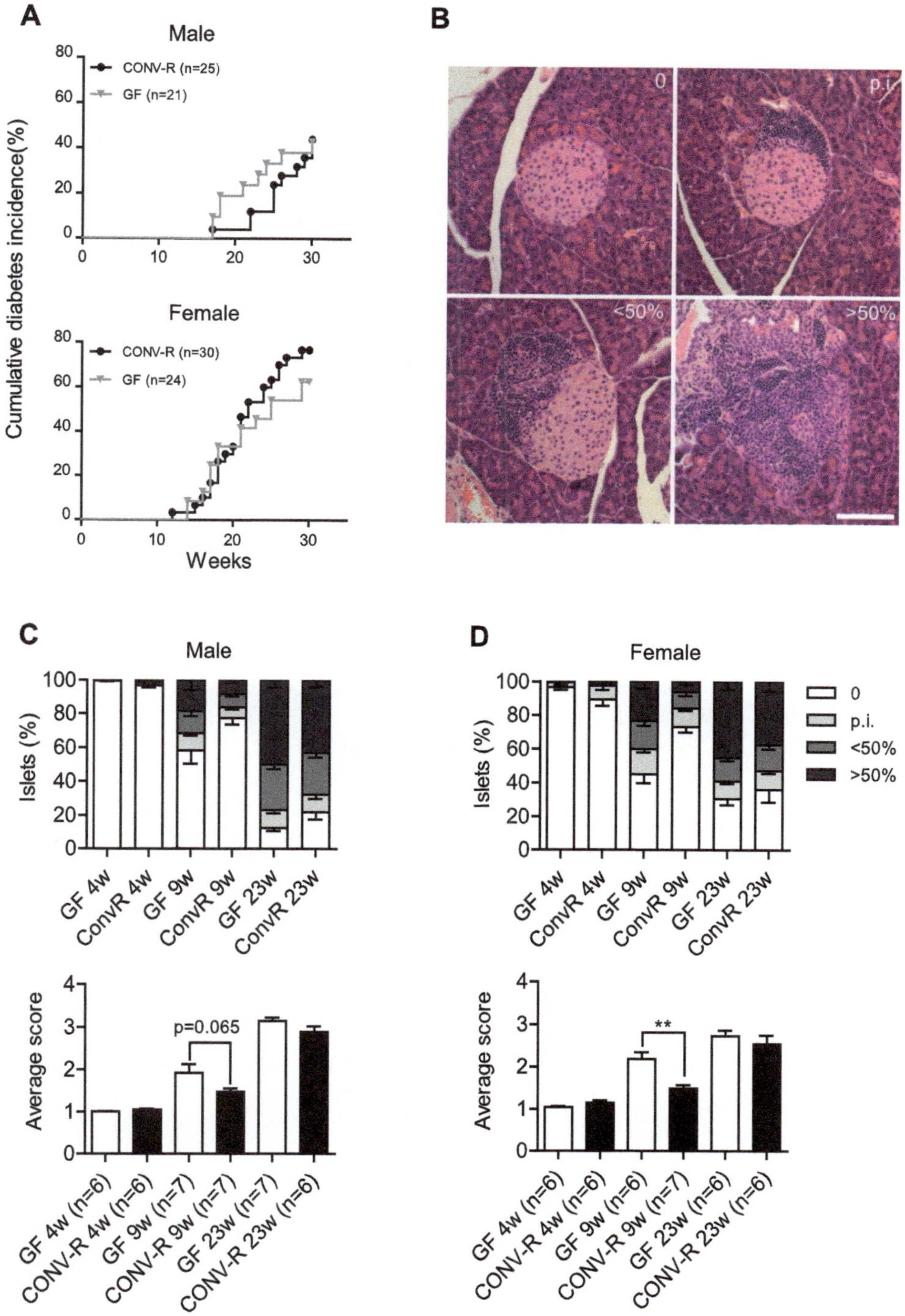

Figure 1. Diabetes incidence and insulitis in NOD mice. (A) Cumulative diabetes incidence in male and female GF and CONV-R mice. (B) Representative images of islets in four insulitis categories: 0 (no infiltration); p.i. (peri-insulitis); <50% destruction; >50% destruction. Scale bar represents 100 μm. (C, D) Distribution of islet scores and average insulitis score in GF and CONVR male (C) and female (D) mice at 4, 9 and 23 weeks (n = 6–7). Data are presented as mean ± s.e.m. **p<0.01 determined by Student's *t*-test.

(Fig. 1C, D). In addition, we did not observe any differences in beta cell area of the pancreas in female NOD mice at 23 weeks (Fig. S1).

We observed that GF NOD mice were significantly more likely to be positive for IAA compared with CONV-R NOD mice at 4 weeks (Table 1) and autoantibody titers were higher in GF compared with CONV-R NOD mice at 9 weeks (Fig. S2).

Colonization status affects serum cytokine levels

To analyse potential changes in immunological parameters in response to the absence of microbiota, we analysed interleukin 10 (IL-10), interferon gamma (IFN-γ) and interleukin 12 (IL-12). At 15 weeks, IL-10 levels were higher in GF versus CONV-R male NOD mice, but no differences were noted for IFN-γ and IL-12 (Fig. 2A–C). However, at 23 weeks, levels of IFN-γ and IL-12 were significantly higher in male and female GF NOD mice compared with their CONV-R counterparts (Fig. 2B, C) and IL-10 levels were reduced in female CONV-R mice (Fig. 2A).

Improved peripheral glucose metabolism in GF NOD mice

We hypothesized that peripheral glucose metabolism is improved in NOD mice lacking a microbiota, which may partly explain why we did not observe an increased rate of diabetes incidence in GF NOD mice despite an increase in IAA and pro-inflammatory cytokines compared with CONV-R NOD mice. At 30 weeks, fasting glucose levels were not different between GF and CONV-R non-progressing male NOD mice, but fasting insulin levels were lower in the GF mice (Fig. 3A, B), indicating an improved peripheral glucose metabolism similar to GF wild-type mice on different genetic backgrounds [29,30]. We also performed an OGTT in GF and CONV-R NOD mice at 17–18 weeks of age (in the total group, i.e. both non-progressors and progressors). We observed a faster glucose clearance in GF versus CONV-R female NOD mice and a tendency towards improved glucose tolerance in GF versus CONV-R male NOD mice (Fig. S3). Insulin levels after an OGTT were not different between GF and CONV-R NOD mice (Fig. S3), indicating that the improved glucose clearance in GF NOD mice was not due to enhanced insulin secretion.

Dysregulation of blood glucose in non-progressing GF NOD mice

Although we did not see any difference in diabetes incidence between GF and CONV-R NOD mice, we observed striking differences when we analysed the non-fasting blood glucose levels in the mice that did not progress to diabetes by 30 weeks of age (Fig. 3C–H). At 12 weeks, blood glucose levels were lower in non-progressing GF NOD male mice compared with their CONV-R counterparts (Fig. 3C). However, from 20 weeks, blood glucose levels were significantly higher in non-progressing GF compared with CONV-R NOD mice (Fig. 3C, D). The mean blood glucose levels and the percent relative standard deviation (%RSD) in blood glucose levels per mouse from 12–30 weeks were higher in non-progressing GF compared with CONV-R NOD mice (Fig. 3E–H),

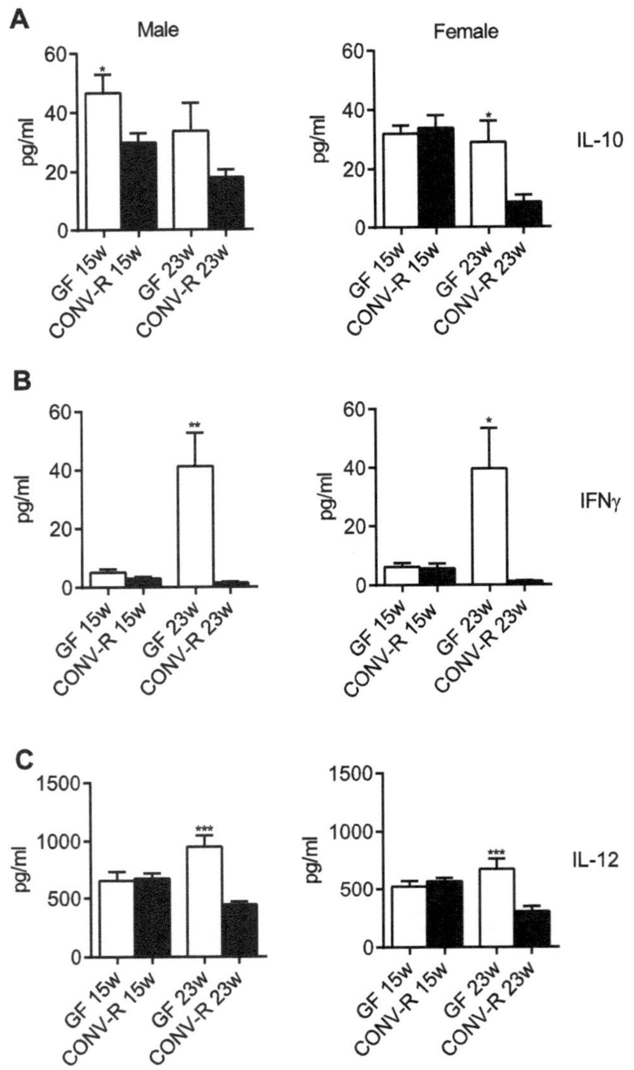

Figure 2. Altered serum levels of pro- and anti-inflammatory cytokines in GF NOD mice. Serum levels of IL-10 (A), interferon gamma (B) and IL-12 (C) in male and female mice at 15 and 23 weeks. Data are presented as mean ± s.e.m. *p<0.05, **p<0.01, ***p<0.001 GF vs CONV-R mice determined by Student's *t*-test. (Female: 15 weeks n = 9; 23 weeks n = 5. Male: 15 weeks n = 6; 23 weeks n = 7.).

Table 1. Proportion of insulin autoantibody (IAA)-positive mice in relation to age.

Age	GF	CONV-R	P value
4 weeks	76.5% (n = 17)	38.9% (n = 18)	0.041
9 weeks	92.9% (n = 14)	61.9% (n = 21)	0.056
23 weeks	90% (n = 20)	75% (n = 16)	0.374

Analysis of serum samples of germ-free (GF) and conventionally raised (CONV-R) NOD mice. Data were analyzed by Fisher's exact test.

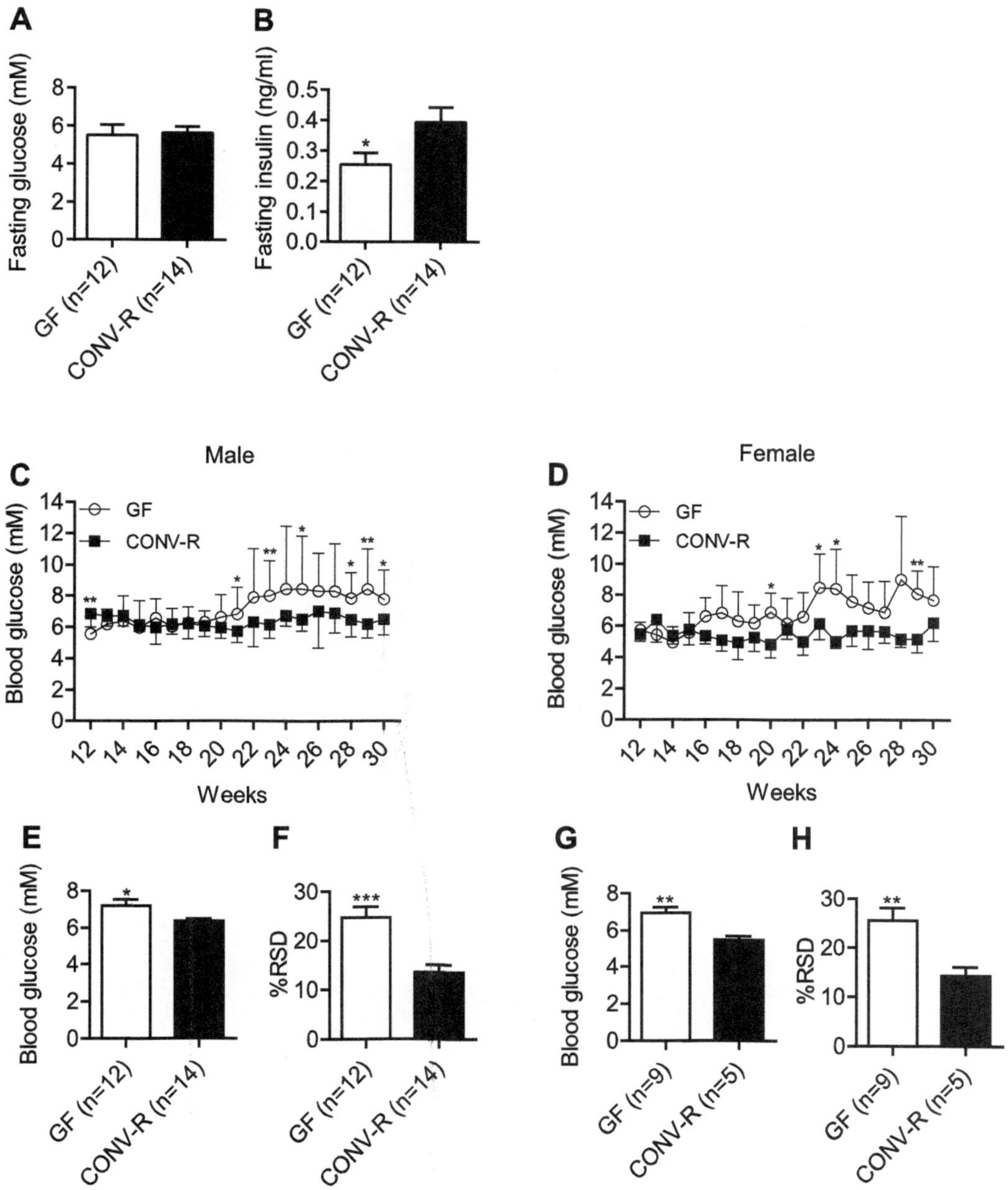

Figure 3. Altered blood glucose control in GF NOD mice. (A,B) Fasting blood glucose (A) and insulin levels (B) in male non-progressing mice 30 weeks of age. (C,D) Non-fasting blood glucose levels in non-diabetic male (GF n = 12, CONV-R n = 14) (C) and female (GF n = 9, CONV-R n = 5) (D) mice from 12–30 weeks. (E–H) Average blood glucose levels per mouse and percent relative standard deviation (RSD) of glucose values per mouse from 12–30 weeks in male (E,F) and female (G,H) mice. Data are presented as mean ± s.e.m. (A, B, E–H) or mean ± s.d. (C,D). *p<0.05, **p<0.01, ***p<0.001 vs CONV-R mice determined by Student's *t*-test.

further demonstrating the decrease in blood glucose control in both male and female GF NOD mice.

Colonization status affects the serum metabolic profile in NOD mice

To investigate whether the early metabolic abnormalities preceding islet autoimmunity in children who progressed to type 1 diabetes observed in a previous human study [22] might be modulated by the gut microbiota, we performed global metabolomic analysis of serum taken from GF and CONV-R NOD mice (both non-progressors and progressors to autoimmune diabetes). Two analytical platforms with broad analytical coverage were applied to all samples: (1) a global lipidomics platform based on UPLC-MS, which covers molecular lipids such as phospholipids, sphingolipids, and neutral lipids; and (2) a platform for global profiling of small polar metabolites based on comprehensive two-dimensional GC×GC-TOFMS, which covers small molecules such as amino acids, free fatty acids, keto-acids, various other organic acids, sterols, and sugars. A total of 358 molecular lipids and 195 polar metabolites were detected and included in the analysis. When observing the significantly altered metabolites in young mice, we found that the colonization status was the dominant factor that affected the clustering of metabolic profiles (Fig. 4), in agreement with recent findings by Markle et al. [21].

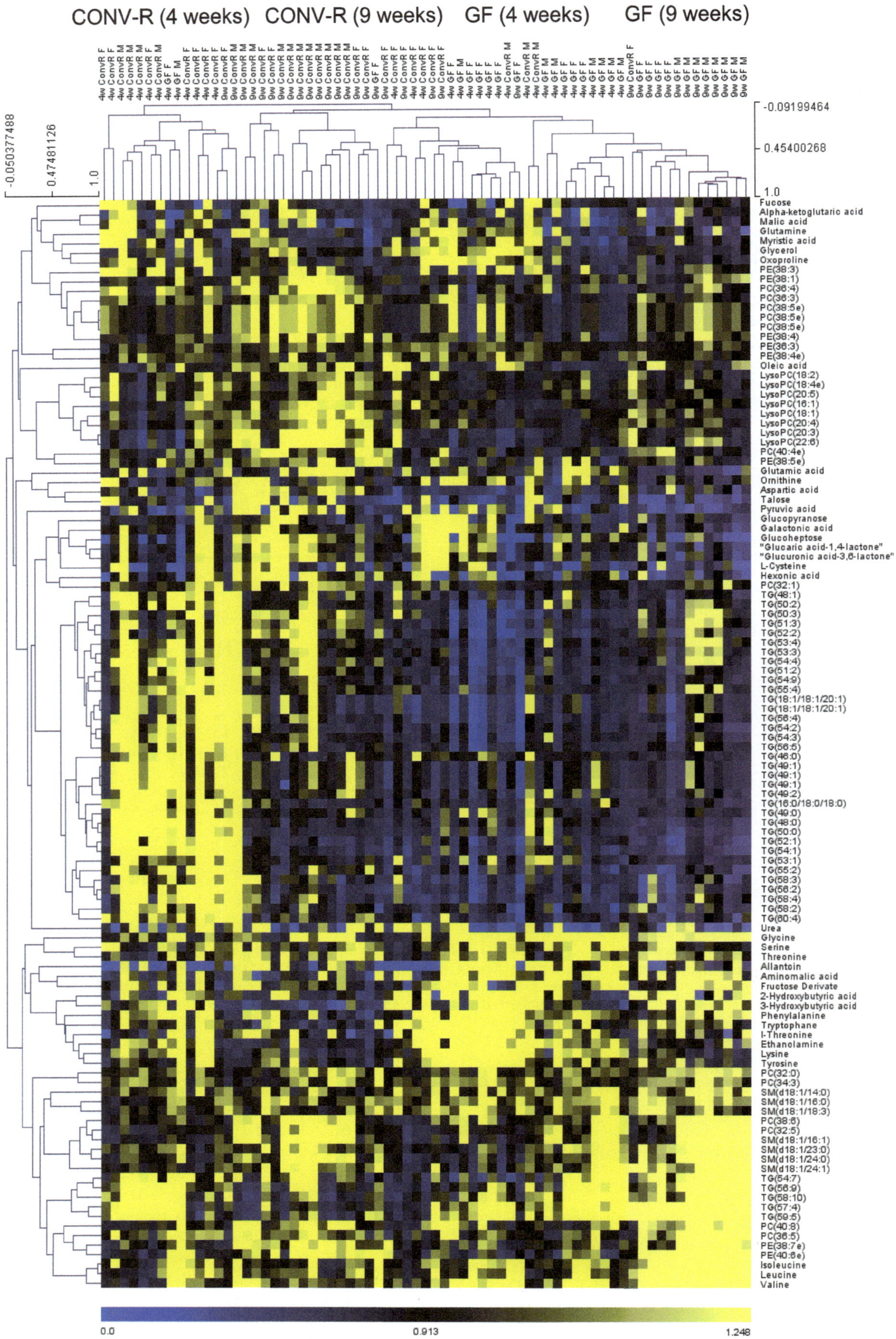
CONV-R (4 weeks)
CONV-R (9 weeks)
GF (4 weeks)
GF (9 weeks)
-0.050377488
0.47481126
1.0
-0.09199464
0.45400268
1.0
Fucose
Alpha-ketoglutaric acid
Malic acid
Glutamine
Myristic acid
Glycerol
Oxoproline
PE(38:3)
PE(38:1)
PC(36:4)
PC(36:3)
PC(38:5e)
PC(38:5e)
PC(38:5e)
PE(38:4)
PE(36:3)
PE(38:4e)
Oleic acid
LysoPC(18:2)
LysoPC(18:4e)
LysoPC(20:5)
LysoPC(16:1)
LysoPC(18:1)
LysoPC(20:4)
LysoPC(20:3)
LysoPC(22:6)
PC(40:4e)
PE(38:5e)
Glutamic acid
Ornithine
Aspartic acid
Talose
Pyruvic acid
Glucopyranose
Galactonic acid
Glucoheptose
"Glucaric acid-1,4-lactone"
"Glucuronic acid-3,6-lactone"
L-Cysteine
Hexonic acid
PC(32:1)
TG(48:1)
TG(50:2)
TG(50:3)
TG(51:3)
TG(52:2)
TG(53:4)
TG(53:3)
TG(54:4)
TG(51:2)
TG(54:9)
TG(55:4)
TG(18:1/18:1/20:1)
TG(18:1/18:1/20:1)
TG(56:4)
TG(54:2)
TG(54:3)
TG(56:5)
TG(46:0)
TG(49:1)
TG(49:1)
TG(49:1)
TG(49:2)
TG(16:0/18:0/18:0)
TG(49:0)
TG(48:0)
TG(50:0)
TG(52:1)
TG(54:1)
TG(53:1)
TG(55:2)
TG(58:3)
TG(56:2)
TG(58:4)
TG(58:2)
TG(60:4)
Urea
Glycine
Serine
Threonine
Allantoin
Aminomalic acid
Fructose Derivate
2-Hydroxybutyric acid
3-Hydroxybutyric acid
Phenylalanine
Tryptophane
l-Threonine
Ethanolamine
Lysine
Tyrosine
PC(32:0)
PC(34:3)
SM(d18:1/14:0)
SM(d18:1/16:0)
SM(d18:1/18:3)
PC(38:6)
PC(32:5)
SM(d18:1/16:1)
SM(d18:1/23:0)
SM(d18:1/24:0)
SM(d18:1/24:1)
TG(54:7)
TG(56:9)
TG(58:10)
TG(57:4)
TG(59:5)
PC(40:8)
PC(36:5)
PE(38:7e)
PE(40:6e)
Isoleucine
Leucine
Valine
0.0
0.913
1.248

Figure 4. Heatmap of significantly altered identified metabolites in GF and CONV-R NOD mice in 4- and 9-week old mice. For each metabolite, the levels in each mouse are normalized to the mean level in CONV-R mice, i.e., yellow and blue indicate increased and decreased levels of the metabolites, respectively, relative to the average level in CONV-R mice. Hierarchical clustering is applied across all metabolites (performed across all n = 69 samples analyzed) and all mice. (Female n = 6–10. Male n = 7–11.).

Within the GF and CONV-R groups, we observed subclustering by age and gender (Fig. 4).

The colonization status had a similar effect on metabolic profiles of 4- and 9-week-old mice ($r = 0.52$, $P<0.001$, for the associations of CONV-R/GF fold changes in 4- and 9-week old mice for the 156 significantly different metabolites). As expected, the metabolites of similar structural class tended to co-cluster (Fig. 4), thus allowing for comparison of metabolic profiles at the class level. GF NOD mice had reduced levels of tricarboxylic acid (TCA) cycle metabolites, sugar derivatives and triglycerides compared with CONV-R mice (Fig. 4). Furthermore, branched chain amino acids (BCAAs) were elevated at 9 and 23 weeks in male GF NOD mice and at 4 and 9 weeks in female GF NOD mice (Figs. 4, 5). There was also an elevated cluster of metabolites in the profile of GF NOD mice that consisted primarily of amino acids including glycine, phenylalanine, tyrosine and 2-hydroxybutyric acid (Fig. 4).

We previously observed that differences between the cord serum metabolomes of newborn infants who progress to type 1 diabetes and their controls are similar to differences found between the 9-week-old GF and CONV-R Swiss Webster mice [31]. To determine whether these similarities were also observed in the NOD mice, we compared previously acquired human data from 15 type 1 diabetes progressors and 24 controls [22] with the metabolomics dataset from 9-week-old GF and CONV-R NOD mice. Triglycerides were excluded from the comparison due to high variability in the clinical dataset. A total of 53 lipids and 25 polar metabolites were matched across the datasets. We found that the difference in the metabolome of type 1 diabetes human progressors compared with controls significantly correlated with that of GF compared with CONV-R NOD mice ($r = 0.43$, $P = 7.0 \times 10^{-5}$, comparing mean concentrations of each of the 78 metabolites in type 1 diabetes progressors and GF mice, scaled by mean concentrations in non-progressors and CONV-R mice, respectively).

Discussion

Here we identified a profound role of the gut microbiota in the regulation of glycaemic control as well as of immunological and metabolic profiles in a mouse model of autoimmune diabetes. The absence of gut microbiota in NOD mice did not affect overall disease incidence, but resulted in increased insulitis and levels of IAA and pro-inflammatory cytokines, and worsened glucose control in mice that did not progress to diabetes. Furthermore, we observed differences in the serum metabolomic profiles between GF and CONV-R NOD mice that resembled the difference between those of newborn infants who later progress to type 1 diabetes and non-progressors, suggesting that the metabolomic changes in infants who later progress to type 1 diabetes may be modulated by the gut microbiota.

The similarity in diabetes incidence in both male and female mice between GF and CONV-R NOD is in agreement with earlier studies [21,32]. We observed an increase in insulitis in GF NOD mice at 9 weeks, again consistent with previous results [32], but the effect was only transient and there was no difference in beta cell area in older mice. Disease incidence is affected by housing conditions [33] and the relatively high disease incidence in our CONV-R mice could be explained by the clean housing conditions in our specific pathogen free facility. IAA positivity was more frequent at 4 weeks of age in GF versus CONV-R NOD mice, which may mirror progressive beta cell autoimmunity [34] and contribute to the enhanced beta cell destruction indicated by the increased insulitis at 9 weeks. The gut microbiota is known to affect B-cell development [35] and B-cells have been shown to be important contributors to diabetes progression in the NOD mouse model [36]. However, the difference in IAA production from B-cells did not contribute to an effect on overall diabetes incidence.

We observed that levels of IFN-γ and IL-12 were higher in GF compared with CONV-R NOD mice at 23 weeks in both male and female mice. These cytokines are known to influence diabetes progression in NOD mice [37], and IL-12-induced secretion of IFN-γ at the effector stage of diabetes development has previously been shown to promote diabetes in NOD mice [38,39]. The increase in IL-12 and IFN-γ at 23 weeks was paralleled by an increase in autoantibody titers in GF NOD mice, consistent with an association between these cytokines and autoimmunity. In addition, we observed a decrease in IL-10 levels in female CONV-R at 23 weeks of age. IL-10 has been shown to protect against diabetes in NOD mice but only when administered from an early age [40], and thus the reduction in IL-10 levels we observed might not have an influence on autoimmunity.

Earlier studies have shown that GF wild-type mice have improved peripheral glucose metabolism compared with their CONV-R counterparts [30]. We therefore tested the hypothesis that the incidence of diabetes is similar in GF and CONV-R NOD mice because improved peripheral glucose metabolism counterbalances the increased autoimmunity in GF NOD mice. In agreement with our hypothesis, we showed that fasting insulin levels in NOD mice that had not progressed to diabetes by 30 weeks were lower in GF versus CONV-R mice despite similar fasting glucose levels. Furthermore, female GF NOD mice had improved glucose clearance at 17–18 weeks. We propose that the GF NOD mice are more resistant to developing diabetes because lower levels of insulin are required to maintain normoglycaemia in these mice. However, the blood glucose levels of the GF NOD mice that had not progressed to diabetes by 30 weeks increased after 20 weeks of age with considerably higher variability compared with CONV-R NOD mice in both male and female mice, suggesting that blood glucose control in the non-fasting state is reduced in GF NOD mice.

We observed differences in the global profiles of polar metabolites and molecular lipids between 9-week-old GF and CONV-R NOD mice that were similar to those reported earlier between GF and CONV-R Swiss Webster mice [31]. Specifically, as previously seen in GF wild-type Swiss Webster mice, GF NOD mice had reduced levels of TCA cycle metabolites, sugar derivatives and triglycerides compared with their CONV-R counterparts. However, in contrast to an increase in only one BCAA (valine) in GF versus CONV-R Swiss Webster mice [31], we observed an increase in all three BCAAs (isoleucine, valine and leucine) in GF versus CONV-R NOD mice irrespective of gender. Increased levels of BCAAs predict both type 1 and 2 diabetes [22,41,42] and have been shown to contribute to insulin resistance [43]. An abnormal insulin response caused by increased levels of

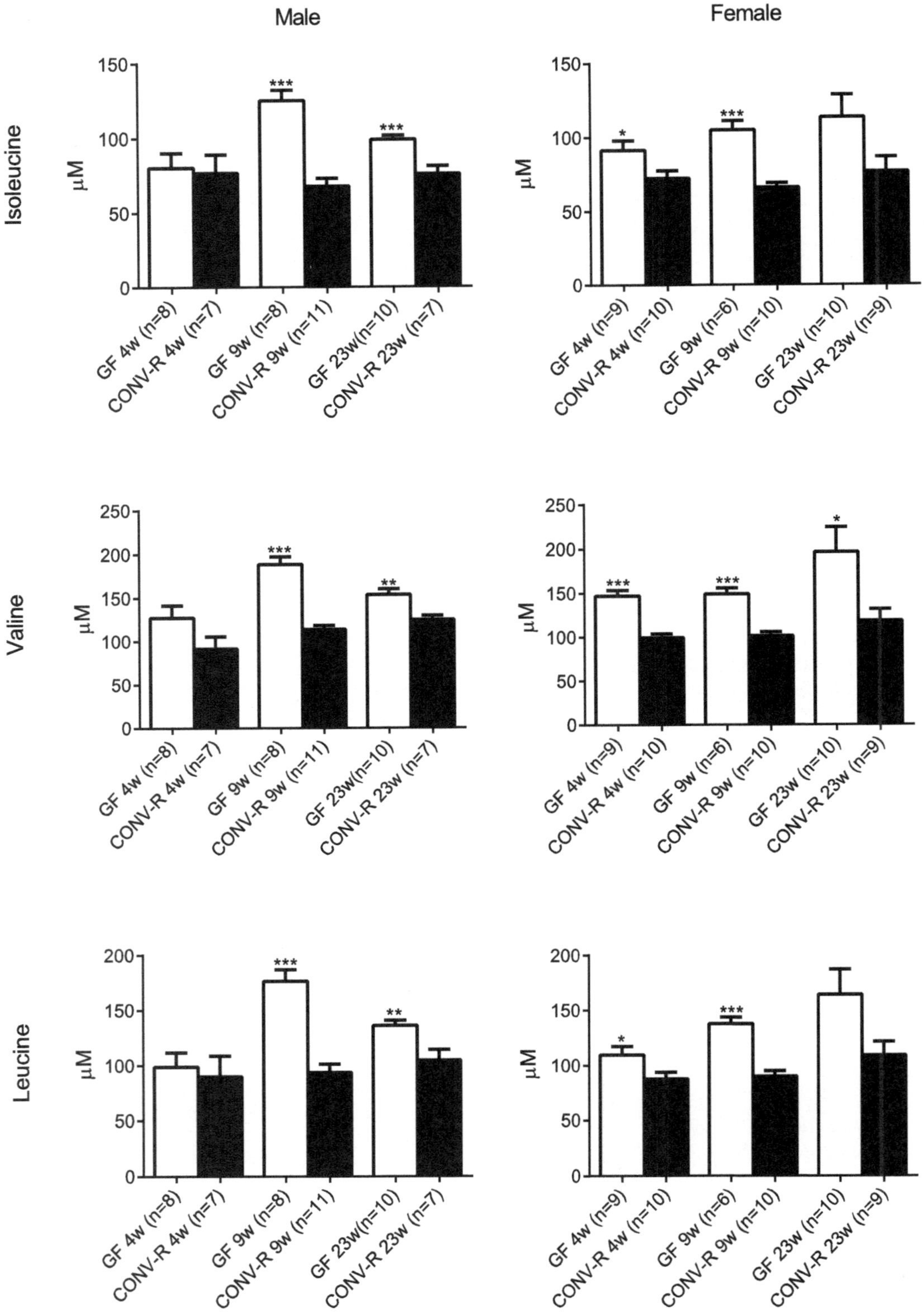

Figure 5. Increased levels of branched chain amino acids in GF NOD mice. Relative concentrations of branched chain amino acids mice at 4, 9 and 23 weeks. (Male n = 7–11. Female n = 9–14.) Data are presented as mean ±s.e.m. *p<0.05, **p<0.01, ***p<0.001 vs CONV-R mice determined by Student's *t*-test.

BCAAs could thus potentially explain the reduced glycaemic control in GF NOD mice.

We also observed an increase in the amino acids glycine, phenylalanine, tyrosine and 2-hydroxybutyric acid in GF versus CONV-R NOD mice, which was not seen in the previous study in GF versus CONV-R Swiss Webster mice [31]. These metabolites are associated with progression to insulin resistance and type 2 diabetes [41,42,44] but it is unclear whether they also affect beta cell function.

The differences in the metabolic profiles between GF and CONV-R NOD mice in our study correlated significantly with differences in the metabolic profiles between newborn infants who later progressed to type 1 diabetes and non-progressors from a previous study [22]. Notably, elevated insulinotropic BCAAs and diminished TCA cycle metabolites had been observed in these pre-diabetic children even before the first seroconversion for islet autoantibodies [22]. These results indicate that the changes in metabolic profiles in infants who later progress to type 1 diabetes could be microbially driven.

In our study, the effects of the microbiota in NOD mice were similar in males and females and thus not likely to be dependent on testosterone levels, in contrast to previous results that identified a gender-dependent protective effect of the microbiota in NOD mice [21]. This is of importance because type 1 diabetes does not have a female bias in humans [3] and suggests that there are microbial effects in addition to those mediated by sex hormones that may protect against autoimmune diabetes.

In conclusion, our results support a role of the gut microbiota as a regulator of diabetic autoimmunity and glucose metabolism and suggest that altered microbial metabolism may contribute to the pathogenesis of type 1 diabetes.

Supporting Information

Figure S1 Beta cell area in 23 week old NOD mice. Insulin area as a percent of total pancreas area was measured in female mice at 23 weeks ($n = 6$ per group). Data are presented as mean ± s.e.m.

Figure S2 Altered IAA titers in GF NOD mice. Scatter plot of relative IAA units (4w GF $n = 17$, CONV-R $n = 18$; 9w GF $n = 14$, CONV-R $n = 21$; 23w GF $n = 20$, CONV-R $n = 16$). Line represents median value $^{**}p<0.01$ determined by Student's *t*-test.

Figure S3 Glucose tolerance in GF NOD mice. Oral glucose tolerance test, average area under the curve (AUC) and serum insulin levels in GF and CONV-R mice at 17–18 weeks of age ($n = 4$–5). Data are presented as mean ±s.e.m. $^{*}p<0.05$ determined by Student's *t*-test.

Acknowledgments

We thank Rosie Perkins for editing the manuscript, Carina Arvidsson and Caroline Wennberg for superb mouse husbandry, and Tuulikki Seppänen-Laakso, Ismo Mattila, Heli Nygren, Vidya Velagapudi and Anna-Liisa Ruskeepää (VTT Technical Research Centre of Finland, Espoo, Finland) for excellent technical assistance in metabolomics analysis.

Author Contributions

Conceived and designed the experiments: TUG FB MO. Performed the experiments: TUG TH. Analyzed the data: TUG TH MK FB MO. Wrote the paper: TUG FB MO.

References

1. Lernmark A, Larsson HE (2013) Immune therapy in type 1 diabetes mellitus. Nat Rev Endocrinol 9: 92–103.
2. Patterson CC, Dahlquist GG, Gyürüs E, Green A, Soltész G (2009) Incidence trends for childhood type 1 diabetes in Europe during 1989–2003 and predicted new cases 2005–20: a multicentre prospective registration study. Lancet 373: 2027–2033.
3. Gale EA, Gillespie KM (2001) Diabetes and gender. Diabetologia 44: 3–15.
4. Barnett AH, Eff C, Leslie RD, Pyke DA (1981) Diabetes in identical twins. A study of 200 pairs. Diabetologia 20: 87–93.
5. Kaprio J, Tuomilehto J, Koskenvuo M, Romanov K, Reunanen A, et al. (1992) Concordance for type 1 (insulin-dependent) and type 2 (non-insulin-dependent) diabetes mellitus in a population-based cohort of twins in Finland. Diabetologia 35: 1060–1067.
6. Knip M, Veijola R, Virtanen SM, Hyöty H, Vaarala O, et al. (2005) Environmental triggers and determinants of type 1 diabetes. Diabetes 54: S125–136.
7. Strachan DP, Taylor EM, Carpenter RG (1996) Family structure, neonatal infection, and hay fever in adolescence. Arch Dis Child 74: 422–426.
8. Ben Nasr M, D'Addio F, Usuelli V, Tezza S, Abdi R, et al. (2014) The rise, fall, and resurgence of immunotherapy in type 1 diabetes. Pharmacol Res.
9. Herold KC, Vignali DA, Cooke A, Bluestone JA (2013) Type 1 diabetes: translating mechanistic observations into effective clinical outcomes. Nat Rev Immunol 13: 243–256.
10. Vergani A, D'Addio F, Jurewicz M, Petrelli A, Watanabe T, et al. (2010) A novel clinically relevant strategy to abrogate autoimmunity and regulate alloimmunity in NOD mice. Diabetes 59: 2253–2264.
11. Bjorksten B (2009) Disease outcomes as a consequence of environmental influences on the development of the immune system. Curr Opin Allergy Clin Immunol 9: 185–189.
12. Greiner T, Backhed F (2011) Effects of the gut microbiota on obesity and glucose homeostasis. Trends Endocrinol Metab 22: 117–123.
13. Karlsson FH, Tremaroli V, Nookaew I, Bergstrom G, Behre CJ, et al. (2013) Gut metagenome in European women with normal, impaired and diabetic glucose control. Nature 498: 99–103.
14. Qin J, Li Y, Cai Z, Li S, Zhu J, et al. (2012) A metagenome-wide association study of gut microbiota in type 2 diabetes. Nature 490: 55–60.
15. Giongo A, Gano KA, Crabb DB, Mukherjee N, Novelo LL, et al. (2011) Toward defining the autoimmune microbiome for type 1 diabetes. ISME J 5: 82–91.
16. de Goffau MC, Luopajarvi K, Knip M, Ilonen J, Ruohtula T, et al. (2013) Fecal Microbiota Composition Differs Between Children With beta-Cell Autoimmunity and Those Without. Diabetes 62: 1238–1244.
17. Kilkkinen A, Virtanen SM, Klaukka T, Kenward MG, Salkinoja-Salonen M, et al. (2006) Use of antimicrobials and risk of type 1 diabetes in a population-based mother-child cohort. Diabetologia 49: 66–70.
18. Koren O, Goodrich JK, Cullender TC, Spor A, Laitinen K, et al. (2012) Host remodeling of the gut microbiome and metabolic changes during pregnancy. Cell 150: 470–480.
19. Wen L, Ley RE, Volchkov PY, Stranges PB, Avanesyan L, et al. (2008) Innate immunity and intestinal microbiota in the development of type 1 diabetes. Nature 455: 1109–1113.
20. Calcinaro F, Dionisi S, Marinaro M, Candeloro P, Bonato V, et al. (2005) Oral probiotic administration induces interleukin-10 production and prevents spontaneous autoimmune diabetes in the non-obese diabetic mouse. Diabetologia 48: 1565–1575.
21. Markle JG, Frank DN, Mortin-Toth S, Robertson CE, Feazel LM, et al. (2013) Sex differences in the gut microbiome drive hormone-dependent regulation of autoimmunity. Science 339: 1084–1088.
22. Oresic M, Simell S, Sysi-Aho M, Nanto-Salonen K, Seppanen-Laakso T, et al. (2008) Dysregulation of lipid and amino acid metabolism precedes islet autoimmunity in children who later progress to type 1 diabetes. J Exp Med 205: 2975–2984.
23. Sysi-Aho M, Ermolov A, Gopalacharyulu PV, Tripathi A, Seppanen-Laakso T, et al. (2011) Metabolic regulation in progression to autoimmune diabetes. PLoS Comput Biol 7: e1002257.
24. Castillo S, Mattila I, Miettinen J, Oresic M, Hyotylainen T (2011) Data analysis tool for comprehensive two-dimensional gas chromatography/time-of-flight mass spectrometry. Anal Chem 83: 3058–3067.
25. Nygren H, Seppanen-Laakso T, Castillo S, Hyotylainen T, Oresic M (2011) Liquid Chromatography-Mass Spectrometry (LC-MS)-Based Lipidomics for Studies of Body Fluids and Tissues. Methods Mol Biol 708: 247–257.
26. Pluskal T, Castillo S, Villar-Briones A, Oresic M (2010) MZmine 2: Modular framework for processing, visualizing, and analyzing mass spectrometry-based molecular profile data. BMC Bioinformatics 11: 395.
27. Saeed AI, Sharov V, White J, Li J, Liang W, et al. (2003) TM4: a free, open-source system for microarray data management and analysis. Biotechniques 34: 374–378.
28. Anderson MS, Bluestone JA (2005) The NOD mouse: a model of immune dysregulation. Annu Rev Immunol 23: 447–485.
29. Backhed F, Ding H, Wang T, Hooper LV, Koh GY, et al. (2004) The gut microbiota as an environmental factor that regulates fat storage. Proc Natl Acad Sci U S A 101: 15718–15723.
30. Caesar R, Reigstad CS, Backhed HK, Reinhardt C, Ketonen M, et al. (2012) Gut-derived lipopolysaccharide augments adipose macrophage accumulation

but is not essential for impaired glucose or insulin tolerance in mice. Gut 61: 1701–1707.
31. Velagapudi VR, Hezaveh R, Reigstad CS, Gopalacharyulu P, Yetukuri L, et al. (2010) The gut microbiota modulates host energy and lipid metabolism in mice. J Lipid Res 51: 1101–1112.
32. Alam C, Bittoun E, Bhagwat D, Valkonen S, Saari A, et al. (2011) Effects of a germ-free environment on gut immune regulation and diabetes progression in non-obese diabetic (NOD) mice. Diabetologia 54: 1398–1406.
33. Bach J-F (2002) The effect of infections on susceptibility to autoimmune and allergic diseases. N Engl J Med 347: 911–920.
34. van Belle TL, Coppieters KT, von Herrath MG (2011) Type 1 diabetes: etiology, immunology, and therapeutic strategies. Physiol Rev 91: 79–118.
35. Sommer F, Backhed F (2013) The gut microbiota–masters of host development and physiology. Nat Rev Microbiol 11: 227–238.
36. Fiorina P, Vergani A, Dada S, Jurewicz M, Wong M, et al. (2008) Targeting CD22 reprograms B-cells and reverses autoimmune diabetes. Diabetes 57: 3013–3024.
37. Shoda LK, Young DL, Ramanujan S, Whiting CC, Atkinson MA, et al. (2005) A comprehensive review of interventions in the NOD mouse and implications for translation. Immunity 23: 115–126.
38. Fujihira K, Nagata M, Moriyama H, Yasuda H, Arisawa K, et al. (2000) Suppression and acceleration of autoimmune diabetes by neutralization of endogenous interleukin-12 in NOD mice. Diabetes 49: 1998–2006.
39. Trembleau S, Penna G, Gregori S, Giarratana N, Adorini L (2003) IL-12 administration accelerates autoimmune diabetes in both wild-type and IFN-gamma-deficient nonobese diabetic mice, revealing pathogenic and protective effects of IL-12-induced IFN-gamma. J Immunol 170: 5491–5501.
40. Yang Z, Chen M, Wu R, Fialkow LB, Bromberg JS, et al. (2002) Suppression of autoimmune diabetes by viral IL-10 gene transfer. J Immunol 168: 6479–6485.
41. Wang TJ, Larson MG, Vasan RS, Cheng S, Rhee EP, et al. (2011) Metabolite profiles and the risk of developing diabetes. Nat Med 17: 448–454.
42. Floegel A, Stefan N, Yu Z, Muhlenbruch K, Drogan D, et al. (2013) Identification of serum metabolites associated with risk of type 2 diabetes using a targeted metabolomic approach. Diabetes 62: 639–648.
43. Newgard CB, An J, Bain JR, Muehlbauer MJ, Stevens RD, et al. (2009) A branched-chain amino acid-related metabolic signature that differentiates obese and lean humans and contributes to insulin resistance. Cell Metab 9: 311–326.
44. Gall WE, Beebe K, Lawton KA, Adam KP, Mitchell MW, et al. (2010) alpha-hydroxybutyrate is an early biomarker of insulin resistance and glucose intolerance in a nondiabetic population. PLoS ONE 5: e10883.

2

Modeling of Hypo/Hyperglycemia and Their Impact on Breast Cancer Progression Related Molecules

Sirin A. I. Adham[1]*, Hasina Al Rawahi[1], Sumaya Habib[1], Mansour S. Al Moundhri[2], Alicia Viloria-Petit[3], Brenda L. Coomber[3]

1 Department of Biology, College of Science, Sultan Qaboos University, P. O. Box 36, 123 Muscat, Oman, **2** Department of Medicine, College of Medicine, Sultan Qaboos University, P.O. Box 35, 123 Muscat, Oman, **3** Department of Biomedical Sciences, Ontario Veterinary College, University of Guelph, Guelph, ON, Canada

Abstract

Breast cancer (BC) arises commonly in women with metabolic dysfunction. The underlying mechanism by which glycemic load can exert its action on tumor metastasis is under investigated. In this study we showed that glycemic microenvironment alters the expression of three classes of proteins, VEGF and its receptors, cell to cell, and cell to extracellular matrix (ECM) adhesion proteins in MDA-MB-231 parental cells and its two metastatic variants to the bone and brain (MDA-MB-231BO and MDA-MB-231BR, respectively). Using western blotting, we showed that VEGFR2 levels were higher in these variant cells and persisted in the cells under extreme hypoglycemia. Hypoglycemia did not alter VEGFR2 expression *per se* but rather suppressed its posttranslational glycosylation. This was reversed rapidly upon the restoration of glucose, and cyclohexamide (CHX) treatment demonstrated that this deglycosylated VEGFR2 was not a product of de-novo protein synthesis. VEGFR2 co-receptor Neuropilin-1 was up-regulated four-fold in all MDA-MB-231 cells (parental and two variants) compared to VEGFR2 expression, and was also susceptible to glycemic changes but resistant to CHX treatment for up to 72 hrs. Hypoglycemia also resulted in a significant decrease in specific catenin, cadherin, and integrin proteins, as well as cellular proliferation and colony forming ability. However, MDA-MB-231BR cells showed a unique sensitivity to hypo/hyperglycemia in terms of morphological changes, colony formation ability, integrin β3 expression and secreted VEGF levels. In conclusion, this study can be translated clinically to provide insight into breast cancer cell responses to glycemic levels relevant for our understanding of the interaction between diabetes and cancer.

Editor: Aamir Ahmad, Wayne State University School of Medicine, United States of America

Funding: Sultan Qaboos university funded this work. The grant number is: IG/Biol/Sci/01/12. The funder had no role in study design, data collection and analysis, decision to publish, or preparation of the manuscript.

Competing Interests: The authors have declared that no competing interests exist.

* Email: sadham@squ.edu.om

Introduction

Worldwide, Breast Cancer (BC) is considered the second most diagnosed type of cancer after lung cancer [1]. Metabolic disruption is an example of a recently described 'emergent hallmark' of cancer which indicates that cancer cells reprogram their metabolism in order to most effectively support their neoplastic proliferation [2]. Diabetes Mellitus (DM) and BC share many risk factors such as obesity, sedentary lifestyle, advanced age, and dietary risk factors (high intake of fat and refined carbohydrates) [3]. The two conditions that arise as a result of treating type II diabetes are hyperglycemia and hypoglycemia, which refer to chronically high and low blood glucose levels, respectively [4]. Metformin is a biguanide derivative which lowers the glucose levels in blood, having a protective effect against BC [5]. An epidemiological study showed that metformin also decreased the risk of BC by 19–66% when compared to non-treated diabetic cases [6]. Further specific studies defining the types and subtypes of BC on the molecular level will give insight into those BC patients who are responding differently to metformin treatment.

There are several hypotheses explaining the mode of how diabetes mellitus (with the coexistence of its complications, hyperglycemia and hypoglycemia), could exert effects on BC. It has been shown that the insulin-like growth factor IGF1 pathway is active in both BC and DM [7]. IGF1 is a mitogenic and anti-apoptotic agent, which activates pro-survival and proliferative pathways in normal breast cells, an action similar to estrogens in BC [8]. In addition to the activation of IGF1, insulin itself has mitogenic and anti-apoptotic effects on breast tissue through its activation of phosphatidylinositol 3-kinase (PI3-K), an important pathway in BC [9]. Recent reports stated the role of vascular endothelial growth factor (VEGF) in regulating cell metabolism. High plasma VEGF concentrations are associated with less carbohydrate intake and lower body mass in type II diabetes, and over expression of VEGF by the adipose tissue protects against diet-induced obesity and insulin resistance. In a recent report, VEGF neutralization resulted in improving the diet induced metabolic dysfunction in a mouse model [10,11,12]. IGF-IR was co-localized along with VEGF receptor 2 (VEGFR2) on circulating epithelial cancer cells of BC patients [13]. In general, breast cancer resistance to hormonal therapy has been linked with high activity/expression of receptor tyrosine kinases. In particular, the VEGF/VEGFR2 pathway supports the growth of estrogen-independent breast cancer cells [14].

Based on these previous observations we hypothesized that VEGFR2 expression in BC cells might be modulated by the changes in the glycemic tumor microenvironment and this modulation would depend on the site of metastasis. Previously we described how glucose concentration acts as a key regulator for VEGF receptor VEGFR2 in epithelial ovarian cancer (EOC) cells, where this protein was degraded by the proteosome under hypoglycemic conditions [15]. In this present study we investigated the effect of hypoglycemia and hyperglycemia on three major classes of proteins: (i) the ligand VEGF and its receptors (VEGFR1, VEGFR2 and co-receptor Neuropilin-1), (ii) cell-cell adhesion proteins, (iii) cell to ECM adhesion proteins. We evaluated these molecules in the MDA-MB-231 cells (MDA-MB-231P), and their metastatic variants to the bone (MDA-MB-231BO) and brain (MDA-MB-231BR) [16]. Unlike our previous findings with EOC cells, we found that VEGFR2 protein is not degraded but rather persists in the BC cells under hypoglycemia with a reduction in its posttranslational glycosylation. Glucose restoration led to its rapid re-glycosylation. The MDA-MB-231BR cells were the most affected by the glycemic changes, showing the most notable changes in protein expression in response to hypo/hyperglycemia and exclusive up-regulation of β3 integrin with higher concentrations of glucose.

Finally, our results show that the VEGF/VEGFR2 axis is differentially modulated by glycemic load among the cells studied. We suggest VEGFR2 modulation by glucose is important for the progression of BC cells. Breast cancer progression, particularly the hormone resistant types represented by MDA-MB-231 cells, might be linked with diabetes mellitus complications (hyper/hypoglycemia) through the VEGF pathway since under extreme hypoglycemic conditions VEGFR2 persisted in the cells, did not degrade and was rapidly switched to its mature functional form upon availability of glucose.

Materials and Methods

Cell lines and Cell Culture

MCF-7, BT-474, and Parental MDA-MB-231 cells were purchased from ATCC USA; bone (MDA-MB-231BO) and brain (MDA-MB-231BR) metastasized BC cell variants of MDA-MB-231 were previously derived and characterized [16] and were kindly provided by Dr. T. Yoneda (M.D. Anderson Cancer Center, Houston, Texas). The cells were grown in complete culture medium DMEM containing 10% fetal bovine serum (FBS, Sigma), 1% sodium pyruvate (Sigma-Aldrich) and 0.5% gentamycin (Invitrogen). They were grown and maintained in 5% CO_2 in a humidified atmosphere at 37°C.

In vitro Hypoglycemia, Hyperglycemia and Normoxia

When the cell lines reached 100% confluency in 10 cm plate, they were washed twice with PBS and the normal growth media was replaced with serum free media as follows: 10 ml special DMEM without glucose (0 mM; hypoglycemia) (Gibco, life technologies, Germany). The hyperglycemic condition was achieved by incubating the cells in 10 ml of usual DMEM-high glucose containing 25 mM of glucose and the normal physiological glucose concentration (5 mM) of DMEM was prepared as a combination of 2 ml from the standard DMEM high glucose (Sigma, Germany) which contains 4500 mg/ml of glucose (25 mM) and 8 ml of the 0 mM DMEM.

Glucose Restoration after 24 h of Hypoglycemia

To study the expression pattern of VEGFR2 after the restoration of glucose the cells were initially grown in DMEM with 0 mM glucose for 24 h. After 24 hours the cells were re-exposed to regular DMEM (25 mM glucose) and samples were collected for western blotting after various times of glucose restoration. The total protein was extracted from the cells in the restored glucose conditions and their respective controls (cells not exposed to hypoglycemia for 24 h) at different time points, including 10, 20, 30, 40 and 50 minutes and 1, 2, 3, 4, 5, 6, 7, 8, and 12 h.

Cyclohexamide Treatment after 24 h of Hypoglycemia and Restoration of Glucose

To check the effects of halting de novo protein synthesis in the cells, the cells were treated with 10 μg/ml of cyclohexamide (CHX; Sigma Aldrich) in two conditions: DMEM with 0 mM glucose (–glu) and DMEM with 25 mM glucose (+glu), and samples collected for western blotting. The respective controls were: +glu–CHX; –glu–CHX; +glu+CHX; –glu+CHX. These conditions were repeated in five different time points: 10 min, 20 min, and 1, 3 and 6 h upon glucose restoration.

SDS-PAGE and Western Blotting

Total protein lysates were loaded equally in the wells of SDS-PAGE, and after electrophoresis, transferred to PVDF membrane (Millipore). Thereafter, the membranes were washed with TBS solution and blocked for 30 min in 5% free fat milk dissolved in 1X TBST (Tris-base, NaCl and 0.001% Tween-20 with pH 7.6). After blocking, the membranes were incubated overnight at 4°C with the corresponding primary antibody (Table S1) diluted in the same blocking solution. POD-conjugated secondary antibody and BM chemiluminescence western blotting substrate (Roche) were used to visualize bands on an X-ray sensitive film (Roche). Western blots were repeated at least three times and a representative blot from consistent triplicates was chosen for the figures. The graphs were prepared to represent the intensity of the bands on the x-Ray films which were quantified using the Image J software and the average of three independent replicates was calculated.

Real -Time qPCR

RNA isolation from the different cell lines under the three different glycemic conditions (0 mM, 5 mM and 25 mM) was done using the Trizol reagent (Sigma-Aldrich, USA). One microgram of RNA was treated with DNaseI (Invitrogen, USA) and converted to cDNA using high-capacity cDNA Reverse Transcription kit (Life technologies, USA). The transcripts were quantified using Real-time qPCR performed on Applied Biosystems 7500 fast Real-Time PCR detection System (Applied Biosystems, life technologies, USA). The reaction mix contained 20 ng of the cDNA template, 2 μl of each primer (10 μM forward and reverse primers) and 10 μl Fast SYBR Green master mix 2X (Life technologies, USA). The primer sequences [17] to amplify E-cadherin were: Sense- 5′-GGAAGTCAGTTCAGACTCCAG-CC-3′ Anti Sense- 5′ AGGCCTTTTGACTGTAATCACACC-3′ and the beta actin primers were also designed based on previously published primers [18]: sense 5′-GCTGTGCTACGT-CGCCCTG-3 and anti sense' 5′-GGAGGAGCTGGAAG-CAGCC-3′. The PCR profile was as follows: 20 seconds at 95°C, followed by 40 cycles of 3 seconds at 95°C and 30 seconds at 60°C. The obtained Ct value of each gene of interest was normalized to the Ct of the reference genes as follows: Delta

$Ct = Ct_{gene\ test} - Ct_{endogenous\ control}$; Delta Delta $Ct = \Delta Ct_{sample1} - \Delta Ct_{calibrator}$; RQ = Relative quantification = $2^{-\Delta\Delta Ct}$ this RQ value represents the fold of increase compared to the reference gene.

Colony Formation Assay

The effect of hypoglycemia on the ability of the cells to form colonies was investigated by growing the MDA-MB-231P, MDA-MB-231BO and MDA-MB-231BR for 24 hours in hypoglycemia (1000 cells in each well of the six well plates). The cells were then washed and re-incubated in regular DMEM for two weeks, then visualized by staining with crystal violet solution (25% methanol and 0.5% crystal violet). The colonies were manually counted and quadruplicates of each dose were performed.

Alamarblue Assay

Cell viability was determined using Alamarblue Assay (Invitrogen, USA), following the manufacturers protocol. Briefly, 25,000 cells were seeded in 96-well dishes in normal growth medium. Twenty-four hours later, cells were washed twice with DMEM, then 100 µl serum-free DMEM with (25 mM) or without (0 mM) glucose were added to each well. After 12 hr, Alamarblue reagent was added to each well in a final concentration of 10%. 4 hours later, the absorbance at 570 and 630 nm was determined, and Alamarblue reduction was calculated based on manufacturer's instructions. Each experiment was repeated at least twice in quadruplicates.

VEGF ELISA

To evaluate the quantity of VEGF secreted by the cells under the two conditions (hypo and hyperglycemia) the cells were seeded in 24 well plates in regular growth media. After 24 h the media was changed to DMEM with 1% FBS with either 0, 5, or 25 mM glucose and cells were grown for another 48 hr. Conditioned media samples were collected and subjected to quantification by ELISA for human-specific VEGF-A following the manufacturer's protocol (R&D Systems, Minneapolis, MN, USA).

Statistical analysis

Statistical analyses were carried out with GraphPad InStat 3 Software for parametric data and statistically significant differences were determined by two-tailed unpaired student's t test or one-way ANOVA. Kruskal-Wallis H test was used for the analysis of the non-parametric data. Significant differences were defined as $p<0.05$.

Results

Different Levels of VEGFR2 in MDA-MB-231P and its Two Variants MDA-MB-231BO MDA-MB-231BR

Growing in DMEM (glucose levels 25 mM-FBS; i.e., hyperglycemia) breast cancer MDA-MB-231P cells expressed the least VEGFR2 when compared to their metastatic derivatives to the bone (MDA-MB-231BO) and brain (MDA-MB-231BR). The highest VEGFR2 expression was detected in the MDA-MB-231BO cell line and MDA-MB-231BR cells showed intermediate expression (**Figure 1A**). The phosphorylated VEGFR2 was detected in all the MDA-MB-231cells (parental and metastatic variants) only when the cells were growing in 25 mM of glucose (**Figure 1A**).

Brain Metastasized Cells (MDA-MB-231BR) Showed a Significant Decrease in VEGF Secretion under Hypoglycemia

In four independent experiments, VEGF (pg/ml) was quantified and showed a non-significant difference in the levels secreted by MDA-MB-231P and MDA-MB-231BO cells under the three growth conditions (0 mM, 5 mM, 25 mM glucose) (**Figure 1B**). In hyperglycemic condition (25 mM of glucose) MDA-MB-231BR secreted significantly higher levels of VEGF ($p = 0.0122$) when compared with its VEGF secretion in hypoglycemia and when compared with the other cells under the same hyperglycemic conditions.

VEGFR2 was Expressed in its Non-glycosylated Isoform after 24 Hours of Glucose Deprivation

The mode of VEGFR2 isoform expression was different among the three cell lines (parental and the two variants). Both the mature glycosylated form of the protein (230 kDa) and the immature unglycosylated form (200 kDa) were detected when all the cell lines were grown under hyperglycemic conditions (25 mM of glucose), (**Figure 1C**). In normal physiological glucose (5 mM) only the parental cells was able to produce the mature 230 kDa form of VEGFR2. The two metastasis derivative cell lines (MDA-MB-231BO, MDA-MB-231BR) produced only the immature glycosylated and unglycosylated forms (200 and 147 kDa, respectively) in DMEM with 5 mM glucose. In hypoglycemic conditions (0 mM) all the cells produced only a 147 kDa VEGFR2 as the unglycosylated form of the protein. All the MDA-MB-231 cells expressed VEGFR1 equally without any significant reduction in amount or molecular weight under hypo or hyperglycemia (**Figure 1C**). In addition to the higher levels of VEGF, MDA-MB-231BR cells also expressed higher levels of GLUT-1 protein when compared with the MDA-MB-231P and MDA-MB-231BO cells and in all the cells tested GLUT-1 protein increased when glucose concentration increased (**Figure 1D**). Finally, we also examined the involvement of the unfolded protein response back up mechanism under hypoglycemia. All cells showed no significant difference in the levels of the unfolded protein response represented by the level of GRP 78 protein which was proportionally increased when glucose concentration decreased (**Figure 1D**).

Mature Glycosylation of VEGFR2 is Restored upon Glucose Re-exposure

Figure 2A shows that within 20 min of glucose re-exposure after 24 h hypoglycemia, the immature glycosylated 200 kDa isoform was detectable in all 3 cell types with the coexistence of the 147 kDa isoform. These two isoforms sustained their levels of expression until 1hr of glucose re-exposure (**Figure 2B**), after which the non-glycosylated (147 kDa) band was gradually lost (**Figure 2C**). With longer glucose re-exposure (approximately 4–6 hrs), the full mature VEGFR2 (230 kDa) and the immature 200 kDa bands were consistently detected (**Figure 2C**).

The Recovery of Glycosylated VEGFR-2 upon Glucose Restoration was not a Product of de-novo Protein Synthesis

We used cycloheximide (CHX) treatment to confirm that VEGFR2 was not degraded during the hypoglycemic period and then re-synthesized upon glucose restoration. Initially, the effectiveness of cyclohexamide to block VEGFR2 synthesis was evaluated by growing the MDA-MB-231BO cells for 24 hrs in hypoglycemia (0 mM) and hyperglycemia (25 mM) in the

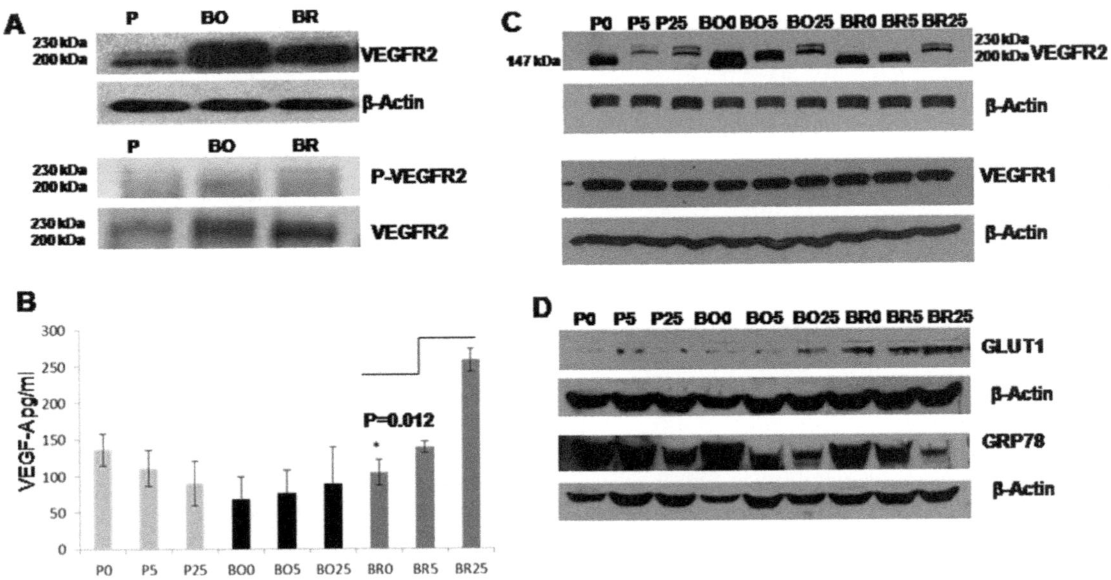

Figure 1. The expression of VEGF and its receptor VEGFR2 in MDA-MB-231 cells and its metastatic variants varies with glycemic conditions. (A) Western blots show the difference in VEGFR2 and phospho-VEGFR2 in MDA-MB-231 parental (P), bone metastatic (BO) and brain metastatic (BR) variants growing in DMEM containing 25 mM glucose. (B) Graph represents the mean of four independent ELISA experiments measuring the total VEGF-A secreted in the conditioned media, (error bars represent ± standard deviation). Statistical analysis showed no significant difference in the amount of VEGF-A secreted when the MDA-MB-231P and MDA-MB-231BO cells were grown under the different glucose concentrations. However, MDA-MB-231BR cells produced significantly higher levels of VEGF-A ($p = 0.012$) when grown in DMEM containing 25 mM of glucose compared to 0 mM of glucose. Figure abbreviations P: MDA-MB-231 Parental, BO: MDA-MB-231Bone and BR: MDA-MB-231Brain; cell lines were grown in DMEM 0, 5 and 25 mM glucose for 24 hrs without FBS. (C) VEGFR2 expression in MDA-MB-231P, MDA-MB-231BO and MDA-MB-231BR cells. The 147 kDa band was the dominant band expressed at 0 mM glucose. The regular double bands (200 kDa and 230 kDa) were detected in all the cells at 25 mM glucose. The cells expressed the bands differentially when placed in 5 mM glucose media. The MDA-MB-231P cells produced the 200 and 230 kDa forms; the MDA-MB-231BO cells produced the 147 and 200 kDa forms while the MDA-MB-231BR cells did not express any of the mature glycosylated bands at 5 mM glucose concentration. The bottom blot shows the expression of VEGFR1 was constant and did not change among the cell lines nor under the different glucose conditions. (D) Blot shows MDA-MB-231BR cells produced higher levels of GLUT-1 protein than the other cell lines. GRP78 had the same expression pattern among the different cells and its expression had an inverse relationship with glucose concentration. Note: β-Actin was used in all the blots as protein loading control.

presence or absence of CHX. CHX resulted in the depletion of VEGFR2 completely from the cells when exposed to 0 mM and 25 mM glucose. In contrast, in control conditions (without CHX) cells expressed the mature and immature glycosylated forms of the protein (230 kDa and 200 kDa, respectively) at 25 mM glucose and only predominantly the 147 kDa form at 0 mM of glucose (**Figure 3A**). VEGFR2 stability was detected after 1 hr and 3 hrs of glucose restoration with or without CHX. The VEGFR2 band intensity was reduced in the samples from CHX exposed cells and the band disappeared in MDA-MB-231P after 3 hrs of glucose restoration grown in the presence of CHX (**Figure 3B**). In control samples in which glucose was restored and CHX was not added, VEGFR2 band size was proportionally increasing with time indicating that the protein was not degraded and only its glycosylation status was altered. This was particularly clear in the two variant cells since they express higher levels of VEGFR2 (**Figure 3B**).

Neuropilin-1 (NRP-1) Expression was Highly Expressed in MDA-MB-231P and its two Variants and was Resistant to CHX Treatment

NRP-1 glycoprotein is a co-receptor for VEGFR2. It was found to be highly expressed in all the MDA-MB-231 cells used as only 25 μg of total protein lysate were loaded in the gel to get a reasonable signal while 100 μg was used to visualize VEGFR2 in the same samples. Under 24 hrs of hypoglycemia and the presence of CHX all cells (parental and variants) showed a decrease in the unglycosylated form of the protein (100 KDa band), however the 140 KDa form persisted. (lane 2 in **Figure 3C**). MDA-MB-231P cells showed a slightly different response to CHX- when the glucose was restored gradually to the cells, CHX resulted in a decrease in NRP-1 band intensity after the third hour of glucose restoration in the presence of CHX (**Figure 3C**). There were no differences in the NRP-1 band intensity when the cells were in hypoglycemia for 24 hrs and when the glucose was restored for another 24 hrs in the presence of CHX in both variant cells (lane 2 and 10, **Figure 3C**). Prolonged treatment of MDA-MB-231BR cells with CHX demonstrated that NRP-1 expression was not susceptible to degradation even after 72 hr of CHX treatment (**Figure 3D**), and the MDA-MB-231BO cells showed the same pattern (data not shown).

Hypoglycemia Results in Changes in MDA-MB-231BR Cell Morphology

The morphology of MDA-MB-231BR variants changed upon glucose deprivation. Most cells lost their normal elongated shape and gained a rounded morphology, and as glucose concentration increased these cells gradually restored their normal shape (**Figure 4A**). The morphology of MDA-MB-231P and MDA-MB-231BO cells was not affected by glucose reduction (**Figure 4A**). The addition of FBS had no effect on cell morphology when cells were grown with 25 mM glucose (data not shown) demonstrating that glucose was the main factor behind this change.

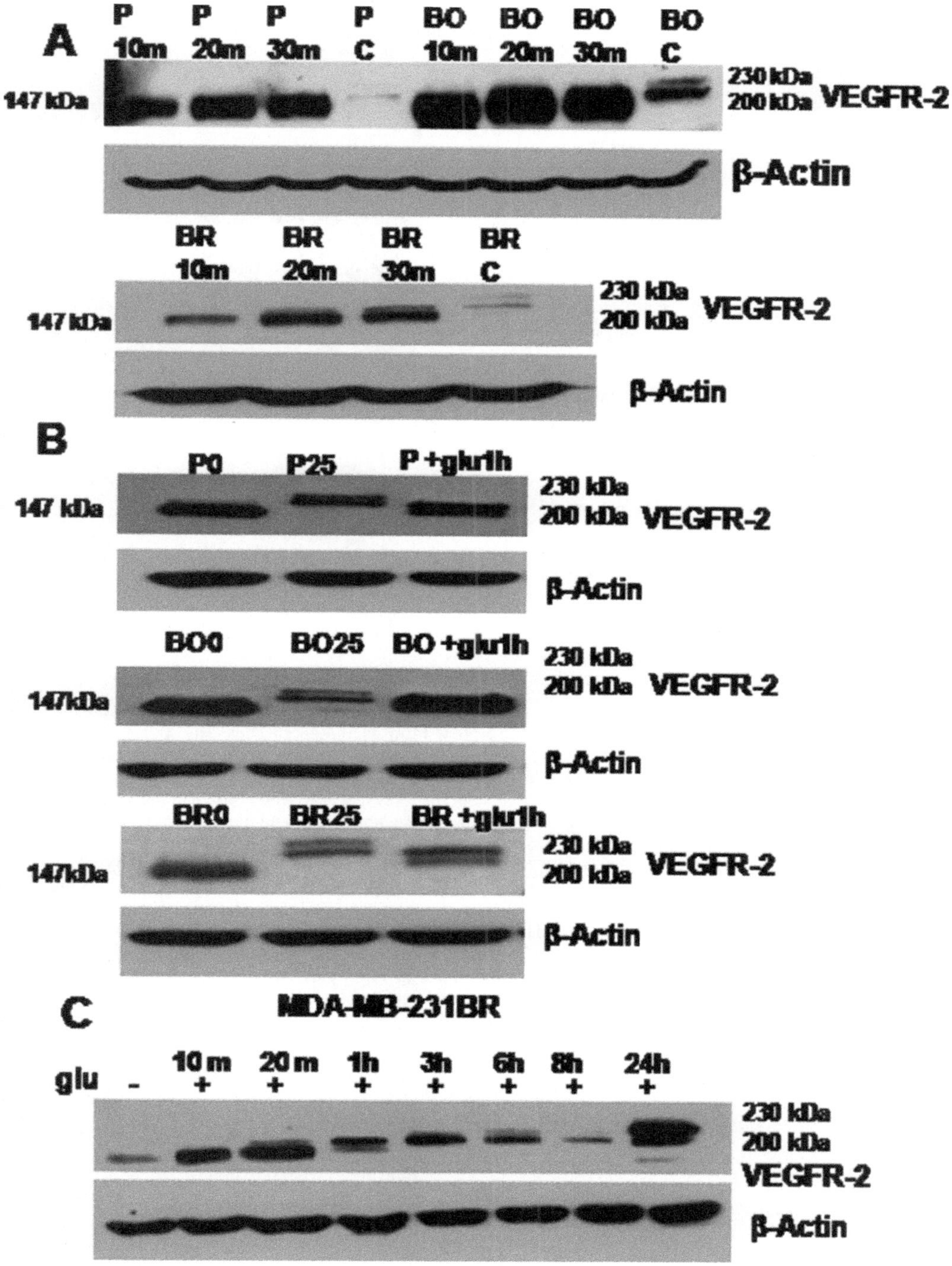

Figure 2. Glucose restoration resulted in a rapid glycosylation of the immature VEGFR2 band. (A) Western blot shows the VEGFR2 expression pattern in the cells exposed to 0 mM glucose media for a period of 24 hrs, followed by glucose restoration for 10, 20, 30 mins and the control cells (cells grown in control regular DMEM (25 mM glucose) without prior hypoglycemic exposure) P: MDA-MB-231P; BO: MDA-MB-231BO and BR: MDA-MB-231BR. The mature VEGFR2 band at 200 kDa was detected after 20 mins of glucose restoration which was more obvious in the MDA-MB-231BR (bottom blot). (B) Western blots showing that glucose restoration for 1 hour (after a period of 24 hrs of hypoglycemia) enhanced the formation of the glycosylated band of VEGFR2 (200 kDa) in all three cell lines MDA-MB-231P (P+glu 1hr), MDA-MB-231BO (BO+glu1h) and MDA-MB-231BR (BR+glu1h). The samples indicated by P25, B25 and BR25 are the samples collected from the cells growing in regular DMEM (25 mM glucose) expressing both mature bands of VEGFR2 (200 kDa and 230 kDa). P0, BO0 and BR0 are the MDA-MB-231P, MDA-MB-231BO and MDA-MB-231BR cells respectively, exposed to hypoglycemia for 24 hrs without glucose restoration. All three cell lines expressed only the unglycosylated band of VEGFR2 (147 kDa) when grown in 0 mM DMEM. (C) Western blots depicting the gradual increase in VEGFR2 band size upon glucose restoration in MDA-MB-231BR cells. Note: β-Actin was used in all the blots as a protein loading control.

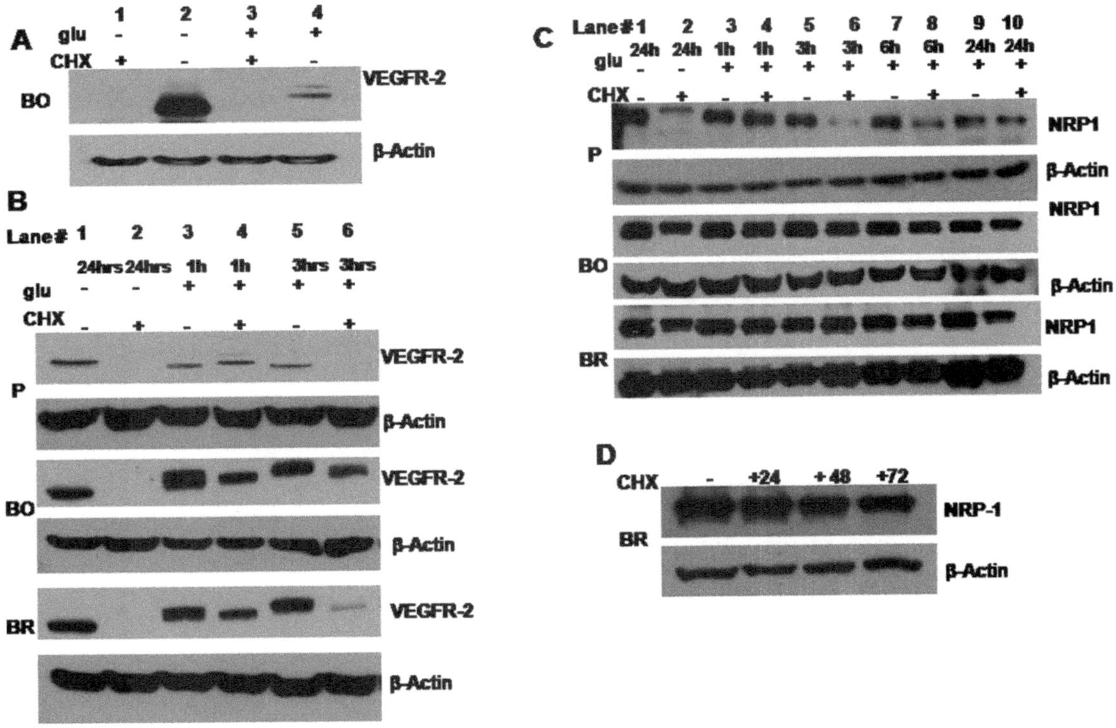

Figure 3. The glycosylated VEGFR2 found upon glucose re-exposure was not a product of a de-novo protein synthesis. (A) Cyclohexamide treatment for a period of 24 hrs depleted VEGFR2 protein from all three cell lines. The blot in this panel demonstrates that cyclohexamide depleted VEGFR2 from the MDA-MB-231BO cells (regularly expressing the highest level of VEGFR2 among the three cell lines) whether they were hypoglycemic or hyperglycemic (lane 1 and 3). The control cyclohexamide negative samples –glu –CHX and +glu -CHX showed detectable VEGFR2 expression (lane 2 and 4). (B) VEGFR2 was completely depleted from the three cell lines when grown in hypoglycemia in the presence of CHX (lane 2). The samples in lanes 3 and 5 are cells exposed to hypoglycemia for 24 hrs without CHX and glucose was restored for 1 hr (lane 3) or 3h (lane 5), respectively. Comparing the former two lanes (3 and 5) shows clearly that the VEGFR2 band was increasing in molecular weight as the time of glucose exposure increased; this is very prominent in the middle (MDA-MB-231BO) and bottom blots (MDA-MB-231BR). The samples in lane 4 and 6 were glucose restored for 1 hr and 3 hrs respectively with CHX added at the time of glucose restoration. After 3 hr of CHX and glucose restoration of MDA-MB-231P cells, the VEGFR2 band was not detectable (lane 6- P), however the MDA-MB-231BO and MDA-MB-231BR cells (lane 6 BO, lane 6 BR) expressed a detectable VEGFR2 band. Note: β-Actin was used in all the blots as a protein loading control. (C) Stability of NRP-1 expression under low glucose and CHX treatment. NRP-1 was detected in the same samples as in the previous panel (B) and it did not show a profound decrease in its expression in both MDA-MB-231BO and MDA-MB-231BR. However in MDA-MB-231P samples the NRP-1 band pattern was changed after 24 hrs of hypoglycemia in the presence of CHX (lane 2). The NRP-1 band was also decreased in the glucose-restored samples with CHX (added at the time of restoration) (lanes 6, 8, and 10). (D) The blot shows that in MDA-MB-231BR cells the NRP-1 protein was resistant to CHX treatment for up to 72 hrs of exposure. Note: β-Actin was used in all the blots as a protein loading control.

Hypoglycemia Reduced the Colony Formation Ability of Breast Cancer Cells

Next, we evaluated the effect of hypoglycemia (24 hrs 0 mM glucose) on the ability of MDA-MB-231 parent cells and variants to form colonies. The colonies formed were different among the three cell lines; MDA-MB-231BO and MDA-MB-231BR cells produced large and well-delimited colonies compared to the MDA-MB-231P cells which formed smaller, disorganized colonies. Glucose deprivation for 24 hrs and its restoration with regular DMEM (25 mM glucose) reduced the ability of all MDA-MB-231 cells to form colonies when compared with the cells not exposed to hypoglycemia (**Figure 4B**). The statistical analysis of four independent experiments showed that a significant decrease in colony number was observed mainly in the MDA-MB-231BR cell line $p = 0.0013$ (**Figure 4B**).

Hypoglycemia Resulted in a Significant Decrease in the Cells Proliferation Ability

The proliferation ability of the MDA-MB-231 cells was determined using the Alamarblue assay. In general, all cells (MDA-MB-231P, MDA-MB-231BO, and MDA-MB-231BR) showed significant decrease in the percentage of reduced Alamarblue when exposed to hypoglycemia; p values were 0.0012, 0.001 and 0.0129 respectively (**Figure 4C**). The results represent the mean of three independent experiments.

Profiling the Expression of Adhesion Molecules under Hypoglycemia

Given the morphological changes observed in the MDA-MB-231BR metastatic variant upon hypoglycemic conditions, we screened all cells for their expression of a panel of cell adhesion molecules, which were previously shown to modulate cellular attachment and cell morphology, and influence metastatic ability. These molecules included the epithelial molecules E-cadherin, α, β and γ catenin, and the mesenchymal marker N cadherin (**Figure 5**). Consistent with previous studies which found that loss of E-cadherin associates with metastatic ability [19], MDA-MB-231P, MDA-MB-231BO and MDA-MB-231BR cells had completely lost E-cadherin expression (**Figure 5A**). N-cadherin was highly expressed in all the studied cells (only 10 μg of total protein lysate was loaded), and was down regulated in the MDA-

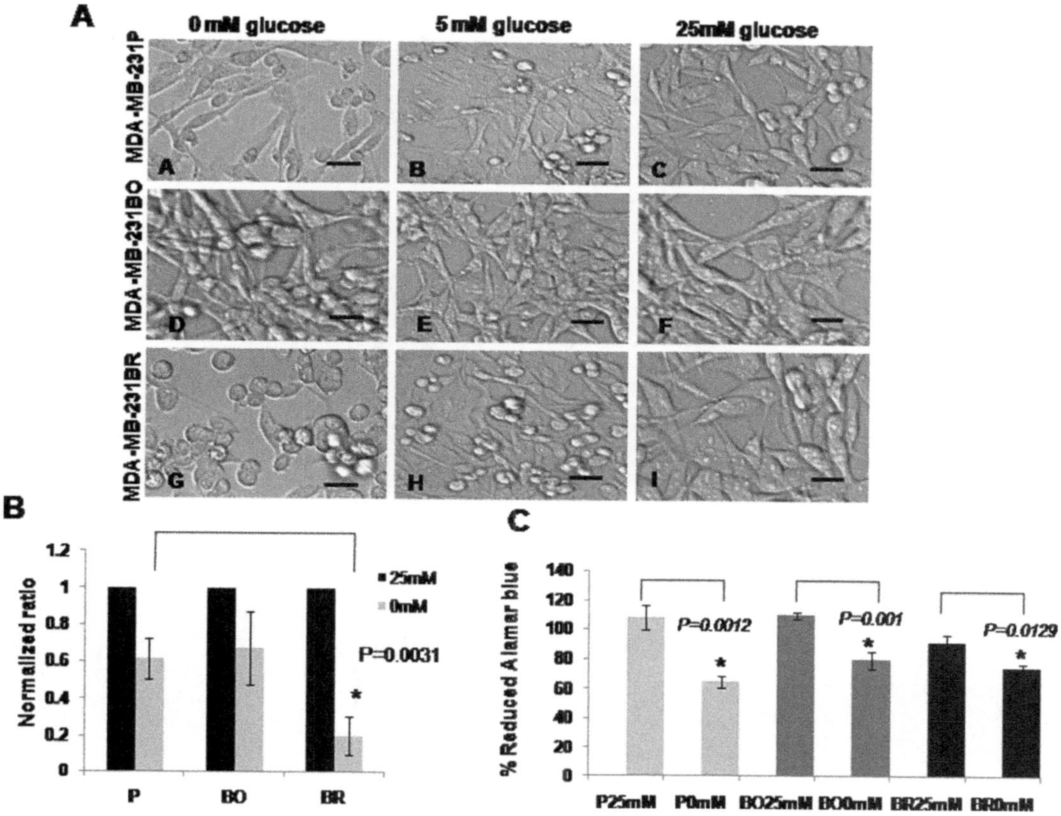

Figure 4. Hypoglycemia caused a change in MDA-MB-231BR cell morphology. Phase contrast images of the three MDA-MB-231 cell lines. Image (A) shows MDA-MB-231P cells grown in DMEM 0 mM glucose images; (B–C) the same cells grown in DMEM with different glucose concentrations: 5 mM and 25 mM. Image (D) represents MDA-MB-231BO cells growing in DMEM 0 mM glucose; images (E–F) are for the same cells grown in the other glucose concentrations. Neither MDA-MB-231P nor MDA-MB-231BO cells were morphologically changed by the various changes in glucose concentration. The MDA-MB-231BR cells grown in the absence of glucose for 24 hrs lost their extended protrusions (G), became rounded and maintained their attachment to the culture plate; images (H and I) show how the shape of the cells was restored upon the increase in glucose concentration. Scale bars = 100 μm. Breast cancer cells formed fewer colonies and had reduced proliferation under hypoglycemic conditions. (B) Graph represents the ratio of the average number of colonies counted in four independent experiments. The y-axis represents the normalized number of colonies counted in the hypoglycemia exposed wells versus the control formed by the cells. MDA-MB-231BR cells produced the least colonies among the three cell lines when exposed to hypoglycemia and this was confirmed by running the non-parametric Kruskal Wallis test $H = 15.66$ and $p = 0.0013$. (C) The graph represents cell growth as the percentage of Alamarblue reduced by the cells under hypo/hyperglycemia. There was a significant decrease in the reduced Alamarblue when the cells were grown in hypoglycemia for 24 hrs (MDA-MB-231P, MDA-MB-231BO, and MDA-MB-231BR) Results are shown as mean ± SD and were statistically analyzed by a two-tailed student's t test ($n = 3$).

MB-231P and MDA-MB-231BO cells under hypoglycemia. The MDA-MB-231BR cells expressed the lowest level of N-cadherin when compared to the other cells (**Figure 5B**; blot on the left and graph on the right of the panel). Expression of the known tumor suppressor γ-catenin was less in the metastatic variant cells when compared to the MDA-MB-231P cells and was also down regulated in hypoglycemia. β-catenin was detected in slightly higher levels in both MDA-MB-231P and MDA-MB-231BO when compared to MDA-MB-231BR, and was not significantly down regulated under hypoglycemia in MDA-MB-231P cells however its expression in both MDA-MB-231BO and MDA-MB-231BR cells was significantly reduced under hypoglycemia ($p = 0.0037$ and $p = 0.0014$) (**Figure 5B**; bottom left graph). α-catenin was the least abundant among the three catenins and was detected in slightly higher amounts in the MDA-MB-231P cells, with no significant change in response to glucose concentrations, however, it showed significant reduction under hypoglycemia in both variant cells (**Figure 5B**; bottom graph to the right).

Integrin β3 was Exclusively up Regulated in the Brain Metastatic Variant Cells

The expression of cell-to-ECM adhesion molecules, namely integrins, β4, αV, α5, and β3 were examined in our cell lines. β4 integrin was detected at higher levels in the MDA-MB-231P cells (with no obvious reduction under hypoglycemia), expressed at very low levels in MDA-MB-231BO cells, and almost not detected in MDA-MB-231BR cells (**Figure 6A**; blot on the left and graph on the right of the panel). Integrin αV expression was lower in MDA-MB-231BO cells as compared to MDA-MB-231P and MDA-MB-231BR cells, and was reduced in all studied cells in response to hypoglycemia however, this reduction was only significant in MDA-MB-231P cells. Integrin α5 was highly expressed in all the cells (**Figure 6A**), MDA-MB-231BR cells exhibited higher levels of integrin β3 as compared to the other two cell variants and the expression of this integrin was significantly reduced under hypoglycemia in MDA-MB-231BR cells $p = 0.005$ (**Figure 6B**; blots on the left and graph on the bottom right).

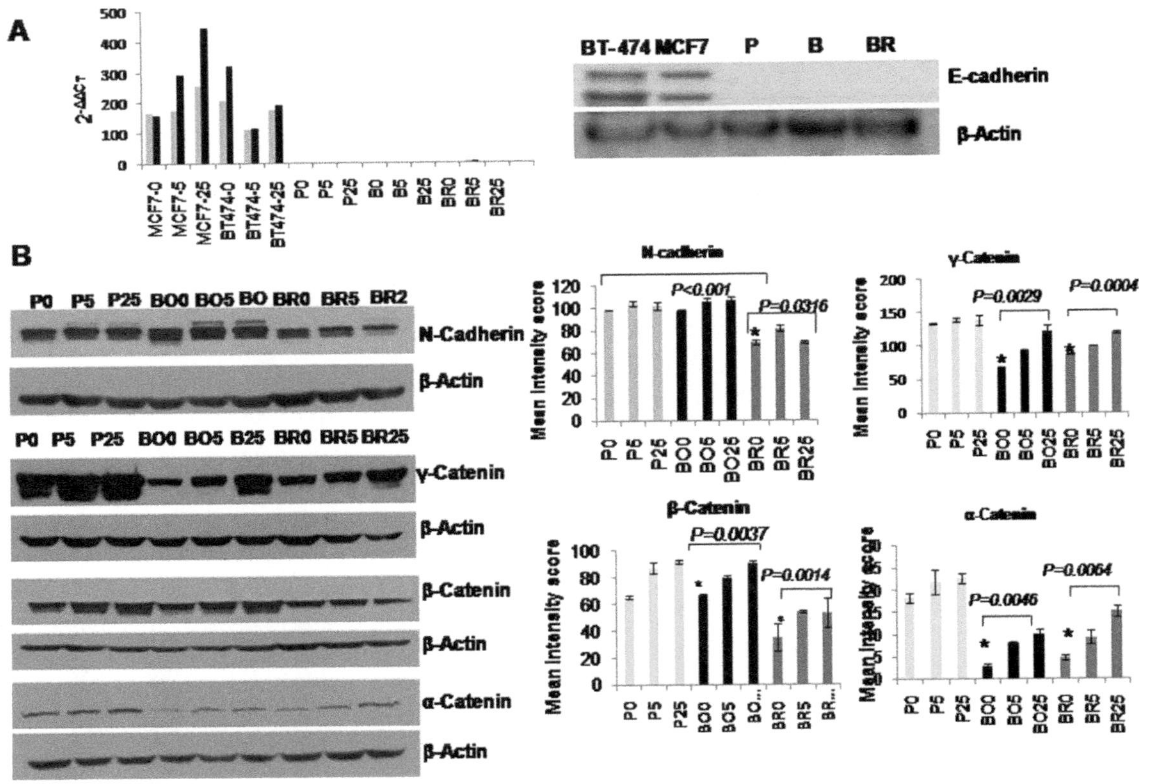

Figure 5. Expression of E-Cadherin, N-Cadherin, γ, β and α-Catenins in response to glucose for 24 hrs. (A) The graph (left) shows real time PCR results for the positive expression of E-cadherin in MCF-7 and BT-474 cell lines; the grey and black bars represent two repeated independent experiments. However, MDA-MB-231P and its two variant cell lines did not express detectable E-cadherin message or protein (right); (B) Representative blots (left) and quantification (right) shows that MDA-MB-231P and MDA-MB-231BO cells expressed higher levels of N-cadherin compared with the MDA-MB-231BR cells, and that N-cadherin in the former cells was significantly reduced under hypoglycemia. γ, β and α-Catenins were all reduced under hypoglycemic conditions and their expression was significantly decreased in the two MDA-MB-231 variant cells only. Error bars represent ± standard deviation. Note: β-Actin was used in all the blots as a protein loading control.

Discussion

Hypoglycemia and hyperglycemia are important states that affect the tumor microenvironment and they usually arise as the manifestation of diabetes mellitus [20]. In this study we aimed to verify the response of MDA-MB-231P, MDA-MB-231BO, and MDA-MB-231BR cells to define special aspects of protein expression patterns in an attempt to determine targets that are affected by the surrounding microenvironment. The results of this study eventually will aid in understanding the mechanisms relating the complications of diabetes mellitus with BC progression and metastasis. In this present *in vitro* comparative study we found that the expression of VEGFR2 in MDA-MB-231P cells was less than that in the metastatic derivatives MDA-MB-231BR and MDA-MB-231BO, respectively. This suggests that VEGFR2 expression may be reflective of the invasion and progression stage of breast cancer [21]. This finding is consistent with our previous report in which we indicated that VEGFR2 expressed by cancer cells supports tumor cell proliferation and cell survival in suspension [22]. According to several reports MDA-MB-231 does not express the receptors for estrogen, progesterone nor human epidermal growth factor receptor 2 (ER, PR, HER2, respectively), and they were isolated from a hormone resistant tumor [23,24] therefore, we investigated the impact of glycemic load on the expression of VEGF/VEGFR2 which is known to support the growth of this molecular subtype of breast cancer cells [14].

VEGFR2 is initially synthesized as a 147 kDa protein, and after posttranslational glycosylation the protein matures to become a 200 kDa molecule with further glycosylation bringing the protein to its full mature size which is 230 kDa; both the 200 and 230 kDa isoforms can be activated by phosphorylation [25]. We show here that hypoglycemia alone is not effective at halting the synthesis of VEGFR2, which was constantly expressed in its immature form under hypoglycemia. Restoration of glucose allows it to develop into its mature state through posttranslational glycosylation. We found the two metastatic variant cells had higher levels of VEGFR2 than the parental cells, and the levels were different between them. The MDA-MB-231BO had more VEGFR2 than the MDA-MB-231BR cells, indicating that the metastatic site may influence expression of VEGFR2 protein by breast cancer cells [26]. We know that this particular molecular subtype of breast cancer expresses high levels of VEGFR2 protein which is proportionally related with hormone resistance [27]. These results might be translated clinically to answer the question why the glucose reducing agent metformin works as a protective agent against breast cancer progression in some patients and not in all. Thus triple negative breast cancer patients who are difficult to treat with hormone therapy might be treated with a combination of anti-VEGF therapy and metformin, which collectively could reduce the burden of these tyrosine kinases.

Neuropilin-1 was highly expressed in all the cells and was more stable than VEGFR2 under hypoglycemia. We previously showed knockdown of VEGFR2 in EOC was accompanied by an increase

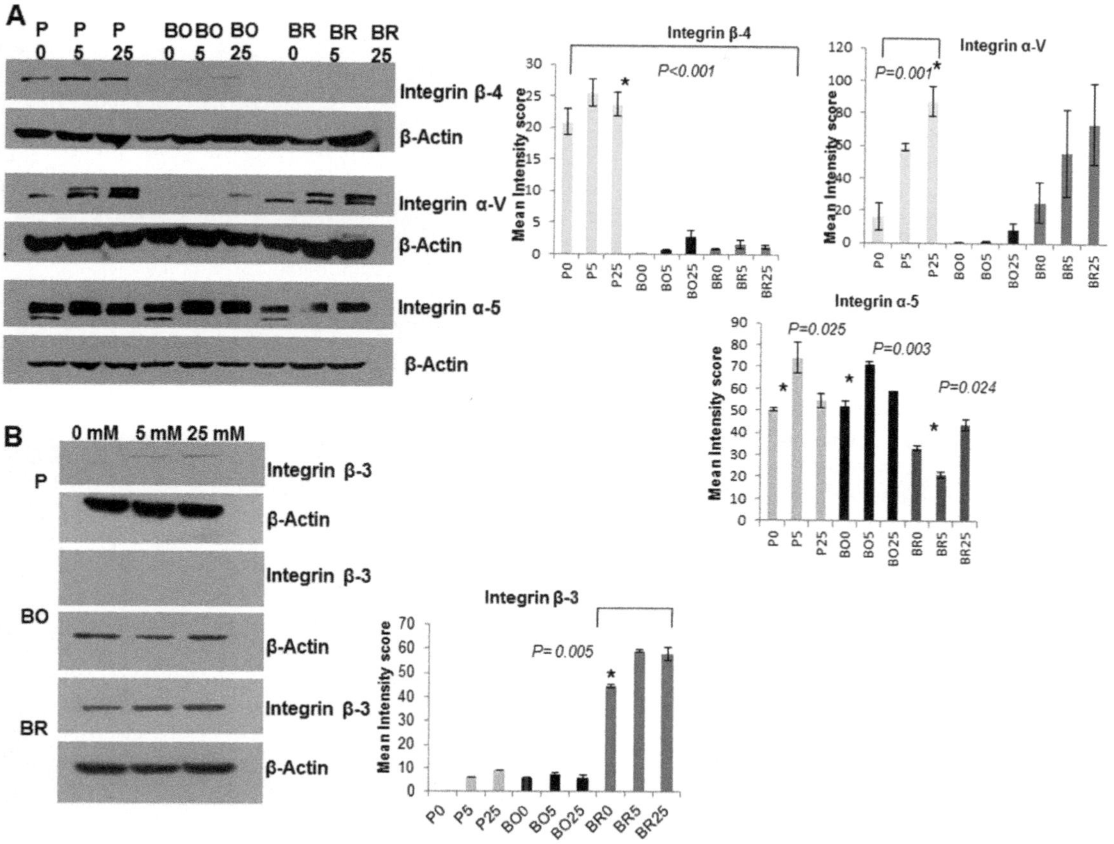

Figure 6. Integrin β4, αV, α5 and β3, were differentially regulated among the three cell lines in response to glucose. (A) Integrin β4 was weakly expressed, or undetectable in the MDA-MB-231BO and MDA-MB-231BR cells respectively however, it was expressed in all glycemic conditions in MDA-MB-231P cells which was significantly higher than the variants cells $p>0.001$ (graph on the right). Integrin αv was down regulated in MDA-MB-231BO and not detected when cells were exposed to DMEM 0 mM glucose (B0) (graph on far right). Integrin α-V was significantly decreased under hypoglycemia only in MDA-MB-231P cells $p = 0.001$. Integrin α5 was expressed in all the three cell lines and was down regulated in the absence of glucose in all the cells in study (bottom graph on the right and lower left panel). Integrin β3 was not detectable in the MDA-MB-231BO cells, and barely detectable in the MDA-MB-231P cells. It was expressed in detectable levels in MDA-MB-231BR cells and was slightly down regulated in reduced glucose. Error bars represent ± standard deviation. Note: β-Actin was used in all the blots as a protein loading control.

in NRP-1 expression and was associated with a more aggressive phenotype [28]. We also showed hypoglycemia resulted in diminishing NRP-1 expression from EOC [15]. The sustained NRP-1 expression under prolonged periods of hypoglycemia in the breast cancer cells used here suggests that this protein may play an important albeit different role in these cells as compared to EOC cells. NRP-1 has a long half-life in the MDA-MB-231 cells; its levels only started to decrease slightly after 72 hrs of CHX exposure, while VEGFR2 was completely degraded after 3 hrs of CHX treatment. This indicates that the two proteins (VEGFR2, NRP-1) are differentially regulated by glucose in MDA-MB-231 cells. Brain metastatic MDA-MB-231 variant cells showed unique features in response to hypoglycemia such as a rounded morphology and an increase in GLUT-1 protein expression. These observations are in agreement with previous findings that alterations in cell morphology accompany changes in the metabolic activity of cancer cells [29]. The changes we observed in MDA-MB-231BR cells suggest that the metabolic and biochemical profile of breast cancer cells might influence which site they are able to colonize. Alternatively, microenvironmental features of different tissue beds may select for cancer cells with specific features to exploit such a niche. A recent finding showed that brain metastasized breast cancer cells express γ-aminobutyric acid (GABA)-related genes which enables breast cancer cells to utilize GABA as an oncometabolite, this represents neuronal like adaptation mechanism by which breast cancer cells transforms to brain [30].

Previous study indicate that hypoglycemia but not hyperglycemia increased glucose transport across blood-brain barrier endothelial cells present in the CNS; this was mainly due to increased GLUT1 on the luminal surface of the cells [31]. MDA-MB-231BR cells were unique in up-regulating the GLUT1 protein in a glucose dependent fashion compared with the other two cell lines, indicating their possible adaptation to the new location where surrounding brain tissue is subjected to high glucose [32]. However, GLUT1 protein expression was slightly down regulated upon hypoglycemia in MDA-MB-231BR cells which contradicts what has been found in endothelial cells [31]. In cancer cells, cell morphology reflects gene expression and patterns of protein expression which correlate with tumor cell invasiveness [33]. In monolayer cultures MDA-MB-231 cells have a bipolar spindle shape with extended protrusions at both ends of the cell body [34]. We found the morphology of MDA-MB-231BR cells was the most sensitive to glucose alteration in the culture media. When glucose was absent, the cells lost their normal morphology and became rounded without the extended protrusions and when glucose was restored the cells reverted to their usual morphology. Similar morphological reversibility was observed in MDA-MB-231 and

MCF-7 cells when treated with inhibitors for β1 integrin, PI3K and MAPK which resulted in nearly complete phenotypic reversion in three dimensional contexts [35].

In MDA-MB-231BR cells we noticed that integrin β3 was exclusively up regulated compared to the other cell lines, and hypoglycemic conditions resulted in its down regulation. This finding can be explained by the previous report which showed that integrin αvβ3 activation in MDA-MB-435 human cancer cells (a highly metastatic cell line to brain) supports the efficient brain metastatic growth through continuous up-regulation of VEGF protein under normoxia [36]. We detected αv protein in both MDA-MB-231P as well as MDA-MB-231BR variant cells and it was regulated by glucose, while MDA-MB-231BO variant cells expressed barely detectable levels under both physiological and hyperglycemic conditions. This result might indicate that although αv and β3 integrins form a heterodimer, integrin β3 alone or in another complex might be enough to drive the metastasis to brain. Further analysis is required to evaluate this observation.

The cell-cell adhesion molecules tested were also differentially regulated in MDA-MB-231 and its variant cells. For instance there was a profound decrease in γ-catenin protein in the metastatic derived cells and its expression was increased in hyperglycemia, while β-catenin had a different response to glucose in the different cells. It has been reported that Wnt/β-catenin pathway and thioredoxin-interacting protein (TXNIP) mediate the "glucose sensor" mechanism in MDA-MB-231 cells, and higher glucose levels resulted in an increase in GSK3β and consequently higher levels of activated β-catenin protein [37]. Thus, our findings open a new avenue to determine the status of Wnt/β-catenin pathway in the MDA-MB-231 and its variants. Among the three cell lines studied, MDA-MB-231BR cells had the lowest capability to reduce Alamarblue and produced the fewest colonies after exposure to hypoglycemia. As a general observation, cancer cells use anaerobic glycolysis for their rapid growth, and thus are sensitive to glucose deprivation [38,39]. It has been shown that the survival of MCF-7/ADR breast cancer cells was decreased exponentially up to 8 hours of their incubation in glucose-free medium due to the induction of c-myc dependent apoptosis [40]. However, in an in vivo breast cancer cell model for brain metastasis in immunodeficient mice, the MDA-MB-231BR cells were 2-fold less sensitive to the glucose analogue 2DG (modeling a glucose deprivation state) when compared to the MDA-MB-231P and MDA-MB-231BO variant cells [41].

We found that in hyperglycemia but not hypoglycemia, MDA-MB-231BR cells secreted higher levels of VEGF, which was different from the expression response of the MDA-MB-231P or MDA-MB-231BO. Another study found that up-regulation of vascular endothelial growth factor (VEGF) lead to activate αvβ3 integrin, which is important for the metastasis of breast cancer cells to the brain under normoxic conditions [36]. This may in part explain our results that MDA-MB-231BR cells produced higher levels of VEGF as well as higher levels of β3-integrin under the regular growth conditions. Our findings open new avenues for further biochemical and metabolic analysis to investigate the pathways that are activated or inactivated in response to glucose deprivation in brain metastasized breast cancer.

Conclusions

The results of this study indicate that these two glycemic (hypo/hyperglycemia) conditions are controlling several pathways in these breast cancer cells differentially depending on their tissue localization preferences. Generally, hypoglycemia caused a negative effect on the proliferation and colony formation ability of MDA-MB-231 breast cancer cells. Hypo/hyperglycemia also had an impact on VEGFR2 and NRP-1 expression which supports the existence of a possible molecular correlation between type II diabetes mellitus and breast cancer progression. Hypoglycemia created a unique expression pattern of some adhesion molecules and tumor growth factors critical for their signaling pathways. Furthermore, the obvious morphological changes in MDA-MB-231BR cell line under hypoglycemia could be a result of lower levels of integrin β3. Finally, this translational research aids in shedding more light on the molecular targets for the different BC stages and tumor microenvironment which impact their progression.

Supporting Information

Table S1 Primary antibodies used with their corresponding manufacturer and working dilution and the species raised in.

Acknowledgments

We thank Jodi Morrison, Najwa Al Balushi, Dr. Vivek Joseph and Dr. Adviti Naik for technical help.

Author Contributions

Conceived and designed the experiments: SA MSA BLC. Performed the experiments: SA HA SH. Analyzed the data: SA AVP BLC. Contributed reagents/materials/analysis tools: SA AVP MSA BLC. Contributed to the writing of the manuscript: SA.

References

1. Ferlay J, Forman D, Mathers CD, Bray F (2012) Breast and cervical cancer in 187 countries between 1980 and 2010. Lancet 379: 1390–1391.
2. Hanahan D, Weinberg RA (2011) Hallmarks of cancer: the next generation. Cell 144: 646–674.
3. Shikata K, Ninomiya T, Kiyohara Y (2013) Diabetes mellitus and cancer risk: Review of the epidemiological evidence. Cancer Sci 104: 9–14.
4. Banarer S, Cryer PE (2004) Hypoglycemia in type 2 diabetes. Med Clin North Am 88: 1107–1116, xii–xiii.
5. Goodwin PJ, Stambolic V (2011) Obesity and insulin resistance in breast cancer–chemoprevention strategies with a focus on metformin. Breast 20 Suppl 3: S31–35.
6. Redaniel MT, Jeffreys M, May MT, Ben-Shlomo Y, Martin RM (2012) Associations of type 2 diabetes and diabetes treatment with breast cancer risk and mortality: a population-based cohort study among British women. Cancer Causes Control 23: 1785–1795.
7. Cohen DH, LeRoith D (2012) Obesity, type 2 diabetes, and cancer: the insulin and IGF connection. Endocr Relat Cancer 19: F27–45.
8. Zeng L, Biernacka KM, Holly JM, Jarrett C, Morrison AA, et al. (2010) Hyperglycaemia confers resistance to chemotherapy on breast cancer cells: the role of fatty acid synthase. Endocr Relat Cancer 17: 539–551.
9. Gliozzo B, Sung CK, Scalia P, Papa V, Frasca F, et al. (1998) Insulin-stimulated cell growth in insulin receptor substrate-1-deficient ZR-75-1 cells is mediated by a phosphatidylinositol-3-kinase-independent pathway. J Cell Biochem 70: 268–280.
10. Hubold C, Oltmanns KM, Schultes B, Jelkmann W, Born J, et al. (2006) High plasma VEGF relates to low carbohydrate intake in patients with type 2 diabetes. Int J Obes (Lond) 30: 1356–1361.
11. Elias I, Franckhauser S, Ferre T, Vila L, Tafuro S, et al. (2012) Adipose tissue overexpression of vascular endothelial growth factor protects against diet-induced obesity and insulin resistance. Diabetes 61: 1801–1813.
12. Wu LE, Meoli CC, Mangiafico SP, Fazakerley DJ, Cogger VC, et al. (2014) Systemic vascular endothelial growth factor-A (VEGF-A) neutralization ameliorates diet induced metabolic dysfunction. Diabetes.
13. Pizon M, Zimon DS, Pachmann U, Pachmann K (2013) Insulin-Like Growth Factor Receptor I (IGF-IR) and Vascular Endothelial Growth Factor Receptor 2 (VEGFR-2) Are Expressed on the Circulating Epithelial Tumor Cells of Breast Cancer Patients. PLoS One 8: e56836.
14. Williams CM, Engler AJ, Slone RD, Galante LL, Schwarzbauer JE (2008) Fibronectin expression modulates mammary epithelial cell proliferation during acinar differentiation. Cancer Res 68: 3185–3192.

15. Adham SA, Coomber BL (2009) Glucose is a key regulator of VEGFR2/KDR in human epithelial ovarian carcinoma cells. Biochem Biophys Res Commun 390: 130–135.
16. Yoneda T, Williams PJ, Hiraga T, Niewolna M, Nishimura R (2001) A bone-seeking clone exhibits different biological properties from the MDA-MB-231 parental human breast cancer cells and a brain-seeking clone in vivo and in vitro. J Bone Miner Res 16: 1486–1495.
17. Corn PG, Smith BD, Ruckdeschel ES, Douglas D, Baylin SB, et al. (2000) E-cadherin expression is silenced by 5′ CpG island methylation in acute leukemia. Clin Cancer Res 6: 4243–4248.
18. Dingemans AM, van den Boogaart V, Vosse BA, van Suylen RJ, Griffioen AW, et al. (2010) Integrin expression profiling identifies integrin alpha5 and beta1 as prognostic factors in early stage non-small cell lung cancer. Mol Cancer 9: 152.
19. Yoshida J, Horiuchi A, Kikuchi N, Hayashi A, Osada R, et al. (2009) Changes in the expression of E-cadherin repressors, Snail, Slug, SIP1, and Twist, in the development and progression of ovarian carcinoma: the important role of Snail in ovarian tumorigenesis and progression. Med Mol Morphol 42: 82–91.
20. Onozuka H, Tsuchihara K, Esumi H (2011) Hypoglycemic/hypoxic condition in vitro mimicking the tumor microenvironment markedly reduced the efficacy of anticancer drugs. Cancer Sci 102: 975–982.
21. Guo S, Colbert LS, Fuller M, Zhang Y, Gonzalez-Perez RR (2010) Vascular endothelial growth factor receptor-2 in breast cancer. Biochim Biophys Acta 1806: 108–121.
22. Sher I, Adham SA, Petrik J, Coomber BL (2009) Autocrine VEGF-A/KDR loop protects epithelial ovarian carcinoma cells from anoikis. Int J Cancer 124: 553–561.
23. Wang K, Xie SM, He JJ, Ren Y, Xia HB, et al. (2011) [Establishment of a bioluminescent MDA-MB-231 cell line for in vivo imaging of human triple-negative breast cancer xenograft]. Nan Fang Yi Ke Da Xue Xue Bao 31: 1812–1818.
24. Freitas VM, do Amaral JB, Silva TA, Santos ES, Mangone FR, et al. (2013) Decreased expression of ADAMTS-1 in human breast tumors stimulates migration and invasion. Mol Cancer 12: 2.
25. Takahashi T, Shibuya M (1997) The 230 kDa mature form of KDR/Flk-1 (VEGF receptor-2) activates the PLC-gamma pathway and partially induces mitotic signals in NIH3T3 fibroblasts. Oncogene 14: 2079–2089.
26. Isowa S, Shimo T, Ibaragi S, Kurio N, Okui T, et al. (2010) PTHrP regulates angiogenesis and bone resorption via VEGF expression. Anticancer Res 30: 2755–2767.
27. Scherbakov AM, Krasil'nikov MA, Kushlinskii NE (2013) Molecular mechanisms of hormone resistance of breast cancer. Bull Exp Biol Med 155: 384–395.
28. Adham SA, Sher I, Coomber BL (2010) Molecular blockade of VEGFR2 in human epithelial ovarian carcinoma cells. Lab Invest 90: 709–723.
29. D'Anselmi F, Valerio M, Cucina A, Galli L, Proietti S, et al. (2011) Metabolism and cell shape in cancer: a fractal analysis. Int J Biochem Cell Biol 43: 1052–1058.
30. Van Swearingen AE, Siegel MB, Anders CK (2014) Breast cancer brain metastases: evidence for neuronal-like adaptation in a 'breast-to-brain' transition? Breast Cancer Research 16: 304.
31. Simpson IA, Appel NM, Hokari M, Oki J, Holman GD, et al. (1999) Blood-brain barrier glucose transporter: effects of hypo- and hyperglycemia revisited. J Neurochem 72: 238–247.
32. Shah K, Desilva S, Abbruscato T (2012) The Role of Glucose Transporters in Brain Disease: Diabetes and Alzheimer's Disease. Int J Mol Sci 13: 12629–12655.
33. Kenny PA, Lee GY, Myers CA, Neve RM, Semeiks JR, et al. (2007) The morphologies of breast cancer cell lines in three-dimensional assays correlate with their profiles of gene expression. Mol Oncol 1: 84–96.
34. Hirsch DS, Shen Y, Wu WJ (2006) Growth and motility inhibition of breast cancer cells by epidermal growth factor receptor degradation is correlated with inactivation of Cdc42. Cancer Res 66: 3523–3530.
35. Wang F, Hansen RK, Radisky D, Yoneda T, Barcellos-Hoff MH, et al. (2002) Phenotypic reversion or death of cancer cells by altering signaling pathways in three-dimensional contexts. J Natl Cancer Inst 94: 1494–1503.
36. Lorger M, Krueger JS, O'Neal M, Staflin K, Felding-Habermann B (2009) Activation of tumor cell integrin alphavbeta3 controls angiogenesis and metastatic growth in the brain. Proc Natl Acad Sci U S A 106: 10666–10671.
37. Vaira S, Friday E, Scott K, Conrad S, Turturro F (2012) Wnt/beta-catenin signaling pathway and thioredoxin-interacting protein (TXNIP) mediate the "glucose sensor" mechanism in metastatic breast cancer-derived cells MDA-MB-231. J Cell Physiol 227: 578–586.
38. Weber G (1977) Enzymology of cancer cells (second of two parts). N Engl J Med 296: 541–551.
39. Weber G (1977) Enzymology of cancer cells (first of two parts). N Engl J Med 296: 486–492.
40. Lee YJ, Galoforo SS, Berns CM, Tong WP, Kim HR, et al. (1997) Glucose deprivation-induced cytotoxicity in drug resistant human breast carcinoma MCF-7/ADR cells: role of c-myc and bcl-2 in apoptotic cell death. J Cell Sci 110 (Pt 5): 681–686.
41. Chen EI, Hewel J, Krueger JS, Tiraby C, Weber MR, et al. (2007) Adaptation of energy metabolism in breast cancer brain metastases. Cancer Res 67: 1472–1486.

3

High Variability in Oral Glucose Tolerance among 1,128 Patients with Cystic Fibrosis: A Multicenter Screening Study

Nicole Scheuing[1*¶], Reinhard W. Holl[1¶], Gerd Dockter[2], Julia M. Hermann[1], Sibylle Junge[3], Cordula Koerner-Rettberg[4], Lutz Naehrlich[5], Christina Smaczny[6], Doris Staab[7], Gabriela Thalhammer[8], Silke van Koningsbruggen-Rietschel[9], Manfred Ballmann[4]

1 Institute of Epidemiology and Medical Biometry, Central Institute for Biomedical Technology, University of Ulm, Ulm, Germany, **2** Cystic Fibrosis Centre, Saarland University Hospital for Pediatric and Adolescent Medicine, Homburg/Saar, Germany, **3** Clinic for Pediatric Pneumology and Neonatology, Hannover Medical School, Hannover, Germany, **4** Department of Pediatric Pulmonology, St. Josef Hospital Pediatric Clinic, Ruhr University Bochum, Bochum, Germany, **5** Department of Pediatrics, Justus-Liebig University Giessen, Giessen, Germany, **6** Medical Clinic I, Pneumology and Allergology, University Hospital Frankfurt/Main, Goethe University, Frankfurt/Main, Germany, **7** Division of Pulmonology and Immunology, Department of Pediatrics, Charité Berlin, Berlin, Germany, **8** Department for Pediatric Pulmonology and Allergology, Medical University of Graz, Graz, Austria, **9** Cystic Fibrosis Centre Cologne, Childrens Hospital, University of Cologne, Cologne, Germany

Abstract

Background: In cystic fibrosis, highly variable glucose tolerance is suspected. However, no study provided within-patient coefficients of variation. The main objective of this short report was to evaluate within-patient variability of oral glucose tolerance.

Methods: In total, 4,643 standardized oral glucose tolerance tests of 1,128 cystic fibrosis patients (median age at first test: 15.5 [11.5; 21.5] years, 48.8% females) were studied. Patients included were clinically stable, non-pregnant, and had at least two oral glucose tolerance tests, with no prior lung transplantation or systemic steroid therapy. Transition frequency from any one test to the subsequent test was analyzed and within-patient coefficients of variation were calculated for fasting and two hour blood glucose values. All statistical analysis was implemented with SAS 9.4.

Results: A diabetic glucose tolerance was confirmed in 41.2% by the subsequent test. A regression to normal glucose tolerance at the subsequent test was observed in 21.7% and to impaired fasting glucose, impaired glucose tolerance or both in 15.2%, 12.0% or 9.9%. The average within-patient coefficient of variation for fasting blood glucose was 11.1% and for two hour blood glucose 25.3%.

Conclusion: In the cystic fibrosis patients studied, a highly variable glucose tolerance was observed. Compared to the general population, variability of two hour blood glucose was 1.5 to 1.8-fold higher.

Editor: Dominik Hartl, University of Tübingen, Germany

Funding: The study was funded by the German and French CF associations (Mukoviszidose e.V. and its regional group Saarland-Pfalz, Vaincre de la Mucoviszidose), and by Novo Nordisk. The funders had no role in study design, data collection and analysis, decision to publish, or preparation of the manuscript.

Competing Interests: The study was partly funded by Novo Nordisk. There are no patents, products in development or marketed products to declare.

* Email: nicole.scheuing@uni-ulm.de

¶ Shared first authorship.

Introduction

Cystic fibrosis (CF) is a life-limiting autosomal recessive illness occurring in about one of 2,500 newborns in Europe. As the life expectancy for CF patients has increased due to earlier diagnosis and improved care, CF-related comorbidities became more frequent over the last decades. A growing comorbidity with impact on the course of CF is cystic fibrosis-related diabetes (CFRD). The latest comprehensive guidelines for CFRD recommend yearly screening for abnormal glucose metabolism by oral glucose tolerance test (OGTT) in CF patients aged ≥10 years [1]. A small study suspected that CF patients have a high variation in glucose tolerance over time [2].

Therefore, we aimed to investigate in this short report the variability of glucose tolerance in a large cohort of CF patients. For the first time, a within-patient coefficient of variation (CV) for 2-hour blood glucose was calculated in CF.

Materials and Methods

Ethics statement

The ethical committees of Ulm University and Hannover Medical School approved the study, and patients or their parents provided written informed consent.

Study subjects

Between 2001 and 2010, 1,778 CF patients aged 10 years or older were screened serially by OGTT in a multicenter screening program carried out by 43 German/Austrian specialized centers (Trial No. NCT00662714). All patients had a physician-based diagnosis of CF according to the latest German guidelines [3]. OGTTs were performed and interpreted in line with recommendations of the World Health Organization modified by the American Diabetes Association as described in detail previously [4,5].

In total, 5,765 OGTTs among clinically stable CF patients were carried out until the end of the study (Figure 1). As mentioned in reference [4], all patients screened had to be without symptoms of acute infections or exacerbations of chronic infections and should not have a reduced carbohydrate intake. Moreover, patients with respiratory failure (FEV1<40%) or with enteral tube feeding were excluded. In case of a confirmed diagnosis of CFRD or the use of anti-hyperglycemic treatment, patients were also excluded from screening.

For the present analysis, only OGTTs of non-pregnant patients with no prior systemic steroid therapy or lung transplantation were considered (Figure 1). If patients awaited lung transplantation, OGTTs were also excluded. Furthermore, at least two OGTTs had to be performed per patient (Figure 1). The final study population comprised 4,643 OGTTs of 1,128 CF patients. For each patient included, test results were classified as normal glucose tolerance (NGT), impaired fasting glucose (IFG), impaired glucose tolerance (IGT), IFG and IGT combined, or diabetic glucose tolerance (DGT). The detailed cut-offs are described in reference [4]. As there are some CF patients with isolated IFG [4] and the pathophysiology between IFG and IGT is at least in part different [6], we introduced an IFG group in this analysis. CFRD was defined as a diabetic OGTT confirmed by a consecutive OGTT in the DGT range [1]. Body mass index standard deviation score (BMI-SDS) was calculated using data from the German Health Interview and Examination Survey for Children and Adolescents (KiGGS study, [7]) as national reference. The KiGGS study was used as a reference in a number of previous publications by our group to calculate BMI-SDS in CF patients [4,8,9] and is the best currently available reference data for healthy German children. Data to calculate BMI-SDS on the basis of CF-specific anthropometric reference percentiles are currently not available.

Statistical analysis

To analyze the variation in glucose tolerance, transition frequency from any one test to the subsequent test was studied. As there is no subsequent test for the last test in each patient, 3,515 pairs of consecutive OGTTs were available in the study population (the number of OGTT pairs therefore equals the total number of OGTTs minus the number of patients). For each pair of OGTTs, the first test was categorized in one of the five glucose

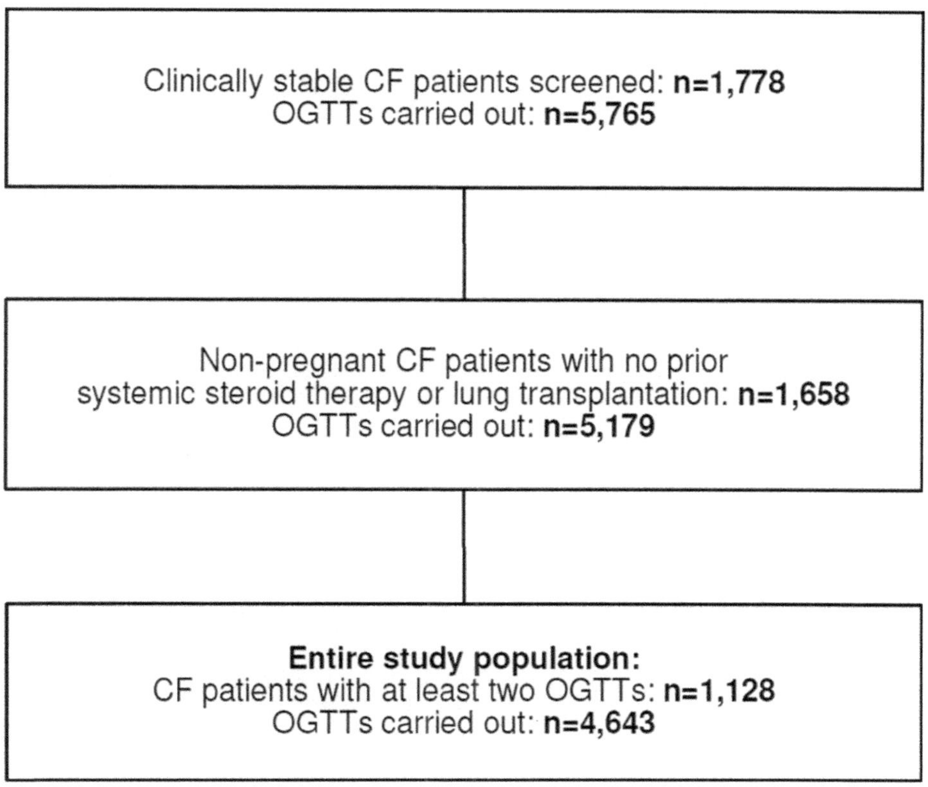

Figure 1. Selection of study population. Abbreviations: *CF* cystic fibrosis, *OGTT* oral glucose tolerance test.

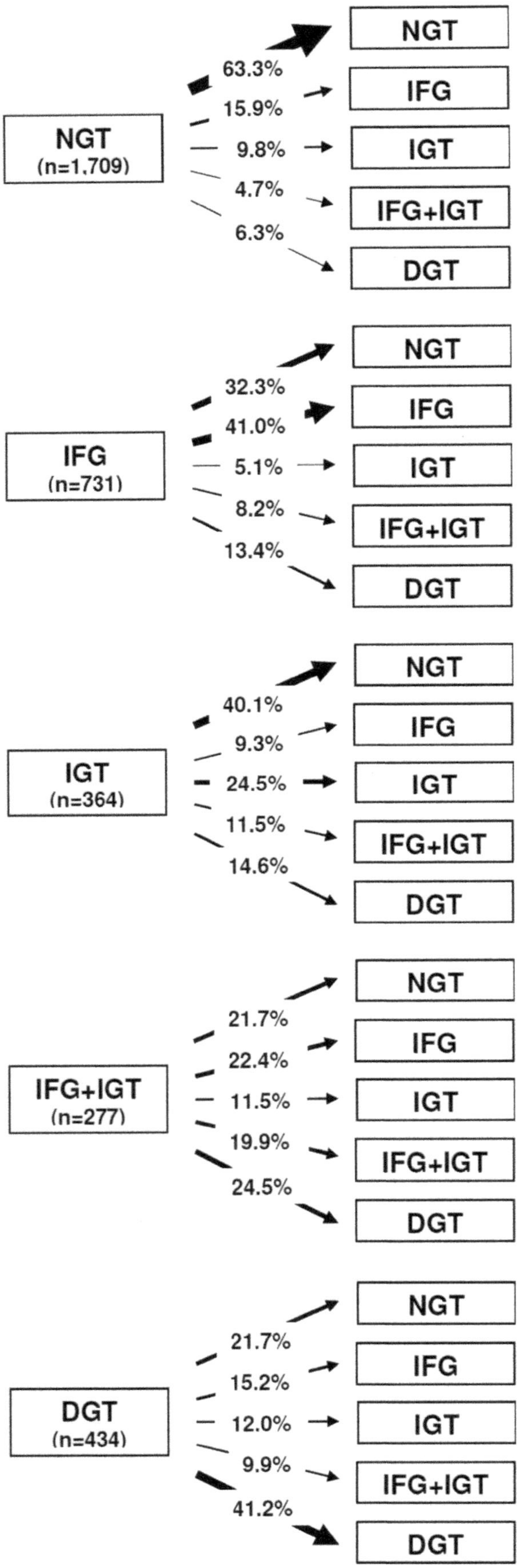

Figure 2. Transition from any one test to a subsequent test. In total, 3,515 pairs of consecutive OGTTs are summarized. For each pair, the first test was categorized in one of the five glucose tolerance classes (NGT, IFG only, IGT only, IFG+IGT, DGT). The figure shows the percentage of subsequent test results for each glucose tolerance category. The number in parentheses indicates the number of OGTTs available for analysis. Abbreviations: *NGT* normal glucose tolerance, *IFG* impaired fasting glucose, *IGT* impaired glucose tolerance, *DGT* diabetic glucose tolerance, *OGTT* oral glucose tolerance test.

tolerance classes (NGT, IFG only, IGT only, IFG+IGT, DGT) and the percentage of subsequent test results was calculated. Moreover, the variation in glucose tolerance is depicted in three individual patients who had seven consecutive OGTTs with at least one diabetic result. To assess the degree of variability of serially measured fasting and 2-hour blood glucose values in CF patients, within-patient CVs (defined as ratio between within-subject standard deviation and mean) were calculated and compared to the general population. CVs were calculated as they are normalized measures of the variability and independent of the mean level.

To evaluate gender or age differences in the deterioration of glucose tolerance from test to test, a logistic mixed regression model was applied. Deterioration of glucose metabolism was defined as worsening of glucose tolerance in a subsequent test compared to the pretest or as confirmation of a diabetic OGTT. Sex and age were entered as independent fixed effects. Age was categorized as 10–<15 years, 15–<20 years and ≥20 years. To account for repeated OGTTs per patient, random effects with first-order autoregressive covariance structure were used. Results are given as odds ratios (OR) with lower and upper confidence limit (CL).

Statistical analyses were performed with SAS 9.4. The level of significance was set at 0.05. To compare demographics between patients included and excluded, Kruskal-Wallis test was applied for continuous parameters and χ^2-test for dichotomous parameters.

Results

48.8% of patients included were female and 28.9% were >20 years. Median [Q_1;Q_3] (mean±SD) age at first OGTT was 15.5 [11.5; 21.5] (18.0±8.4) years and at last OGTT 18.6 [15.3; 25.4] (21.3±8.5) years. At baseline OGTT, the youngest patient aged 10.0 years and the oldest patient 63.9 years. On average, median (mean) duration between two consecutive OGTTs was 1.0 [0.7; 1.2] (1.1±0.7) year. A diabetic OGTT was repeated within a median (mean) time of 6.9 [4.9; 12.9] (9.1±6.2) weeks. As published previously [4], the median duration between two consecutive OGTTs in the DGT range (confirmed diagnosis of CFRD) was 8.1 [5.1; 27.9] weeks. All patients with suspected CFRD (i.e. one OGTT in the DGT range) at the end of the study were followed-up outside the context of the screening study. Each patient with a confirmed diagnosis of CFRD was invited to participate in a randomized controlled trial investigating the use of repaglinide in comparison to insulin therapy. CFRD patients not participating in the clinical trial received insulin therapy and CF-specific nutritional counseling as recommended by guidelines.

Baseline characteristics of the 650 patients excluded are depicted in table 1. Excluded patients were older and had on average a lower BMI-SDS.

Figure 2 displays the transition frequency from any one test to a subsequent test. For example, an OGTT in the DGT range was confirmed in 41.2% by the subsequent test.

Table 1. Demographics of patients included and patients excluded at baseline OGTT.

	Patients included	Patients excluded	p-value
Number, n	1,128	650	-
Age, years	15.5 [11.5; 21.5] (18.0±8.4)	17.4 [12.3; 25.2] (20.0±9.3)	<0.001
Female sex, %	48.8	45.1	NS
Weight, kg	47.8 [34.5; 57.8] (47.8±15.4)	50.2 [35.5; 59.0] (49.0±15.2)	0.04
Height, cm	160.0 [145.6; 170.0] (157.8±15.6)	162.0 [147.0; 172.0] (159.8±15.9)	0.008
BMI, kg/m^2	18.4 [16.2; 20.4] (18.6±3.3)	18.6 [16.2; 20.7] (18.7±3.3)	NS
BMI-SDS	−0.76 [−1.42;−0.11] (−0.80±1.08)	−0.87 [−1.65;−0.18] (−0.99±1.26)	0.005

Data are given as median with quartiles (mean with standard deviation) or as percentage. Abbreviations: *BMI* body mass index, *SDS* standard deviation score, *NS* not significant.

Until the end of the screening study, a total of 136 CF patients revealed a confirmed diagnosis of CFRD i.e. two consecutive OGTTs revealing DGT. Despite the fact that two consecutive OGTTs in the DGT range are sufficient to diagnose CFRD, 54 out of the 136 patients had additional OGTTs. In 42.6% (n = 23) of patients, all subsequent tests were diabetic. In 20.4% (n = 11) of cases, at least one of the subsequent tests revealed NGT.

Figure 3 indicates that independent of age, glucose tolerance varied highly from test to test in three individual patients.

Overall, in CF patients the average within-patient CV for fasting blood glucose values was 11.1% and for 2-hour blood glucose 25.3%. Analyzing patients with (n = 339) and without (n = 789) at least one OGTT in the DGT range separately, patients without an OGTT in the diabetic range had lower CVs for both fasting and 2-hour blood glucose values (fasting: 8.9 vs. 16.1%, $p<0.001$; 2-hour: 22.2 vs. 32.4%, $p<0.001$).

Logistic regression analysis revealed for girls a 1.18-fold [lower CL: 1.03; upper CL: 1.36] higher risk for the deterioration of

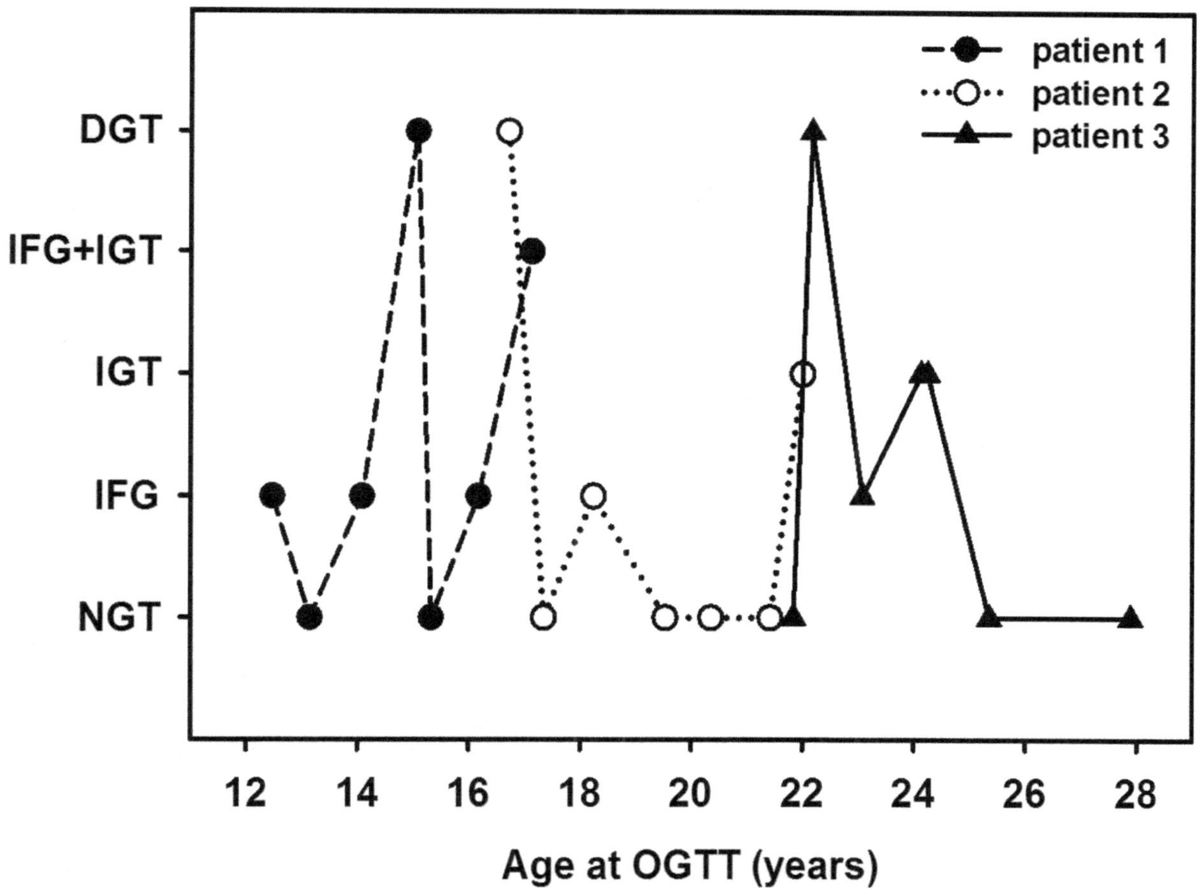

Figure 3. Variation of glucose tolerance in three patients of different age. Each patient had seven consecutive OGTTs with at least one diabetic result. Abbreviations: *DGT* diabetic glucose tolerance, *IFG* impaired fasting glucose, *IGT* impaired glucose tolerance, *NGT* normal glucose tolerance, *OGTT* oral glucose tolerance test.

glucose tolerance compared to boys ($p = 0.015$). In addition, patients aged 15–<20 years (OR: 1.23 [1.04; 1.47], $p = 0.019$) or ≥20 years (OR: 1.22 [1.03; 1.44], $p = 0.024$) had a higher risk than patients aged 10–<15 years. In 15 to <20 year old patients, risk was comparable to patients aged ≥20 years (OR: 1.01 [0.86; 1.19], $p = 0.867$).

Analyzing the influence of sex in the subgroup of older patients (>20 years at baseline OGTT; n = 326 patients with 1,276 OGTTs), revealed also an increased risk in females compared to males, even though the influence was no longer significant due to the lower number of patients studied (OR: 1.23 [0.92; 1.63], $p = 0.162$).

Discussion

Our analysis among asymptomatic CF patients revealed a high variability in glucose tolerance over time, even though patients without DGT seem to be more stable with respect to glucose tolerance. Compared to the general population [10–12], overall within-patient variability of 2-hour blood glucose is 1.5 to 1.8-fold higher in CF. The NHANES III Second Examination revealed a within-patient CV of 16.6% for 2-hour blood glucose [12] and the Hoorn study of 16.7% [11]. In a general practice [10], a within-patient CV of 14.3% was observed. Fluctuating levels of insulin resistance due to acute and chronic infections or CF-related inflammatory cytokines may explain the highly variable glucose tolerance in CF.

The fluctuation in glucose tolerance observed in this study implicates regular control of glucose metabolism in CF. Future guidelines should provide recommendations regarding an adequate time frame for repeating OGTTs in patients with abnormal glucose tolerance as well as for the confirmation interval of a diabetic test result. As outlined by the study protocol and described previously [4], a diabetic OGTT had to be repeated within 4 to 6 weeks in the present study and an OGTT revealing IFG or IGT after 6 months. According to guidelines, all patients with a confirmed CFRD diagnosis or with a diabetic OGTT and classical symptoms of diabetes should receive insulin treatment immediately [1]. Oral antidiabetic agents are not advised until sufficient data become available regarding their efficiency.

Reasons for performing additional OGTTs in patients with already confirmed CFRD are unknown. Maybe patients requested an additional OGTT in the context of intensifying therapy. Especially, asymptomatic CF patients often have problems starting insulin treatment besides numerous CF-related therapies. Another possibility might be that patients with a confirmed CFRD diagnosis were not totally clinically stable at the time of the confirmation test and the medical team therefore decided to repeat the test at a later time point. As OGTT results depend also on the supplementation of pancreatic enzymes, the medical team may have repeated the confirmation test after adjusting pancreatic enzyme substitution.

Although the OGTT revealed a high degree of within-patient variance in CF, it is the best screening tool for abnormalities in glucose tolerance currently available. Fasting plasma glucose, hemoglobin A1c or other classical methods applicable for type 1 or type 2 diabetes are not recommended in CF [1]. In the future, continuous glucose monitoring or standardized test meals might be a useful alternative to OGTT. However, there are no reference values for continuous glucose monitoring so far. To minimize the variability of OGTTs in CF patients, CF-adapted standardization might be one possibility. At the moment, criteria for the performance and interpretation of OGTT are identical to other diabetes types. However, pancreatic enzyme substitution and the grade of inflammation (e.g. C-reactive protein measurement) should be considered before performing an OGTT in CF, and when interpreting OGTT results. More advanced interpretation criteria that take into account dynamics in oral glucose challenge in CF patients might be appropriate. As CFRD is less common compared to the more frequent type 1 or type 2 diabetes, other measures of ß-cell function (e.g. C-peptide) or calculation of indices for insulin secretion and sensitivity might be practicable in clinical settings that may result in better assessment of glucose tolerance in CF patients.

The higher risk for deterioration of glucose tolerance in girls confirms previous studies indicating an earlier onset and a higher prevalence of CFRD in females [4,13,14]. The lower risk in patients younger than 15 years compared to older patients might be explained by the rare occurrence of CFRD in patients <10 years and the increasing prevalence of abnormal glucose tolerance with age [4,15,16].

Selection biases might be one limitation of the present study. Not all centers or CF patients participated, although all German/Austrian medical facilities providing care for CF patients were invited for participation in written form. Moreover, some CF-related therapies (e.g. steroids, lung transplantation) led to exclusion of patients and the complexity of CF itself made study participation often difficult. The higher age and the lower BMI-SDS of patients excluded may point to a more severe progression of the disease compared to patients included. Exclusion criterion for the majority of the 650 patients not analyzed was the availability of solely one OGTT. This might be due to termination of the study or occurrence of exclusion criteria after the first OGTT. Moreover, each patient could withdraw from the study at any time.

In summary, in the asymptomatic CF patients studied, one diabetic OGTT seems not sufficient to diagnose CFRD due to the existing high variability of glucose tolerance. A normal glucose tolerance after a confirmed CFRD diagnosis (i.e. two consecutive OGTTs revealing DGT) cannot be excluded. Despite improvement of glucose tolerance, these patients are classified as diabetic [1], although this labelling may be contra-intuitive for patients and physicians. It is still a debate whether solely a persistently diabetic glucose tolerance is associated with an increased risk of clinical decline in CF or even a pre-diabetic condition.

Acknowledgments

The authors thank all participating centers for performing OGTTs and providing data for the present analysis. A detailed list of centers was recently published [4].

Author Contributions

Conceived and designed the experiments: RWH MB. Performed the experiments: GD SJ CKR LN CS DS GT SVKR MB. Analyzed the data: NS JMH RWH. Contributed reagents/materials/analysis tools: GD SJ CKR LN CS DS GT SVKR MB. Contributed to the writing of the manuscript: NS. Revision of manuscript: RWH GD JMH SJ CKR LN CS DS GT SVKR MB. Final approval of the version to be published: NS RWH GD JMH SJ CKR LN CS DS GT SVKR MB.

References

1. Moran A, Brunzell C, Cohen RC, Katz M, Marshall BC, et al. (2010) Clinical care guidelines for cystic fibrosis-related diabetes: A position statement of the American Diabetes Association and a clinical practice guideline of the Cystic Fibrosis Foundation, endorsed by the Pediatric Endocrine Society. Diabetes Care 33: 2697–2708.

2. Sterescu AE, Rhodes B, Jackson R, Dupuis A, Hanna A, et al. (2010) Natural history of glucose intolerance in patients with cystic fibrosis: Ten-year prospective observation program. J Pediatr 156: 613–617.
3. Naehrlich L, Stuhrmann-Spangenberg M, Barben J, Bargon J, Blankenstein O, et al. (June 2013) S2 consensus-guideline: diagnostic of mucoviscidosis. AWMF 026–023.Available: www.awmf.org/uploads/tx_szleitlinien/026-023 m_S2k_Diagnostik_der_Mukoviszidose_ 2013-07.pdf. Accessed 2014 June 4.
4. Scheuing N, Holl RW, Dockter G, Fink K, Junge S, et al. (2013) Diabetes in cystic fibrosis: Multicenter screening results based on current guidelines. PLoS One 8: e81545.
5. Schmid K, Fink K, Holl RW, Hebestreit H, Ballmann M (2014) Predictors for future cystic fibrosis-related diabetes by oral glucose tolerance test. J Cyst Fibros 13: 80–85.
6. Nathan DM, Davidson MB, DeFronzo RA, Heine RJ, Henry RR, et al. (2007) Impaired fasting glucose and impaired glucose tolerance: implications for care. Diabetes Care 30: 753–759.
7. Rosario AS, Kurth BM, Stolzenberg H, Ellert U, Neuhauser H (2010) Body mass index percentiles for children and adolescents in Germany based on a nationally representative sample (KiGGS 2003–2006). Eur J Clin Nutr 64: 341–349.
8. Scheuing N, Berger G, Bergis D, Gohlke B, Konrad K, et al. (2014) Adherence to clinical care guidelines for cystic fibrosis-related diabetes in 659 German/Austrian patients. J Cyst Fibros [Epub]. DOI:10.1016/j.jcf.2014.05.006.
9. Scheuing N, Badenhoop K, Borkenstein M, Konrad K, Lilienthal E, et al. (2014) Why is insulin pump treatment rarely used in adolescents and young adults with cystic fibrosis-related diabetes? Pediatr Diabetes [Epub]. DOI:10.1111/pedi.12158.
10. Feskens EJ, Bowles CH, Kromhout D (1991) Intra- and interindividual variability of glucose tolerance in an elderly population. J Clin Epidemiol 44: 947–953.
11. Mooy JM, Grootenhuis PA, de Vries H, Kostense PJ, Popp-Snijders C, et al. (1996) Intra-individual variation of glucose, specific insulin and proinsulin concentrations measured by two oral glucose tolerance tests in a general Caucasian population: The Hoorn study. Diabetologia 39: 298–305.
12. Selvin E, Crainiceanu CM, Brancati FL, Coresh J (2007) Short-term variability in measures of glycemia and implications for the classification of diabetes. Arch Intern Med 167: 1545–1551.
13. Ode KL, Frohnert B, Laguna T, Phillips J, Holme B, et al. (2010) Oral glucose tolerance testing in children with cystic fibrosis. Pediatr Diabetes 11: 487–492.
14. Konrad K, Thon A, Fritsch M, Fröhlich-Reiterer E, Lilienthal E, et al. (2013) Comparison of cystic fibrosis-related diabetes with type 1 diabetes based on a German/Austrian pediatric diabetes registry. Diabetes Care 36: 879–886.
15. Lanng S, Thorsteinsson B, Lund-Andersen C, Nerup J, Schiøtz PO, et al. (1994) Diabetes mellitus in Danish cystic fibrosis patients: prevalence and late diabetic complications. Acta Paediatr 83: 72–77.
16. Moran A, Dunitz J, Nathan B, Saeed A, Holme B, et al. (2009) Cystic fibrosis-related diabetes: current trends in prevalence, incidence, and mortality. Diabetes Care 32: 1626–1631.

4

Access to Diagnostic Tests and Essential Medicines for Cardiovascular Diseases and Diabetes Care: Cost, Availability and Affordability in the West Region of Cameroon

Ahmadou M. Jingi[1], Jean Jacques N. Noubiap[2*], Arnold Ewane Onana[3], Jobert Richie N. Nansseu[4], Binhuan Wang[5], Samuel Kingue[1], André Pascal Kengne[6]

1 Department of Internal Medicine and Specialties, Faculty of Medicine and Biomedical Sciences, University of Yaoundé I, Yaoundé, Cameroon, **2** Internal Medicine Unit, Edéa Regional Hospital, Edéa, Cameroon, **3** National Obesity Center, Yaoundé Central Hospital, Yaoundé, Cameroon, **4** Sickle Cell Unit, Mother and Child Centre, Chantal Biya Foundation, Yaoundé, Cameroon, **5** Department of Population Health, Division of Biostatistics, New York School of Medicine, New York, United States of America, **6** Non-communicable Disease Research Unit, South African Medical Research Council and University of Cape Town, Cape Town, South Africa

Abstract

Objective: To assess the availability and affordability of medicines and routine tests for cardiovascular disease (CVD) and diabetes in the West region of Cameroon, a low-income setting.

Methods: A survey was conducted on the availability and cost of twelve routine tests and twenty medicines for CVD and diabetes in eight health districts (four urban and four rural) covering over 60% of the population of the region (1.8 million). We analyzed the percentage of tests and medicines available, the median price against the international reference price (median price ratio) for the medicines, and affordability in terms of the number of days' wages it would cost the lowest-paid unskilled government worker for initial investigation tests and procurement for one month of treatment.

Results: The availability of tests varied between 10% for the ECG to 100% for the fasting blood sugar. The average cost for the initial investigation using the minimum tests cost 29.76 days' wages. The availability of medicines varied from 36.4% to 59.1% in urban and from 9.1% to 50% in rural settings. Only metformin and benzathine-benzylpenicilline had a median price ratio of ≤1.5, with statins being largely unaffordable (at least 30.51 days' wages). One month of combination treatment for coronary heart disease costs at least 40.87 days' wages.

Conclusion: The investigation and management of patients with medium-to-high cardiovascular risk remains largely unavailable and unaffordable in this setting. An effective non-communicable disease program should lay emphasis on primary prevention, and improve affordable access to essential medicines in public outlets.

Editor: Gianpaolo Reboldi, University of Perugia, Italy

Funding: The authors have no support or funding to report.

Competing Interests: The authors have declared that no competing interests exist.

* Email: noubiapjj@yahoo.fr

Introduction

Hypertension, diabetes and consequential cardiovascular diseases (CVD), have reached epidemic proportions worldwide, and disproportionately affect low- and middle-income countries (LMICs) [1]. Nearly 80% of deaths from CVD and diabetes occur in LMICs, resulting in non-communicable diseases (NCDs) overtaking communicable diseases as the major leading cause of disease and death in LMICs [1]. Moreover, the economic and societal impact of CVD on individuals, households and countries is enormous. These effects are particularly important in LMICs, where CVD more often affects individuals in their working age, and therefore contributes disproportionately to losses of potential years of healthy and active life, which can impair economic growth [2–4]. Indeed, it has been demonstrated that through their combined impact on economies, health systems, households and families, diabetes and CVD are major threats to the current and future economic development and prosperity of individuals and societies in Africa [5].

Timely interventions including early detection, lifestyle changes and use of effective and affordable medicines, have been shown to reduce morbidity and mortality associated to CVD [6]. Unfortunately, studies have shown that these essential interventions for CVD and diabetes are not always available and accessible in the public sector in LMICs [7,8]. Although there is a better availability of these interventions including medicines for CVD and diabetes in the private sector, the end-user cost is a major deterrent to access to the large segment of the population in LMICs. Moreover, because prevention and treatment interventions for CVD and diabetes are mostly purchased through out-of-pocket

Table 1. Availability of medicines and test per site and the population served.

Survey site	Area	Population served 2012 estimates	Availability of Medicines	Availability of WHO recommended tests	Availability of all tests
Foumban	Urban	170,571	36.4%	83.3%	91.7%
Dschang	Urban	211,818	45.5%	100%	100.0%
Mifi	Urban	254,123	59.1%	66.7%	58.3%
Foumbot	Rural	59,223	45.5%	66.7%	50.0%
Bangourain	Rural	29,694	50.0%	33.3%	25.0%
Balessing[a]	Rural	NA	18.2%	50.0%	41.7%
Penka Michel	Rural	88,338	22.7%	83.3%	75.0%
Mbouda	Urban	250,967	50.0%	83.3%	83.3%
Batcham	Rural	90,271	9.1%	50.0%	41.7%
Salvia[b]	Urban	NA	100%	16.7%	NA
Market[b]	Urban	NA	63.6%	NA	NA

NA: Not Applicable.
[a]Found in Penka-Michel health district.
[b]Found in the Mifi health district.

payments in LMIC, treatment for NCDs is largely unaffordable in these settings [4,9].

In Cameroon where more than 50% of the population live below the poverty line and where there is no effective health insurance system [10,11], out-of-pocket payments represented 94.5% of private health expenditures in 2011 [12]. CVD and diabetes are growing public health concerns in Cameroon [13]. Major deficiencies exist in both the quality and access to care such that these NCDs and their risk factors are diagnosed infrequently and managed inadequately. Interestingly however, CVD and diabetes are increasingly receiving more from the Cameroon government [13]. Since 2001, a number of health policies on NCDs including CVD and diabetes have been formulated and adopted by the National Ministry of Public Health. The recognition of hypertension and diabetes as emerging public health threats has led to the creation of the National Diabetes-Hypertension Control Program which aims to promote equitable access to quality health services in order to reduce the morbidity and mortality from these conditions [14]. To achieve this goal, making essential medicines for CVD and diabetes available and affordable is paramount. Therefore, data on the current access to CVD and diabetes care are crucial for shaping and improving strategies to combat CVD and diabetes.

In May 2003, the World Health Organization (WHO) in collaboration with Health Action International developed a standardized method for surveying medicine prices, availability, affordability, and price components in LMIC [15]. Using this standardized method, the present study aimed to assess the prices, availability and affordability of selected routine tests and common essential medicines for CVD and diabetes care in Cameroon.

Methods

Ethics statement

The study was approved by the Regional Office of the Ministry of Public Health (MOH) for the West region, acting as Ethics Committee. Signed authorization was obtained from the head of each participating outlet, who also identified the relevant informant. All informants interviewed in the study provided a verbal consent to take part in the study. Verbal consent was approved by the Ethics Committee and found to be appropriate since this study did not involve data collection on individual subject. The consent was documented by a tick of boxes in our data collection log book. Each of them was individually informed on the intended use of the data collected and the confidentially surrounding the exploitation of the data. They were further advised that they were under no obligation to take part in the study, and that by accepting to respond to our questionnaire they were consenting to take part in the study and allowing the collected data to serve the intended purpose.

Setting

We conducted a survey in the West Region of Cameroon which, had in 2010 a population of 1,785,285 inhabitants (9.2% of the country's total population), with a density of 128.5 inhabitants/km^2 (2nd most densely populated region) [16]. The region is divided into 20 health districts, and has a total of 530 health facilities, both public and private. Public outlets acquire medicines from the state owned Regional Centre for the Essential Drug Program and sell them to the public on a cost-recovery basis following the national guidelines. Private outlets acquire medicines from a private accredited supplier, LABOREX and sell them to the public at prices different from those recommended by the national guidelines.

Selection of medicine outlets

Facilities were selected based on study feasibility, whether urban or rural and the size of the population served, with the aim of sufficiently representing the region. We selected 6 urban and 5 rural outlets. The main hospital of the capital of the region was included, as well as one pharmacy selected as the private outlet. This pharmacy is a popular medicine outlet with the highest anticipated chance of getting all the needed medicines. It served as the reference medicine outlet. One market vendor was also sampled in the regional capital main market to serve as a reference outlet in the informal circuit. The remaining 3 urban and 5 rural outlets selected were those reachable within one-day's drive from the capital; they were all public outlets (state administered), district hospitals or a sub-divisional hospital. In total, there were 2 private outlets (one in the formal sector and one in the informal circuit),

Table 2. Availability, affordability and median price of selected tests in the investigation of cardiovascular disease and diabetes.

Test	Availability			Median price		Number of days' wage for investigation
	Rural	Urban	All sites	Local (FCFA)	US Dollar	
Glycaemia	100%	100%	100%	1,250	2.38	1.34
Creatinemia	80%	100%	80%	3,000	5.72	3.21
Urea	80%	100%	80%	3,000	5.72	3.21
Total cholesterol	20%	75%	40%	3,350	6.39	3.59
HDL cholesterol	20%	75%	40%	3,350	6.39	3.59
Triglyceride	20%	75%	40%	2,850	5.43	3.05
Proteinuria	100%	100%	90%	1,000	1.91	1.07
Kaliemia	40%	100%	60%	3,000	5.72	3.21
HbA1c	0%	50%	20%	11,750	22.40	12.58
Uric acid	0%	100%	40%	3,100	5.91	3.32
Full blood count	80%	100%	80%	3,750	7.15	4.02
ECG	0%	25%	10%	10,000	19.07	10.7

and 9 public outlets. In all, the selected sites served over 60% of the population of the region, distributed in eight health districts, four rural and four urban (Table 1).

Selection of medicines and diagnostic tests to be surveyed

The survey collected information on 20 medicines used to treat CVD and diabetes. Medicines were selected in line with a previous work by a WHO team on selected essential medicines for chronic diseases in six low and middle-income countries [7], their potential impact on the burden of disease and their availability in standard formulations. The majority of these medicines are included in the WHO model list of essential medicines [17]. Diagnostic tests for CVD and diabetes included the minimal WHO workup, and other tests that were considered relevant for assessment and management of cardiovascular risk as recommended by the WHO [18]. The selection was finalized after consultation with local experts.

Data collection

Data were collected by a single trained investigator in all the sites during a one week period in 2012, using a pre-conceived questionnaire, based on the standardized method for surveying medicine prices, availability, affordability, and price components in LMICs developed by the WHO and Health Action International [15]. For each medicine and at each outlet, information included the availability of any drug dosage of the cheapest form (originator brand or generic) and the cost per tablet or vial paid by clients. The price collected from each outlet was the price charged directly to clients. Data on tests were equally collected on the same checklist. These data on tests were collected in the hospitals surveyed. In the absence of social security system in Cameroon, medications and tests covered in the current study are paid for essentially from out-of-pocket money.

Data analysis

This was a pilot study based on a convenient sample, and accordingly no formal power estimation. We assessed the availability of medicines in two ways: 1) by estimating the percentage (%) of the 20 medicines available in each site and 2) by estimating the percentage (%) of outlets in which any dose or form of the medicine was found. Availability less than 30% is considered very low and greater than 80% is considered high [19]. We similarly determined the availability of tests as the percentage of outlets in which a test was found and the percentage of tests found at each site. We also estimated the median price ratio (MPR) of each medicine. This ratio compares a medicine's median local price to its international reference price (IRP) in the Management Sciences for Health (MSH) 2012 Price Indicator Guide [20]. MSH international reference prices, which are generally offered by both not-for-profit and for-profit suppliers to developing countries, are recommended as the most useful standard. When no supplier prices were available, buyer prices were used. The MPR is used to express how much greater or less the median local medicine price is than the IRP. For example, an MPR of 2 would mean that the local medicine price is twice the IRP. Generally, a MPR of one or less indicates an efficient public sector procurement system. For patients' medicine prices, MPR ≤ 1.5 were considered reasonable for all medicine forms (usually higher for innovator medicines) [7].

Affordability was estimated using the median medicine prices of public medicine outlets, or private outlet when this was not available in the public outlet, and the salary of the lowest-paid unskilled government worker which was 28,000 FCFA/month (USD 53) at the time of the survey, and calculating the number of days' wages required to pay for investigation tests and to purchase a one-month course of treatment. Treatments costing one day's wage or less (for a 30-day supply of medicine) were considered affordable.

Results

Availability of tests and medicines

The profile of the survey sites is described in Table 1. The availability of investigation tests is summarized in Table 2; ranging from 10% for the ECG to 100% for fasting blood sugar. It was markedly higher in the urban setting. Across study sites, the availability of investigation tests ranged from 58.3% to 100% for urban sites and 41.7% to 75% for rural sites (Table 1).

Tables 1 and 3 show the availability of medicines used to treat cardiovascular disease and diabetes. Only 9 medicines surveyed had availability greater than 50%. This was higher in urban

Table 3. Availability, affordability, median price and ratios of Medicines.

Drug presentation	Availability				Median price (per tablet or vial)				Defined daily dose	Cost of Daily treatment (USD)	Cost of 30 days' treatment (USD)	Number of days' wage for 1 month
	Rural	Urban	Reference (Pharmacy)	All sites	Local price (FCFA)	Local price (USD)	WHO price (USD)	Ratio*				
Acetylsalicylic acid 500 mg	40%	100%	100%	70%	5.0	0.01	0.0045	2.22	100 mg	0.002	0.06	0.03
Atenolol 50 mg	0%	0%	100%	10%	78.1	0.15	0.0106	14.15	75 mg	0.23	6.75	3.92
Benzathine-benzylpenicilline 2.4MIU	100%	100%	100%	100%	210.0	0.40	0.3241	1.23	2MIU	0.40	12.00	6.74
Captopril 25 mg	0%	50%	100%	30%	100.0	0.19	0.0216	9.80	50 mg	0.38	11.40	6.41
Ramipril 5 mg	0%	25%	100%	20%	240.1	0.46	NA	NA	5 mg	0.84	25.20	14.16
Hydrochlorothiazide 50 mg	20%	50%	100%	40%	10.0	0.02	0.0050	4.00	25 mg	0.01	0.30	0.17
Furosemide 40 mg	100%	100%	100%	100%	5.0	0.01	0.0061	1.64	40 mg	0.01	0.30	0.17
Isosorbide dinitrate 5 mg	0%	0%	100%	10%	81.6	0.16	0.0142	11.27	20 mg	0.64	19.20	10.79
Losartan 50 mg	0%	0%	100%	10%	685.4	1.31	0.0185	70.81	50 mg	0.76	22.80	12.81
Simvastatin 20 mg	0%	0%	100%	10%	295.0	0.56	0.0252	22.22	20 mg	1.81	54.30	30.51
Methyldopa 250 mg	40%	75%	100%	60%	30.0	0.06	0.0295	2.03	1 g	0.24	7.20	4.10
Nifedipine 10 mg	20%	75%	100%	10%	20.0	0.04	0.0130	3.08	30 mg	0.12	3.60	2.02
Nifedipine 20 mg SR	0%	25%	100%	20%	42.3	0.08	0.0233	3.43	30 mg	0.12	3.60	2.02
Phenoxymethylpenincilline 250 mg	60%	50%	100%	60%	15.0	0.03	0.0158	1.90	3MIU	0.18	5.40	3.03
Propranolol 40 mg	20%	0%	100%	20%	26.9	0.05	0.0059	8.47	160 mg	0.20	6.00	3.37
Spironolactone 50 mg	0%	0%	100%	10%	156.7	0.30	0.0338	8.87	75 mg	0.45	13.50	7.58
Heparine 5000 UI	0%	0%	100%	10%	2 835.0	5.41	0.9055	5.97	10000 IU	10.82	324.60	182.36
Glibenclamide 5 mg	60%	100%	100%	80%	5.0	0.01	0.0042	2.38	10 mg	0.02	0.60	0.34
Metformine 500 mg	60%	100%	100%	80%	7.5	0.01	0.0168	0.59	2 g	0.04	1.20	0.67
Actrapid 100 IU/ml	60%	100%	100%	80%	3,000.0	5.72	0.7723	7.41	40 IU	0.23	6.86	3.85
Insulatard 100 IU/ml	0%	0%	100%	10%	3,000.0	5.72	0.7723	7.41	40 IU	0.23	6.86	3.85
Mixtard 100 IU/ml	60%	100%	100%	80%	14,500.0	27.65	0.6143	45.01	40 IU	1.11	33.30	18.70

*Ratio: Local price/WHO price.
NA: Data not available in the 2012 edition.

Table 4. Estimated costs of managing cardiovascular risk profile.

Purpose		Components	Cost of tests (days' wages)	Costs of drugs (days' wages)	Total cost (days' wages)
Diagnosis and stratification	Absolute risk	Minimal WHO recommended tests	29.76	NA	29.76
Primary prevention	<10% Risk	Lifestyle changes and 12-monthly risk monitoring	1.05	NA	1.05
	10–20% Risk	Lifestyle changes and 6-monthly risk monitoring	2.11	NA	2.11
	20–30% Risk	Statin/Antihypertensive/6-monthly risk monitoring	2.11	30.67	32.78
	≥30% Risk	Statin/Antihypertensive/Acetylsalicylic acid/3-monthly risk monitoring	4.22	30.70	34.92
Secondary prevention		β-Blocker, ACEI, Statin, Acetylsalicylic acid/3-monthly risk monitoring	4.22	37.11	41.33

Minimal WHO recommended tests include fasting blood sugar, cholesterol, potassium levels, proteinuria and ECG.
Risk monitoring includes lipid profile, fasting blood sugar and proteinuria. It cost 12.6 days' wages. As this cumulates over the months, 12-monthly monitoring and 6-monthly monitoring cost 1.05 days' wages and 2.11 days' wages.
NA: not applicable.
WHO: World Health Organization; ACEI: Angiotensin Converting Enzyme Inhibitor.

settings except for propranolol and Methyl-penicillin which was higher in the rural settings (Table 3). Up to 7 of the surveyed medicines were found only in private medicine outlets. Medicines' availability across public pharmacies in different sites ranged between 36.4% and 59.1% in urban sites and between 9.1% and 50% in rural sites (Table 1). Medicines' availability was higher in the urban informal sector where up to 63.6% of the medicines were available.

Median prices and affordability of tests and medicines

The affordability of investigation tests and treatment was estimated as the number of days' wages the lowest-paid government worker would be required to pay for the initial tests and one-month course of treatment from the public sector, and when this is not available, from the private sector. This is summarized in Tables 2 and 3. Of all the medicines surveyed, only the oral antidiabetics, hydrochlorothiazide and acetylsalicylic acid cost less than 1 day's wage. Statins remained largely unaffordable. Only metformin and benzathine-benzylpenicilline had an acceptable median price ratio of 0.59 and 1.23 respectively.

Table 4 depicts the minimum estimated cost of management and monitoring of different CVD risk profiles. The minimum number of tests to investigate a newly diagnosed hypertensive patient including a fasting blood sugar, cholesterol, potassium levels, proteinuria and ECG cost 29.76 days' wages. Risk monitoring which comprises lipid profile, fasting blood sugar and proteinuria cost 12.6 days' wages. As this cumulates over the months, 12-monthly monitoring and 6-monthly monitoring cost 1.05 days' wages and 2.11 days' wages. Treating a patient with ischemic heart disease with a drug combination comprising a β-blocker (atenolol), Angiotensin Converting Enzyme Inhibitor (captopril), statin (simvastatin) and acetylsalicylic acid will cost at least 41.33 days' wage. This was largely unaffordable.

Comprehensive analysis of medicine availability and price

Figure 1 presents the availability and price of medicines surveyed. The availability score for each medicine is depicted on the x-axis, while the y-axis shows the value of the number of days' wage required to purchase a one-month course of treatment. The figure can be divided roughly into four quadrants. The upper left quadrant (quadrant I) contains drugs with high number of days' wage and low availability. In the case of these medicines, heparine and simvastatin for instance, patients face both high costs and high difficulty in obtaining them.

The lower right quadrant (quadrant IV) contains drugs with low number of days' wage and high availability. Furosemide had the highest availability (100%) and one of the lowest number of days' wage (0.17). Acetylsalicylic acid was the most affordable medicine, with a 0.03 day's wage, and had an availability of 70%.

Discussion

This survey is the first of this nature in Cameroon and in a large number of low-income countries using standard methods developed and validated by the WHO [15], and with emphasis on two common NCDs in LMICs. We focused on what patients pay for available tests and medicines at the end of the spectrum and thus, did not look at markups, taxes, other distribution costs and different drug forms or conditionings, which explained differences in prices observed in surveys carried out in geographically diverse sites [7,8]. We carried out the survey in a geographically limited site. However, key aspects of availability and affordability of essential medicines are similar to other studies and are thus, comparable.

The investigation and management of patients with medium-to-high cardiovascular risk remains largely unavailable and unaffordable in this low income setting. The minimum recommended tests by the WHO (blood sugar, potassium, creatinemia and proteinuria) had a satisfactory availability of 80% or more, and comparably between rural and urban settings. Lower availabilities of these tests have been found in Benin and Sudan [21]. Lipid profile had low availability, especially in rural settings, and ECG which was seen only in few urban facilities was largely unavailable. HbA1c, a key-test in the monitory of diabetic patients also had very low availability, and was very unaffordable. Only two tests (blood sugar and proteinuria) cost less than 2 days' wages and could therefore be considered affordable. Overall, the cost of minimal WHO recommended tests for initial diagnosis and

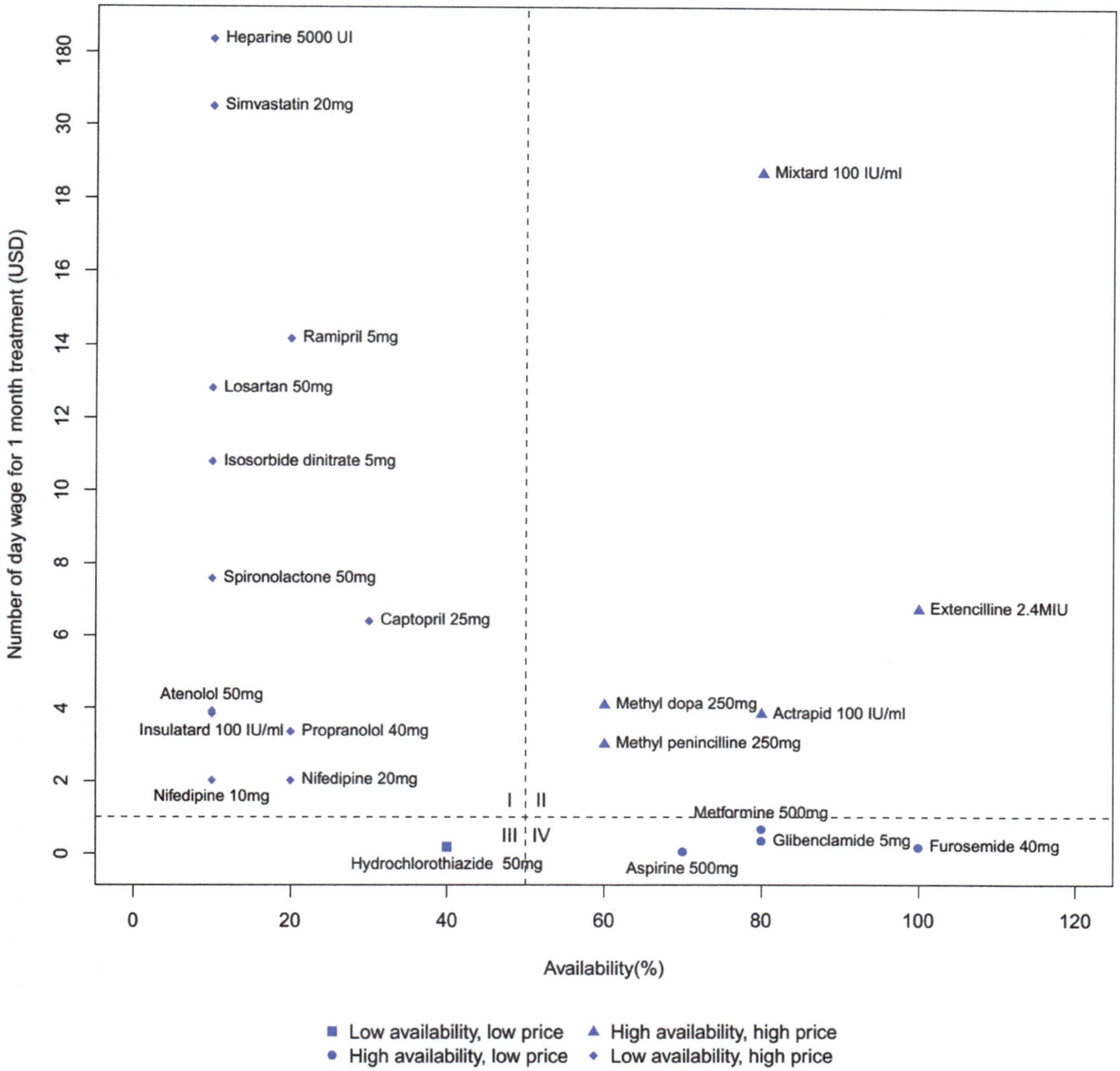

Figure 1. Comprehensive analysis of medicine availability and affordability. The availability (%) each drug is depicted on the x-axis, while the y-axis shows the price (days' wages).

cardiovascular risk stratification was very unaffordable, representing one month salary for the lowest-paid unskilled government worker.

The availability of medicines in our study, although higher than that reported in six LMICs [7], was not always optimal, therefore indicating the existing scope of improvement. The lessons learned from the HIV/antiretroviral experience could be applied in order to improve access to essential medicines for NCDs [22,23]. A recent study evaluating the preparedness of a representative sample of 24 public and not-for-profit Tanzanian health facilities to provide routine care for hypertension and diabetes, has shown that compared with care for HIV, health facilities at all levels were ill-prepared to address the diagnosis, treatment, and ongoing monitoring needs of patients with NCDs. These results suggest that primary-care system for HIV could serve as both model and foundation to improve CVDs and diabetes care including access to essential medicines [24]. Practically, to improve the availability of essentials medicines for CVDs and diabetes in LMICs like Cameroon, ministries of health should optimize the local procurement practices and organize an efficient supply chain all over the country [22]. To assure a continuous availability of these medicines, good monitoring systems for stock levels and use are crucial. The use of wireless communication technologies, such as short message service (SMS), has been shown to increase procurement efficiency and monitoring. Community volunteers can track the availability of medicines in local facilities, and their SMS messages can feed into a website that helps to identify underperforming districts and start corrective action [22,23].

Similar approaches for first-line antimalarial drugs have resulted in a 50% decrease in facility stock-outs in a pilot project to improve drug supply management in rural Tanzania [25].

Despite the relatively good availability of the surveyed medicines, affordability was also very low with only six of the surveyed medicines that cost less than a day's wage. In a similar recent study in China, these costs were much lower than those found in our study: 0.1 days' wages for captopril 25 mg, 0.3 days' wages for metformine 500 mg, 1.4 days' wages for nifedipine 20 mg and 6.6 days' wages for losartan 50 mg [26]. A 1-month course of combination therapy for the secondary prevention of coronary heart disease cost 40.87 days' wages in our setting compared to 18 days' wages in Malawi and 1.5 days' wages in Sri Lanka [7]. The unaffordability of most of medicines would be majored if additional costs of consultation and diagnostic tests were accounted for. A study among Cameroonian informal sector workers which represent the vast majority of the active population in the country, found that only 4.4% of them had health insurance [11]. It has been shown that catastrophic payments and impoverishment due to cardiovascular diseases are more common in people with no health insurance than in those with health insurance [27]. Scaling up the health insurance coverage of the Cameroonian population is therefore crucial to improve access to CVD and diabetes care. Generally, medicines on the national essential medicines list (NEML) are the highest priority for coverage by the health insurance program in sub-Saharan Africa [22]. In the national health insurance system in Rwanda, for example, members are eligible to receive NEML drugs for outpatient treatment with a 10% copayment [28].

Policy options to improve access to affordable medicines through cost containment and promotion of generics have been suggested. Some which could be implemented in the Cameroonian context include: involvement of reputed organizations and of patients associations and consumers groups to raise awareness on the benefit of good quality generics; reliable quality assurance capacity to demonstrate the bioequivalence between generics and originator brands; encouraging generic prescribing and influencing the patient to request for prescription of cheaper version of medicines [29–31]. Generic substitution could lead to significant financial savings. In France for instance, implementation of a general generic substitution strategy saved nearly US$2 billion in 2008 alone [32]. Nonetheless, assurance of generic medicine quality is crucial to protect the population from potentially harmful effects or inefficient medicines and reduce waste of resources. Because of inadequate regulation and insufficient penalization, substandard medicines are common in developing countries [23]. In Rwanda, 20% of hypertensive medicines purchased on the market were of substandard content and 70% were of insufficient stability [33].

Prices of medicines could be reduced by improving purchasing efficiency, eliminating taxes and regulating markups. The analysis of the MPR of the surveyed medicines shows that the local procurement and retail system was inefficient, with most of the MPR greater than 1.5. MPR was acceptable only for metformin and benzathine-benzylpenicilline, and was as high as 70.81 for losartan. Comparatively, a recent study in New Delhi, India, has shown that procurement prices of surveyed medicines were reasonable [34].

The present study has some limitations. First, sampling of survey sites was not random with a risk of sampling bias. However, for equity, strength and feasibility, we surveyed 8 health districts, urban and rural, that served the majority of the population of the region. Second, data on availability were collected at a particular point in time and thus, they do not reflect fluctuations in the availability over time. Third, our study present limited data from the private sector. However, as medicines are usually cheaper in the public sector [7], our study which mainly focuses on data from the public sector present the "best case scenario" of the affordability of drugs surveyed.

Conclusion

This study has provided some insight on issues relating to access to cardiovascular and diabetes care in Cameroon. The investigation and management of patients with medium-to-high cardiovascular risk remains largely unavailable and unaffordable in this low income setting. An effective NCD program should lay emphasis on primary prevention, and improve access to affordable generic essential medicines in public outlets.

Author Contributions

Conceived and designed the experiments: AMJ JJNN AEO. Performed the experiments: AMJ. Analyzed the data: AMJ JJNN BW. Contributed reagents/materials/analysis tools: AMJ JJNN. Wrote the paper: JJNN AMJ APK AEO JRNN BW SK.

References

1. World Health Organization (2010) Global Status Report on Non-communicable Diseases 2010. Geneva: World Health Organization.
2. Abegunde D, Mathers CD, Adam T, Ortegon M, Strong K (2007). The burden and costs of chronic diseases in low-income and middle income countries. Lancet 370: 1929–38.
3. Joshi R, Jan S, Wu Y, MacMahon S (2008) Global inequalities in access to cardiovascular health care: our greatest challenge. J Am Coll Cardiol 52(23): 1817–25.
4. Kankeu HT, Saksena P, Xu K, Evans DB (2013) The financial burden from non-communicable diseases in low- and middle-income countries: a literature review. Health Res Policy Syst 11: 31.
5. Kengne AP, June-Rose McHiza, Amoah AG, Mbanya JC (2013) Cardiovascular diseases and diabetes as economic and developmental challenges in Africa. Prog Cardiovasc Dis 56(3): 302–13.
6. World Health Organization (2013) Prevention of recurrent heart attacks and strokes in low- and middle-income populations: evidence based recommendations for policy makers and health professionals. Geneva: World Health Organization.
7. Mendis S, Fukino K, Cameron A, Laing R, Filipe A Jr et al. (2007) The availability and affordability of selected essential medicines for chronic diseases in six low and middle-income countries. Bull World Health Organ 85: 279–88.
8. Cameron A, Ewen M, Ross-Degnan D, Ball D, Laing R (2009) Medicine prices, availability, and affordability in 36 developing and middle income countries: a secondary analysis. Lancet 373 (9659): 240–9.
9. World Health Organization (2004) Equitable access to essential medicines: a framework for collective action. WHO Policy Perspectives on Medicines n° 8. Geneva: World Health Organization.
10. Ministère de la Santé Publique du Cameroun (2006) Plan stratégique pour la promotion et le développement des mutuelles de santé au Cameroun.
11. Noubiap JJ, Joko WY, Obama JM, Bigna JJ (2013) Community-based health insurance knowledge, concern, preferences, and financial planning for health care among informal sector workers in a health district of Douala, Cameroon. Pan Afr Med J 16: 17.
12. World Health Organization (2011) Global Health Observatory Data Repository. Health financing: health expenditure ratios by country. Available: http://apps.who.int/gho/data/node.main.75?lang=en. Accessed April 10, 2014.
13. Echouffo-Tcheugui JB, Kengne AP (2011) Chronic non-communicable diseases in Cameroon - burden, determinants and current policies. Global Health 7: 44.
14. Njamnshi A, Hiag AB, Mbanya JC (2006) From research to policy: the development of a national diabetes programme in Cameroon. Diabetes Voice 51(3): 18–21.
15. World Health Organization, Health Action International (2008) Measuring medicine prices, availability, affordability and price components 2nd edition. Available: http://www.haiweb.org/medicineprices/surveys.php. Accessed 04 April 2014.
16. eme recensement general de la population humaine (2010) La population du Cameroun en 2010. Available: http://www.statistics-cameroon.org/downloads/La_population_du_Cameroun_2010.pdf. Accessed April 4, 2014.

17. World Health Organization (2007) AFRO Essential medicines price indicator: WHO model list, 2007 edition.
18. World Health Organization (2007) Prevention of cardiovascular disease. Pocket guidelines for assessment and management of cardiovascular risk. Available: http://www.who.int/cardiovascular_diseases/guidelines/PocketGL.ENGLISH.AFR-D-E.rev1.pdf. Accessed 04 April 2014.
19. Gelders S, Ewen M, Noguchi N, Laing R (2006) Price, availability and affordability. An international comparison of chronic disease medicines. Cairo: World health Organization and Health Acton International; 2006. Available: http://www.haiweb.org/GlobalDatabase/Main.htm. Accessed 12 April 2014.
20. Management Sciences for Health (2012) International Drug Price Indicator Guide. Available: http://erc.msh.org/dmpguide/pdf/DrugPriceGuide_2012_en.pdf. Accessed 12 April 2014.
21. Mendis S, Al Bashir I, Dissanayake L, Varghese C, Fadhil I et al. (2012) Gaps in capacity in primary care in low-resource settings for implementation of essential non communicable disease interventions. Int J Hypertens 2012: 584041.
22. Kishore SP, Vendanthan R, Fuster V (2011) Promoting global cardiovascular health ensuring access to essential cardiovascular medicines in low- and middle-income countries. J Am Coll Cardiol 57(20): 1980–7.
23. Hogerzeil HV, Liberman J, Wirtz VJ, Kishore SP, Sevaraj S et al. (2013) Promotion of access to essential medicines for non-communicable diseases: practical implications of the UN political declaration. Lancet 381(9867): 680–9.
24. Peck R, Mghamba J, Vanobberghen F, Kavishe B, Rugarabamu V et al. (2014) Preparedness of Tanzanian health facilities for outpatient primary care of hypertension and diabetes: a cross-sectional survey. Lancet Glob Health. published online April 14. http://dx.doi.org/10.1016/S2214-109X(14)70033-6.
25. Barrington J, Wereko-Brobby O, Ward P, Mwafongo W, Kungulwe S (2010) SMS for Life: a pilot project to improve anti-malaria drug supply management in rural Tanzania using standard technology. Malar J 9: 298.
26. Jiang M, Yang S, Yan K, Liu J, Zhao J et al. (2013) Measuring Access to Medicines: A Survey of Prices, Availability and Affordability in Shaanxi Province of China. PLoS One 8(8): e70836.
27. Heeley E, Anderson CS, Huang Y, Jan S, Li Y et al. (2009) Role of health insurance in averting economic hardship in families after acute stroke in China. Stroke 40: 2149–2156.
28. Vialle-Valentin CE, Ross-Degnaan D, Ntaganira J, Wagner AK (2008) Medicines coverage and community-based health insurance in low-income countries. Health Res Policy Syst 6: 11.
29. Quick JD (2003) Ensuring access to essential medicines in the developing countries: a framework for action. Clin Pharmacol Ther 73(4): 279–283.
30. Kanavos P, Costa-Font J, Seeley E (2008) Competition in off-patent drug markets: Issues regulation and evidence. Economic Policy 23: 499–544.
31. Joncheere K, Rietveld AH, Huttin C (2002) Experiences with generics. In Drugs and Money.7th edition. Edited by Dukes FM, Haaijer-Ruskamp CP, Joncheere A, Rietveld H. The Netherlands: Published on behalf of WHO-Europe: 101–110. IOS Press.
32. World Health Organization (2010) The world health report-health systems fi nancing: the path to universal coverage. Geneva: World Health Organization.
33. Twagirumukiza M, Cosijns A, Pringels E, Remon J, Vervaet C et al. (2009) Influence of tropical climate conditions on the quality of antihypertensive drugs from Rwandan pharmacies. Am J Trop Med Hyg 81: 776–781.
34. Kotwani A (2013) Where are we now: assessing the price, availability and affordability of essential medicines in Delhi as India plans free medicine for all. BMC Health Serv Res 13: 285.

5

Decrease in Urinary Creatinine Excretion in Early Stage Chronic Kidney Disease

Elena Tynkevich[1,2]*, Martin Flamant[3], Jean-Philippe Haymann[4,5,6], Marie Metzger[1,2], Eric Thervet[7,8], Jean-Jacques Boffa[5,6,9], François Vrtovsnik[10], Pascal Houillier[11,12], Marc Froissart[1], Bénédicte Stengel[1,2] and on behalf of the NephroTest Study Group¶

1 CESP, Centre for Epidemiology and Population Health, INSERM Unit 1018, Villejuif, France, **2** University Paris-Sud 11, UMRS 1018, Villejuif, France, **3** AP-HP, Hôpital Bichat, Department of Physiology, Paris, France, **4** AP-HP, Hôpital Tenon, Department of Physiology, Paris, France, **5** INSERM UNIT 702, Paris, France, **6** University Pierre et Marie Curie-Paris 6, UMRS 702, Paris, France, **7** AP-HP, Hôpital Européen Georges Pompidou, Department of Nephrology, Paris, France, **8** AP-HP, Hôpital Européen Georges Pompidou, DHU Common and Rare Arterial Diseases, Paris, France, **9** AP-HP, Hôpital Tenon, Department of Nephrology, Paris, France, **10** AP-HP, Hôpital Bichat, Department of Nephrology, Paris, France, **11** University Paris Descartes-Paris 5, UMRS 775, Paris, France, **12** AP-HP, Hôpital Européen Georges Pompidou, Department of Physiology, Paris, France

Abstract

Background: Little is known about muscle mass loss in early stage chronic kidney disease (CKD). We used 24-hour urinary creatinine excretion rate to assess determinants of muscle mass and its evolution with kidney function decline. We also described the range of urinary creatinine concentration in this population.

Methods: We included 1072 men and 537 women with non-dialysis CKD stages 1 to 5, all of them with repeated measurements of glomerular filtration rate (mGFR) by ^{51}Cr-EDTA renal clearance and several nutritional markers. In those with stage 1 to 4 at baseline, we used a mixed model to study factors associated with urinary creatinine excretion rate and its change over time.

Results: Baseline mean urinary creatinine excretion decreased from 15.3±3.1 to 12.1±3.3 mmol/24 h (0.20±0.03 to 0.15±0.04 mmol/kg/24 h) in men, with mGFR falling from ≥60 to <15 mL/min/1.73 m^2, and from 9.6±1.9 to 7.6±2.5 (0.16±0.03 to 0.12±0.03) in women. In addition to mGFR, an older age, diabetes, and lower levels of body mass index, proteinuria, and protein intake assessed by urinary urea were associated with lower mean urinary creatinine excretion at baseline. Mean annual decline in mGFR was 1.53±0.12 mL/min/1.73 m^2 per year and that of urinary creatinine excretion rate, 0.28±0.02 mmol/24 h per year. Patients with fast annual decline in mGFR of 5 mL/min/1.73 m^2 had a decrease in urinary creatinine excretion more than twice as big as in those with stable mGFR, independent of changes in urinary urea as well as of other determinants of low muscle mass.

Conclusions: Decrease in 24-hour urinary creatinine excretion rate may appear early in CKD patients, and is greater the more mGFR declines independent of lowering protein intake assessed by 24-hour urinary urea. Normalizing urine analytes for creatininuria may overestimate their concentration in patients with reduced kidney function and low muscle mass.

Editor: Jaap A. Joles, University Medical Center Utrecht, Netherlands

Funding: The NephroTest CKD cohort study is supported by the following grants: INSERM GIS-IReSP AO 8113LS TGIR (B.S.), French Ministry of Health AOM 09114 (M.Fr.), INSERM AO 8022LS (B.S.), Agence de la Biomédecine R0 8156LL (B.S.), AURA (M.Fr.), and Roche 2009-152-447G (M.Fr.). The funders had no role in study design, data collection and analysis, decision to publish, or preparation of the manuscript.

Competing Interests: The authors have the following interests. This study was partly supported by Roche. B.S. has received consulting or lecture fees from AbbVie, Amgen, Fresenius, and MSD; M.F. has received research funds from Hoffmann-La Roche; M.F. has been employed by Amgen since January 1, 2011, but was a full-time academic associate professor during the time of study conception and data collection. There are no patents, products in development, or marketed products to declare.

* Email: elena.tynkevich@inserm.fr

¶ Membership of the NephroTest study group is provided in the Acknowledgments.

Introduction

Protein-energy wasting (PEW) is a state of decreased body stores of protein and energy fuels, assessed by biochemical and clinical measures [1–4]. Nutritional disorders are common in patients with end-stage chronic kidney disease (CKD) [1,5–8] and are often associated with inflammation [7,9–12]. Both conditions are known to be associated with high cardiovascular [10,11,13] and all-cause [5,10,14–17] mortality. While nutritional disorders have previously been studied in patients with end-stage CKD [1,6,14,16,18–24] or coronary heart disease [13,25], and in the general population [26–29], little is known about the timing of PEW in non-end-stage CKD [17,30].

Muscle wasting is one of the most valid markers of PEW [2,8,14]. Loss of muscle mass results from an imbalance between protein synthesis and degradation and is worsened by inactivity [22,31] and loss of appetite [9,32,33]. A variety of conditions, including diabetes mellitus [21,24], metabolic acidosis [34,35], and inflammation [19,31,36,37], may promote an increase in protein breakdown. Muscle mass may be assessed by biochemical [2,3,38,39], anthropometric [2,3], or bioelectrical measurements [40,41]. In steady state, urinary creatinine excretion is one of the most specific indexes of total body muscle mass, because creatine originates almost exclusively (98%) from skeletal muscle[39,42]. The amount of both filtered and secreted creatinine excreted in the urine represents the difference between creatinine generation and its extrarenal elimination. The former is proportional to muscle mass but also affected by meat intake [3,39,42], and the latter is known to increase in patients with severely reduced kidney function [42,43]. Several studies reported the normal range and determinants of urinary creatinine concentration in the general population[27]. Very few, however, have investigated its relation to kidney function decline, while taking into account the determinants of muscle mass, including reduced protein intake [17,30]. Moreover, most studies which investigated the association between urinary excretion of creatinine and renal function were based on glomerular filtration rate (GFR) estimated from plasma creatinine concentration, which is itself determined by muscular production of creatinine (and hence its urinary excretion). Thus, using a gold standard GFR measurement method, which is independent of plasma creatinine concentration, is methodologically crucial to study the correlation between urinary creatinine excretion and renal function decline.

We therefore studied the determinants of low urinary creatinine excretion as well as of the evolution of its rate over time, in a large cohort of patients with all stages of CKD and measured glomerular filtration rate (mGFR) from the NephroTest study. In addition, we document the range of urinary creatinine concentrations by age, gender, ethnicity and mGFR level.

Methods

Ethics statement

All patients signed written informed consents before inclusion in the cohort. The NephroTest study design was approved by an ethics committee (Direction générale pour la recherche et l'innovation. Comité consultatif sur le traitement de l'information en matière de recherche dans le domaine de la santé (CCTIRS). Ref: DGRI CCTIRS MG/CP09.503, 9th July 2009).

Patients and study design

The NephroTest study is a prospective hospital-based cohort that began in 2000; by the end of 2010, it had enrolled 1827 adult patients with all stages of CKD and all nephropathy types referred by nephrologists to any of three departments of physiology for annual extensive workups. Eligible patients were ≥18 years of age at inclusion and had neither started dialysis nor received a kidney transplant. Pregnant women were excluded.

Information

Data were recorded during a 5-hour in-person visit for a complete nephrological workup comprising a large set of clinical and laboratory measurements, including blood pressure, body mass index (BMI), and treatments received. Diabetes was defined as either fasting glycemia ≥7 mmol/L or HbA1c ≥6.5% or antidiabetic treatment, hypertension by either a systolic or diastolic blood pressure >140/90 mm Hg or antihypertensive treatment, metabolic acidosis as venous CO_2 <22 mmol/L or alkaline treatment.

Laboratory measurements

At each visit, mGFR was measured concurrently for all patients by ^{51}Cr-EDTA renal clearance and fractional creatinine clearance. Subjects also provided 24-hour urine collection, which enabled us to measure 24-hour creatinine clearance as well as creatininuria with the Jaffe method. Because 24-hour urine collection may be inaccurate, we primarily used 24-hour urinary creatinine extrapolated from fractional creatinine clearance in this study, on the assumption that creatinine excretion is stable over the 24-hour period. Moreover, the analysis of consistency between the two measures of creatinine clearance and that of mGFR enabled us to exclude outliers and to assess the completeness of the 24-hour urine collection. Thus, in addition to 84 patients with missing urinary creatinine, we excluded 78 patients with missing data for fractional creatinine clearance and 56 outliers for mGFR or for fractional or 24-hour creatinine clearance or both, leaving 1609 patients for the analysis of baseline data (Figure 1).

Gender-specific thresholds for low urinary creatinine excretion were defined as values <10th percentile of the distribution in patients with mGFR ≥60 mL/min/1.73 m^2, i.e., 11.4 mmol/24 h in men and 7.2 in women. Several markers of inflammation-malnutrition were also measured and studied, with the following cutoffs to define abnormal values: serum albumin <35 g/L, prealbumin <0.30 g/L, total cholesterol <5.5 mmol/L, triglycerides ≥1.7 mmol/L, transferrin <2 g/L, white blood cells (WBC) ≥7.5×10^3/mm^3, C-reactive protein (CRP) ≥10 mg/L, haptoglobin ≥90th percentile, orosomucoid ≥90th percentile, and plasma fibrinogen ≥5 g/L. Gender-specific thresholds were used to define high-density lipoprotein (HDL) cholesterol cutoff points: 1.0 mmol/L in men and 1.3 mmol/L in women. Urinary urea (mmol/24-hour), reflecting protein intake, and 24-hour proteinuria, were analyzed in quartiles.

Missing values accounted for less than 5% of most indicators. Mean imputation was used for those included in the multivariate analysis. A missing category was created for the indicators with > 5% of values missing, including prealbumin (24%), orosomucoid (37%), and haptoglobin (21%).

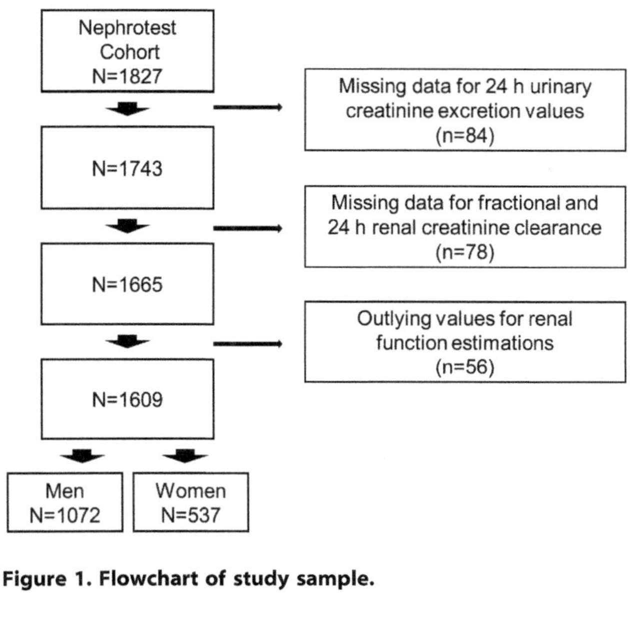

Figure 1. Flowchart of study sample.

Table 1. Patient characteristics according to mGFR level in 1609 patients.

	mGFR (ml/min per1.73 m²)					p Value
	≥60	45–60	30–44	15–29	<15	
	(n = 282)	(n = 321)	(n = 472)	(n = 435)	(n = 99)	
Demographic parameters						
Men	188 (66.7)	233 (72.6)	321 (68.0)	274 (63.0)	56 (56.6)	0.01
Age (years)	52.0±15.1	58.7±14.4	61.0±15.0	61.0±15.0	60.9±15.2	<0.0001
African origin	53 (18.8)	48 (15.0)	56 (11.9)	44 (10.1)	8 (8.1)	<0.0001
Body mass index (kg/m²)	25.9±4.9	26.3±4.9	26.6±4.8	26.6±5.0	27.0±6.0	0.19
Diabetes[a]	62 (22.0)	83 (25.9)	150 (31.8)	136 (31.3)	25 (25.3)	0.02
Metabolic acidosis[b]	6 (2.1)	11 (3.4)	47 (10.0)	100 (23.0)	46 (46.5)	<0.0001
Hypertension[c]	225 (79.8)	284 (88.5)	447 (94.7)	415 (95.4)	98 (99.0)	<0.0001
Any antihypertensive treatment	216 (76.6)	272 (84.7)	435 (92.2)	408 (93.8)	96 (97.0)	<0.0001
Laboratory parameters						
eGFR	75.9±19.6	54.3±12.1	39.5±9.8	25.4±8.5	13.7±5.6	<0.0001
HDL cholesterol (mmol/L)	1.36±0.40	1.35±0.42	1.30±0.44	1.24±0.39	1.29±0.50	0.001
Triglycerides (mmol/L)	1.1 (0.82–1.6)	1.2 (0.87–1.6)	1.4 (0.94–2.0)	1.4 (1.0–2.1)	1.5 (1.1–2.3)	<0.0001
Serum albumin (g/L)	40.2±3.7	40.3±3.9	39.3±4.5	38.8±4.6	38.9±5.0	<0.0001
Prealbumin (g/L)	0.29±0.07	0.30±0.06	0.30±0.07	0.33±0.0.8	0.34±0.08	<0.0001
Transferrin (g/L)	2.4±0.42	2.3±0.37	2.3±0.41	2.2±0.40	2.13±0.36	<0.0001
Homocysteine (umol/L)	13.5±4.3	16.9±6.1	19.1±6.3	21.7±7.6	24.0±7.8	<0.0001
Urinary urea (mmol/24h)	405.6±118.9	381.2±110.7	373.3±124.7	354.4±113.7	297.4±100.8	<0.0001
WBC count (10³/mm³)	6.1±1.8	6.2±2.0	6.5±2.3	6.8±2.2	6.7±1.9	0.0001
Plasma fibrinogen (g/L)	3.4±0.81	3.5±0.88	3.8±0.93	4.2±1.00	4.4±0.99	<0.0001
CRP>*10* mg/L	15 (5.3)	23 (7.2)	43 (9.1)	50 (11.5)	8 (8.1)	0.20
Orosomucoid (g/L)	0.79±0.21	0.85±0.22	0.92±0.25	1.0±0.31	1.1±0.23	<0.0001
Haptoglobin (g/L)	1.2±0.58	1.2±0.58	1.4±0.61	1.5±0.67	1.5±0.69	<0.0001
Proteinuria (g/24h)	0.16 (0.10–0.50)	0.17 (0.11–0.40)	0.26 (0.13–0.93)	0.65 (0.23–1.8)	1.3 (0.55–2.3)	<0.0001

Abbreviations: BP, blood pressure; mGFR, measured glomerular filtration rate; HDL, high-density lipoprotein; WBC, white blood cells; CRP, C-reactive protein.
Values are reported as %, mean ± SD or median (interquartile range).
[a] Fasting glucose ≥7 mmol/L or HbA1c ≥6.5 or antidiabetic treatment or reported diabetes.
[b] Venous CO2 <22 mmol/L or alkaline treatment.
[c] Any antihypertensive treatment or systolic BP>140 or diastolic BP>90 mm Hg.

Statistical analyses

Variables were expressed as percentages, means ± SD, or medians (IQR: interquartile range), as appropriate. We first described patients' characteristics according to mGFR classes defined as follows: ≥ 0, 45-59, 30–44, 15–29, and <15 mL/min/1.73 m². Differences across mGFR classes were tested with ANOVA for continuous variables and with Chi-square test for categorical variables. We also provided urinary creatinine mean values and 10th, 25th, 75th, and 90th percentiles expressed in both mmol/24-h and mmol/kg/24-h, according to mGFR classes, overall and by age (< or ≥60 years), gender, and ethnicity (non-African *vs* African origin).

Crude and adjusted odds ratios (ORs) and 95% confidence intervals (95% CI) for low baseline urinary creatinine excretion according to clinical and laboratory parameters were estimated by logistic regression. To be included in the multivariate analysis, factors had to be significantly associated with low urinary creatinine excretion in the crude analysis with $p<0.20$ and uncorrelated with each other ($-0.50<r<0.50$). Well-established risk factors for muscle mass loss, such as diabetes, were also included regardless of their statistical significance in the crude analysis. We studied three models: one crude, one adjusted only for age (treated continuously), gender, ethnicity, center, and mGFR, and another fully adjusted. These analyses were also carried out by replacing mGFR by estimated GFR (eGFR) using the CKD-EPI equation[44], and by sub-group defined by diabetes status.

Finally, we used a linear mixed model with random intercepts and slopes to estimate mean differences in urinary creatinine excretion rate according to covariates shown to be statistically significant in the logistic regression, as well as its annual slope associated with changes in mGFR and 24-hour urinary urea. In this analysis, we excluded 99 patients with CKD stage 5 at baseline and 37 with missing urinary urea, leaving 1473 patients with a median follow-up of 1.43 years (0–3.34, maximum 5 years). Median interval between visits was 1.12 year (1.00–1.69) for the 855 patients with at least two visits. This analysis was based on a total of 3268 observations. Interactions with time were tested for all covariates. In the final mixed model, we only included interaction terms which were statistically significant using Wald test and improved the model according to Akaike information criteria (AIC).

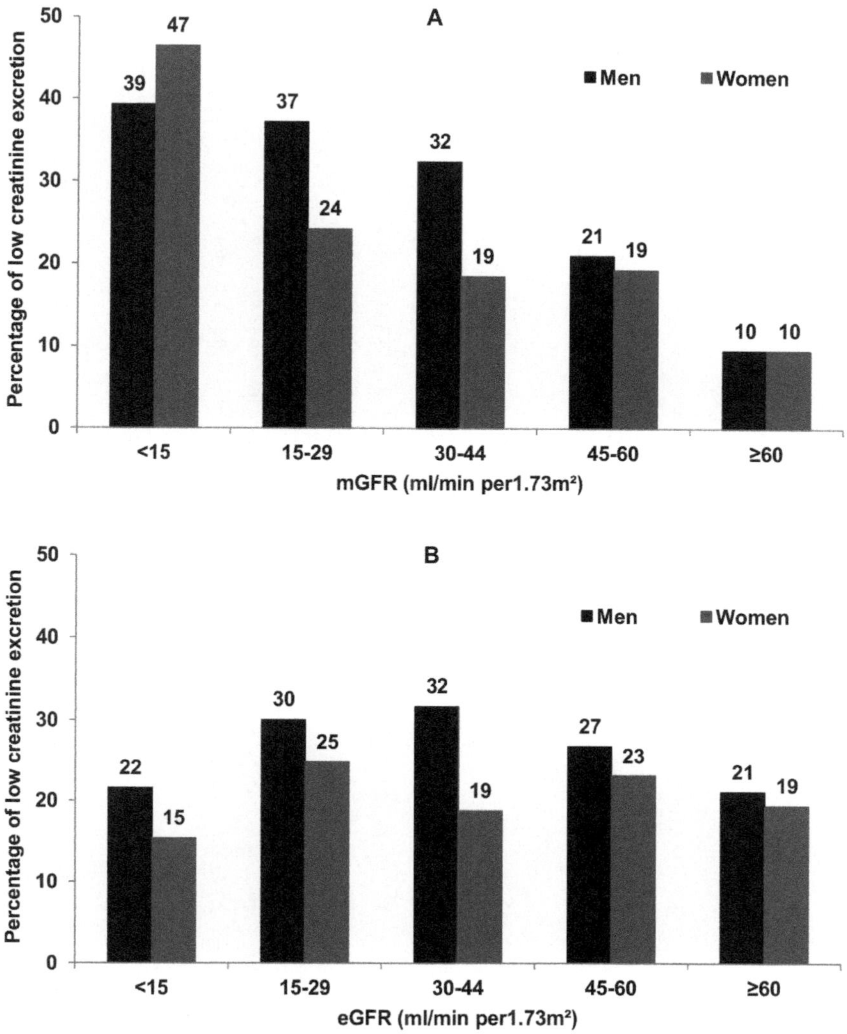

Figure 2. Percentages of low urinary creatinine excretion according to mGFR and eGFR level, by gender. Figure shows the percentage of patients with low creatinine excretion rates according to both measured (2A) and estimated (2B) glomerular filtration rate classes in men and women. Gender-specific thresholds were defined as the 10th percentile of the urinary creatinine distribution in patients with mGFR ≥60 mL/min/1.73 m^2.

A two-sided P-value <0.05 indicated statistical significance. Statistical analyses were performed with SAS software, version 9.3 (SAS institute, Cary, NC).

Results

Patient characteristics according to mGFR level

Patients' age increased and the percentage of those from sub-Saharan Africa or the French West Indies decreased with decreasing mGFR (Table 1). The level of all nutritional factors, except prealbumin, significantly decreased with mGFR decline, while that of inflammation factors (except CRP) as well as the prevalence of metabolic acidosis significantly increased.

Urinary creatinine excretion rate according to GFR level, by gender, age, and ethnicity

Urinary creatinine excretion was normally distributed. Mean urinary creatinine excretion rate decreased as mGFR decreased from ≥60 to <15 mL/min/1.73 m^2 in all categories defined by age, gender, and ethnicity (Table 2). It was higher in men and women with than without African origin. The percentage of patients with low creatinine excretion rates increased as mGFR decreased, reaching about four times the level of the reference category in those with mGFR less than 15 mL/min/1.73 m^2 in both genders (Figure 2A). Of note, this percentage was twice as high in patients with GFR ≥ 0 mL/min/1.73 m^2 when using eGFR instead of mGFR, and did not increase with decreasing eGFR (Figure 2B).

Factors associated with low urinary creatinine excretion rate at baseline

Odds ratios of low urinary creatinine excretion significantly and gradually increased as BMI decreased, both before and after adjusting for demographic variables and mGFR (Table 3). Urinary creatinine excretion was not significantly associated with diabetes and metabolic acidosis. Lower prealbumin and urinary urea levels were significantly associated with higher ORs of low urinary creatinine excretion. In contrast, there was no significant association with serum albumin. Triglycerides were inversely and significantly associated with urinary creatinine excretion. Inflam-

Table 2. Urinary creatinine excretion rate according to mGFR level, by gender, age, and ethnicity.

Ethnic origin, age, mGFR (mL/min per1.73m²)	Men (n = 1072)											Women (n = 537)										
		Urinary creatinine excretion rate											Urinary creatinine excretion rate									
		mmol/kg/24h					mmol/24h						mmol/kg/24h					mmol/24h				
	N	m± sd	10th	25th	75th	90th	m± sd	10th	25th	75th	90th	N	m± sd	10th	25th	75th	90th	m± sd	10th	25th	75th	90th
Total							*n* = 1072											*n* = 537				
≥ 60	**188**	0.20±0.03	0.15	0.17	0.22	0.24	15.3±3.1	11.4	13.0	17.0	19.4	**94**	0.16±0.03	0.12	0.14	0.17	0.19	9.6±1.9	7.2	8.3	10.8	12.2
45–60	**233**	0.18±0.03	0.14	0.15	0.20	0.22	13.9±3.0	10.6	11.8	15.5	17.9	**88**	0.15±0.03	0.11	0.13	0.16	0.18	9.2±2.1	6.8	7.7	10.6	11.7
30–44	**321**	0.17±0.03	0.13	0.14	0.19	0.21	13.2±3.2	9.3	11.0	15.2	17.3	**151**	0.15±0.03	0.10	0.12	0.17	0.19	9.3±2.2	6.8	7.5	10.6	12.3
15–29	**274**	0.17±0.04	0.12	0.14	0.19	0.22	12.7±3.2	9.0	10.5	14.6	17.0	**161**	0.13±0.03	0.09	0.11	0.15	0.18	8.8±2.1	6.1	7.3	10.6	11.5
<15	**56**	0.15±0.04	0.11	0.13	0.18	0.20	12.1±3.3	7.7	9.2	14.0	16.8	**43**	0.12±0.03	0.08	0.09	0.14	0.15	7.6±2.5	5.0	5.5	8.9	10.8
Non-African origin																						
<60 years							*n* = 377											*n* = 219				
≥ 60	**92**	0.20±0.03	0.16	0.18	0.22	0.24	15.3±2.9	11.7	13.0	16.9	19.1	**45**	0.16±0.03	0.12	0.14	0.19	0.22	9.7±1.8	7.6	8.9	10.8	11.9
45–60	**78**	0.18±0.03	0.15	0.17	0.20	0.22	14.5±3.0	11.4	12.5	16.0	18.5	**35**	0.16±0.03	0.13	0.13	0.18	0.20	9.4±2.3	6.8	7.8	10.8	11.9
30–44	**96**	0.19±0.03	0.15	0.17	0.21	0.22	14.6±3.4	11.0	12.3	16.8	18.6	**61**	0.16±0.04	0.12	0.13	0.18	0.22	9.7±2.4	7.0	8.1	11.0	12.8
15–29	**91**	0.17±0.03	0.13	0.15	0.19	0.22	13.2±2.6	10.3	11.4	14.8	16.7	**61**	0.14±0.03	0.10	0.11	0.16	0.19	8.9±2.3	6.0	7.4	10.9	12.0
<15	**20**	0.17±0.03	0.13	0.14	0.20	0.21	13.8±3.0	9.2	12.4	15.1	17.5	**17**	0.13±0.03	0.09	0.11	0.13	0.15	7.9±2.5	5.3	6.1	8.9	11.6
≥60 years							*n* = 524											*n* = 215				
≥60	**50**	0.18±0.03	0.14	0.15	0.20	0.21	14.3±2.7	10.7	12.5	15.8	17.4	**27**	0.15±0.02	0.13	0.14	0.15	0.18	8.6±1.4	6.4	7.7	9.5	10.3
45–60	**113**	0.17±0.03	0.13	0.15	0.18	0.20	12.9±2.7	10.1	11.2	14.4	16.6	**41**	0.14±0.02	0.11	0.12	0.15	0.16	8.5±1.7	6.7	7.1	9.6	10.6
30–44	**186**	0.16±0.03	0.12	0.14	0.18	0.20	12.2±2.6	8.9	10.3	13.9	15.4	**60**	0.13±0.03	0.09	0.11	0.15	0.16	8.3±1.7	6.4	7.0	9.2	10.5
15–29	**147**	0.15±0.04	0.11	0.13	0.18	0.20	11.9±3.2	8.3	9.8	13.8	15.7	**73**	0.13±0.03	0.09	0.10	0.14	0.16	8.6±1.8	6.2	7.3	9.8	11.0
<15	**28**	0.14±0.03	0.11	0.12	0.15	0.18	10.9±2.6	7.5	8.5	13.4	14.4	**14**	0.10±0.03	0.07	0.08	0.14	0.15	6.7±2.3	4.0	4.8	8.4	10.0
African origin																						
<60 years							*n* = 112											*n* = 43				
≥60	**35**	0.21±0.08	0.18	0.19	0.24	0.25	17.4±3.1	13.0	15.7	19.7	20.8	**11**	0.15±0.02	0.12	0.13	0.17	0.17	11.7±1.6	9.8	10.6	12.9	13.1
45–60	**28**	0.21±0.04	0.16	0.19	0.23	0.27	16.1±3.2	11.8	14.1	18.3	20.0	**3**	0.17±0.01	0.16	0.16	0.18	0.18	11.6±1.1	10.8	10.8	12.9	12.9
30–44	**23**	0.20±0.03	0.16	0.18	0.22	0.24	15.6±3.8	10.5	12.9	18.6	19.8	**14**	0.16±0.03	0.13	0.14	0.18	0.20	10.5±1.7	8.0	9.1	11.7	13.3
15–29	**23**	0.22±0.04	0.16	0.19	0.24	0.27	16.4±3.2	12.4	13.2	18.9	19.9	**12**	0.16±0.04	0.10	0.12	0.19	0.20	10.6±1.6	9.8	10.2	11.4	11.5
<15	**3**	0.18±0.03	0.09	0.09	0.24	0.24	14.1±8.0	5.1	5.1	20.0	20.0	**3**	0.12±0.02	0.11	0.11	0.14	0.14	10.1±3.8	7.2	7.2	14.4	14.4
≥60 years							*n* = 37											*n* = 17				
≥60	**6**	0.19±0.02	0.16	0.16	0.20	0.22	14.3±0.42	10.8	11.5	17.9	18.6	**1**	-	-	-	-	-	-	-	-	-	-
45–60	**11**	0.17±0.04	0.15	0.15	0.19	0.21	13.4±1.7	10.4	11.0	14.8	16.6	**6**	0.14±0.02	0.12	0.12	0.15	0.17	10.0±1.3	8.4	9.1	11.4	11.5
30–44	**13**	0.16±0.03	0.13	0.14	0.17	0.20	12.9±1.8	11.7	11.8	13.8	15.2	**6**	0.14±0.03	0.10	0.13	0.17	0.20	10.1±3.6	7.4	7.6	10.3	17.0

Table . Cont.

Ethnic origin, age, mGFR (mL/min per1.73m^2)	Men (n = 1072)											Women (n = 537)										
		Urinary creatinine excretion rate											Urinary creatinine excretion rate									
		mmol/kg/24h					mmol/24h						mmol/kg/24h					mmol/24h				
	N	m± sd	10th	25th	75th	90th	m± sd	10th	25th	75th	90th	N	m± sd	10th	25th	75th	90th	m± sd	10th	25th	75th	90th
15–29	5	0.16±0.01	0.15	0.16	0.16	0.17	10.9±2.6	8.8	9.8	12.2	13.1	4	0.16±0.04	0.11	0.13	0.19	0.20	10.3±2.3	7.8	8.4	12.3	12.5
<15	2	0.14±0.02	0.13	0.13	0.15	0.15	10.8±3.4	10.6	10.6	11.2	11.2	0	-	-	-	-	-	-	-	-	-	-

Abbreviations: mGFR, measured glomerular filtration rate.

mation, reflected by either higher WBC, plasma fibrinogen or haptoglobin levels, was also inversely and significantly associated with low urinary creatinine excretion after adjusting for confounders, but no such association was observed with CRP and orosomucoid. The higher the quartile of 24-hour proteinuria, the lower the ORs of low urinary creatinine excretion rate.

Fully adjusted ORs for low urinary creatinine excretion increased significantly as mGFR decreased (Table 4), but did not with eGFR: ORs were 0.95 (0.59–1.5), 0.90 (0.57–1.4), 0.94 (0.57–1.5), and 0.62 (0.29–1.3) for eGFR of 45–60, 30–44, 15–29, and <15 as compared with ≥60 mL/min/1.73 m^2. Other factors significantly associated with low creatinine excretion in the multivariate model were age, gender, ethnicity, BMI, 24-hour urinary urea and proteinuria. While the association with metabolic acidosis remained nonsignificant (data not shown), it is noteworthy that diabetes became strongly associated with low urinary creatinine excretion after adjustment for the other risk factors. Similar associations were observed in patients with and without diabetes except for pre-albumin, which was related to low urinary creatinine excretion only in those with diabetes.

Factors associated with baseline rate and annual change in urinary creatinine excretion

As expected, factors associated with lower mean creatinine excretion rate at baseline were similar to those found above with the logistic model. Each 10 mL/min/1.73 m^2 decrease in mGFR was associated with 0.23±0.03 mmol/24 h decrease in urinary creatinine excretion rate, and each 10 mmol/24h decrease in urinary urea with 0.09±0.00 mmol/24 h (Table 5). Patients with proteinuria in the highest quartile had a higher rate of 0.80±0.16 mmol/24 h than those in the lowest quartile.

Mean annual decline in mGFR was 1.53±0.12 mL/min/ 1.73 m^2 and mean annual decrease in urinary urea was 7.42±1.22 mmol/24 h. Mean change in urinary creatinine excretion rate was 0.28±0.02 mmol/24 h per year and did not differ according to baseline characteristics except gender: women had slower mean annual decrease than men. Patients with a fast annual decline in mGFR of 5 mL/min/1.73 m^2 (about 3 times the mean level) had a decrease in urinary creatinine excretion more than twice as big than those with stable mGFR, independent of changes in protein intake assessed by urinary urea as well as of other determinants.

Discussion

This study showed that decrease in urinary creatinine excretion may occur early in CKD independent of nutritional factors and protein intake. As expected, the study confirmed the impact of age, ethnicity and nutritional factors on urinary creatinine excretion, but also found a graded relationship with proteinuria and no significant association with inflammation. Together with the range of urinary creatinine excretion provided by age, gender, ethnicity as well as by mGFR, these findings have important clinical implications regarding management of muscle mass loss and validation of urine collection in CKD patients.

Very few studies have investigated the relation between muscle loss and kidney function decline. Foley *et al.* [28] reported a high prevalence (27.2%) of reduced muscle mass assessed by bioimpedance in community-dwelling adults. Although its prevalence increased as estimated glomerular filtration rate (eGFR) decreased, the association was no longer significant after adjustment for age and comorbidity. Nevertheless, these results are difficult to compare with ours, because bioimpedance measures not only muscle mass but also body water [38,45]. In the Modification of

Table 3. Factors associated with low urinary creatinine excretion rate at baseline, n = 1609.

	Crude OR (95% CI)	Age, gender, ethnicity, centre and mGFR-adjusted OR (95% CI)
BMI group (kg/m^2)		
<18.5	4.0 (2.1-7.8)	7.5 (3.5–16.3)
18.5–25	1	1
25–30	0.53 (0.41–0.69)	0.29 (0.21–0.39)
30–35	0.45 (0.31–0.65)	0.22 (0.15–0.34)
≥35	0.20 (0.09–0.44)	0.11 (0.05–0.26)
Diabetes[a] (yes *vs* no)	1.3 (0.98–1.6)	0.84 (0.65–1.1)
Metabolic acidosis[b] (yes *vs* no)	1.3 (0.96–1.8)	0.91 (0.63–1.3)
Nutritional markers		
HDL cholesterol <*vs* ≥ 1.3/1.0 mmol/L*	0.73 (0.57–0.93)	0.62 (0.48–0.81)
Triglycerides ≥ *vs* <1.7 mmol/L	0.91 (0.71–1.2)	0.68 (0.52–0.89)
Serum albumin <*vs* ≥ 35 g/L	1.1 (0.79–1.5)	0.90 (0.62–1.3)
Prealbumin <*vs* ≥ 0.30 g/L	1.3 (1.03–1.7)	1.5 (1.1–1.9)
Urinary urea by quartiles (mmol/24h)		
lower	14.0 (9.2–21.2)	16.4 (10.5–25.7)
2nd	4.4 (2.9–6.8)	5.0 (3.2–7.9)
3nd	1.9 (1.2–3.0)	2.2 (1.4–3.5)
upper	1	1
Inflammation markers		
WBC count ≥ *vs* <7.5 10^3/mm^3	0.97 (0.75–1.3)	0.74 (0.56–0.98)
Plasma fibrinogen ≥ *vs* <5 g/L	1.1 (0.80–1.6)	0.68 (0.47–0.99)
Haptoglobin ≥ *vs* <90th percentile	0.91 (0.60–1.4)	0.60 (0.38–0.95)
Orosomucoid ≥ *vs* <90th percentile	1.6 (1.0–2.4)	1.1 (0.72–1.8)
CRP ≥ *vs* <10 mg/L	1.3 (0.89–1.9)	0.96 (0.63–1.4)
Proteinuria by quartiles (g/24h)		
lower	1	1
2nd	0.65 (0.48–0.89)	0.50 (0.35–0.71)
3nd	0.74 (0.54–1.0)	0.46 (0.32–0.66)
upper	0.56 (0.40–0.77)	0.29 (0.19–0.43)

Abbreviations: OR (95% CI), odds-ratios and 95% confidence interval; mGFR, measured glomerular filtration rate; BMI, body mass index; HDL, high-density lipoprotein; WBC, white blood cells; CRP, C-reactive protein.
Cut-off points of urinary urea were: <312.8 mmol/24h, 312.8–382.5 mmol/24h, 382.5–456.3 mmol/24h,>456.3 mmol/24 in men; <252.0 mmol/24h, 252.0–302.1 mmol/24h, 302.1–375.0 mmol/24h,>375.0 mmol/24h in women. Cut-off points of proteinuria urea were: <0.14 g/24h, 0.14–0.35 g/24h, 0.35–1.1 g/24,>1.1 g/24h in men; <0.12 g/24g, 0.12–0.21 g/24h, 0.21–0.89 g/24h,>0.89 g/24h in women.
*Gender-specific thresholds were used to define high-density lipoprotein cholesterol cut-off points: 1.0 mmol/L in men and 1.3 mmol/L in women.
[a] Fasting glucose ≥ 7 mmol/L or HbA1c ≥6.5 or antidiabetic treatment or reported diabetes.
[b] Venous CO2 <22 mmol/L or alkaline treatment.

Diet in Renal Disease (MDRD) study [30], several nutritional parameters, including urinary creatinine, showed lower values for patients with mGFR <21 ml/min/1.73 m^2 than for those with mGFR>37 ml/min/1.73 m^2. The associations, however, were strongly attenuated after controlling for protein and energy intakes leading the authors to conclude that they were mediated by the lower dietary intake associated with kidney function decline. In contrast, *Micco et al* [17] showed an inverse cross-sectional association between urinary creatinine excretion and CKD stages from 3 to 5 independent of nutritional factors as well as a decrease over time in urinary creatinine excretion independent of eGFR decline. The NephroTest study extends these findings to earlier CKD stages, showing that low creatinine excretion rate was indeed twice as common in stage 3a (GFR within 45–60 mL/min/1.73 m^2) than in stages 1–2 (GFR ≥60 mL/min/1.73 m^2), independent of both nutritional parameters and protein intake assessed by urinary urea. Although an increase in extrarenal excretion of creatinine, including its conversion to other metabolites and its breakdown by gut bacteria [39,43] cannot be ruled out as an explanation of the above association, this is unlikely because it is usually significant in the latest stage of CKD. Similarly, while it is well-known that the relative participation of tubular secretion in creatinine excretion increases with kidney function decline, this has definitely no impact on the overall urinary creatinine excretion in steady state such as that of patients with CKD.

As expected and in line with other studies[13,18,26–28,30,39] age, gender and ethnicity were major determinants of urinary creatinine excretion rate. Moreover, the large sample size of the NephroTest study enabled for the first time to document the range of urinary creatinine excretion rate not only according to these variables as previously reported, but also according to mGFR

Table 4. Multivariate analysis of factors associated with low urinary creatinine excretion rate at baseline, by diabetes status.

OR (95% CI)	Overall population (n = 1609)	Without diabetes (n = 1153)	With diabetes (n = 456)
Age, year	1.05 (1.04–1.06)	1.05 (1.04–1.07)	1.05 (1.02–1.07)
Gender (men vs women)	2.1 (1.5–2.9)	1.9 (1.3–2.9)	2.1 (1.1–3.9)
African vs non-African origin	0.28 (0.16–0.49)	0.42 (0.22–0.80)	0.15 (0.05–0.44)
mGFR (ml/min per1.73m2)			
≥60	1	1	1
45–60	2.4 (1.3–4.2)	2.1 (1.1–4.2)	2.5 (0.79–7.9)
30–44	3.6 (2.1–6.2)	3.2 (1.7–6.2)	3.8 (1.3–11.0)
15–29	5.2 (2.9–9.2)	5.0 (2.5–10.0)	4.7 (1.6–14.5)
<15	9.2 (4.3–19.6)	8.2 (3.3–20.5)	11.9 (2.6–55.4)
Diabetes mellitus			
no	1	-	-
yes	1.8 (1.3-2.6)	-	-
BMI group (kg/m²)			
<18.5	9.6 (4.2–21.9)	9.7 (4.1–22.9)	
18.5–25	1	1	5.0 (2.4–10.4)
25–30	0.29 (0.20–0.41)	0.32 (0.21–0.48)	1
30–35	0.24 (0.15–0.39)	0.12 (0.06–0.26)	1.6 (0.81–3.0)
≥35	0.12 (0.05–0.32)	0.12 (0.03–0.53)	0.51 (0.15–1.8)
Prealbumin *(g/L)*			
>0.30	1	1	1
<0.30	1.2 (0.84–1.7)	0.83 (0.54–1.3)	2.3 (1.3–4.2)
Urinary urea (mmol/24h)			
lowest	13.6 (8.3–22.1)	17.8 (9.0–35.5)	10.6 (4.8–23.4)
2nd	4.2 (2.6–6.9)	5.1 (2.5–10.2)	3.7 (1.7–7.8)
3rd	2.0 (1.2–3.4)	2.5 (1.2–5.2)	1.6 (0.75–3.5)
highest	1	1	1
Proteinuria (g/24h)			
lowest	1	1	1
2nd	0.63 (0.42–0.94)	0.65 (0.40–1.0)	0.58 (0.25–1.4)
3rd	0.52 (0.34–0.81)	0.51 (0.30–0.86)	0.63 (0.27–1.4)
highest	0.37 (0.23–0.60)	0.38 (0.21–0.69)	0.37 (0.16–0.86)

Abbreviations: OR (95% CI), odds-ratios and 95% confidence interval; mGFR, measured glomerular filtration rate; BMI, body mass index.
Cut-off points of urinary urea were: <312.8 mmol/24h, 312.8–382.5 mmol/24h, 382.5–456.3 mmol/24h,>456.3 mmol/24 in men; <252.0 mmol/24h, 252.0–302.1 mmol/24h, 302.1–375.0 mmol/24h,>375.0 mmol/24h in women. Cut-off points of proteinuria urea were: <0.14 g/24h, 0.14–0.35 g/24h, 0.35–1.1 g/24,>1.1 g/24h in men; <0.12 g/24g, 0.12–0.21 g/24h, 0.21–0.89 g/24h,>0.89 g/24h in women.
*Multivariate adjustment, including center.

level. These values could thus be used by clinicians to validate 24-hour urine collection in patients with reduced kidney function.

A large set of nutritional measures were available in this study. BMI has been reported to be significantly associated with muscle mass in both transplanted [20] and dialysis patients [14,19]. In line with other studies of CKD [13,17,18,25] and non CKD populations [26,27], we observed that urinary creatinine excretion was significantly lower with lower BMI. Prealbumin is also considered as an important nutritional marker [1,2,6,9,14,37,46]. We found that lower urinary creatinine levels were significantly associated with a low prealbumin level in patients with diabetes, but not in those without. The number of missing data for prealbumin, however, may have weakened the latter association. In contrast, serum albumin was not associated with urinary creatinine excretion. Although it has been shown to be positively associated with total muscle mass estimated from X-ray absorptiometry [29], its usefulness as a nutritional marker has been challenged in end-stage renal disease (ESRD) patients[3,47,48]. Similarly, we failed to find that urinary creatinine excretion was significantly associated with transferrin, homocysteine, total and HDL cholesterol or triglycerides. As expected, urinary urea was significantly and positively associated with creatininuria in our study. Indeed, protein intake is an important determinant of muscle mass [28,39]. Our finding that the decrease in urinary creatinine excretion over time is associated with mGFR decline independent of both nutritional measurements and lowering

Table 5. Linear mixed model analysis of factors associated with mean differences in the level (in mmol/24h) and change over time (in mmol/24h per year) in urinary creatinine excretion rate.

	Mean difference in urinary creatinine excretion (95% Confidence Interval)
Intercept, mmol/24h *	12.68(12.39,12.98)
Factors associated with baseline urinary creatinine	
Age, year	−0.06(−0.07,−0.05)
Women vs men	−3.57(−3.83,−3.32)
African vs non African origin	1.87(1.57,2.18)
mGFR, per each 10 ml/min/1.73 m^2 decrease	−0.23(−0.29,−0.17)
Diabetes	−0.38(−0.63,−0.13)
BMI, kg/m^2	
<18.5	−1.54(−2.21,−0.88)
18.5–25	0 (ref)
25–30	1.11(0.87,1.34)
30–35	1.71(1.39,2.02)
>35	1.91(1.41,2.42)
Urinary urea, per each 10 mmol/day decrease	−0.09(−0.10,−0.08)
Proteinuria	
lowest	0 (ref)
2nd	0.42(0.13,0.71)
3rd	0.66(0.36,0.96)
highest	0.80(0.48,1.12)
Slope, mmol/24h per year**	−0.19(−0.24,−0.14)
Factors associated with changes in urinary creatinine	
Women vs Men	0.16(0.08,0.25)
mGFR, per each 5 ml/min/1.73m^2 per yr decrease†	−0.29(−0.34,−0.25)
Urinary urea, per each 25 mmol/24h per yr decrease†	−0.15(−0.17,−0.14)

*mean predicted level in urinary creatinine excretion rate in mmol/24h for 60-yr old non-African and non-diabetic men, with normal BMI (within 18.5 to 25 kg/m^2), baseline mGFR of 40 ml/min/1.73 m^2, urinary urea of 400 mmol/d and proteinuria in the lowest quartiles.
** mean predicted change in urinary creatinine excretion rate in mmol/24h per year in men with stable mGFR and urinary urea, i.e., with no change in level from baseline.
† 5 ml/min/1.73 m^2 per yr decrease in mGFR and 25 mmol/24h per yr decrease in urinary urea correspond to about three times the mean annual decrease for each variable.

protein intake suggests that other mechanisms than reduced dietary intakes may explain muscle wasting in CKD.

Only sparse data are available about the potential impact of diabetes on muscle mass loss. *Cano et al.* [24] reports lower lean body mass estimated from creatinine generation in diabetic *vs* nondiabetic patients on hemodialysis. *Pupim et al.* [21] also showed that the loss of lean body mass accelerates in dialysis patients with diabetes. Mechanisms related to diabetes mellitus [32,37] have been suggested to explain this relation. *Siew et al.* [33] demonstrated a significant association between skeletal muscle protein breakdown and insulin resistance in nondiabetic chronic hemodialysis patients. In agreement with other studies [18,27], we found significantly lower urinary creatinine excretion in CKD patients with than without diabetes mellitus. Metabolic acidosis has also been shown to be associated with malnutrition-inflammation in end-stage CKD [35]. Its occurrence in the very late stages of CKD[49] may explain why we found no relation between low muscle mass and acidosis.

Although inflammation frequently accompanies poor nutritional status [1,7,14,31,36,48,50] and plays an important role in the pathophysiology of muscle wasting [36,50], there are conflicting results about the association of inflammatory status with muscle mass loss [36]. The elevated CRP levels often observed in CKD patients [7,8,11,12] reflect the generation of proinflammatory cytokines, which may contribute to muscle wasting by stimulating protein catabolism. In disagreement with some [14,19], but not all studies [18,28], inflammation defined by CRP ≥10 mg/L was not significantly associated with urinary creatinine excretion rate after adjusting for nutritional factors in this study. Importantly, there was no association with either of the other available inflammatory markers, including orosomucoid, haptoglobin, plasma fibrinogen, or WBC after multivariate adjustment. In contrast, there was a graded and independent relationship with 24-hour proteinuria which, to our knowledge, has not been described before. The complex associations of proteinuria with protein wasting and inflammation may explain the observed association. Further studies are needed to elucidate whether muscle wasting is related to inflammation in non-end-stage CKD or whether it depends on the type of malnutrition, as suggested in dialysis patients [48].

The strengths of this study include the use of a gold-standard method to measure renal function (mGFR), the ability to assess urinary creatinine excretion based on both carefully collected urine during a 5-hour visit and 24-hour urine collection as well as the availability of repeated measurements of these markers as well as of several potential determinants of muscle wasting that may have confounded the association of interest. It is worth noting that we found no association of urinary creatinine excretion with GFR estimated from the CKD-EPI equation, which is explained by the impact of creatinine generation on both serum and urinary creatinine resulting in overestimation of eGFR as compared with mGFR in patients with low urinary creatinine, and conversely, underestimation in those with high urinary creatinine. This study also has limitations. First, we had no information about physical activity [22,28,31], which might have explained some of our findings. Second, although no direct measure of muscle mass exists, it might be considered a limitation that we used urinary creatinine excretion as a measure of muscle mass instead of reference methods such as computerized tomography (CT) or magnetic resonance imaging (MRI) [40,41]. However, the time and money required for these methods make them impractical in large-scale clinical studies. Finally, demographic- and anthropometric parameter-based equations [51–53] used to estimate muscle mass in individuals with normal kidney function are inappropriate in the CKD population because they do not take into account the decrease in urinary creatinine excretion with reduced kidney function.

Conclusions

Our findings suggest that decrease in urinary creatinine excretion rate may appear early in CKD patients, independent of decreased protein intake assessed by urinary urea excretion, as well as of other determinants of muscle mass loss including gender, an older age, non-African origin, diabetes, lower BMI and 24-h proteinuria levels. Urinary creatinine concentration is a useful tool, easy to apply routinely. Reference values provided by age, gender, and GFR level might help clinicians to identify individuals who may need both special interventions, including nutritional or exercise advice, and monitoring of their response to these interventions. The decrease of urinary creatinine excretion with GFR decline also questions the accuracy of normalizing for creatininuria when estimating urine analytes concentration which may be overestimated in CKD patients with reduced muscle mass.

Acknowledgments

We thank Jo-Ann Cahn for the English revision of this manuscript.

The NephroTest study group: Bichat Univ Hospital (Paris): François Vrtovsnik, Eric Daugas (Nephrology) and Martin Flamant, Emmanuelle Vidal-Petiot (Physiology); European Georges Pompidou Univ Hospital (Paris): Christian Jacquot, Alexandre Karras, Eric Thervet, Christian d'Auzac (Nephrology) and P. Houillier, M. Courbebaisse, D. Eladari et G. Maruani (Physiology); Tenon Univ Hospital (Paris): Jean-Jacques Boffa, Pierre Ronco, H. Fessi, Eric Rondeau (Nephrology) and Emmanuel Letavernier, Jean Philippe Haymann (Physiology); Landy Clinic (Saint-Ouen): P. Urena-Torres (Nephrology); Bordeaux Univ Hospital: Christian Combe (Nephrology), and Inserm (Villejuif): M. Metzger, B. Stengel, France.

Author Contributions

Analyzed the data: E. Tynkevich M. Flamant MM M. Froissart BS. Wrote the paper: E. Tynkevich M. Flamant M. Froissart BS. Contributed to concept and design of the work, interpretation of data, and the critical revision and final approval of the version to be published: E. Tynkevich M. Flamant JH MM E. Thervet JB FV PH M. Froissart BS.

References

1. Kalantar-Zadeh K, Ikizler TA, Block G, Avram MM, Kopple JD (2003) Malnutrition-inflammation complex syndrome in dialysis patients: causes and consequences. Am J Kidney Dis Off J Natl Kidney Found 42: 864–881.
2. Fouque D, Kalantar-Zadeh K, Kopple J, Cano N, Chauveau P, et al. (2008) A proposed nomenclature and diagnostic criteria for protein-energy wasting in acute and chronic kidney disease. Kidney Int 73: 391–398. doi: 10.1038/sj.ki.5002585.
3. Blumenkrantz MJ, Kopple JD, Gutman RA, Chan YK, Barbour GL, et al. (1980) Methods for assessing nutritional status of patients with renal failure. Am J Clin Nutr 33: 1567–1585.
4. Mak RH, Ikizler AT, Kovesdy CP, Raj DS, Stenvinkel P, et al. (2011) Wasting in chronic kidney disease. J Cachexia Sarcopenia Muscle 2: 9–25. doi: 10.1007/s13539-011-0019-5.
5. Kalantar-Zadeh K, Kopple JD (2001) Relative contributions of nutrition and inflammation to clinical outcome in dialysis patients. Am J Kidney Dis Off J Natl Kidney Found 38: 1343–1350. doi: 10.1053/ajkd.2001.29250.
6. Aparicio M, Cano N, Chauveau P, Azar R, Canaud B, et al. (1999) Nutritional status of haemodialysis patients: a French national cooperative study. French Study Group for Nutrition in Dialysis. Nephrol Dial Transplant 14: 1679–1686. doi: 10.1093/ndt/14.7.1679.
7. Stenvinkel P, Heimbürger O, Paultre F, Diczfalusy U, Wang T, et al. (1999) Strong association between malnutrition, inflammation, and atherosclerosis in chronic renal failure. Kidney Int 55: 1899–1911. doi: 10.1046/j.1523-1755.1999.00422.x.
8. Qureshi AR, Alvestrand A, Danielsson A, Divino-Filho JC, Gutierrez A, et al. (1998) Factors predicting malnutrition in hemodialysis patients: A cross-sectional study. Kidney Int 53: 773–782. doi: 10.1046/j.1523-1755.1998.00812.x.
9. Fouque D, Pelletier S, Mafra D, Chauveau P (2011) Nutrition and chronic kidney disease. Kidney Int 80: 348–357. doi: 10.1038/ki.2011.118.
10. Qureshi AR, Alvestrand A, Divino-Filho JC, Gutierrez A, Heimbürger O, et al. (2002) Inflammation, Malnutrition, and Cardiac Disease as Predictors of Mortality in Hemodialysis Patients. J Am Soc Nephrol 13: S28–S36.
11. Zimmermann J, Herrlinger S, Pruy A, Metzger T, Wanner C (1999) Inflammation enhances cardiovascular risk and mortality in hemodialysis patients. Kidney Int 55: 648–658. doi: 10.1046/j.1523–1755.1999.00273.x.
12. Ortega O, Rodriguez I, Gallar P, Carreño A, Ortiz M, et al. (2002) Significance of high C-reactive protein levels in pre-dialysis patients. Nephrol Dial Transplant Off Publ Eur Dial Transpl Assoc - Eur Ren Assoc 17: 1105–1109.
13. Ix JH, de Boer IH, Wassel CL, Criqui MH, Shlipak MG, et al. (2010) Urinary creatinine excretion rate and mortality in persons with coronary artery disease: the Heart and Soul Study. Circulation 121: 1295–1303. doi: 10.1161/CIRCULATIONAHA.109.924266.
14. Honda H, Qureshi AR, Axelsson J, Heimburger O, Suliman ME, et al. (2007) Obese sarcopenia in patients with end-stage renal disease is associated with inflammation and increased mortality. Am J Clin Nutr 86: 633–638.
15. Kovesdy CP, George SM, Anderson JE, Kalantar-Zadeh K (2009) Outcome predictability of biomarkers of protein-energy wasting and inflammation in moderate and advanced chronic kidney disease. Am J Clin Nutr 90: 407–414. doi: 10.3945/ajcn.2008.27390.
16. Noori N, Kopple JD, Kovesdy CP, Feroze U, Sim JJ, et al. (2010) Mid-Arm Muscle Circumference and Quality of Life and Survival in Maintenance Hemodialysis Patients. Clin J Am Soc Nephrol 5: 2258–2268. doi: 10.2215/CJN.02080310.
17. Micco LD, Quinn RR, Ronksley PE, Bellizzi V, Lewin AM, et al. (2013) Urine Creatinine Excretion and Clinical Outcomes in CKD. Clin J Am Soc Nephrol: CJN.01350213d oi: 10.2215/CJN.01350213.
18. Oterdoom LH, van Ree RM, de Vries APJ, Gansevoort RT, Schouten JP, et al. (2008) Urinary creatinine excretion reflecting muscle mass is a predictor of mortality and graft loss in renal transplant recipients. Transplantation 86: 391–398. doi: 10.1097/TP.0b013e3181788aea.
19. Carrero JJ, Chmielewski M, Axelsson J, Snaedal S, Heimbürger O, et al. (2008) Muscle atrophy, inflammation and clinical outcome in incident and prevalent dialysis patients. Clin Nutr Edinb Scotl 27: 557–564. doi: 10.1016/j.clnu.2008.04.007.
20. Molnar MZ, Streja E, Kovesdy CP, Bunnapradist S, Sampaio MS, et al. (2011) Associations of body mass index and weight loss with mortality in transplant-waitlisted maintenance hemodialysis patients. Am J Transplant Off J Am Soc Transplant Am Soc Transpl Surg 11: 725–736. doi: 10.1111/j.1600-6143.2011.03468.x.
21. Pupim LB, Heimbürger O, Qureshi AR, Ikizler TA, Stenvinkel P (2005) Accelerated lean body mass loss in incident chronic dialysis patients with diabetes mellitus. Kidney Int 68: 2368–2374. doi: 10.1111/j.1523-1755.2005.00699.x.
22. Anand S, Chertow GM, Johansen KL, Grimes B, Kurella Tamura M, et al. (2011) Association of self-reported physical activity with laboratory markers of nutrition and inflammation: the Comprehensive Dialysis Study. J Ren Nutr Off J Counc Ren Nutr Natl Kidney Found 21: 429–437. doi: 10.1053/j.jrn.2010.09.007.

23. Kovesdy CP, Shinaberger CS, Kalantar-Zadeh K (2010) Epidemiology of dietary nutrient intake in ESRD. Semin Dial 23: 353–358. doi: 10.1111/j.1525-139X.2010.00745.x.
24. Cano NJM, Roth H, Aparicio M, Azar R, Canaud B, et al. (2002) Malnutrition in hemodialysis diabetic patients: evaluation and prognostic influence. Kidney Int 62: 593–601. doi: 10.1046/j.1523-1755.2002.00457.x.
25. Bansal N, Hsu C, Zhao S, Whooley MA, Ix JH (2011) Relation of body mass index to urinary creatinine excretion rate in patients with coronary heart disease. Am J Cardiol 108: 179–184. doi: 10.1016/j.amjcard.2011.03.020.
26. Oterdoom LH, Gansevoort RT, Schouten JP, de Jong PE, Gans ROB, et al. (2009) Urinary creatinine excretion, an indirect measure of muscle mass, is an independent predictor of cardiovascular disease and mortality in the general population. Atherosclerosis 207: 534–540. doi: 10.1016/j.atherosclerosis.2009.05.010.
27. Barr DB, Wilder LC, Caudill SP, Gonzalez AJ, Needham LL, et al. (2005) Urinary Creatinine Concentrations in the U.S. Population: Implications for Urinary Biologic Monitoring Measurements. Environ Health Perspect 113: 192–200. doi: 10.1289/ehp.7337.
28. Foley RN, Wang C, Ishani A, Collins AJ, Murray AM (2007) Kidney Function and Sarcopenia in the United States General Population: NHANES III. Am J Nephrol 27: 279–286. doi: 10.1159/000101827.
29. Baumgartner RN, Koehler KM, Romero L, Garry PJ (1996) Serum albumin is associated with skeletal muscle in elderly men and women. Am J Clin Nutr 64: 552–558.
30. Kopple JD, Greene T, Chumlea WC, Hollinger D, Maroni BJ, et al. (2000) Relationship between nutritional status and the glomerular filtration rate: results from the MDRD study. Kidney Int 57: 1688–1703. doi: 10.1046/j.1523-1755.2000.00014.x.
31. Evans WJ (2010) Skeletal muscle loss: cachexia, sarcopenia, and inactivity. Am J Clin Nutr 91: 1123S–1127S. doi: 10.3945/ajcn.2010.28608A.
32. Workeneh BT, Mitch WE (2010) Review of muscle wasting associated with chronic kidney disease. Am J Clin Nutr 91: 1128S–1132S. doi: 10.3945/ajcn.2010.28608B.
33. Siew ED, Pupim LB, Majchrzak KM, Shintani A, Flakoll PJ, et al. (2007) Insulin resistance is associated with skeletal muscle protein breakdown in non-diabetic chronic hemodialysis patients. Kidney Int 71: 146–152. doi: 10.1038/sj.ki.5001984.
34. Bailey JL, Wang X, England BK, Price SR, Ding X, et al. (1996) The acidosis of chronic renal failure activates muscle proteolysis in rats by augmenting transcription of genes encoding proteins of the ATP-dependent ubiquitin-proteasome pathway. J Clin Invest 97: 1447–1453. doi: 10.1172/JCI118566.
35. Kalantar-Zadeh K, Mehrotra R, Fouque D, Kopple JD (2004) Poor Nutritional Status and Inflammation: Metabolic Acidosis and Malnutrition-Inflammation Complex Syndrome in Chronic Renal Failure. Semin Dial 17: 455–465. doi: 10.1111/j.0894-0959.2004.17606.x.
36. Avesani CM, Carrero JJ, Axelsson J, Qureshi AR, Lindholm B, et al. (2006) Inflammation and wasting in chronic kidney disease: Partners in crime. Kidney Int 70: S8–S13. doi: 10.1038/sj.ki.5001969.
37. Mak RH, Ikizler TA, Kovesdy CP, Raj DS, Stenvinkel P, et al. (2011) Erratum to: Wasting in chronic kidney disease. J Cachexia Sarcopenia Muscle 2: 119. doi: 10.1007/s13539-011-0026-6.
38. Bhatla B, Moore H, Emerson P, Keshaviah P, Prowant B, et al. (1995) Lean body mass estimation by creatinine kinetics, bioimpedance, and dual energy x-ray absorptiometry in patients on continuous ambulatory peritoneal dialysis. ASAIO J Am Soc Artif Intern Organs 1992 41: M442–446.
39. Heymsfield SB, Arteaga C, McManus C, Smith J, Moffitt S (1983) Measurement of muscle mass in humans: validity of the 24-hour urinary creatinine method. Am J Clin Nutr 37: 478–494.
40. Mitsiopoulos N, Baumgartner RN, Heymsfield SB, Lyons W, Gallagher D, et al. (1998) Cadaver validation of skeletal muscle measurement by magnetic resonance imaging and computerized tomography. J Appl Physiol 85: 115–122.
41. Kaysen GA, Zhu F, Sarkar S, Heymsfield SB, Wong J, et al. (2005) Estimation of total-body and limb muscle mass in hemodialysis patients by using multifrequency bioimpedance spectroscopy. Am J Clin Nutr 82: 988–995.
42. Wyss M, Kaddurah-Daouk R (2000) Creatine and Creatinine Metabolism. Physiol Rev 80: 1107–1213.
43. Jones JD, Burnett PC (1974) Creatinine Metabolism in Humans with Decreased Renal Function: Creatinine Deficit. Clin Chem 20: 1204–1212.
44. Levey AS, Stevens LA, Schmid CH, Zhang YL, Castro AF, et al. (2009) A New Equation to Estimate Glomerular Filtration Rate. Ann Intern Med 150: 604.
45. Proctor DN, O'Brien PC, Atkinson EJ, Nair KS (1999) Comparison of techniques to estimate total body skeletal muscle mass in people of different age groups. Am J Physiol 277: E489–495.
46. Chertow GM, Ackert K, Lew NL, Lazarus JM, Lowrie EG (2000) Prealbumin is as important as albumin in the nutritional assessment of hemodialysis patients. Kidney Int 58: 2512–2517. doi: 10.1046/j.1523-1755.2000.00435.x.
47. Gama-Axelsson T, Heimbürger O, Stenvinkel P, Bárány P, Lindholm B, et al. (2012) Serum albumin as predictor of nutritional status in patients with ESRD. Clin J Am Soc Nephrol CJASN 7: 1446–1453. doi: 10.2215/CJN.10251011.
48. Stenvinkel P, Heimbürger O, Lindholm B, Kaysen GA, Bergström J (2000) Are there two types of malnutrition in chronic renal failure? Evidence for relationships between malnutrition, inflammation and atherosclerosis (MIA syndrome). Nephrol Dial Transplant 15: 953–960. doi: 10.1093/ndt/15.7.953.
49. Moranne O, Froissart M, Rossert J, Gauci C, Boffa JJ, et al. (2009) Timing of Onset of CKD-Related Metabolic Complications. J Am Soc Nephrol 20: 164–171. doi: 10.1681/ASN.2008020159.
50. Carrero JJ, Stenvinkel P (2009) Persistent inflammation as a catalyst for other risk factors in chronic kidney disease: a hypothesis proposal. Clin J Am Soc Nephrol CJASN 4 Suppl 1: S49–55. doi: 10.2215/CJN.02720409.
51. Ix JH, Wassel CL, Stevens LA, Beck GJ, Froissart M, et al. (2011) Equations to Estimate Creatinine Excretion Rate: The CKD Epidemiology Collaboration. Clin J Am Soc Nephrol 6: 184–191. doi: 10.2215/CJN.05030610.
52. De Keyzer W, Huybrechts I, Dekkers ALM, Geelen A, Crispim S, et al. (2012) Predicting urinary creatinine excretion and its usefulness to identify incomplete 24 h urine collections. Br J Nutr 108: 1118–1125. doi: 10.1017/S0007114511006295.
53. Rule AD, Bailey KR, Schwartz GL, Khosla S, Lieske JC, et al. (2009) For estimating creatinine clearance measuring muscle mass gives better results than those based on demographics. Kidney Int 75: 1071–1078. doi: 10.1038/ki.2008.698.

6

HLA Class I and Class II Associations with ESRD in Saudi Arabian Population

Nuha Mahmoud Hamdi[1], Fadel Hassan Al-Hababi[2]*, Amr Ekhlas Eid[3]

1 Immunology Department, Riyadh Regional Laboratory, King Saud Medical Complex, Riyadh, Kingdom of Saudi Arabia, 2 Virology Department, Riyadh Regional Laboratory, King Saud Medical Complex, Riyadh, Kingdom of Saudi Arabia, 3 Nephrology Department, Riyadh Medical Complex, King Saud Medical Complex, Riyadh, Kingdom of Saudi Arabia

Abstract

Background: Chronic renal failure (CRF) leads in the majority of instances to end stage renal disease (ESRD) requiring renal replacement therapy. Our interest was to evaluate the possible associations of HLA class I and class II antigens with ESRD independent of other factors, in Saudi Arabia population.

Methodology: A retrospective study to determine the HLA class I and class II polymorphisms and their association with ESRD, was performed on 350 patients with ESRD, and 105 healthy unrelated control. Patients and control groups were typed by SSOP lumenix techniques. The alleles positively associated to the ESRD were: HLA-B*15, B*18, B*49 - DRB1*03, negatively associated alleles were A*26, HLA-B*39, B*50. The haplotypes positively associated with ESRD were: HLA-A*01-DRB1*13 and HLA-A*30-DRBI*03. The negatively associated haplotypes were: HLA-A*02-B*39, A*02-B*50, A*24-B*35, A*24-B*58, A*24-DRB1*16, A*68-DRB1*04, A*02-DQB1*03, A*29-DQB1*02, A*29-DOB1*05 and B*27-DRB1*07 and the last one is the most significant protective haplotypes.

Conclusion: The high Relative Risk (RR) observed and its statistical correlation reflect the strength of the described association between HLA antigens and ESRD.

Editor: Xiao-Feng Yang, Temple University School of Medicine, United States of America

Funding: King Saud Medical City's funding division has supported lab technicians and staff nurses. The funders had no role in study design, data collection and analysis, decision to publish, or preparation of the manuscript.

Competing Interests: The authors have declared that no competing interests exist.

* Email: fadelhh@hotmail.com

Introduction

Chronic Kidney Disease (CKD) is now one of the major health problems globally and early diagnosis is vital to prevent the development of end-stage renal failure (ESRD) which is defined as the need for renal replacement therapy such as dialysis or Kidney Transplant [1]. Various factors have been shown to be associated with ESRD such as age, gender, genetics, race, hypertension, and smoking etc. [2]. Although, the exact reasons for the growth of the ESRD program are unknown, it is postulated that changes in the demographics of the population, differences in disease burden among racial groups and under-recognition of earlier stages of CKD and of risk factors for CKD may partially explain this growth [3]. Genome-wide strategies have been used to pinpoint genes that contribute to the risks of development of these disorders [4].

In a recent systemic review based on 44 studies from Gulf Cooperation Council (GCC) showed that the incidence of ESRD has increased while the prevalence and mortality rate of ESRD in the GCC has not been reported sufficiently. The leading primary causes of ESRD recorded in the countries of GCC is diabetes which co-morbid conditions being hypertension and hepatitis C virus infection, the most common death was cardio vascular disease and sepsis [5]. The prevalence of CKD in the young Saudi population is around 5.7% [1]. According to the Saudi Center for Organ Transplantation (SCOT) annual report in 2012, the incidence of dialysis in the Kingdom of Saudi Arabia was 129 new cases per million population (PMP) with 3666 new patients in 2012 [6].

This compares to 360 PMP, 585 PMP and in the United States and Europe, respectively [7,8]. While the prevalence of dialysis patients in the Kingdom of Saudi Arabia in 2012 was 499 new cases PMP with 14,171 dialysis patients [6]. This country showed higher prevalence that other developing countries which, it is vary from less than 100 PMP and 163 PMP in sub-Saharan Africa and India respectively, to about 330 PMP in Jordan and 360 PMP in Iran [9–11].

The rising prevalence is due largely to two main factors; the ageing of the population and the global epidemic of diabetes. An increasing prevalence of the most common causes of ESRD in the GCC: the prevalence of obesity that is associated with multi-chronic diseases have been reported, which exceeds that in the developed countries because of their rapid economic growth and associated changes in lifestyle [12,13]. The International Diabetes Federation reports that five of the countries of the GCC ranked globally among the top ten countries in the world for diabetes prevalence [14].

The most common causes in Saudi Arabia is diabetic nephropathy (DN) prevalence as a cause of ESRD is 17.27%, glomerulonephritis 12.68%, hypertensive nephropathy prevalence is 7.75%, Secondary glomerulonephritis/Vasculitis haemolyticureamic syndrome (HUS) is 1.7%, uncertain aetiology, and other conditions, that are rarely reported as causes of ESRD, such as schistosomiasis, tuberculosis, sickle cell nephropathy and contrast nephropathy 19.59% [15]. Co-morbidities associated with ESRD diabetes prevalence is 47.85%, hypertension prevalence is 77.88%, cardiovascular disease prevalence is 14.51% and vascular disease as a co-morbidity condition as 11.7% [15].

Genes of human leukocyte antigens (HLA) (major histocompatability complex (MHC)) are located on short arm of chromosome six which are inherited in a co-dominant manner from parents to the offspring [16]. The HLA system is being paid more and more attention because it is very significant in polymorphous immunological reactions [17]. Histocompatibility testing has great importance in the selection of kidney recipient candidates and donors for transplantation, particularly HLA-DRB1, HLA-A, and HLA-B alleles, which code for molecules with a central role in the immune response and an essential role in the control of self recognition and consequently defense against microorganisms [18]. Previous studies have shown that certain polymorphisms of HLA class I and class II may influence the susceptibility to ESRD [19].

This study was conducted to determine protective and susceptible role of HLA class I and class II alleles and haplotypes in end stage renal disease patients.

Materials and Methods

Population Samples

This study investigated 350 unrelated Saudi patients were diagnosed with End Stage Renal disease (226 men/124 women, mean age ± SD, 43.2±16.67 years. For statistical comparison 105 healthy donors were recruited as control (58 men, 47 women, 30.3±15.43) from King Saud Medical City, King Fahad dialysis Center (table 1). HLA typing was performed in Department of immunology at Riyadh Regional Laboratory. Before launching into research, the research and clinical trials committee clearance from King Saud Medical City (KSMC).

DNA extraction and DNA typing of HLA loci

10 mL of blood was collected from the patients and normal donors after obtaining prior informed consent. DNA was isolated from blood samples by a fully automated system (MagNA Pure Compact, Roche) according to the manufacturer's instructions. The isolated DNA was stored at −80°C to be used for PCR. HLA-A, HLA-B HLA-DRB1 and DQRB1genotyping was performed by using LABType polymerase chain reaction reversed sequence-specific oligonucleotide (PCR-rSSO) (Luminex, One Lambda, Canoga Park, CA, USA) according to the manufacturer's instructions. Briefly, target DNA was amplified using specific primer sets that are biotinylated at 5 terminus for labeling the PCR product to allow its detection by R-Phycoerythrin-conjugated Streptavidine (SAPE). PCR product was denatured, neutralized, and rehybridized to oligonucleotide probes bound to fluorescently coded microbeads. Then biotinylated hybridized amplicons on microbeads were allowed to be labeled with SAPE. Luminex 100 flow analyzer detected the fluorescent intensities of Phycoerythrin (PE) on each microbeads. The retrieved output was analyzed by HLA Fusion software (ONE LAMBDA, INC, USA) for allele identification.

Statistical analysis

HLA alleles and haplotype frequencies were estimated by direct counting in patients and in healthy controls to compare the differences between the allele frequencies in the control and ESRD groups, a 2×2 contingency table analysis was performed using the Fisher exact test. The strength of association between HLA alleles was estimated by Relative Risk (RR) and 95% confidence intervals (CI). $P<0.05$ was considered to be statistically significant and was considered sufficient to reject the null hypothesis. Values with relative risk higher than 1 were considered positive association with ESRD risk. Other alleles which express relative risk lowers than 1 were considered negative association with ESRD protection (A line on the software used for statistical analysis like SPSS, OpenEpi with Version no. 20).

Results and Discussion

Since the mid-1980's, there has been marked increase in the incidence and prevalence of ESRD around the world [20]. Various pathologies may be associated to HLA alleles and/or haplotypes such as idiopathic membranous nephropathy, minimal change nephritic syndrome, immunoglobulin A (IgA) nephropathy, post-streptococcal glomerulonephritis and familiar focal glomerulonephritis [21,22]. Family studies of the HLA class II system in acute post-streptococcal glomerulonephritis in the population of Zulia State confirm in the association between HLA alleles and the disease [23].

Idiopathic membranous glomerulonephritis is associated with HLA-DR2 in Japanese patients and with HLA-DR3 in Caucasians [24]. Similarly, compared to the Greek population, a higher frequency of HLA-DRB1*0301 has been reported in British patients with idiopathic membranous nephropathy [25]. Also anti-glomerular basement membrane nephritis in Japanese patients has a strong association with DRB1*1501 [26]. Although the presence of certain HLA alleles may be associated with increased susceptibility to renal disease, other HLA alleles may be protective, for example, DRB1*07 is negatively associated with membranous glomerulonephritis in Caucasians [27].

The present study showed that class I HLA-A*02 (ESRD 25.86% vs. con 26.67%) is the most frequent allele in ESRD and control groups of Saudi Arabian population. Other common alleles include A*01 (ESRD 10% vs. con 7.14%) (%), A*03 (ESRD 7.86% vs. con 6.19%), A*24 (ESRD 25.86% vs. con 26.67%), A*31 (ESRD 6.29% vs. con 7.62%), A*30 (ESRD 7% vs. con 4.76) and A*68 (ESRD 8.14% vs. con 10.48%) were the most frequent detected, with no significant difference between the ESRD patient

Table 1. Characteristic of ESRD cases and controls for age and sex.

	ESRD	Controls
Gender (male/female)	226/124	58/47
Mean age ± SD	43.2±16.67	30.3±15.43

Table 2. The frequency and associations of HLA A* alleles in ESRD patients and healthy controls.

Allele	ESRD N = 700	F	CON N = 210	F	P	RR	95% CI
HLA A*01	70	10.00	15	7.14	0.227	1.4	0.8192 to 2.3926
HLA A*02	181	25.86	56	26.67	0.8578	0.969643	0.7499 to 1.2538
HLA A*03	55	7.86	13	6.19	0.4588	1.269231	0.7075 to 2.2770
HLA A*06	1	0.14	0	0	1	0.903	0.0369 to 22.0856
HLA A*08	1	0.14	0	0	1	0.903	0.0369 to 22.0857
HLA A*11	13	1.86	7	3.33	0.2794	0.557143	0.2252 to 1.3784
HLA A*14	0	0	1	0.48	1	0.1003	0.0041 to 2.4540
HLA A*23	36	5.14	10	4.76	1	1.08	0.5453 to 2.1391
HLA A*24	58	8.29	17	8.10	1	1.023529	0.6097 to 1.7183
HLA A*26	36	5.14	20	9.52	0.0318	0.54	0.3196 to 0.9123
HLA A*29	10	1.43	5	2.38	0.3561	0.6	0.2074 to 1.7360
HLA A*30	49	7.00	10	4.76	0.3369	1.47	0.7579 to 2.8510
HLA A*31	44	6.29	16	7.62	0.526	0.825	0.4755 to 1.4314
HLA A*32	29	4.14	8	3.81	1	1.0875	0.5048 to 2.3426
HLA A*33	29	4.14	6	2.86	0.5393	1.45	0.6103 to 3.4452
HLA A*34	4	0.57	0	0.00	0.5789	2.709	0.1464 to 50.1147
HLA A*36	2	0.29	0	0	1	1.505	0.0725 to 31.2277
HLA A*62	1	0.14	0	0	1	0.903	0.0369 to 22.0856
HLA A*66	6	0.86	0	0.00	0.3547	3.913	0.2213 to 69.1773
HLA A*68	57	8.14	22	10.48	0.3275	0.777273	0.4872 to 1.2401
HLA A*69	2	0.29	0	0.00	1	1.505	0.0725 to 31.2277
HLA A*74	12	1.71	4	1.90	0.7714	0.9	0.2933 to 2.7613
HLA A*80	4	0.57	0	0	1	2.709	0.1464 to 50.1147
TOTAL	700	100.00	210	100.00			

N = number of individuals, ESRD = End Stage Renal Disease, control = healthy donors, F = alleles frequency, p = Fisher's exact p value, RR = Relative Risk.

and the control group. On the other hand HLA-A*26 (ESRD 5.14% vs. con 9.52%, p = 0.0318, RR = 0.54, CI = 0.3196 to 0.9123), showed a significant negative association with ESRD and emerged as a protective allele in ESRD (Table2).

The most common alleles in class I HLA B* alleles were B*07, (ESRD 8.29% vs. con 6.67%), B*08 (ESRD 8.86% vs. con 8.57), B*15 (ESRD 9.86% vs. con 3.81%, p = 0.0044), B*18 (ESRD 4.14% vs. con 0.95, p = 0.0277, B*35 (ESRD 6.43% vs. con 8.57%), B*39 (ESRD n = 11, 1.57%, vs. con 5.24%, p = 0.0076), B*49 (ESRD 4.29% vs. con 0.95%, p = 0.0181, RR = 4.5, CI = 1.0844 to 18.6739), B*50 (ESRD 11.57% vs. con 17.62% p = 0.026, and 51*(ESRD 15.86% vs. con 19.05%) in both ESRD patient and control group (Table 3). Positive significant difference for B*15 (RR = 2.5875, CI = 1.2650 to 5.2925), B*18 (RR = 4.35, CI = 1.0466 to 18.0795), B*49 as risk factor for ESRD and negative significant difference for B*39 (RR = 0.3, CI = 0.1319 to 0.6821), B*50 (RR = 0.656757, CI = 0.4596 to 0.9386) as a protective factor for ESRD were observed (Table 3).

In a study at the King Khalid University Hospital, which investigated 235 Saudi patients with ESRD and 60 normal, healthy individuals, the most common alleles in both groups were HLA-A2, A68, A24, A3, HLA-B51, B50, B7, B8 with no any significant difference between the two groups [20] [20]. Another report from the Azerbaijan republic, which investigated 26 patients with ESRD and 51 healthy controls, HLA-A2, A3, A24, and HLA-B35, B51 and B18 were the most frequently detected HLA antigens in all subjects. A significant association was found between susceptibility to ESRD and HLA-A11, A33 and HLA-B49 (P<0.05) [28].

In another study from Zulia and Venezuela on 188 patients with ESRD and 107 controls, HLA-B38, B51, B53 and B62 were positively associated with ESRD andHLA-A9, B12, B17, B40 and B48 were negatively associated with ESRD [23].

Diabetic nephropathy (DN) is leading cause of ESRD worldwide. It affects approximately 30% of patients with long-standing type 1 diabetes mellitus (T1DM) and type 2 diabetes mellitus (T2DM). Also familiar clustering of DN suggests genetic predisposition factor plays a role in the pathogenesis of this disease [29] [29]. Of the 12844 Saudi patients on dialysis, about 24% are in the active waiting list for transplantation with another 20% being evaluated for inclusion in the waiting list. The data showed that 31% of the dialysis patients are hypertensive, 14% are diabetic in addition to 30% suffer of both diabetes and hypertension [6].

For class II HLA-DRB1 our study showed that the most frequent alleles were DRB1*03 (ESRD n = 121, 17.29% vs. con n = 22, 10.48%), 04 (ESRD n = 99, 14.14% vs. con n = 40, 19.05), DRB1*07 (ESRD n = 110, 15.71 vs. con n = 43, 20.48), DRB1*11 (ESRD n = 71, 10.14% vs. con n = 15, 7.14%), DRB1*13 (ESRD n = 114, 16.29% vs. con n = 28, 13.33%) and DRB1*15 (ESRD n = 78, 11.14% vs. control, n = 27, 12.86%) in ESRD and control groups with no significant difference between the two group, except for DRB1*03 (p = 0.0173, RR = 1.65, CI = 1.0762 to 2.5296) as a risk factor for ESRD (Table 4). In HLA-DQB1 alleles showed common frequencies for DQB1*02 (ESRD n = 232, 33.14% vs. control n = 64, 30.77%), DQB1*03 (ESRD n = 167, 23.86% vs. control n = 61, 29.33%), DQB1*05 (ESRD n = 82, 11.71% vs. con n = 28, 13.46%) and DQB1*06 (ESRD n = 201, 28.71% vs. con n = 54, 25.96%) in ESRD and control groups with no significant difference (Table 5).

This is in contrast to a study on Saudi population, which showed that in HLA-DRB1 *04, 07, 13, 03 (17), as the most frequently occurring class II alleles of both groups. While in HLA-DQB1 *02 and HLA-DQB1*06 were the most frequent alleles, with no significant difference between the groups except in DQB1*03 (8) (P = 0.04), which showed a positive association with ESRD [20].

The antigen frequencies were then compared to other studies on populations with close ethnicity Arab population. A recent study with Sudanese subjects showed that for the HLA-A loci, HLA-A2, 30, 3, 24, 1 and A68 were the most frequent antigens and for HLA-B loci HLA-B51, B41, B39, B57, B35, B50 and B52, were the most frequent antigens. HLA-DR13 and DR15 showed the highest antigen frequencies in the DR alleles. In HLA-DQ, DQ1 showed the highest gene frequency [30] [30]. In the Jordanian population A*0201 and B*0713, were the most frequent HLA class I alleles found and DRB1*0704, DRB1*0401 and DRB1*1501 were the most frequent [31] [31]. Another study on the HLA distribution in Egyptian patients with ESRD (n = 100) and normal healthy controls (n = 100), showed that the highest frequency for class I HLA-B35 (28%), B21 (18%) and class II HLA-DRB1*03 (29%) and DRB1*04 (29%). The number of individuals with HLA-B35 was significantly higher in the patient group (P = 0.025), whereas individuals with HLA-B5, B18 were significantly lower in the patient group (P = 0.044 and 0.048 respectively) [32].

This study was carried out without regard to primary renal disease leading to ESRD and focused on the final outcomes. This would help to avoid unexplained causes contributed by many known or unknown diseases. However, several studies provided the evidence that genetic polymorphism and epigenetic variations determine the individual susceptibility of patients to develop rapid progressive kidney disease [33]. A negative association between most A locus antigens and chronic glomerulonephritis and hypertensive nephrosclerosis were found In Turkish patients. And positive association were found between the HLA-B58 and HLA-DRB1*03 with amyloidosis and diabetic nephropathy, respectively [27]. Another Egyptian study among 457 individuals comprising 207 ESRD patients and 250 healthy controls showed that HLA-A2, -B8 and DRB1*3 and HLA-DRB1*11 were significantly correlated with diabetic nephropathy, in addition the B8-DR3 haplotype was shown to be susceptible to DM [34].

There is large variability in the frequency of HLA alleles present in the population ethnic groups. These differences in the results published by different authors are due to the variability in the frequency of HLA alleles present in the population ethnic groups. Also, may be due to the difference in the linkage disequilibrium between the HLA alleles and genes within or flanking the MHC region involved in immune response may play a role in ESRD progression. For instance the polymorphism in genes encoding the cytokines IL-6, IL-4 TNF-α and INF- γ have been shown that may be involved in the progression to ESRD [35–37].

Our study represents an expanded analysis for HLA haplotype among Saudi healthy population and its association in ESRD cases. Two loci heterogeneity haplotype, HLA A*02-B*51 (ESRD 4.58% vs. 6.03%) was the most common. A02- B50 (ESRD 3.35% vs. con 6.58%) and A02-B07 (ESRD 2.86% vs. con 2.47%) were less frequent, A02-DRB113 (ESRD 4.33% vs. con 2.48%) and A02-DRB1 03 (ESRD 4.08% vs. con 6.61%), A02-DQB102 (ESRD 8.49% vs. con 9.64%) and A02-DQB1 06 (ESRD 7.35% vs. con 7.44%) (Tables: 6, 7 and 8). Furthermore, B08-DRB1 03 (ESRD 3.67% vs. con 2.53%) and B51-DRB1 13 (ESRD 3.29% vs. con 3.93%) are the common haplotypes (Tables 9 and 10). However, no significant difference between the ESRD patients and control haplotypes were observed.

However, the haplotypes that showed statistically significant values with negative association with ESRD protection were A2-B50 (p = 0.0098, RR = 0.5098, CI = 0.3123 to 0.8322), A24-B35 (p = 0.0441, RR = 0.3731, CI = 0.1483 to 0.9383), A*68-DRB1*04

Table 3. The frequency and associations of HLA B* alleles in ESRD patients and healthy controls.

Allele	ESRD N=700	F	CON N=210	F	P	RR	95% CI
HLA B*07	58	8.29	14	6.67	0.5598	1.242857	0.7079 to 2.1821
HLA B*08	62	8.86	18	8.57	1	1.033333	0.6257 to 1.7064
HLA B*13	14	2	5	2.38	0.7832	0.84	0.3061 to 2.3050
HLA B*14	14	2	3	1.43	0.775	1.4	0.4062 to 4.8253
HLA B*15	69	9.86	8	3.81	0.0044	2.5875	1.2650 to 5.2925
HLA B*18	29	4.14	2	0.95	0.0277	4.35	1.0466 to 18.0795
HLA B*27	8	1.14	6	2.86	0.1039	0.4	0.1404 to 1.1399
HLA B*31	1	0.14	0	0.00	1	0.903	0.0369 to 22.0856
HLA B*32	1	0.14	0	0.00	1	0.903	0.0369 to 22.0857
HLA B*35	45	6.43	18	8.57	0.2805	0.75	0.4439 to 1.2671
HLA B*37	5	0.71	1	0.48	1	1.5	0.1762 to 12.7686
HLA B*38	10	1.43	1	0.48	0.4725	3	0.3863 to 23.3007
HLA B*39	11	1.57	11	5.24	0.0076	0.3	0.1319 to 0.6821
HLA B*40	14	2	3	1.43	0.775	1.4	0.4062 to 4.8253
HLA B*41	18	2.57	9	4.29	0.2435	0.6	0.2736 to 1.3157
HLA B*42	11	1.57	1	0.48	0.3147	3.3	0.1540 to 0.8729
HLA B*44	19	2.71	6	2.86	1	0.95	0.3844 to 2.3479
HLA B*45	3	0.43	1	0.48	1	0.9	0.0941 to 8.6071
HLA B*47	3	0.43	0	0.00	1	2.107	0.1093 to 40.6298
HLA B*48	1	0.14	0	0.00	1	0.903	0.0369 to 22.0856
HLA B*49	30	4.29	2	0.95	0.0181	4.5	1.0844 to 18.6739
HLA B*50	81	11.57	37	17.62	0.026	0.656757	0.4596 to 0.9386
HLA B*51	111	15.86	40	19.05	0.2906	0.8325	0.6004 to 1.1544
HLA B*52	10	1.43	7	3.33	0.0839	0.428571	0.1652 to 1.1121
HLA B*53	25	3.57	5	2.38	0.5111	1.5	0.5814 to 3.8698
HLA B*55	3	0.43	1	0.48	1	0.9	0.0941 to 8.6071
HLA B*57	14	2	3	1.43	0.775	1.4	0.4062 to 4.8253
HLA B*58	26	3.71	6	2.86	0.6723	1.3	0.5424 to 3.1161
HLA B*73	2	0.29	1	0.48	1	0.6	0.0547 to 6.5845
HLA B*81	1	0.14			1	0.903	0.0369 to 22.0856
HLA B*92	1	0.14			1	0.903	0.0369 to 22.0856

N= number of individuals, ESRD = End Stage Renal Disease, control = healthy donors, F= alleles frequency, p= Fisher's exact p value, RR= Relative Risk.

Table 4. The frequency and associations of HLA DRB1 alleles in ESRD patients and healthy controls.

Allele	ESRD N=700	F	CON N=210	F	P	RR	95% CI
DRB1*01	27	3.86	9	4.29	0.839	0.9	0.4301 to 1.8835
DRB1*02	1	0.14	0	0.00	1	0.903	0.0369 to 22.0856
DRB1*03	121	17.29	22	10.48	0.0173	1.65	1.0762 to 2.5296
DRB1*04	99	14.14	40	19.05	0.1003	0.7425	0.5321 to 1.0362
DRB1*05	1	0.14	0	0.00	1	0.903	0.0369 to 22.0856
DRB1*06	1	0.14	0	0.00	1	0.903	0.0369 to 22.0856
DRB1*07	110	15.71	43	20.48	0.1147	0.767442	0.5590 to 1.0537
DRB1*08	16	2.29	1	0.48	0.1416	4.8	0.6403 to 35.9829
DRB1*09	3	0.43	2	0.95	0.3266	0.45	0.0757 to 2.6753
DRB1*10	21	3	6	2.86	1	1.05	0.4294 to 2.5674
DRB1*11	71	10.14	15	7.14	0.2265	1.42	0.8315 to 2.4250
DRB1*12	5	0.71	1	0.48	1	1.5	0.1762 to 12.7686
DRB1*13	114	16.29	28	13.33	0.3304	1.221429	0.8323 to 1.7924
DRB1*14	7	1	3	1.43	0.7048	0.7	0.1826 to 2.6833
DRB1*15	78	11.14	27	12.86	0.538	0.866667	0.5754 to 1.3054
DRB1*16	25	3.57	13	6.19	0.1142	0.576923	0.3005 to 1.1076
TOTAL	**700**	**100**	**210**	**100**			

N= number of individuals, ESRD = End Stage Renal Disease, control = healthy donors, F= alleles frequency, p= Fisher's exact p value, RR= Relative Risk.

Table 5. The frequency and associations of HLA DQB1 alleles in ESRD patients and healthy controls.

Allele	ESRD N = 700	F	CON N = 210	F	P	RR	95% CI
DQB1*01	1	0.14	0	0	1	0.903	0.0369 to 22.0856
DQB1*02	232	33.14	64	30.77	0.5559	1.077143	0.8563 to 1.3549
DQB1*03	167	23.86	61	29.33	0.1216	0.813489	0.6342 to 1.0435
DQB1*04	13	1.86	1	0.48	0.21	3.862857	0.5107 to 29.4978
DQB1*05	82	11.71	28	13.46	0.545	0.870204	0.5832 to 1.2983
DQB1*06	201	28.71	54	25.96	0.4824	1.106032	0.8550 to 1.4308
DQB1*08	1	0.14	0	0	1	0.903	0.0369 to 22.0856
DQB1*20	1	0.14	0	0	1	0.903	0.0369 to 22.0856
DQB1*50	2	0.29	0	0	1	0.903	0.0369 to 22.0856
TOTAL	700	100.00	210	100			

N = number of individuals, ESRD = End Stage Renal Disease, control = healthy donors, F = alleles frequency, p = Fisher's exact p value, RR = Relative Risk.

($p = 0.049$, RR = 0.4696, CI = 0.2301 to 0.9581), A*02-DQB1*03 ($p = 0.0429$, RR = 0.6146, CI = 0.3942 to 0.9582). The A01-DRB1 13 ($p = 0.0123$, RR = 12.1829, CI = 0.7386 to 200.9482) and A30 -DRB1 03 ($p = 0.0123$, RR = 12.1829, CI = 0.7386 to 200.9482) showed statistically significant values with positive association with ESRD risk.

The haplotypes investigation of ESRD from Zulia, Venezuela population showed positive association with ESRD in: A2-B51, A2-B53, A23-B38 and A68-B38. The A42-B12, A9-B35 and A28-B40 haplotypes were negatively associated with ESRD, expressing relative risk lower than 1 [16]. On the correlations between HLA haplotype and various forms of glomerulopathy, HLA-A2, -B8 and DRB1*3 and HLA-DRB1*11 significantly correlated with diabetic nephropathy, respectively. B8-DR3 haplotype is susceptible to DM [34].

A study investigating the incidence of kaposi's sarcoma after renal transplantation reported a remarkably high frequency of HLA-A2 (83.3%) among patients compared to normal individuals (43.6%) [38]. In addition, a Canadian study found a higher percentage (69%) of the HLA-A2 allele in young patients with diabetic ESRD compared to normal, healthy individuals (36%), with the majority of patients showing either the HLA-A2-DR4 or HLA-DR8 haplotypes.

In developing countries like Saudi Arabia and other Gulf Cooperation Council (GCC) countries, which share a similar cultural background, ethnicity, socio-demographic distributions and socioeconomic development, many reports, has been shown evidence of increasing prevalence of the most common causes of ESRD [5]. Also there is increasing in the prevalence of obesity in these countries and its associated multichronic diseases, exceeds that in the developed countries because of their rapid economic growth and associated changes in lifestyle [12,13]. Since certain haplotypes particularly two loci and three loci are common to some of the racial groups, it would be possible to find small disparity between population within these countries in the HLA frequencies and haplotype. Hence, there is a need to compare haplotype frequencies among the populations from different regions of Saudi Arabia and GCC. This would be important for creating a national registry and organ-sharing network for GCC people.

In conclusion, this study throws light on the frequency and distribution of HLA class I and class II alleles and haplotypes that confer susceptibility and protection in the Saudi Arabian patients with end stage renal disease (ESRD). However a larger study encompassing more number of patients and controls would be needed to assess the clinical relevance of the results obtained. In the future, molecular diagnostics on HLA polymorphisms may serve to identify patients with survival advantages and could be used by physicians to plan their treatment in the GCC.

Recommendation

The association of HLA alleles and/or haplotype could be used as a risk classification marker and thereby progression to much more severe disease could be protected or diagnosed earlier. This would require further investigation with larger number of patients and healthy individuals and with every disease may cause ESRD. A great need to compare haplotype frequencies among the populations from different regions of Saudi Arabia and GCC populations to develop a national registry and organ-sharing network for GCC people.

Table 6. Main high-frequency HLA A–B haplotype and their frequencies in ESRD patients and healthy controls (haplotype frequency ≥1.5%).

Haplotype	ESRD	ESRD %	CONT	CONT %	P value	RR	95% CI
A1-B51	24	1.96	6	1.64	0.8285	1.1938	0.4917 to 2.8981
A2-B07	35	2.86	9	2.47	0.8559	1.1606	0.5632 to 2.3919
A2-B15	20	1.64	2	0.55	0.1978	2.9845	0.7009 to 12.7087
A2-B35	18	1.47	8	2.19	0.074	0.6715	0.2944 to 1.5317
A2-B39	7	0.57	7	1.92	0.0242	0.2984	0.1054 to 0.8453
A2-B50	41	3.35	24	6.58	0.0098	0.5098	0.3123 to 0.8322
A2-B51	56	4.58	22	6.03	0.2701	0.7597	0.4705 to 1.2266
A3-B50	19	1.55	3	0.82	0.4435	1.8902	0.5625 to 6.3516
A24-B08	21	1.72	4	1.1	0.482	1.5668	0.5413 to 4.5354
A24-B35	10	0.82	8	2.19	0.0441	0.3731	0.1483 to 0.9383
A24-B08	19	1.55	9	2.47	0.258	0.6301	0.2875 to 1.3806
A24-B58	1	0.08	4	1.1	0.0113	0.0746	0.0084 to 0.6655
A31-B50	11	0.9	7	1.92	0.1528	0.469	0.1831 to 1.2011
A31-B51	20	1.64	12	3.29	0.0566	0.4974	0.2455 to 1.0078
A68-B51	20	1.64	6	1.64	1	0.9948	0.4025 to 2.4587

Table 7. Main high-frequency HLA A – DRB1 haplotype and their frequencies in ESRD patients and healthy controls (haplotype frequency ≥1.5%).

HAPLOTYPE	ESRD	ESRD %	CONT	CONsT %	P value	RR	95% CI
A*01-DRB1*03	19	1.55	3	0.83	0.6261	1.8783	0.5590 to 6.3115
A*01-DRB1*07	21	1.72	6	1.65	0.4432	1.038	0.4221 to 2.5523
A*01-DRB1*13	20	1.63	0	0	0.0123	12.1829	0.7386 to 200.9482
A*01-DRB1*15	15	1.23	6	1.65	0.6002	0.7414	0.2898 to 1.8971
A*02 -DRB1*03	45	3.68	8	2.2	0.1872	1.6682	0.7936 to 3.5065
A*02 -DRB1*04	40	3.27	18	4.96	0.1507	0.659	0.3826 to 1.1352
A*02 -DRB1*07	50	4.08	24	6.61	0.064	0.6179	0.3852 to 0.9910
A*02 -DRB1*11	22	1.8	6	1.65	1	1.0874	0.4443 to 2.6615
A*02 -DRB1*13	53	4.33	9	2.48	0.1238	1.7465	0.8700 to 3.5059
A*02 -DRB1*15	36	2.94	17	4.68	0.1324	0.628	0.3570 to 1.1047
A*02 -DRB1*16	16	1.31	7	1.93	0.4512	0.628	0.3570 to 1.1047
A*03 -DRB1*03	19	1.55	3	0.83	0.6261	1.8783	0.5590 to 6.3115
A*03 -DRB1*04	12	0.98	6	1.65	1	0.5965	0.2255 to 1.5783
A*24 -DRB1*03	30	2.45	4	1.1	0.1486	2.2243	0.7888 to 6.2721
A*24 -DRB1*04	20	1.63	7	1.93	0.6495	0.8473	0.3612 to 1.9879
A*24 -DRB1*16	3	0.25	6	1.65	0.0061	0.1483	0.0373 to 0.5900
A*26 -DRB1*03	19	1.55	11	3.03	0.0793	0.5123	0.2461 to 1.0665
A*26 -DRB1*04	15	1.23	7	1.93	0.311	0.6355	0.2611 to 1.5467
A*30 -DRB1*03	20	1.63	0	0	0.0123	12.1829	0.7386 to 200.9482
A*31-DRB1*13	28	2.29	10	2.75	0.5631	0.8304	0.4072 to 1.6932
A*68-DRB1*04	19	1.55	12	3.31	0.049	0.4696	0.2301 to 0.9581
A*68-DRB1*07	18	1.47	7	1.93	0.4821	0.7626	0.3210 to 1.8115
A*68-DRB1*15	10	0.82	6	1.65	0.2255	0.4943	0.1809 to 1.3508

Table 8. Main high-frequency HLA A – DQB1 haplotype and their frequenciesin ESRD patients and healthy controls (haplotype frequency ≥1.5%).

HAPLOTYPE	ESRD	ESRD %	CONT	CONT %	P value	RR	95% CI
A*01-DQB1*02	36	2.94	6	1.65	0.2620	1.6438	0.6981 to 3.8707
A*01-DQB1*03	31	2.53	10	2.75	0.8505	0.8493	0.4204 to 1.7159
A*01-DQB1*06	38	3.1	6	1.65	0.2005	1.8767	0.7997 to 4.4042
A*02-DQB1*02	104	8.49	35	9.64	0.5257	0.8805	0.6115 to 1.2680
A*02-DQB1*03	56	4.57	27	7.44	0.0429	0.6146	0.3942 to 0.9582
A*02-DQB1*05	35	2.86	10	2.75	1.0000	1.0371	0.5187 to 2.0739
A*02-DQB1*06	90	7.35	27	7.44	1.0000	0.9878	0.6530 to 1.4941
A*03-DQB1*02	24	1.96	5	1.38	0.6552	1.4224	0.5466 to 3.7014
A*03-DQB1*03	23	1.88	8	2.2	0.6684	0.8519	0.3844 to 1.8883
A*03-DQB1*06	21	1.71	6	1.65	1.0000	1.0371	0.4218 to 2.5502
A*11-DQB1*02	24	1.96	5	1.38	0.6552	1.4224	0.5466 to 3.7014
A*11-DQB1*03	20	1.63	4	1.1	0.6262	1.4816	0.5097 to 4.3071
A*24-DQB1*02	43	3.51	9	2.48	0.4028	1.4158	0.6969 to 2.8764
A*24-DQB1*03	27	2.2	10	2.75	0.5531	0.8001	0.3910 to 1.6372
A*24-DQB1*05	13	1.06	8	2.2	0.1140	0.4815	0.2011 to 1.1527
A*24-DQB1*06	18	1.47	7	1.93	0.4818	0.762	0.3208 to 1.8100
A*26-DQB1*02	25	2.04	14	3.86	0.0549	0.5292	0.2780 to 1.0072
A*26-DQB1*03	19	1.55	9	2.48	0.2412	0.6256	0.2855 to 1.3707
A*26-DQB1*06	16	1.31	7	1.93	0.4511	0.6773	0.2808 to 1.6337
A*29-DQB1*02	4	0.33	5	1.38	0.0337	0.2371	0.0640 to 0.8782
A*29-DQB1*05	1	0.08	5	1.38	0.0030	0.0593	0.0069 to 0.5057
A*30-DQB1*02	29	2.37	8	2.2	1.0000	1.0742	0.4954 to 2.3291
A*30-DQB1*03	21	1.71	3	0.83	0.3267	2.0743	0.6222 to 6.9149
A*30-DQB1*05	13	1.06	2	0.55	0.5422	1.9261	0.4367 to 8.4962
A*30-DQB1*06	29	2.37	3	0.83	0.0864	2.8645	0.8776 to 9.3493
A*31-DQB1*02	23	1.88	8	2.2	0.6684	0.8519	0.3844 to 1.8883
A*31-DQB1*03	14	1.14	8	2.2	0.1308	0.5186	0.2193 to 1.2264
A*31-DQB1*06	44	3.59	14	3.86	0.8734	0.9313	0.5163 to 1.6799
A*32-DQB1*02	23	1.88	4	1.1	0.4867	1.7039	0.5931 to 4.8951
A*32-DQB1*03	15	1.22	7	1.93	0.3107	0.635	0.2609 to 1.5455
A*33-DQB1*02	21	1.71	2	0.55	0.1334	3.1114	0.7330 to 13.2073
A*68-DQB1*02	33	2.69	8	2.2	0.7087	1.2223	0.5697 to 2.6228
A*68-DQB1*03	30	2.45	14	3.86	0.1490	0.635	0.3404 to 1.1845
A*68-DQB1*06	25	2.04	10	2.75	0.4174	0.7408	0.3592 to 1.5280

Table 9. Main high-frequency HLA B– DRB1 haplotype and their frequencies in ESRD patients and healthy controls (haplotype frequency ≥1.5%).

HAPLOTYPE	ESRD	ESRD %	CONT	CONT%	P value	RR	95% CI
B*07-DRB1*13	23	1.76	3	0.84	0.333	2.0882	0.6306 to 6.9154
B*07-DRB1*15	25	1.91	8	2.25	0.669	0.8512	0.3873 to 1.8708
B*08-DRB1*03	48	3.67	9	2.53	0.3289	1.4527	0.7198 to 2.9319
B*08-DRB1*04	13	0.99	6	1.69	0.2671	0.5902	0.2259 to 1.5417
B*14-DRB1*03	23	1.76	3	0.84	0.333	2.0882	0.6306 to 6.9154
B*14-DRB1*13	34	2.6	7	1.97	0.5684	1.323	0.5915 to 2.9592
B*27-DRB1*07	0	0	5	1.4	0.0004	0.0248	0.0014 to 0.4477
B*35-DRB1*04	18	1.38	9	2.53	0.1528	0.5448	0.2469 to 1.2022
B*35-DRB1*16	3	0.23	6	1.69	0.0043	0.1362	0.0342 to 0.5419
B*50-DRB1*04	21	1.61	13	3.65	0.0316	0.44	0.2225 to 0.8700
B*50-DRB1*07	66	5.05	28	7.87	0.0513	0.642	0.4192 to 0.9833
B*50-DRB1*13	24	1.84	2	0.56	0.0948	3.2686	0.7762 to 13.7646
B*51-DRB1*03	20	1.53	5	1.4	1	1.0895	0.4118 to 2.8826
B*51-DRB1*04	36	2.75	12	3.37	0.5991	0.8171	0.4297 to 1.5539
B*51-DRB1*07	26	1.99	6	1.69	0.8302	1.1803	0.4896 to 2.8454
B*51-DRB1*13	43	3.29	14	3.93	0.5153	0.8366	0.4630 to 1.5116
B*51-DRB1*15	31	2.37	11	3.09	0.447	0.7676	0.3897 to 1.5119
B*52-DRB1*15	7	0.54	7	1.97	0.0165	0.2724	0.0962 to 0.7715
B*52-DRB1*03	16	1.22	3	0.84	0.7793	1.4527	0.4256 to 4.9579

Table 10. Main high-frequency HLA B– DQB1 haplotype and their frequencies in ESRD patients and healthy controls (haplotype frequency ≥1%).

HAPLOTYPE	ESRD	ESRD %	CONT	CONT %	P value	RR	95% CI
B*07-DQB1*02	22	2.83	6	1.69	1	0.9987	0.4081 to 2.4444
B*07-DQB1*03	29	1.3	8	2.25	1	0.9874	0.4554 to 2.1409
B*07-DQB1*06	37	0.31	10	2.82	1	1.0078	0.5062 to 2.0066
B*08-DQB1*02	48	4.29	13	3.67	1	1.0057	0.5511 to 1.8353
B*08-DQB1*03	22	1	6	1.69	1	0.9987	0.4081 to 2.4444
B*08-DQB1*06	33	2.14	9	2.54	1	0.9987	0.4824 to 2.0676
B*15-DQB1*02	11	2.22	3	0.85	1	0.9987	0.2801 to 3.5607
B*15-DQB1*06	33	3.6	9	2.54	1	0.9987	0.4824 to 2.0676
B*35-DQB1*02	15	1.91	4	1.13	1	1.0214	0.3411 to 3.0585
B*35-DQB1*03	55	2.07	15	4.24	1	0.9987	0.5712 to 1.7463
B*35-DQB1*05	30	0.31	8	2.26	1	1.0214	0.4724 to 2.2084
B*35-DQB1*06	18	1.84	5	1.41	1	0.9806	0.3666 to 2.6228
B*39-DQB1*02	22	0.31	6	1.69	1	0.9987	0.4081 to 2.4444
B*41-DQB1*03	22	1.61	6	1.69	1	0.9987	0.4081 to 2.4444
B*50-DQB1*02	122	5.44	33	9.32	1	1.007	0.6981 to 1.4524
B*50-DQB1*03	44	2.07	12	3.39	1	0.9987	0.5333 to 1.8705
B*50-DQB1*06	22	2.76	6	1.69	1	0.9987	0.4081 to 2.4444
B*51-DQB1*02	48	3.83	13	3.67	1	0.9987	0.5333 to 1.8705
B*51-DQB1*03	74	3.98	20	5.65	1	1.0927	0.6757 to 1.7672
B*51-DQB1*05	18	1.99	5	1.41	1	0.9806	0.3666 to 2.6228
B*51-DQB1*06	96	5.67	26	7.34	1	1.0057	0.6627 to 1.5263
B*52-DQB1*06	26	0.69	7	1.98	1	1.0117	0.4428 to 2.3116
B*58-DQB1*02	15	2.14	4	1.13	1	1.0214	0.3411 to 3.0585

Acknowledgments

We are very grateful for Mr Khalid Abdulrahman, Director of Riyadh regional laboratory, for his encouragement and support. And we thank our staff and technicians in Riyadh regional laboratory.

Author Contributions

Wrote the paper: NMH FHA AE. Made substantial contributions to the analysis and interpretations of data: NMH FHA AE. Responsible for overall experiments: NMH FHA AE.

References

1. Alsuwaida AO, Farag YM, Al Sayyari AA, Mousa D, Alhejaili F, et al. (2010) Epidemiology of chronic kidney disease in the Kingdom of Saudi Arabia (SEEK-Saudi investigators) - a pilot study. Saudi J Kidney Dis Transpl 21: 1066–1072.
2. McClellan W, Speckman R, McClure L, Howard V, Campbell RC, et al. (2007) Prevalence and characteristics of a family history of end-stage renal disease among adults in the United States population: Reasons for Geographic and Racial Differences in Stroke (REGARDS) renal cohort study. J Am Soc Nephrol 18: 1344–1352.
3. Obrador GT, Pereira BJG (2008) Epidemiology of chronic kidney disease and screening recommendations.
4. Braunwald E (2001) Harrison's principles of internal medicine. New York: McGraw-Hill, Medical Publishing Division.
5. Hassanien AA, Al-Shaikh F, Vamos EP, Yadegarfar G, Majeed A (2012) Epidemiology of end-stage renal disease in the countries of the Gulf Cooperation Council: a systematic review. JRSM Short Rep 3: 38.
6. The Saudi Center for Organ Transplantation (SCOT) (2012) The annual report of The Saudi Center for Organ Transplantation (SCOT).
7. U.S. Renal Data System (2008) USRDS Annual Data Report: Atlas of Chronic Kidney Disease and End-Stage Renal Disease in the United States.
8. Grassmann A, Gioberge S, Moeller S, Brown G (2005) ESRD patients in 2004: global overview of patient numbers, treatment modalities and associated trends. Nephrol Dial Transplant 20: 2587–2593.
9. Modi GK, Jha V (2006) The incidence of end-stage renal disease in India: a population-based study. Kidney Int 70: 2131–2133.
10. Barsoum RS (2006) Chronic kidney disease in the developing world. N Engl J Med 354: 997–999.
11. Aghighi M, Mahdavi-Mazdeh M, Zamyadi M, Heidary Rouchi A, Rajolani H, et al. (2009) Changing epidemiology of end-stage renal disease in last 10 years in Iran. Iran J Kidney Dis 3: 192–196.
12. Ng SW, Zaghloul S, Ali HI, Harrison G, Popkin BM (2011) The prevalence and trends of overweight, obesity and nutrition-related non-communicable diseases in the Arabian Gulf States. Obes Rev 12: 1–13.
13. Al-Nozha MM, Al-Mazrou YY, Al-Maatouq MA, Arafah MR, Khalil MZ, et al. (2005) Obesity in Saudi Arabia. Saudi Med J 26: 824–829.
14. Federation ID (2010) Latest diabetes figures paint grim global picture.
15. Al-Sayyari AA, Shaheen FA (2011) End stage chronic kidney disease in Saudi Arabia. A rapidly changing scene. Saudi Med J 32: 339–346.
16. Shiina T, Inoko H, Kulski JK (2004) An update of the HLA genomic region, locus information and disease associations: 2004. Tissue Antigens 64: 631–649.
17. Stanevicha V, Eglite J, Zavadska D, Sochnevs A, Shantere R, et al. (2007) HLA class II DR and DQ genotypes and haplotypes associated with rheumatic fever among a clinically homogeneous patient population of Latvian children. Arthritis Res Ther 9: R58.
18. Fudenberg HH (1984) Basic immunogenetics. New York: Oxford University Press. 302 pp.
19. Crispim JC, Mendes-Junior CT, Wastowski IJ, Palomino GM, Saber LT, et al. (2008) HLA polymorphisms as incidence factor in the progression to end-stage renal disease in Brazilian patients awaiting kidney transplant. Transplant Proc 40: 1333–1336.
20. Almogren A, Shakoor Z, Hamam KD (2012) Human leucocyte antigens: their association with end-stage renal disease in Saudi patients awaiting transplantation. Br J Biomed Sci 69: 159–163.
21. Barocci S, Fiordoro S, Santori G, Valente U, Mossa M, et al. (2004) Alport syndrome: HLA association and kidney graft outcome. Eur J Immunogenet 31: 115–119.
22. Layrisse Z, Rodriguez-Iturbe B, Garcia-Ramirez R, Rodriguez A, Tiwari J (1983) Family studies of the HLA system in acute post-streptococcal glomerulonephritis. Hum Immunol 7: 177–185.
23. Sergio Rivera P, Márquez G, Cipriani AM, Hassanhi M, Villalobos CC, et al. (2012) HLA class I association with progression to end-stage renal disease in patients from Zulia, Venezuela. J Immunologia 31: 37–42.
24. Ogahara S, Naito S, Abe K, Michinaga I, Arakawa K (1992) Analysis of HLA class II genes in Japanese patients with idiopathic membranous glomerulonephritis. Kidney Int 41: 175–182.
25. Vaughan RW, Tighe MR, Boki K, Alexoupolos S, Papadakis J, et al. (1995) An analysis of HLA class II gene polymorphism in British and Greek idiopathic membranous nephropathy patients. Eur J Immunogenet 22: 179–186.
26. Kitagawa W, Imai H, Komatsuda A, Maki N, Wakui H, et al. (2008) The HLA-DRB1*1501 allele is prevalent among Japanese patients with anti-glomerular basement membrane antibody-mediated disease. Nephrol Dial Transplant 23: 3126–3129.
27. Karahan GE, Kekik C, Oguz FS, Onal AE, Bakkaloglu H, et al. (2010) Association of HLA phenotypes of end-stage renal disease patients preparing for first transplantation with anti-HLA antibody status. Ren Fail 32: 380–383.
28. Davood PP, Farhadi N, Najafizadeh M (2008) Protective and susceptible HLA class I Genes in Patients with End-Stage Renal Disease. Research Journal of Biological Sciences 3: 1344–1346.
29. Ma ZJ, Sun P, Guo G, Zhang R, Chen LM (2013) Association of the HLA-DQA1 and HLA-DQB1 Alleles in Type 2 Diabetes Mellitus and Diabetic Nephropathy in the Han Ethnicity of China. J Diabetes Res 2013: 452537.
30. Dafalla AM, McCloskey DJ, Alemam AA, Ibrahim AA, Babikir AM, et al. (2011) HLA polymorphism in Sudanese renal donors. Saudi J Kidney Dis Transpl 22: 834–840.
31. Sanchez-Velasco P, Karadsheh NS, Garcia-Martin A, Ruiz de Alegria C, Leyva-Cobian F (2001) Molecular analysis of HLA allelic frequencies and haplotypes in Jordanians and comparison with other related populations. Hum Immunol 62: 901–909.
32. Shaheen Noha FT, El . Khashab Saheer (2013) HLA Association in Egyptian patients with End-Stage Renal Disease. The World Congress of Nephrology 2013. Hong Kong.
33. Tampe B, Zeisberg M (2014) Contribution of genetics and epigenetics to progression of kidney fibrosis. Nephrol Dial Transplant 29 Suppl 4: iv72–79.
34. El-Gezawy EM, Baset HA, Nasif KA, Osama A, AbdelAzeem HG, et al. (2011) Human leukocyte antigens as a risk factor for the primary diseases leading to end stage renal disease in Egyptian patients. Egypt J Immunol 18: 13–21.
35. Ranganath P, Tripathi G, Sharma RK, Sankhwar SN, Agrawal S (2009) Role of non-HLA genetic variants in end-stage renal disease. Tissue Antigens 74: 147–155.
36. Bloudickova S, Kuthanova L, Hubacek JA (2011) Polymorphisms in IFN-gamma, TNF-alpha and IL-10 in patients on maintenance haemodialysis. Folia Biol (Praha) 57: 30–34.
37. Monos DS, Kamoun M, Udalova IA, Csanky E, Cizman B, et al. (1995) Genetic polymorphism of the human tumor necrosis factor region in insulin-dependent diabetes mellitus. Linkage disequilibrium of TNFab microsatellite alleles with HLA haplotypes. Hum Immunol 44: 70–79.
38. Qunibi W, Akhtar M, Sheth K, Ginn HE, Al-Furayh O, et al. (1988) Kaposi's sarcoma: the most common tumor after renal transplantation in Saudi Arabia. Am J Med 84: 225–232.

7

Regional Differences of Undiagnosed Type 2 Diabetes and Prediabetes Prevalence Are Not Explained by Known Risk Factors

Teresa Tamayo[1,10]*, Sabine Schipf[2,10], Christine Meisinger[3,10], Michaela Schunk[4,10], Werner Maier[4,10], Christian Herder[5,8], Michael Roden[5,6,8], Matthias Nauck[7,10], Annette Peters[3,8,9], Henry Völzke[2,9,10], Wolfgang Rathmann[1,10]

1 Institute of Biometrics and Epidemiology, German Diabetes Center, Leibniz Center for Diabetes Research at Heinrich-Heine-University, Düsseldorf, Germany, **2** Institute for Community Medicine, University Medicine Greifswald, Greifswald, Germany, **3** Helmholtz Zentrum München, German Research Center for Environmental Health, Institute of Epidemiology II, Neuherberg, Germany, **4** Helmholtz Zentrum München, German Research Center for Environmental Health, Institute of Health Economics and Health Care Management, Neuherberg, Germany, **5** Institute for Clinical Diabetology, German Diabetes Center, Leibniz Center for Diabetes Research at Heinrich-Heine-University, Düsseldorf, Germany, **6** Department of Endocrinology and Diabetology, University Hospital Düsseldorf, Düsseldorf, Germany, **7** Institute of Clinical Chemistry and Laboratory Medicine, University Medicine Greifswald, Greifswald, Germany, **8** German Center for Diabetes Research (DZD e.V.), Sites Düsseldorf and Munich, Germany, **9** German Center of Cardiovascular Research (DZHK e.V.), Sites Munich and Greifswald, Germany, **10** Competence Network Diabetes mellitus (Federal Ministry of Education and Research, Germany), Sites Düsseldorf, Munich and Greifswald, Germany

Abstract

Background: We have previously found regional differences in the prevalence of known type 2 diabetes between northeastern and southern Germany. We aim to also provide prevalence estimates for prediabetes (isolated impaired fasting glucose (i-IFG), isolated glucose intolerance (i-IGT), combined IFG and IGT) and unknown type 2 diabetes for both regions.

Methods: Prevalence (95%CI) of prediabetes (i-IFG: fasting glucose 5.6–6.9 mmol/l; i-IGT: 2 h postchallenge gluose 7.8–11.0 mmol/l, oral glucose tolerance test (OGTT), ≥8 h overnight fasting) and unknown diabetes were analyzed in two regional population-based surveys (age group 35–79 years): SHIP-TREND (Study of Health in Pomerania (northeast), 2008–2012) and KORA F4 (Cooperative Health Research in the region of Augsburg (south), 2006–2008). Both studies used similar methods, questionnaires, and identical protocols for OGTT. Overall, 1,980 participants from SHIP-TREND and 2,617 participants from KORA F4 were included.

Results: Age-sex-standardized prevalence estimates (95%CI) of prediabetes and unknown diabetes were considerably higher in the northeast (SHIP-TREND: 43.1%; 40.9–45.3% and 7.1%; 5.9–8.2%) than in the south of Germany (KORA F4: 30.1%; 28.4–31.7% and 3.9%; 3.2–4.6%), respectively. In particular, i-IFG (26.4%; 24.5–28.3% vs. 17.2%; 15.7–18.6%) and IFG+IGT (11.2%; 9.8–12.6% vs. 6.6%; 5.7–7.5%) were more frequent in SHIP-TREND than in KORA. In comparison to normal glucose tolerance, the odds of having unknown diabetes (OR, 95%CI: 2.59; 1.84–3.65) or prediabetes (1.98; 1.70–2.31) was higher in the northeast than in the south after adjustment for known risk factors (obesity, lifestyle).

Conclusions: The regional differences of prediabetes and unknown diabetes are in line with the geographical pattern of known diabetes in Germany. The higher prevalences in the northeast were not explained by traditional risk factors.

Editor: Massimo Pietropaolo, University of Michigan Medical School, United States of America

Funding: The project was funded by a grant of the Competence Network for Diabetes mellitus of the Federal Ministry of Education and Research (support code 01GI1110D). The KORA research platform (KORA, Cooperative Health Research in the Region of Augsburg) was initiated and financed by the Helmholtz Zentrum München - German Research Center for Environmental Health, which is funded by the German Federal Ministry of Education and Research and by the State of Bavaria. The KORA Diabetes Study was partly funded by a German Research Foundation (DFG) grant to WR from the German Diabetes Center. The German Diabetes Center is funded by grants of the German Federal Ministry of Health, and the Ministry of School, Science and Research of the State of North-Rhine-Westphalia. The Study of Health in Pomerania (SHIP-TREND) is part of the Community Medicine Research net (CMR) at the University of Greifswald, Germany. The CMR encompasses several research projects, which share data from the population-based SHIP project (http://ship.community-medicine.de). Oral glucose tolerance tests were funded by grants given to WR (German Diabetes Center, Düsseldorf, Germany). The funders had no role in study design, data collection, analysis, decision to publish or preparation of the manuscript.

Competing Interests: The authors have declared that that no competing interests exist.

* Email: teresa.tamayo@ddz.uni-duesseldorf.de

Introduction

According to the sixth edition of the IDF Diabetes atlas [1], considerable regional differences in the prevalence of type 2 diabetes (age-adjusted) exist between European nations ranging from 2.4% in Moldova to more than 14% in Turkey [2]. While geographic variations in diabetes prevalence between nations are well known, regional differences within countries are rarely analyzed. Especially, information on regional variation of prediabetes and unknown (undiagnosed) diabetes is lacking. In the USA, the Behavioral Risk Factor Surveillance System identified higher prevalence estimates of known (diagnosed) type 2 diabetes of 11.7% in the adult population of the southeastern area ("diabetes belt") while the comparative estimate was 8.5% for the rest of the country [3]. In a meta-analysis of regional surveys in the Diabetes Collaborative Research of Epidemiologic Studies (DIAB-CORE consortium) we found a high prevalence of known type 2 diabetes in the northeastern regions of Germany with 10.9% in Pomerania (Vorpommern) and a comparatively low prevalence of 5.8% in the south [4]. However, it remained unclear whether a higher awareness and screening for the disease among general practitioners and in the population led to a lower frequency of undiagnosed diabetes, or whether a higher morbidity itself may have contributed to higher prevalence estimates in the northeast. Therefore, we compared age- and sex-specific estimates for prediabetes and unknown diabetes in two German regions – one in the northeast (Pomerania, SHIP-TREND) and one in the south (Augsburg region, KORA F4) using oral glucose tolerance tests (OGTT, ADA criteria) [5]. The study sampling and standard operating procedures of SHIP-TREND were largely similar to KORA F4 (including OGTT) in order to provide a high comparability between the two studies.

Methods

Study population SHIP-TREND (northeastern Germany)

A sample of 8,826 adults aged 20–79 years with German nationality was drawn from the central population registry of Western Pomerania (212,157 inhabitants living in Greifswald, Stralsund, Anklam and surrounding counties). A two-stage cluster sampling method was adopted from the WHO Multinational Monitoring of Trends and Determinants in Cardiovascular Disease (MONICA) Project in Augsburg, Germany. Stratification variables were age, sex, and city/county of residence [6]. Of all persons invited, 4,420 (50.1%) individuals participated in the examinations (2008–2012). All participants provided written informed consent and the medical ethics committee of the University of Greifswald approved the study protocol. Further information on the study design of the SHIP-TREND survey has been published elsewhere [6,7].

Study population KORA F4 (southern Germany)

The KORA F4 study is the follow-up of the KORA S4 survey which was carried out in 1999–2001 in the city of Augsburg and 16 municipalities from the surrounding counties (about 600,000 inhabitants). The re-investigation took place in 2006–2008 (KORA F4). A two-stage cluster sampling method was used which followed the WHO MONICA project method in the Augsburg region. For Augsburg city, a simple random sampling was performed. In the surrounding rural districts, 16 counties were selected with probabilities proportional to their size [8]. Of 6,640 participants with German nationality aged 25–74 years, 4,261 participated at the baseline examinations S4. In KORA F4, 3,080 (72%) S4 participants were re-investigated. At baseline, an oral glucose tolerance test (OGTT) was administered to all 1,353 non-diabetic subjects in the age group 55–74 years [9]. Younger participants were not screened for undiagnosed diabetes. At follow-up, OGTT measurements were carried out without age restriction after exclusion of individuals with known diabetes [9,10]. For the current study, the cross-sectional data of KORA F4 was analyzed only. The OGTT-based screening for unknown diabetes in KORA S4 in age group 55–74 years at baseline, (62–82 years at follow-up) might have resulted in an early diagnosis of diabetes and therefore in a lower number of unknown diabetes at follow-up. Because of this methodological difference to SHIP-TREND, we report results for younger (<60 years) and older participants separately. All study participants gave written informed consent to the study, which was approved by the Ethics Committee of the Bavarian Medical Association.

Laboratory analyses including glucose measurements

In both studies, blood was collected without stasis after an overnight fast of ≥8 hours. After blood withdrawal the blood samples were immediately centrifuged and kept cool (4°C) until analysis of blood glucose in the central laboratory. Measurements of fasting glucose and 2 h glucose were based on plasma in SHIP-TREND and on serum in KORA F4. In order to determine whether both samples were comparable, duplicate measurements were carried out using serum samples of all SHIP-TREND participants. Both measurements (plasma and serum glucose) were highly correlated ($r = 0.99$; $p < 0.0001$). In Passing Bablok regression analysis of serum versus plasma glucose (mmol/l) an intercept of −0.10 (95%CI −0.10; −0.10) and a slope of 1 were observed concluding that plasma values in SHIP-TREND might be only slightly lower than serum values. Furthermore, 30 serum blood glucose samples were drawn at random from KORA F4 and re-assessed in the SHIP-TREND laboratory, yielding a correlation coefficient of $r = 0.94$ ($p < 0.0001$). On average, these original 30 KORA F4 measurements were only slightly lower (mean − 0.06 mmol/l; SD 0.17) when they were re-analyzed in the SHIP-TREND laboratory. Thus, serum glucose from KORA F4 and plasma glucose from SHIP-TREND were considered as comparable for the current analysis.

HDL-, LDL- and total cholesterol, and triglycerides were measured as described elsewhere [6,11].

Ascertainment of diabetes and prediabetes in SHIP-TREND and KORA F4

Oral glucose tolerance tests followed concordant standardized operating procedures (SOP) in both studies [9]. Participants were asked to fast for ≥8 hours except for water (eg. from 22:00 p.m.) and should not smoke or consume caffeine containing drinks, such as coffee and avoid sports before the examination. In SHIP-TREND and KORA F4, OGTTs were completed during morning hours. Fasting glucose was sampled, and 75 grams of anhydrous glucose (Dextro OGT; Boehringer Mannheim, Mannheim Germany) was given to participants without known diabetes (SHIP-TREND: known diabetes or current use of glucose-lowering agents; KORA F4: current use of glucose-lowering agents or unknown (newly study-diagnosed) diabetes at baseline (S4), validated by a physician). Fasting glucose and 2 h postload glucose were measured using a hexokinase method. In SHIP-TREND, Dimension Vista by Siemens Healthcare Diagnostics (Eschborn, Germany) and in KORA F4, GLU flex by Dade Behring (Marburg, Germany) were used.

Participants with fasting glucose values <5.6 mmol/l (< 100 mg/dl) and 2 h glucose <7.8 mmol/l (<140 mg/dl) were defined as having normal glucose tolerance (NGT) (5). Fasting glucose values ≥7.0 mmol/l (≥126 mg/dl) or 2 h glucose ≥ 11.1 mmol/l (≥200 mg/dl) were classified as unknown diabetes. Prediabetes was diagnosed if fasting glucose values ranged between 5.6 and 6.9 mmol/l (100–125 mg/dl, i-IFG) and/or 2 h postload glucose values between 7.8 and 11.0 mmol/l (140–199 mg/dl, i-IGT). Participants were categorized to three groups of prediabetes (glucose disturbances): isolated impaired fasting glucose (i-IFG), isolated impaired glucose tolerance (i-IGT), and combined IFG and IGT (IFG+IGT).

Anthropometry, interviews and medical information in SHIP-TREND and KORA F4

In both studies, trained and certified personnel collected information on sociodemographic variables, lifestyle habits and medical history by the following common standardized personal interviews. Participants were asked to bring original packaging of their medications that were taken during the last 7 days before the examination date. Unique identifiers and drug names were recorded according to the Anatomical Therapeutical Chemical (ATC) classification system.

Trained staff measured height and weight of participants wearing lightweight clothing without shoes. Blood pressure was measured in sitting position using a validated automatic device (SHIP-TREND and KORA F4: OMRON HEM 705-CP). Three independent measurements were taken in three-minute-intervals after an initial rest of at least 5 minutes. The mean of the second and third blood pressure measurement was calculated in both studies and used for the analysis.

Lifestyle and socioeconomic indicators

Physical activity level was based on self-reported time per week spent on sports during leisure time in summer and winter. Low exercise level activities such as stepping stairs or walking were not assessed. Participants were considered as inactive if their leisure time exercise comprised <1 h per week in summer or winter.

Participants were classified as smokers if they smoked at least one cigarette per day and as non-smokers if they were either never smoking or stopped smoking at least 12 month ago. Alcohol consumption (in g/day) was calculated from self-reported consumption of beer, wine, and liquors per week.

Educational level was assessed by highest self-reported schooling degree achieved. Low education was defined as ≤9 years of schooling either with school leaving certificate (completed lower secondary education level) or without.

Study population

The study is based on participants aged 35 to 79 years (SHIP-TREND: n = 3,624; KORA F4: n = 2,929). Participants were excluded from the analyses of pre-diabetes states if one of the following criteria was met: self-reported, known diabetes, or diabetes treatment (SHIP-TREND: n = 430; KORA F4: n = 225), missing information on known diabetes (SHIP-TREND: n = 12; KORA F4: n = 86), or missing or implausible values in glucose measurements (SHIP-TREND: n = 536; KORA = 1).

All participants who underwent glucose challenge testing were required to be in the fasting state (≥8 hours overnight fasting). In SHIP-TREND, however, 666 participants without known diabetes were not fasting for 8 hours. Therefore, estimates for known diabetes are reported for the complete sample including non-fasting participants (SHIP-TREND: n = 3,624; KORA F4: n = 2,928). For the estimation of unknown diabetes or prediabetes, participants who did not meet fasting criteria were excluded from analysis. These "non-fasting" 666 participants from SHIP-TREND had a lower proportion of women (43.5% vs. 54.6%; p<0.0001), lower HDL-cholesterol (1.4 mmol/l vs. 1.5 mmol/l; p = 0.001) and higher triglycerides (median 1.6 vs. 1.3 mmol/l; p<0.0001) than the 1,980 participants with 8 h overnight fasting. However, both groups from SHIP-TREND – fasting versus non-fasting participants – did not differ in age, body mass index, total cholesterol, LDL-cholesterol, blood pressure, fasting and 2 h glucose. Therefore, the additional analyses on regional differences in known diabetes include all 3,491 participants from SHIP-TREND and 2,928 participants from KORA F4, whereas the main analyses on prediabetes and unknown diabetes are based on 1,980 participants from SHIP-TREND and 2,617 participants from KORA F4.

Statistical analysis

For descriptive analyses, mean (SD) were calculated for continuous variables and proportions for categorical variables. Differences between study regions were calculated using Wilcoxon-Test for metric and Fisher's exact test for dichotomous variables. Statistical significance was set at p<0.05. Prevalence estimates for prediabetes and unknown diabetes were directly standardized to the German adult population (31st December 2007). Logistic regression models were carried out to determine factors associated with either unknown diabetes or prediabetes. Models were fitted adjusting for age, sex, BMI, physical activity, smoking, alcohol consumption, and formal schooling. Analyses were performed using SAS statistical software version 9.3 (SAS Institute Inc., Cary, NC, USA). Distribution of fasting glucose and 2 h glucose were plotted with RStudio (*RStudio*, Inc., Boston, USA) using the kernel density estimation as a method to estimate the probability density function.

Results

In the complete sample of both studies including individuals with known diabetes and non-fasting individuals aged 35–79 years, age-sex-standardized prevalence of known diabetes was 11.9% (95%CI: 10.8–13.0%) in the northeast and 6.5% (5.2–7.8%) in the south. Individuals with type 2 diabetes from the northeast were younger (63 vs. 67 years; p<0.0001), had higher fasting glucose levels (8.7 vs. 7.7 mmol/l, p = 0.01), a higher body mass index (32.4 vs. 31.3 kg/m^2; p = 0.02), higher blood pressure (systolic: 137.8 vs. 132.3 mmHg, p<0.001; diastolic: 78.3 vs. 74.4 mmHg; p<0.001), and higher triglycerides (median: 2.0 vs. 1.6 mmol/l; p = <0.001), but slightly lower cholesterol levels (total: 5.1 vs. 5.3 mmol/l; p = 0.07; HDL-Cholesterol: 1.26 vs. 1.27 mmol/l, p = 0.28; LDL-C: 3.1 vs. 3.3 mmol/l, p = 0.011) (Table S1).

For the analysis of prediabetes and unknown diabetes, participants with known diabetes and with a fasting period of < 8 hours were excluded, leaving 1,980 participants from SHIP-TREND (1,080 women; 900 men) and 2,617 participants (1,379 women; 1,239 men) from KORA F4. The characteristics of these participants are shown in Table 1. SHIP-TREND participants were slightly younger, but had a higher body mass index, higher blood pressure values, increased triglycerides and elevated fasting and 2 h glucose. The participants of both regions did not differ in cholesterol levels (HDL-cholesterol, LDL-cholesterol and total cholesterol).

The age- and sex-specific distributions of fasting and 2 h glucose values are shown for both study regions in Figures 1 and 2. The distributions were shifted towards generally higher levels both for fasting and 2 h glucose in SHIP-TREND compared to KORA F4. This shift was more pronounced in those with NGT, in particular in the age-group 35–59 years. In this group, the mean difference between the two regional populations for 2 h glucose was

Table 1. Characteristics of the two population-based regional surveys: SHIP-TREND (northeast) and KORA F4 (south)*.

	SHIP-TREND	KORA F4	p-value
N	1,980	2,617	
Female sex (%)	54.6	52.7	0.221
Age (years)	54.0 (11.4)	55.5 (12.2)	<0.001
Fasting glucose (mmol/l)	5.6 (0.8)	5.3 (0.6)	<0.001
2 h glucose (mmol/l)	6.7 (2.4)	6.2 (2.1)	<0.001
Body mass index (kg/m^2)	28.1 (4.8)	27.4 (4.6)	<0.001
Systolic blood pressure (mmHg)	126.6 (17.3)	121.6 (18.3)	<0.001
Diastolic blood pressure (mmHg)	77.6 (9.8)	75.4 (9.8)	<0.001
Total cholesterol (mmol/l)	5.6 (1.1)	5.6 (1.0)	0.901
HDL-cholesterol (mmol/l)	1.5 (0.4)	1.5 (0.4)	0.571
LDL-cholesterol (mmol/l)	3.5 (0.9)	3.5 (0.9)	0.105
Triglycerides (mmol/l), median (IQR)	1.3 (0.9–1.8)	1.3 (0.9–1.8)	<0.001

*Results are means (SD), proportions (%) or median (IQR). P-values are calculated using Wilcoxon-Test for metric and Fisher's exact test for dichotomous variables.
Abbreviations: SHIP-TREND: Study of Health in Pomerania (2008–2012); KORA F4: Cooperative Health Research in the Region of Augsburg;
The sample was restricted to participants without known diabetes and to participants who were fasting for ≥8 hours.

0.3 mmol/l (95%CI: 0.2–0.4 mmol/l). In older individuals with NGT, this mean difference was similar, with slightly wider confidence intervals (0.3; 0.1–0.4 mmol/l). In participants with prediabetes and undiagnosed diabetes this pattern was less clear and differences did not reach statistical significance.

After age- and sex-standardization to the German population (31.12.2007), the prevalence (95%CI) of unknown diabetes was almost twofold higher in the northeast than in the south (7.1%; 5.9–8.2% vs. 3.9%; 3.2–4.6%). Overall, prediabetes (IFG, IGT or both) was also more prevalent in the northeast (43.0%; 40.8–45.1%) than in the south (30.1%; 28.4–31.7%) (Figure 3).

After stratification for age and sex, the crude estimates of prediabetes were significantly higher in the northeast than in the south in the younger age-groups 35–44 years, 45–54 years, and 55–64 years (Table 2). Prediabetes prevalence was also 2.2-fold higher in males and 2.7-fold higher in women aged 35–44 years. This sex-difference leveled off with increasing age-group and was reversed in men aged 75–79 years, however, not reaching statistical significance.

With respect to the three subgroups of prediabetes, regional differences in age- and sex-standardized prevalence were significant both for i-IFG and combined IFG+IGT, but did not reach level of statistical significance for i-IGT (SHIP-TREND: i-IFG

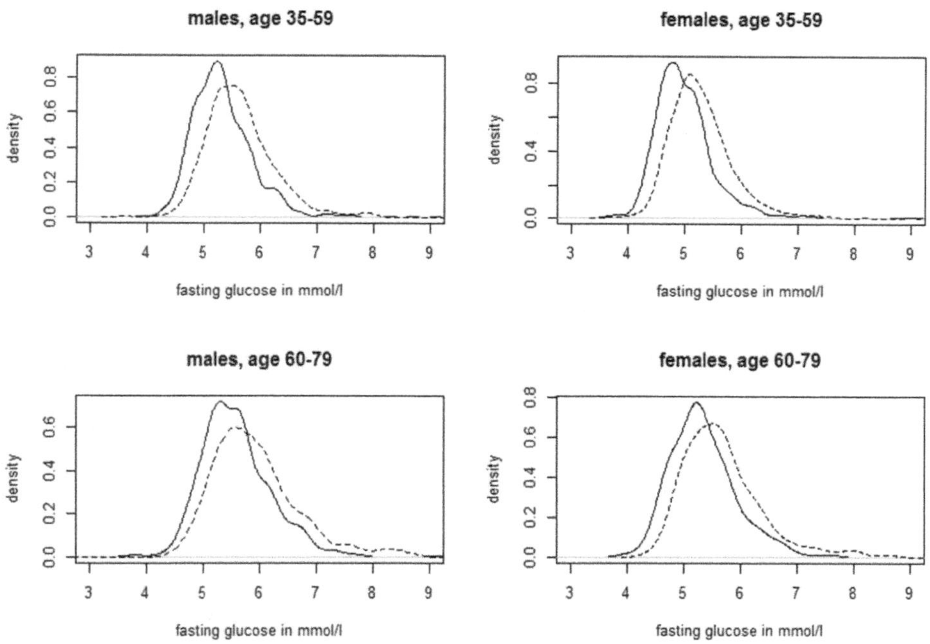

Figure 1. Kernel densities for fasting glucose in mmol/l per study region stratified for age group and sex. Solid line: KORA F4; dashed line: SHIP-TREND.

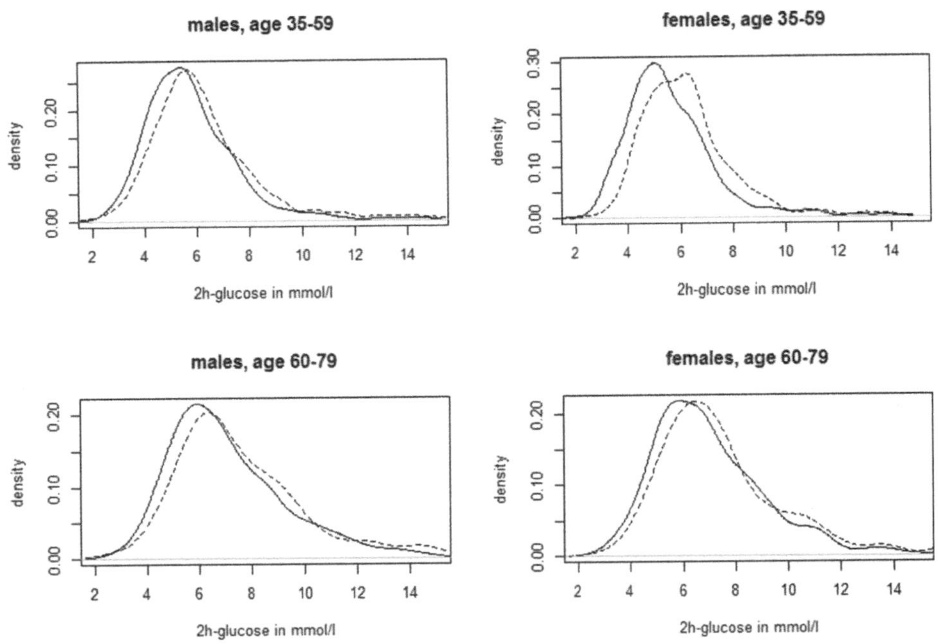

Figure 2. Kernel densities for 2 h glucose in mmol/l per study region stratified for age group and sex. Solid line: KORA F4; dashed line: SHIP-TREND.

26.4% (24.5–28.3%); combined IFG+IGT 11.2% (9.8–12.6%); KORA F4: i-IFG; combined IFG+IGT 17.2% (15.7–18.6%) and 6.6% (5.7–7.5%)).

Table 3 shows age- and sex-specific prevalence estimates for i-IFG, i-IGT, and combined IFG+IGT and unknown diabetes. I-IFG was the most common glucose disturbance in both regions. Prevalence of i-IFG was more than two-fold increased in the northeast in men aged 35–44 years and in women aged 45–54 years compared to the south (Table 3). Among individuals with i-IGT no significant regional differences were found in any age group. In combined IFG and IGT, prevalence was increased in the northeast in comparison to the south in both sexes only in the

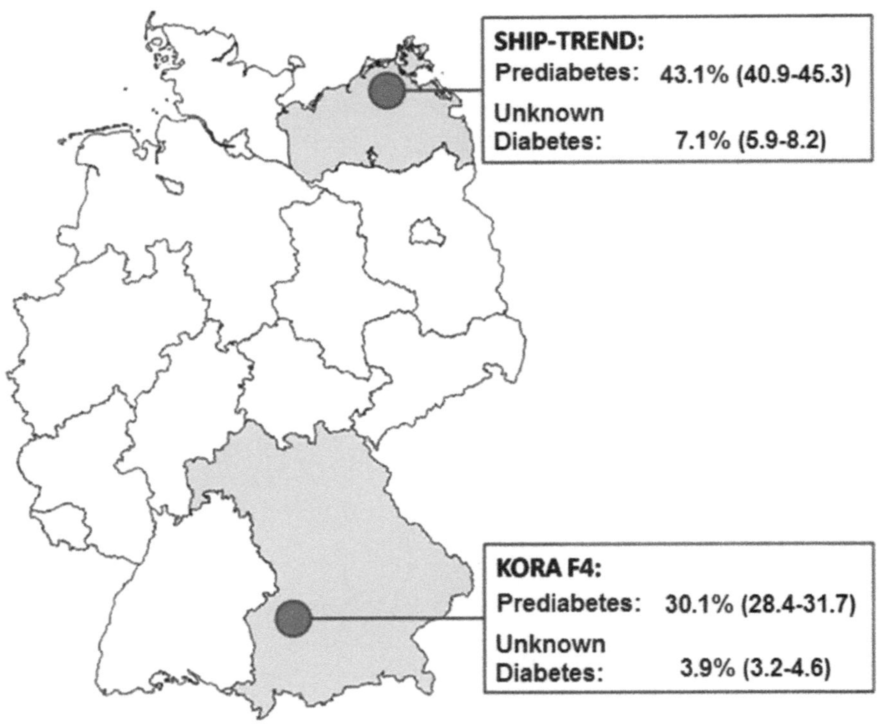

Figure 3. Prevalence of prediabetes (Pre-DM = i-IFG, i-IGT or combined IFG+IGT) and unknown diabetes (New-DM) in two German regions, standardized to the German population (31/12/2007).

Table 2. Prevalence of prediabetes (i-IFG, i-IGT or combined IFG+IGT) in the northeast (SHIP-TREND) and south (KORA F4) of Germany*.

Age (years)	SHIP-TREND	KORA F4
N	1,980	2,617
Men		
35–44	**43.5 (36.8–50.4)**	**20.2 (15.8–25.2)**
45–54	**50.4 (44.0–56.8)**	**35.2 (29.7–41.1)**
55–64	**57.8 (51.2–64.3)**	**44.3 (38.7–50.1)**
65–74	58.2 (50.1–66.0)	52.3 (46.0–58.6)
75–79	43.8 (29.5–58.8)	52.7 (42.1–63.1)
Women		
35–44	**19.9 (15.4–25.1)**	**7.3 (4.7–10.6)**
45–54	**30.9 (25.8–36.4)**	**14.7 (11.2–18.9)**
55–64	**45.5 (39.6–51.4)**	**30.7 (25.7–36.1)**
65–74	49.2 (41.7–56.7)	44.1 (38.2–50.0)
75–79	48.5 (30.8–66.5)	41.9 (31.3–52.9)

*The sample was restricted to participants without known diabetes and to participants who were fasting for ≥8 hours. Results are crude prevalence estimates (%) and 95% confidence intervals. Significant regional differences ($p<0.05$) are highlighted in bold.
Abbreviations: SHIP-TREND: Study of Health in Pomerania (2008–2012); KORA F4: Cooperative Health Research in the Region of Augsburg (2006–2008). I-IFG (isolated impaired fasting glucose: 5.6–6.9 mmol/l (100–125 mg/dl), fasting); i-IGT (impaired glucose tolerance: 7.8–11.0 mmol/l (140–199 mg/dl), 2 hour postload).

complete sample aged 35–79 years. Furthermore, prevalence of undiagnosed diabetes was significantly increased in men aged 35–79 years from northeast, while the difference was not significant in women.

Finally, the odds of having unknown diabetes or prediabetes were about twofold increased in the northeast in comparison to the south (univariate OR: unknown diabetes vs. NGT: 2.12, 1.67–2.82; univariate OR: prediabetes vs. NGT: 1.78, 1.57–2.01). The association of glucose disorders with region was not explained by traditional risk factors and became even stronger after controlling for age, sex, BMI, physical activity, smoking, alcohol consumption and education. ($OR_{adj.}$: unknown diabetes vs. NGT: 2.59, 1.84–3.65; $OR_{adj.}$: prediabetes vs. NGT: 1.98, 1.70–2.31).

Discussion

Our study shows that age-sex-standardized prevalence of unknown diabetes is considerably higher in the northeast than in the south of Germany (age group 35–79 years). Regional differences in prediabetes followed a similar northeast-south gradient and were more pronounced in the younger (35–59 years) than in the older age group (60–79 years). Thus, the prevalence of prediabetes in individuals from the northeast was largely comparable with that from individuals from the south, who were about 10 (women) to 20 years (men) older. Overall, regional differences were not explained by traditional risk factors such as BMI, physical activity, smoking, or low education.

This regional variation is in line with previous data on known type 2 diabetes prevalence in five regional population-based studies (DIAB-CORE), in nationwide health insurance data, and in a nationwide telephone survey (GEDA 2010) [4,12,13]. The increased prevalence of prediabetes and undiagnosed diabetes in the northeast in comparison to the south suggests that different diabetes screening activities are not likely to explain the regional differences in diabetes prevalence in Germany. Furthermore, a recent study based on the follow-up examinations in the DIAB-CORE consortium found that type 2 diabetes incidence (per 1,000 person-years) was also higher in the northeast than in the south of Germany (northeast: 13.2 (95%CI 10.9–16.1); south: 9.3 (7.7–11.3)) [14]. The present finding of a higher (pre)diabetes risk is in line with earlier reports on increased waist circumference levels, higher blood pressure and an increased (cardiovascular) mortality in Northeastern than in Southern Germany [15–17].

Previous results from our DIAB-CORE consortium suggested that regional deprivation, in particular the unemployment rate on municipality and neighborhood level partially explained the regional differences in known type 2 diabetes [18,19]. These relationships were independent of obesity or individual socioeconomic status [18,19]. Regional deprivation may also contribute to the regional differences in unknown diabetes and prediabetes. In this context, it is conceivable that relocation of healthier inhabitants to wealthier regions, which offer more jobs and a better overall infrastructure, may leave behind inhabitants with a generally higher morbidity and less healthy lifestyle.

It might also be of importance that the two study areas have been part of two different states during the years 1949–1990. The northeastern region of SHIP-TREND was part of the German Democratic Republic (GDR) and the southern region of KORA F4 was part of the Federal Republic of Germany (FRG). Both states differed considerably in their legislation, governmental, health care, and economic systems. Almost 25 years after reunification, persisting diversities have been reported which might be relevant for the different (pre)diabetes risk. First, in 1998, nutrition still differed between both regions [20]. As an example, tea, coffee and drinking water consumption was significantly lower in the former GDR than in the former FRG states, while the situation was inverse for soft drinks [20]. Furthermore, fruits were consumed more frequently in the territories of the former GDR, while leafy greens and other vegetables were predominantly consumed in the FRG [20]. Similar nutritional differences were found in a comparison of the EPIC-Potsdam (northeast) with the EPIC-Heidelberg (southwest) study [21]. Second, fetal and infant growth plays a role in the development of type 2 diabetes [22]. During the first years after reunification, combined statistics

Table 3. Age- and sex-specific prevalence of glucose disorders in the northeast (SHIP-TREND) and south (KORA F4) of Germany*.

Age (years)	i-IFG		i-IGT		IFG+IGT		Unknown diabetes	
	SHIP-TREND	KORA F4	SHIP-TREND	KORA F4	SHIP-TREND	KORA F4	SHIP-TREND	KORA F4
	n = 526	n = 458	n = 109	n = 173	n = 214	n = 185	n = 140	n = 110
Men								
35–44	**34.3 (28.0–41.0)**	**16.5 (12.5–21.2)**	2.8 (1.0–5.9)	1.7 (0.5–3.9)	6.5 (3.6–10.6)	2.0 (0.7–4.3)	2.3 (0.8–5.3)	1.0 (0.2–2.9)
45–54	**38.7 (32.6–45.1)**	**24.6 (19.6–30.0)**	4.0 (2.0–7.3)	5.7 (3.3–9.1)	7.7 (4.7–11.7)	5.0 (2.8–8.2)	5.6 (3.1–9.3)	1.8 (0.6–4.1)
55–64	37.0 (30.7–43.5)	29.1 (24.1–34.5)	3.5 (1.5–6.7)	4.9 (2.7–7.9)	17.4 (12.7–22.9)	10.4 (7.2–14.3)	13.0 (8.9–18.1)	7.4 (4.8–11.0)
65–74	31.0 (23.9–38.8)	28.7 (23.2–34.6)	4.4 (1.8–8.9)	7.0 (4.2–10.8)	22.8 (16.5–30.1)	16.7 (12.3–21.8)	13.9 (8.9–20.3)	7.8 (4.8–11.7)
75–79	18.8 (8.9–32.6)	22.6 (14.6–32.6)	8.3 (2.3–20.0)	16.1 (9.3–25.2)	16.7 (7.5–30.2)	14.0 (7.7–22.7)	16.7 (7.5–30.2)	12.9 (6.8–21.5)
35–79	**34.8 (31.7–38.0)**	**24.5 (22.1–27.0)**	3.9 (2.7–5.4)	5.6 (4.4–7.0)	**13.0 (10.9–15.4)**	**8.7 (7.2–10.4)**	**8.8 (7.0–10.8)**	**5.1 (3.9–6.5)**
women								
35–44	8.7 (5.7–12.7)	3.8 (2.0–6.4)	8.1 (5.1–11.8)	2.9 (1.4–5.3)	3.3 (1.5–6.1)	0.6 (0.1–2.1)	0.0 (0.0–1.3)	0.6 (0.1–2.1)
45–54	**18.1 (13.9–22.9)**	**8.1 (5.4–11.5)**	6.6 (4.1–10.0)	5.2 (3.1–8.1)	6.3 (3.8–9.6)	1.4 (0.5–3.3)	3.9 (2.1–6.8)	1.7 (0.6–3.7)
55–64	**28.7 (25.5–34.3)**	**14.7 (11.0–19.1)**	6.6 (4.0–10.2)	6.6 (4.1–9.9)	10.1 (6.9–14.2)	9.4 (6.4–13.2)	8.4 (5.4–12.2)	4.7 (2.7–7.6)
65–74	**26.5 (20.2–33.6)**	**19.2 (14.8–24.3)**	5.5 (2.7–9.9)	13.6 (9.9–18.2)	17.1 (11.9–23.4)	11.2 (7.8–15.4)	11.6 (7.3–17.2)	5.2 (3.0–8.5)
75–79	12.2 (3.4–28.2)	14.0 (7.4–23.1)	9.1 (1.9–24.3)	18.6 (11.0–28.4)	27.3 (13.3–45.5)	9.3 (4.1–17.5)	12.1 (3.4–28.2)	10.5 (4.9–18.9)
35–79	**19.7 (17.4–22.2)**	**11.2 (9.6–13.0)**	6.8 (5.4–8.5)	7.5 (6.2–9.1)	**9.0 (7.3–10.8)**	**5.6 (4.4–6.9)**	5.6 (4.3–7.2)	3.4 (2.5–4.5)

*The sample was restricted to participants without known diabetes and to participants who were fasting for ≥8 hours. Data of 2,557 participants with normal glucose tolerance were included but not shown (SHIP: n = 991; KORA: n = 1,618). Results are crude prevalences(%) and 95% confidence intervals if not otherwise specified. Significant regional differences ($p<0.05$) are highlighted in bold. Abbreviations: SHIP-TREND: Study of Health in Pomerania (2008–2012); KORA F4: Cooperative Health Research in the Region of Augsburg (2006–2008); i-IFG: isolated impaired fasting glucose: 5.6–6.9 mmol/l (100–125 mg/dl, fasting); i-IGT: isolated impaired glucose tolerance: 7.8–11.0 mmol/l (140–199 mg/dl, 2 hour postload).

showed that perinatal mortality was increased in the territories of the former GDR in comparison to the federal states of the FRG [23]. It is conceivable that the perinatal mortality was also increased in the Northeast during the time when the study population of SHIP-TREND was born [23]. However, since 2000, perinatal mortality has declined in both regions and is currently lower in the territories of the former GDR. It is noteworthy, that a recent analysis of the German Perinatal Survey (2007–2011) reported a lower body length at birth for the neonates in the territories of the former GDR while there was no clear geographic pattern for preterm birth rate, birth weight, or the percentage of neonates with birth weight ≥4,500 g [24]. However, whether infant growth patterns, pancreas and liver development, may contribute to the regional differences in diabetes and prediabetes remains unclear.

There are few studies available on regional differences in diabetes prevalence from other countries. In China, regional differences in known and unknown type 2 diabetes seemed to arise from differences in urban and rural lifestyles [25]. While type 2 diabetes (known and unknown combined) was more frequent in urban areas (6.9% vs. 5.6%), the proportion of undiagnosed type 2 diabetes in total diabetes was higher in rural areas (70.5% vs. 58.0%). Urban-rural differences might not be relevant in our study because both regions have a similar geographic distribution of towns and rural areas. Therefore, novel risk factors for diabetes such as traffic-related air pollution (e.g. particle pollution, nitrogen oxides), job strain, emotional stress, anxiety or depressive disorders and the potential mediating role of inflammation need to be considered in future studies [26–29].

Regional differences in undiagnosed (pre)diabetes have important implications for health care planning. A meta-analysis demonstrated that individuals with prediabetes were 5–10 times more likely to develop diabetes annually than normoglycaemic individuals [30]. It has been estimated that up to 70% of individuals with prediabetes will develop diabetes over the course of life [31]. Furthermore, undiagnosed diabetes is associated with an increased mortality [32,33]. In individuals with prediabetes an increased risk for neuropathy, nephropathy, retinopathy, and macrovascular disease has been described [31,34]. In line with these observations, drug treatment costs were already increased in persons with prediabetes and unknown type 2 diabetes, when compared to individuals with normal glucose tolerance [35].

From a public health perspective, diabetes prevention strategies should take into account these regional characteristics [36,37]. Our results indicate that type 2 diabetes prevention in Germany potentially needs to start at fairly young age (at least before the age of 35) in the northeast, whereas prevention in the south – especially in females - may possibly focus more on middle-aged populations.

Some limitations of the study have to be mentioned. First, in SHIP-TREND plasma glucose has been examined, while in KORA F4 serum glucose was analyzed. However, fasting plasma glucose and fasting serum glucose were compared in SHIP-TREND showing a high agreement between both methods. Second, KORA F4 is a follow-up survey and examinations have been carried out seven years after baseline examinations. At baseline, OGTTs were administered to all participants aged 55 years and older. Thus, exclusion of individuals with type 2 diabetes in this age group encompassed unknown diabetes and known diabetes, while only persons with known diabetes were excluded in SHIP-TREND. This might have influenced the results in older age groups. Therefore, we report results for younger and older participants separately. Furthermore, the SHIP-TREND study started examinations in 2008 (lasting until 2012) when the examinations in KORA F4 were already finished. The difference of four years on average in data collection might have influenced the results, however, probably only to a small degree.

The strength of the study is the large number of well-characterized participants that underwent OGTTs following common standardized protocols.

In conclusion, men and women in the northeast of Germany have a considerably higher prevalence of prediabetes (IFG, IGT or both) and unknown type 2 diabetes than their counterparts in the south of Germany. In particular, prediabetes is more prevalent at younger age in the northeast. Therefore, prevention strategies and health care policy need to take into account these regional differences in morbidity and diabetes risk. Further studies are warranted to examine the risk factors underlying these regional differences, in particular, the impact of individual and regional socioeconomic indicators.

Supporting Information

Table S1 Characteristics of excluded participants with type 2 diabetes in SHIP-TREND and KORA F4*. *Results are means (SD), proportions (%) or Median (IQR). P-values were calculated using Wilcoxon-Test for metric and fisher exact test for dichotomous variables. Missing values in KORA: 14 for fasting glucose, 5 in BMI, 1 for BP and lipids. Missing values in SHIP-TREND: 1 for FPG and BMI, 3 for BP and lipids. Abbreviations: SHIP-TREND: Study of Health in Pomerania (2008–2012); KORA F4: Cooperative Health Research in the Region of Augsburg (2006–2008).

Acknowledgments

The authors thank Klaus Strassburger (German Diabetes Center, Düsseldorf) for his statistical advice.

Author Contributions

Conceived and designed the experiments: WR TT. Analyzed the data: TT. Contributed reagents/materials/analysis tools: CM AP CH SS MN HV MR WR. Contributed to the writing of the manuscript: TT. Harmonization of data from KORA F4 and SHIP-TREND: TT SS MS WM. Contributed to the discussion, reviewed and edited the manuscript: TT SS CM MS WM CH MR MN AP HV WR.

References

1. IDF Diabetes Atlas (2013) IDF Diabetes Atlas, 6th ed. Brussels, Belgium: International Diabetes Federation.
2. Tamayo T, Rosenbauer J, Wild SH, Spijkerman AM, Baan C, et al. (2014). Diabetes in Europe: an update. Diabetes Res Clin Pract 103: 206–217.
3. Barker LE, Kirtland KA, Gregg EW, Geiss LS, Thompson TJ. (2011) Geographic distribution of diagnosed diabetes in the U.S.: a diabetes belt. Am J Prev Med 40: 434–439.
4. Schipf S, Werner A, Tamayo T, Holle R, Schunk M., et al. (2012) Regional differences in the prevalence of known Type 2 diabetes mellitus in 45–74 years old individuals: results from six population-based studies in Germany (DIAB-CORE Consortium). Diabet Med 29: e88–95.
5. American Diabetes Association. (2012) Standards of medical care in diabetes-2012. Diabetes Care; 35 Suppl 1: S11–63.
6. Völzke H, Alte D, Schmidt CO, Radke D, Lorbeer R, et al. (2011) Cohort Profile: The Study of Health in Pomerania. Int J Epidemiol 40: 294–307.
7. John U, Greiner B, Hensel E, Lüdemann J, Piek M, et al. (2001) Study of Health In Pomerania (SHIP): a health examination survey in an east German region: objectives and design. Soz Praventivmed 46: 186–194.

8. Chambless L, Cairns V, Herbold M, Döring A, Filipiak B, et al. (1987) MONICA-Augsburg: Survey Sampling. Munich, Germany: Gesellschaft für Strahlen- und Umweltforschung. GSF-Bericht 31/86.
9. Rathmann W, Haastert B, Icks A, Löwel H, Meisinger C, et al. High prevalence of undiagnosed diabetes mellitus in southern Germany: target populations for efficient screening. The KORA survey 2000. Diabetologia 2003; 46: 182–189.
10. Meisinger C, Strassburger K, Heier M, Thorand B, Baumeister SE, et al. (2010) Prevalence of undiagnosed diabetes and impaired glucose regulation in 35–59-year-old individuals in southern Germany: the KORA F4 Study. Diabet Med 27: 360–362.
11. Meisinger C, Döring A, Stöckl D, Thorand B, Kowall B, et al. (2012) Uric Acid is more strongly associated with impaired glucose regulation in women than in men from the general population : the KORA F4-Study. PLOS One; 7: e37180.
12. Wilke T, Ahrendt P, Schwartz D, Linder R, Ahrens S, et al. (2013) Incidence and prevalence of type 2 diabetes mellitus in Germany: an analysis based on 5,43 Million patients. Dtsch Med Wochenschr 138: 69–75. Article in German.
13. Robert Koch-Institut (Hrsg) (2012) Daten und Fakten: Ergebnisse der Studie »Gesundheit in Deutschland aktuell 2010«. Beiträge zur Gesundheitsberichterstattung des Bundes, 2012. RKI, Berlin. [Article in German] Available: http://edoc.rki.de/documents/rki_fv/remDCCtjOJxI/PDF/21TgKGZEOWNCY.pdf. Accessed 2014 April 28.
14. Schipf S, Ittermann T, Tamayo T, Holle R, Schunk M, et al. (2014) Regional differences in the incidence of self-reported type 2 diabetes in Germany: results from five population-based studies in Germany (DIAB-CORE Consortium). J Epidemiol Community Health. [Epub ahead of print].
15. Stang A, Döring A, Völzke H, Moebus S, Greiser KH, et al. (2011) Regional differences in body fat distributions among people with comparable body mass index: a comparison across six German population-based surveys. Eur J Cardiovasc Prev Rehabil 18: 106–114.
16. Meisinger C, Heier M, Völzke H, Löwel H, Mitusch R, et al. (2006) Regional disparities of hypertension prevalence and management within Germany. J Hypertens 24: 293–299.
17. Wiesner G, Bittner EK (2004) Life expectancy, potential years of life lost (PYLL), an avoidable mortality in an East/West comparison. Bundesgesundheitsbl. Gesundheitsforsch Gesundheitsschutz 47: 266–278.
18. Maier W, Holle R, Hunger M, Peters A, Meisinger C, et al.; DIAB-CORE Consortium. (2013) The impact of regional deprivation and individual socio-economic status on the prevalence of Type 2 diabetes in Germany. A pooled analysis of five population-based studies. Diabet Med 30: e78–86.
19. Müller G, Kluttig A, Greiser KH, Moebus S, Slomiany U, et al. (2013) Regional and neighborhood disparities in the odds of type 2 diabetes: Results from 5 population-based studies in Germany (DIAB-CORE Consortium). Am J Epidemiol 178: 221–230.
20. Mensink GBM, Beitz R (2004) Food and nutrient intake in East and West Germany, 8 years after the reunification. European Journal of Clinical Nutrition 58, 1000–1010.
21. Schulze MB, Brandstetter BR, Kroke A, Wahrendorf J, Boeing H (1999) Quantitative Food Intake in the EPIC-Germany Cohorts. Ann Nutr Metab 43: 235–245.
22. Hales CN, Barker DJ (2013) Type 2 (non-insulin-dependent) diabetes mellitus: the thrifty phenotype hypothesis. Int J Epidemiol. 42: 1215–22.
23. Robert Koch-Institut (2004) GBE-Schwerpunktbericht: Gesundheit von Kindern und Jugendlichen. Gesundheitsberichterstattung des Bundes. RKI, Berlin.
24. Voigt M, Wittwer-Backofen U, Scholz R, Schneider KTM, Straube S, et al. (2013) Analysis of the German Perinatal Survey of the Years 2007–2011 and Comparison with Data from 1995–1997: Neonatal Characteristics and Duration of Pregnancy. Z Geburtsh Neonatol 217: 211–214.
25. Dong Y, Gao W, Nan H, Yu H, Li F, et al. (2005) Prevalence of Type 2 diabetes in urban and rural Chinese populations in Qingdao, China. Diabet Med. 22: 1427–1433.
26. Rajagopalan S, Brook RD (2012) Air pollution and type 2 diabetes: mechanistic insights. Diabetes 61: 3034–3037.
27. Fransson EI, Heikkilä K, Nyberg ST, Zins M, Westerlund H, et al. (2012) Job strain as a risk factor for leisure-time physical inactivity: an individual-participant meta-analysis of up to 170,000 men and women: the IPD-Work Consortium. Am J Epidemiol 176: 1078–1089.
28. Rotella F, Mannucci E (2013) Depression as a risk factor for diabetes: a meta-analysis of longitudinal studies. J Clin Psychiatry 74: 31–37.
29. Herder C, Kowall B, Tabak AG, Rathmann W (2013) The potential of novel biomarkers to improve risk prediction of type 2 diabetes. Diabetologia 57: 16–29.
30. Gerstein HC, Santaguida P, Raina P, Morrison KM, Balion C, et al. (2007) Annual incidence and relative risk of diabetes in people with various categories of dysglycemia: a systematic overview and meta-analysis of prospective studies. Diabetes Res Clin Pract 78: 305–312.
31. Tabák AG, Herder C, Rathmann W, Brunner EJ, Kivimäki M (2012) Prediabetes: a high-risk state for diabetes development. Lancet 379: 2279–2290.
32. Kowall B, Rathmann W, Heier M, Giani G, Peters A, et al. (2011) Categories of glucose tolerance and continuous glycemic measures and mortality. Eur J Epidemiol 26: 637–645.
33. DECODE Study Group, European Diabetes Epidemiology Group (2002) Is the current definition for diabetes relevant to mortality risk from all causes and cardiovascular and non-cardiovascular diseases? Diabetes Care 26: 688–696.
34. Bongaerts BW, Rathmann W, Kowall B, Herder C, Stöckl D, et al. (2012) Postchallenge hyperglycemia is positively associated with diabetic polyneuropathy: the KORA F4 study. Diabetes Care 2012; 35: 1891–1893.
35. Icks A, Claessen H, Strassburger K, Tepel M, Waldeyer R, et al. (2013) Drug costs in prediabetes and undetected diabetes compared with diagnosed diabetes and normal glucose tolerance: results from the population-based KORA Survey in Germany. Diabetes Care 36: e53–4.
36. Knowler WC, Barrett-Connor E, Fowler SE, Hamman RF, Lachin JM, et al.; Diabetes Prevention Program Research Group. (2002) Reduction in the incidence of type 2 diabetes with lifestyle intervention or metformin. N Engl J Med. 346: 393–403.
37. Tuomilehto J, Lindström J, Eriksson JG, Valle TT, Hämäläinen H, et al.; Finnish Diabetes Prevention Study Group. (2001) Prevention of type 2 diabetes mellitus by changes in lifestyle among subjects with impaired glucose tolerance. N Engl J Med. 344: 1343–1350.

8

Lifestyle Factors Associated with Type 2 Diabetes and Use of Different Glucose-Lowering Drugs

Sinna P. Ulrichsen[1], Anil Mor[1]*, Elisabeth Svensson[1], Finn B. Larsen[2], Reimar W. Thomsen[1]

1 Department of Clinical Epidemiology, Faculty of Health, Aarhus University Hospital, Aarhus, Denmark, **2** Centre for Public Health and Quality Improvement, Central Denmark Region, Aarhus, Denmark

Abstract

Aims: To examine the lifestyle profile among persons with and without Type 2 diabetes mellitus (DM) and among users of different glucose-lowering drugs.

Methods: We used questionnaire data from a Danish health survey and identified presence of Type 2 DM and use of medications through medical databases. We calculated age- and gender-standardized prevalence ratios (PRs) of lifestyle factors according to Type 2 DM and different glucose-lowering drugs.

Results: Of 21,637 survey participants aged 25–79 years, 680 (3%) had Type 2 DM (median age 63 years) with a median diabetes duration of 5 years. Participants with Type 2 DM had a substantially higher prevalence of obesity (36% vs. 13%, PR: 3.1, 95% confidence interval (CI): 2.8–3.6), yet more reported to eat a very healthy diet (25% vs. 21%, PR: 1.2, 95% CI: 1.0–1.4) and to exercise regularly (67% vs. 53%, PR: 1.3, 95% CI: 1.2–1.4). Also, fewer were current smokers or had high alcohol intake. When compared with metformin users, obesity was substantially less prevalent in users of sulfonylurea (PR: 0.5, 95% CI: 0.4–0-8), and insulin and analogues (PR: 0.4, 95% CI: 0.3–0.7). Tobacco smoking was more prevalent in sulfonylurea users (PR: 1.4, 95% CI: 0.9–2.1) compared with metformin users. We found no material differences in physical exercise, diet or alcohol intake according to type of glucose-lowering drug.

Conclusions: Type 2 DM patients are substantially more obese than other individuals, but otherwise report to have a healthier lifestyle. Metformin use is strongly associated with obesity, whereas sulfonylurea use tends to be associated with tobacco smoking.

Editor: Victor Sanchez-Margalet, Virgen Macarena University Hospital, School of Medicine, University of Seville, Spain

Funding: This research was supported by the Clinical Epidemiology Research Foundation, Aarhus University Hospital, Aarhus, Denmark. The Department of Clinical Epidemiology, Aarhus University Hospital, receives funding for other studies from companies in the form of research grants to (and administered by) Aarhus University. The funders had no role in study design, data collection and analysis, decision to publish, or preparation of the manuscript.

Competing Interests: The authors have declared that no competing interests exist.

* Email: anil.mor@clin.au.dk

Introduction

Type 2 diabetes mellitus (DM) and its complications are an increasing challenge to health care systems worldwide [1,2]. Diabetes confers a 1.8-fold increased risk of death from any cause, including a 2.3-fold increased risk of death from vascular causes, but also markedly increased risk of death from renal disease, liver disease, infections, mental disorders, and cancer [3–7]. Much of our knowledge on these associations is based on large observational registry-based studies, lacking information on lifestyle factors. Thus, it is unclear to which extent these associations (e.g. diabetes and increased risk of cancer) are related to unhealthier lifestyle in diabetes [6–8]. Similarly, comparative effectiveness studies of different glucose-lowering therapies in diabetes, as well as studies of important side effects or beneficial pleiotropic effects of these therapies, often rely on observational designs that also may be hampered by uncontrolled confounding by lifestyle factors [9]. Even in prospective studies with primary data collection, potential confounding often persists owing to unmeasured data on lifestyle factors, such as details about dietary habits and physical activity, associated with Type 2 DM [3].

Sensitivity analysis and external adjustment for unmeasured confounding by lifestyle factors allow for bias assessment, and therefore, detailed information about lifestyle behaviour associated with Type 2 DM and its treatment is needed [10].

We therefore aimed to examine lifestyle differences among persons with and without Type 2 DM and among users of different glucose-lowering drugs based on data from a Danish public health survey.

Materials and Methods

Setting

We conducted this population-based cross-sectional study in Central Denmark region, encompassing about 1.2 million inhabitants. Denmark is a welfare state with tax-funded universal access to health care, providing primary and secondary care without out-of-pocket expenses and partial reimbursement for most prescribed medications, including glucose-lowering drugs [11]. Individual-level data from all Danish registries can be linked via a unique personal identifier, the CPR number, assigned at birth and registered in the Danish Civil Registration system [12].

Study population

In 2006, the Central Denmark Region conducted a public health survey called "*Hvordan har du det?*" (English: "How are you?"). This region consists of 19 municipalities. The authorities decided to randomly select and invite 1500 participants from each municipality, except for one municipality encompassing the capital city of the region where 4500 participants were selected. A total of 31,500 Danish citizens between 25 and up to 79 years of age, living in the Central Denmark Region with at least one parent born in Denmark, were selected and invited to participate in the survey. In total, 21,708 (69%) invited persons agreed and gave their informed consent to participate in the survey. Following this, a detailed questionnaire with approximately 400 questions on self-rated health, occurrence of chronic diseases, socioeconomic factors, and lifestyle factors were sent to all respondents who agreed to participate. Furthermore, three reminders were sent to those who did not respond to the questionnaire to increase the response rate [13]. Finally, 21,637 participants returned valid questionnaire data. Figure 1 shows the selection process of the study.

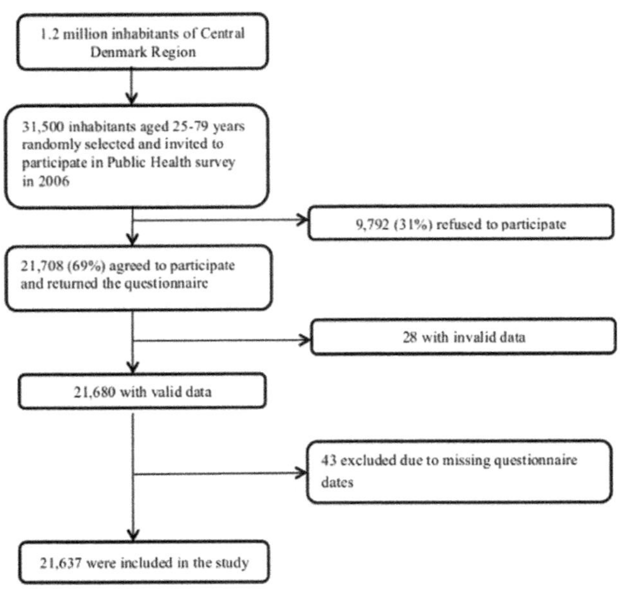

Figure 1. Selection of participants for the survey.

For our present analyses based on the "How are you" data, approval by the Danish Scientific Ethical Committee was not needed according to Danish legislation, as our study was registry-based and did not include human biological material. The questionnaire was prepared in the Danish language and the study design, including the questionnaire and sampling method, has been described in more detail elsewhere [11,14].

Data on lifestyle factors

Lifestyle factors included in the questionnaire were body mass index (BMI), physical activity, diet, smoking status, and alcohol intake. BMI (kg/m^2) was categorized according to the World Health Organization's (WHO) criteria as underweight (<18.5), normal weight (18.5–24.9), overweight (25.0–29.9) and obese (≥ 30.0) [15]. Regular physical exercise was defined as the participation in leisure sports or other regular physical exercise (yes, no). Based on 30 detailed questions about fruit, vegetables, fish, and fat intake, a validated diet score was calculated, and categorized into very healthy (high amount of fruit, vegetables, fish, and low amount of saturated fat), reasonably healthy (moderately high intake of fruit, vegetables, fish, and saturated fat), or unhealthy (low intake of fruit, vegetables, fish, and high amount of saturated fat) [16]. Smoking status was defined as current (daily or occasionally), former, or never tobacco smoking. Alcohol intake was categorized as above or within the recommended maximum intake at the time of the survey (≤14/≤ 21 weekly drinks for women/men, respectively).

Patients with Type 2 DM

We defined Type 2 DM as persons who were at least 30 years of age at the time of first hospital contact with diabetes or who received any oral glucose-lowering drug at any time. Diabetes duration was defined as years between the first diabetes diagnosis or drug prescription and the date of filling the questionnaire. We identified all individuals with any diabetes-related hospital contact in the Danish National Registry of Patients (DNRP) (see codes in the appendix S1), and identified glucose-lowering drug prescription using Anatomical Therapeutic Chemical (ATC) codes in the Aarhus University Prescription Database (AUPD) (see the appendix S1 for ATC codes). The DNRP contains complete hospitalization history of all Danish residents since 1977 with one primary discharge diagnosis and up to 20 secondary discharge diagnosis coded according to the International Classification of Diseases (ICD) 8th revision (ICD-8) until the end of 1993, and 10th revision (ICD-10) thereafter [17]. The AUPD include information on all reimbursed prescriptions since 1996 from former Aarhus County, and since 1998 from former Viborg and Ringkjøbing Counties [18].

Glucose-lowering drugs

We categorized Type 2 DM patients according to filled glucose-lowering drug prescriptions in the AUPD within 100 days before and 100 days after the date of returning the questionnaire. This period was chosen to capture most current users of glucose-lowering drugs, as most glucose-lowering drug prescriptions are expected to last for 90 or 100 days in Denmark. Patients reimbursing only one type of glucose-lowering drug were categorized according to the following categories (codes in the appendix S1): metformin, sulfonylureas, insulin and insulin analogues, and other glucose-lowering drugs. Patients with prescriptions for more than one of the above types of glucose-lowering drugs or with combination tablets

Table 1. Characteristics of 21,637 participants according to type 2 diabetes and glucose-lowering drug use.

	Type 2 diabetes		Glucose-lowering drugs					
	No	Yes	Metformin	Combination*	Sulfonylureas	Insulin and analogues	Other glucose-lowering drugs	No glucose-lowering drug
	n = *20,957* (%)	*n* = *680* (%)	*n* = *106* (%)	*n* = 191 (%)	*n* = 94 (%)	*n* = 113 (%)	*n* = 4 (%)	*n* = 172 (%)
Gender								
Women	11172 (53)	336 (49)	56 (53)	97 (51)	46 (49)	47 (42)	2 (50)	88 (51)
Men	9785 (47)	344 (51)	50 (47)	94 (49)	48 (51)	66 (58)	2 (50)	84 (49)
Age, median (IQR)	51 (40, 62)	63 (56, 70)	65 (57, 69)	62 (54, 70)	68 (60, 73)	61 (55, 71)	61 (53, 65)	62 (55, 70)
<45 years	7585 (36)	56 (8)	12 (11)	14 (7)	1 (1)	10 (9)	0 (0)	19 (11)
45–64 years	9434 (45)	312 (46)	38 (36)	98 (51)	35 (37)	56 (50)	3 (75)	82 (48)
65–80 years	3938 (19)	312 (46)	56 (53)	79 (41)	58 (62)	47 (42)	1 (25)	71 (41)
Diabetes duration, median (IQR)	–	5 (2, 10)	3 (1, 5)	7 (4, 9)	4 (2, 7)	12 (8, 18)	6 (3, 9)	4 (2, 8)
0–2 years	–	204 (30)	52 (49)	35 (18)	36 (38)	11 (10)	1 (25)	69 (40)
3–5 years	–	154 (23)	32 (30)	43 (23)	26 (28)	12 (11)	1 (25)	41 (24)
6–10 years	–	192 (28)	17 (16)	89 (47)	25 (27)	27 (24)	2 (50)	34 (20)
11–15 years	–	66 (10)	5 (5)	15 (8)	5 (5)	29 (26)	0 (0)	12 (7)
16–20 years	–	38 (6)	0 (0)	6 (3)	2 (2)	19 (17)	0 (0)	11 (6)
21–30 years	–	23 (3)	0 (0)	3 (2)	0 (0)	15 (13)	0 (0)	5 (3)
CCI score								
0	18292 (87)	434 (64)	76 (72)	137 (72)	60 (64)	67 (59)	3 (75)	91 (53)
1–2	2355 (11)	198 (29)	25 (24)	47 (25)	23 (24)	33 (29)	1 (25)	69 (40)
3+	310 (2)	48 (7)	5 (5)	7 (4)	11 (12)	13 (12)	0 (0)	12 (7)
Myocardial infarction	286 (1)	46 (7)	6 (6)	3 (2)	6 (6)	12 (11)	1 (25)	18 (10)
Congestive heart failure	147 (1)	45 (7)	3 (3)	8 (4)	11 (12)	12 (11)	0 (0)	11 (6)

CCI = Charlson comorbidity index, IQR = inter-quartile range.
*Patients using more than one type of glucose-lowering drug or using combination tablets.

Table 2. Age-and gender-standardized prevalence differences (PDs) and prevalence ratios (PRs) of lifestyle factors according to type 2 diabetes.

	Type 2 diabetes		PDs comparing T2DM patients vs. other individuals	PRs comparing T2DM patients vs. other individuals
	No	Yes		
	n = 20,957 (%)	*n* = *680* (%)	PDs (95% CIs)	PRs (95% CIs)
BMI (kg/m²)				
<18.5	308 (1)	4 (1)	−1.0 (−1.5 to −0.5)	0.3 (0.1 to 0.9)
18.5–24	9979 (48)	163 (24)	−23.8 (−28.3 to −19.3)	0.5 (0.4 to 0.6)
25–29	7490 (36)	234 (34)	−4.8 (−9.5 to 0.0)	0.9 (0.7 to 1.0)
≥30	2708 (13)	243 (36)	27.6 (22.6 to 32.6)	3.1 (2.8 to 3.6)
Missing	472 (2)	36 (5)	-	-
Diet*				
Unhealthy	2809 (13)	71 (10)	−1.3 (−5.1 to 2.6)	0.9 (0.7 to 1.3)
Reasonably healthy	13320 (64)	404 (59)	−3.1 (−8.4 to 2.2)	1.0 (0.9 to 1.0)
Very healthy	4363 (21)	170 (25)	3.4 (−1.0 to 7.8)	1.2 (1.0 to 1.4)
Missing	465 (2)	35 (5)	-	-
Smoking				
Current	6170 (29)	162 (24)	−1.8 (−6.7 to 3.2)	0.9 (0.8 to 1.1)
Former	5261 (25)	223 (33)	−0.7 (−4.6 to 3.2)	1.0 (0.8 to 1.1)
Never	8803 (42)	235 (35)	−0.6 (−5.9 to 4.7)	1.0 (0.9 to 1.1)
Missing	723 (3)	60 (9)	-	-
Alcohol intake†				
High	1234 (6)	33 (5)	−1.8 (−3.6 to 0.0)	0.7 (0.5 to 1.1)
Low	19211 (92)	620 (91)	0.6 (−2.1 to 3.2)	1.0 (1.0 to 1.0)
Missing	512 (2)	27 (4)	-	-
Regular physical exercise‡				
Yes	11031 (53)	455 (67)	15.6 (10.7 to 20.6)	1.3 (1.2 to 1.4)
No	9489 (45)	200 (29)	−15.6 (−20.5 to −10.6)	0.7 (0.6 to 0.8)
Missing	437 (2)	25 (4)	-	-

T2DM = type 2 diabetes mellitus, BMI = body mass index, CI = confidence interval.
*Diet: very healthy (high amount of fruit, vegetables, fish and low amount of saturated fat), reasonably healthy (moderately high amount of fruit, vegetables, fish and saturated fat) or unhealthy (low amount of fruit, vegetables, fish and high amount of saturated fat).
†Alcohol intake: High (above the recommended limit of ≤14/≤21 weekly drinks for women/men) or low (within the recommended limit).
‡Regular exercise: participation in leisure sports or other regular physical activity (yes/no).

were categorized as combination users. Patients not filling any prescription within the 200 days were categorized as Type 2 DM patients with no medical treatment.

Data on comorbidity

Based on hospital diagnosis codes from the DNRP we computed the Charlson comorbidity index (CCI) score for each person defining three comorbidity levels: low (CCI score of 0), medium (CCI score of 1–2), and high (CCI score of 3+) [19]. The two diabetes categories were left out of the CCI score as diabetes defined our index disease [20].

Statistical analyses

We estimated the prevalence of different lifestyle factors, demographic variables, and comorbidity level according to Type 2 DM status and use of different glucose-lowering drugs. We calculated age- and gender-standardized prevalence differences (PDs) and prevalence ratios (PRs) for lifestyle factors, comparing Type 2 DM patients with other survey participants standardized to the cohort of all participants, and comparing users of different glucose-lowering drugs standardized to the cohort of Type 2 DM patients. For the analysis of glucose-lowering drug users, we used metformin monotherapy as reference. We repeated the analyses with restriction to newly diagnosed Type 2 DM patients, i.e. those who had been diagnosed within three years of the survey.

All statistical analyses were performed using Statistical Analysis System (SAS) software (version 9.2, SAS Institute, Cary, NC). This project was approved by the Danish Data Protection Agency (record number 2013-41-1924).

Results

A total of 680 (3.1%) of the 21,637 persons aged between 25 and 80 years were identified as having Type 2 DM. Regarding glucose-lowering drugs, 16% (106/680) patients were treated with metformin, 28% (191/680) with combination therapy, 14% (94/680) with sulfonylureas, 17% (113/680) with insulin and analogues, <1% (4/680) with other glucose-lowering drugs (all were repaglinide users), and 25% (172/680) received no glucose-

Table 3. Age-and gender-standardized prevalence differences (PDs) and prevalence ratios (PRs) of lifestyle factors among newly diagnosed# type 2 diabetes patients.

	Type 2 diabetes		PDs comparing T2DM patients vs. other individuals	PRs comparing T2DM patients vs. other individuals
	No	Yes		
	n = *20,957* (%)	*n* = *204* (%)	PDs (95% CIs)	PRs (95% CIs)
BMI (kg/m²)				
<18.5	308 (1)	0 (0)	–	–
18.5–24	9979 (48)	40 (20)	−29.0 (−35.1 to −22.8)	0.4 (0.3 to 0.5)
25–29	7490 (36)	65 (32)	−5.0 (−12.5 to 2.4)	0.9 (0.7 to 1.1)
≥30	2708 (13)	83 (41)	31.0 (23.2 to 38.8)	3.4 (2.8 to 4.1)
Missing	472 (2)	16 (8)	–	–
Diet*				
Unhealthy	2809 (13)	22 (11)	−2.3 (−7.5 to 3.0)	0.8 (0.5 to 1.3)
Reasonably healthy	13320 (64)	118 (58)	−3.6 (−11.5 to 4.3)	0.9 (0.8 to 1.1)
Very healthy	4363 (21)	51 (25)	4.1 (−2.9 to 11.2)	1.2 (0.9 to 1.6)
Missing	465 (2)	13 (6)	–	–
Smoking				
Current	6170 (29)	51 (25)	−1.7 (−9.1 to 5.8)	0.9 (0.7 to 1.2)
Former	5261 (25)	77 (38)	6.1 (−0.9 to 13.2)	1.2 (1.0 to 1.6)
Never	8803 (42)	60 (29)	−7.9 (−15.7 to 0.0)	0.8 (0.7 to 1.1)
Missing	723 (3)	16 (8)	–	–
Alcohol intake†				
High	1234 (6)	12 (6)	−1.9 (−4.2 to 0.4)	0.7 (0.4 to 1.2)
Low	19211 (92)	184 (90)	1.1 (−2.4 to 4.6)	1.0 (1.0 to 1.1)
Missing	512 (2)	8 (4)	–	–
Regular physical exercise‡				
Yes	11031 (53)	141 (69)	19.5 (12.7 to 26.4)	1.4 (1.3 to 1.5)
No	9489 (45)	57 (28)	−18.7 (−25.6 to −11.9)	0.6 (0.5 to 0.8)
Missing	437 (2)	6 (3)	–	–

T2DM = type 2 diabetes mellitus, BMI = body mass index, CI = confidence interval.
#Newly diagnosed were all the patients diagnosed within 3 years of the survey date.
*Diet: very healthy (high amount of fruit, vegetables, fish and low amount of saturated fat), reasonably healthy (moderately high amount of fruit, vegetables, fish and saturated fat) or unhealthy (low amount of fruit, vegetables, fish and high amount of saturated fat).
†Alcohol intake: High (above the recommended limit of ≤14/≤21 weekly drinks for women/men) or low (within the recommended limit).
‡Regular exercise: participation in leisure sports or other regular physical activity (yes/no).

lowering drugs. Among the 191 combination users, 180 (94%) were treated with metformin in combination, 118 (66%) with sulfonylureas in combination, and 73 (38%) with insulin and analogues in combination.

Patient characteristics

Type 2 DM patients were older than other survey participants (median age 63 years (interquartile range (IQR), 56–70 years) vs 51 years (IQR, 40–62 years)) (*Table 1*). The median duration of diabetes in the Type 2 DM population was 5 years (IQR, 2–10 years) and 36% had a history of hospital-diagnosed comorbidity included in the CCI, compared with 13% of the other survey participants.

Table 1 shows demographic and clinical characteristics according to glucose-lowering drug groups. Sulfonylurea users tended to be older compared with users of any other glucose-lowering drugs. Users of insulin and analogues had longest diabetes history (median duration 12 years, IQR, 8–18), followed by combination therapy users (7 years, IQR, 4–9). Metformin users had a comparably short history of diabetes (median duration 3 years, IQR, 1–5), and also had lower prevalence of comorbidities as compared with other drug groups.

Lifestyle behavior according to Type 2 DM status

Table 2 shows the distribution of lifestyle factors according to diabetes status. Compared with other survey participants, a substantially higher proportion of individuals with Type 2 DM were obese (36% vs. 13%, PR: 3.1, 95% CI: 2.8–3.6). However, more reported eating a very healthy diet (25% vs. 21%, PR: 1.2, 95% CI: 1.0–1.4), and more were engaged in regular physical exercise (67% vs. 53%, PR: 1.3, 95% CI: 1.2–1.4). Type 2 DM patients were also less likely to be current smokers (24% vs. 29%, PR: 0.9, 95% CI: 0.8–1.1) and a slightly lower proportion had alcohol intake over the recommended limits (5% vs. 6%, PR: 0.7, 95% CI: 0.5–1.1) (*Table 2*). After restricting the analyses to newly diagnosed Type 2 DM patients, we did not find any material difference from the complete cohort estimates (*Table 3*).

Table 4. Distribution of lifestyle factors according to glucose-lowering drug use among 680 individuals with type 2 diabetes participating in the Danish "How are you?" public health survey in 2006.

	Type 2 diabetes	Metformin	Combination[δ]	Sulfonylureas	Insulin and analogues	No glucose-lowering drug
	n = 680 (%)	*n* = 106 (%)	*n* = 191 (%)	*n* = 94 (%)	*n* = 113 (%)	*n* = 172 (%)
BMI (kg/m²)						
<18.5	4 (1)	0 (0)	1 (1)	1 (1)	2 (2)	0 (0)
18.5–24	161 (24)	12 (11)	26 (14)	27 (29)	48 (43)	48 (28)
25–29	232 (34)	35 (33)	65 (34)	37 (39)	31 (27)	64 (37)
≥30	243 (36)	52 (49)	92 (48)	24 (26)	22 (19)	53 (31)
Missing	36 (5)	7 (7)	7 (4)	5 (5)	10 (9)	7 (4)
Diet*						
Unhealthy	71 (11)	11 (10)	15 (08)	10 (11)	14 (12)	21 (12)
Reasonably healthy	401 (59)	59 (56)	126 (66)	54 (57)	60 (53)	59 (59)
Very healthy	169 (25)	32 (30)	41 (21)	25 (27)	34 (30)	37 (22)
Missing	35 (5)	4 (4)	9 (5)	5 (5)	5 (4)	12 (7)
Smoking						
Current	160 (24)	23 (22)	36 (19)	28 (30)	29 (26)	44 (26)
Former	223 (33)	35 (33)	70 (37)	29 (31)	37 (33)	52 (30)
Never	233 (35)	40 (38)	64 (34)	30 (32)	40 (35)	59 (34)
Missing	60 (9)	8 (8)	21 (11)	7 (7)	7 (6)	17 (10)
Alcohol intake[†]						
High	32 (05)	7 (7)	6 (3)	4 (4)	7 (06)	8 (5)
Low	617 (91)	94 (89)	179 (94)	85 (90)	102 (90)	157 (91)
Missing	27 (4)	5 (5)	6 (3)	5 (5)	4 (4)	7 (4)
Regular physical exercise[‡]						
Yes	453 (67)	69 (65)	128 (67)	63 (67)	79 (70)	114 (66)
No	198 (29)	36 (34)	53 (28)	27 (29)	29 (26)	53 (31)
Missing	25 (4)	1 (1)	10 (5)	4 (4)	5 (4)	5 (3)

BMI = body mass index.
Note: out of total 680 Type 2 DM patients, 4 patients used other glucose lowering drugs and were excluded due to very less number.
[δ]Combination: Patients using more than one type of glucose-lowering drug or using combination tablets.
*Diet: very healthy (high amount of fruit, vegetables, fish and low amount of saturated fat), reasonably healthy (moderately high amount of fruit, vegetables, fish and saturated fat) or unhealthy (low amount of fruit, vegetables, fish and high amount of saturated fat).
[†]Alcohol intake: High (above the recommended limit of ≤14/≤21 weekly drinks for women/men) or low (within the recommended limit).
[‡]Regular exercise: participation in leisure sports or other regular physical activity (yes/no).

Lifestyle behavior according to glucose-lowering drug use

BMI. The crude prevalence of obesity ranged from 19% (insulin and analogues users) to 49% (metformin users). Patients using insulin and analogues were more likely (43%) to have a normal BMI (18.5–24 kg/m2) than any other drug users (*Table 4*). After standardizing for gender and age, the prevalence of obesity was clearly lower in users of sulfonylureas, insulin and analogues, and in those with no glucose-lowering drug use as compared with metformin users (PR: 0.5, 95% CI: 0.4–0-8; PR: 0.4, 95% CI: 0.3–0.7; PR: 0.6, 95% CI: 0.5–0.8, respectively). Prevalence differences for all medication categories as compared with metformin are shown in *Table 5*.

Diet. In general, more metformin users reported eating reasonably healthy diet, compared with other Type 2 DM individuals. After standardizing for gender and age, the PRs for very healthy diet were decreased in users of combination therapy or no glucose-lowering drugs (PR: 0.7, 95% CI: 0.5–1.0) as compared with metformin therapy and were below 1 for other drug groups (*Table 6*).

Alcohol intake. Only 5% of all Type 2 DM patients reported high alcohol intake, and risk estimates associated with drugs were imprecise. However, standardized PRs for high alcohol intake were lower for all medication categories compared with metformin users, ranging from 0.5 (combination users and sulfonylurea users) to 0.8 (inulin and analogue users) (*Table 6*).

Smoking. The overall prevalence of current smokers ranged from 19% (combination therapy users) to 30% (sulfonylurea users). Standardized PRs for smoking were rather similar and close to 1 for most drug users, except for sulfonylurea users among whom smoking tended to be more prevalent (PR: 1.4, 95% CI: 0.9–2.1) compared to metformin users.

Physical exercise. The proportion with no regular physical exercise ranged from 26% (insulin and analogue users) to 34% (metformin users). After standardization, slightly smaller proportions without regular physical exercise were observed among all medication categories as compared with metformin users (PDs

Table 5. Age- and gender-standardized prevalence differences (PDs) of lifestyle factors according to glucose-lowering drugs.

	Metformin	Combination[δ]	Sulfonylureas	Insulin and analogues	No glucose-lowering drug
	PD% (95% CI)	PD% (95% CI)	PD% (95% CI)	PD% (95% CI)	PD% (95% CI)
BMI (kg/m²)					
<18.5	Ref. (1.0)	–	–	–	–
18.5–24	Ref. (1.0)	2.8 (−5.0 to 10.6)	13.0 (3.0 to 23.0)	29.7 (18.8 to 40.6)	16.4 (7.4 to 25.4)
25–29	Ref. (1.0)	0.5 (−10.4 to 11.3)	6.9 (−5.8 to 19.6)	−7.0 (−18.7 to 4.7)	4.7 (−6.5 to 15.9)
≥30	Ref. (1.0)	−1.3 (−13.1 to 10.5)	−22.6 (−35.4 to −9.8)	−27.9 (−40.1 to −15.6)	−19.2 (−30.9 to −7.6)
Diet*					
Unhealthy	Ref. (1.0)	−1.6 (−8.5 to 5.3)	−0.6 (−8.4 to 7.2)	2.3 (−5.9 to 10.6)	2.8 (−4.7 to 10.3)
Reasonably healthy	Ref. (1.0)	9.6 (−2.2 to 21.3)	1.1 (−12.3 to 14.5)	−1.6 (−14.9 to 11.8)	3.3 (−8.8 to 15.5)
Very healthy	Ref. (1.0)	−9.8 (−20.4 to 0.8)	−4.7 (−17.1 to 7.6)	−2.3 (−14.4 to 9.8)	−10.0 (−20.8 to 0.9)
Alcohol†					
High	Ref. (1.0)	−3.8 (−9.4 to 1.9)	−3.5 (−9.6 to 2.6)	−1.2 (−7.7 to 5.3)	−2.3 (−8.2 to 3.6)
Low	Ref. (1.0)	6.2 (−1.5 to 13.8)	1.6 (−6.7 to 9.9)	2.9 (−5.8 to 11.6)	4.4 (−3.4 to 12.2)
Smoking					
Current	Ref. (1.0)	−5.2 (−14.6 to 4.2)	9.4 (−2.1 to 21.0)	2.9 (−8.5 to 14.2)	1.3 (−8.7 to 11.2)
Former	Ref. (1.0)	4.6 (−6.2 to 15.5)	−5.8 (−18.0 to 6.3)	−0.6 (−12.8 to 11.6)	−1.4 (−12.5 to 9.7)
Never	Ref. (1.0)	−3.7 (−14.1 to 6.7)	−5.6 (−17.6 to 6.3)	−1.9 (−13.8 to 10.1)	−3.4 (−14.1 to 7.3)
Regular physical exercise‡					
Yes	Ref. (1.0)	1.8 (−9.5 to 13.1)	−3.0 (−15.8 to 9.9)	5.1 (−7.4 to 17.7)	1.9 (−9.7 to 13.4)
No	Ref. (1.0)	−6.5 (−17.6 to 4.7)	−2.7 (−15.4 to 9.9)	−9.2 (−21.3 to 3.0)	−4.0 (−15.4 to 7.4)

BMI = body mass index, CI = confidence interval.
[δ]Combination: Patients using more than one type of glucose-lowering drug or using combination tablets.
*Diet: very healthy (high amount of fruit, vegetables, fish and low amount of saturated fat), reasonably healthy (moderately high amount of fruit, vegetables, fish and saturated fat) or unhealthy (low amount of fruit, vegetables, fish and high amount of saturated fat).
†Alcohol intake: High (above the recommended limit of ≤14/≤21 weekly drinks for women/men) or low (within the recommended limit).
‡Regular exercise: participation in leisure sports or other regular physical activity (yes/no).

ranging from −2.7 to −9.2) (*Table 5*), with all PRs below 1 (*Table 6*).

Discussion

Main findings

This questionnaire-based public health survey contributes to the knowledge of how lifestyle choices differ according to use of glucose-lowering drugs. Patients with prevalent Type 2 DM were substantially more obese than individuals without diabetes, but otherwise reported to have a healthier lifestyle. Lifestyle characteristics appeared to differ between users of different glucose-lowering drugs. Metformin use was associated with adverse lifestyle factors, including higher obesity prevalence than other drugs user, and with a tendency towards higher alcohol intake and less physical exercise. Additionally, sulfonylurea use was associated with more current tobacco smoking, whereas insulin use was associated with less adverse lifestyle factors, including lowest BMI and highest physical exercise rates among the different glucose-lowering drug users.

Comparison with other studies

Our results are partly in line with previous findings. Concerning obesity, Cichosz *et al.* reported higher BMI in 100 newly diagnosed Danish Type 2 DM patients compared to 100 age- and gender-matched population controls (30 kg/m^2 vs. 26 kg/m^2) [21]. Recently, 87% of newly diagnosed Danish Type 2 DM patients (median age at diagnosis: 59 years) were found to be either overweight or obese in the prospective DD2 study during 2010–2011, and 65% were obese [22]. Our age- and gender-standardized PR for obesity of 3.2 (95% CI: 2.8–3.6) associated with Type 2 DM versus other individuals is much in line with these figures, thus underlining the reliability of our results.

Results are conflicting from few available studies on other lifestyle habits comparing Type 2 DM and persons without diabetes. Magas *et al.* reported healthier nutritional habits among Type 2 DM patients compared with individuals without diabetes, corroborating the findings from our study [23]. In contrast, Murray *et al.* found that patients with Type 2 DM had lower dietary quality than general population controls as assessed by the Healthy Diet Indicator [24]. Concerning physical activity, we found increased self-reported levels among Type 2 DM patients, which is against the study by Cichosz *et al.* who reported less time spent on moderate to vigorous physical activity among Type 2 DM patients compared with controls without diabetes (34 minutes vs. 62 minutes) [21]. The discrepancies may be related to selection of hospital-based patients with relatively severe Type 2 DM, and/or recruitment of relatively healthy controls, in previous studies as compared with our population-based survey. Alternatively, our study may be hampered by potential information bias among Type 2 DM individuals, as e.g. physical activity was measured by questionnaires whereas Cichosz *et al.* measured it with electronic

Table 6. Age- and gender-standardized prevalence ratios (PRs) of lifestyle factors according to glucose-lowering drugs.

	Metformin	Combination[δ]	Sulfonylureas	Insulin and analogues	No glucose-lowering drug
	PR (95% CI)	PR (95% CI)	PR (95% CI)	PR (95% CI)	PR (95% CI)
BMI (kg/m²)					
<18.5	Ref. (1.0)	–	–	–	–
18.5–24	Ref. (1.0)	1.3 (0.7 to 2.4)	2.2 (1.2 to 4.0)	3.6 (2.0 to 6.5)	2.5 (1.4 to 4.4)
25–29	Ref. (1.0)	1.0 (0.7 to 1.4)	1.2 (0.9 to 1.7)	0.8 (0.5 to 1.2)	1.1 (0.8 to 1.6)
≥30	Ref. (1.0)	1.0 (0.8 to 1.2)	0.5 (0.4 to 0.8)	0.4 (0.3 to 0.7)	0.6 (0.5 to 0.8)
Diet*					
Unhealthy	Ref. (1.0)	0.8 (0.4 to 1.8)	0.9 (0.4 to 2.1)	1.2 (0.6 to 2.6)	1.3 (0.6 to 2.6)
Reasonably healthy	Ref. (1.0)	1.2 (1.0 to 1.4)	1.0 (0.8 to 1.3)	1.0 (0.8 to 1.2)	1.1 (0.9 to 1.3)
Very healthy	Ref. (1.0)	0.7 (0.5 to 1.0)	0.9 (0.6 to 1.3)	0.9 (0.6 to 1.4)	0.7 (0.5 to 1.0)
Alcohol[†]					
High	Ref. (1.0)	0.5 (0.2 to 1.3)	0.5 (0.2 to 1.7)	0.8 (0.3 to 2.3)	0.7 (0.3 to 1.8)
Low	Ref. (1.0)	1.1 (1.0 to 1.2)	1.0 (0.9 to 1.1)	1.0 (0.9 to 1.1)	1.1 (1.0 to 1.2)
Smoking					
Current	Ref. (1.0)	0.8 (0.5 to 1.2)	1.4 (0.9 to 2.1)	1.1 (0.7 to 1.8)	1.1 (0.7 to 1.6)
Former	Ref. (1.0)	1.1 (0.8 to 1.6)	0.8 (0.6 to 1.2)	1.0 (0.7 to 1.4)	1.0 (0.7 to 1.4)
Never	Ref. (1.0)	0.9 (0.7 to 1.2)	0.9 (0.6 to 1.2)	1.0 (0.7 to 1.3)	0.9 (0.7 to 1.2)
Regular physical exercise[‡]					
Yes	Ref. (1.0)	1.0 (0.9 to 1.2)	1.0 (0.8 to 1.2)	1.1 (0.9 to 1.3)	1.0 (0.9 to 1.2)
No	Ref. (1.0)	0.8 (0.6 to 1.2)	0.9 (0.6 to 1.4)	0.7 (0.5 to 1.1)	0.9 (0.6 to 1.3)

BMI = body mass index, CI = confidence interval, Ref = reference.
[δ]Combination: Patients using more than one type of glucose-lowering drug or using combination tablets.
*Diet: very healthy (high amount of fruit, vegetables, fish and low amount of saturated fat), reasonably healthy (moderately high amount of fruit, vegetables, fish and saturated fat) or unhealthy (low amount of fruit, vegetables, fish and high amount of saturated fat).
[†]Alcohol intake: High (above the recommended limit of ≤14/≤21 weekly drinks for women/men) or low (within the recommended limit).
[‡]Regular exercise: participation in leisure sports or other regular physical activity (yes/no).

devices [21]. Finally, when comparing different Type 2 DM populations it must be kept in mind that population levels of obesity, smoking, alcohol intake etc. vary substantially between European countries [25], which is likely to affect proportions of unhealthy lifestyle habits in people with Type 2 DM as well.

Our findings corroborate previous findings of metformin users having the highest obesity prevalence and higher occurrence of several other unhealthy traits than other Type 2 DM patients do. Metformin is the recommended first-line drug for Type 2 DM patients with obesity [26], and many of our metformin users had a short history of diabetes with relatively little time for effective lifestyle changes. Our results are similar to the prevalence of obesity (54%) observed in metformin users in the United Kingdom Prospective Diabetes Study (UKPDS) [27], and slightly lower than the current obesity prevalence of about 60% in newly diagnosed Type 2 DM patients enrolled in the Danish DD2 study [22] of whom 59% are started with metformin monotherapy within the first year [28]. A large study based on the Swedish National Diabetes Register involving more than 51,000 Type 2 DM patients reported similar observation, with users of metformin-containing therapies having shortest duration of diabetes and higher mean BMI (30 to 32 kg/m^2) than users of other oral glucose-lowering drugs or insulin (27 to 28 kg/m^2) [29]. Of note, the Swedish study found much lower Type 2 DM smoking prevalence during 2004–2010 (14%) than observed in our data in 2006 (24%) [24]. In another Danish study of patients hospitalized with ischemic stroke, Horsdal *et al.* [9] reported a smoking prevalence of 27% in patients who had diabetes diagnosis, with patients on metformin therapy smoking most. An Italian study reported no substantial difference in the prevalence of smokers in metformin users (21%), sulfonylurea users (21%) and insulin users (22%) [30]. In contrast to our results, the study from Sweden found lower prevalence of smokers (12%) in sulfonylurea users as compared with metformin users (17%) [24], whereas the UKPDS reported higher prevalence of smokers in insulin users (39%) compared with metformin users (25%) [27].

Concerning alcohol intake, the distribution and pattern seen in our study was similar to findings in a recent Danish study of diabetes patients with ischemic stroke by Horsdal *et al.* [9], who reported 5.2% of all Type 2 DM patients and 7.5% of metformin users having higher alcohol consumption than recommended. Concerning physical exercise, we did not find any material difference between level of physical exercise among different medication users, which is in contrast to results reported by Ekstrom *et al.*, who reported higher prevalence of physical activity (≥3 hrs/week) in patients using metformin (76%), compared to sulfonylurea users (70%) [29].

Strengths and limitations

Strengths of this study include the availability of detailed lifestyle data for a large and randomly selected population-based sample included in a public health survey; and availability of additional information from independent population-based and highly valid medical registries [14,16] for assessment of drug use and comorbidity, reducing the risk of recall or investigator bias. The response rate of 69% in the "How are you?" survey is rather high for a questionnaire study, and the 3.2% prevalence of Type 2 DM in our survey population is close to the national prevalence of 3.9% for diabetes in Denmark reported for the year of the survey in The Danish National Diabetes Register [31]. National public health surveys similar to the "How are you" are consecutively carried out every four years in all regions of Denmark, and are generally considered valid and of high quality [32]. As in most similar survey studies, people who choose to participate in a survey may have a different risk profile and may be in better health than those who decline. However, this probably applies for both Type 2 DM patients with different therapies and other individuals and is unlikely to bias the relative estimates in our study. Furthermore, as information on lifestyle factors was self-reported, we cannot rule out social desirability bias and it is possible that unhealthy lifestyles were underreported, which may potentially have led to an underestimation of unhealthy lifestyle in Type 2 DM. For instance, energy intake is underreported in persons with obesity and Type 2 DM [33], potentially due to external pressure to confirm to nutritional recommendations [34], and this might also hold true for other lifestyle risk behaviors. On the other hand, self-administered surveys are generally considered to be more suitable for sensitive questions on health status, as compared with direct interview surveys [35]. Additionally, in the questionnaire, the survey administrators aimed to minimise social desirability bias by asking several questions on the same topic, but from different perspectives. Another limitation of our study is its cross-sectional design, which implies uncertainty whether diagnosis of Type 2 DM or use of specific glucose-lowering drugs preceded lifestyle changes or vice versa. But, the main objective of our study was to describe differences in lifestyle behavior among people with and without Type 2 DM, and its association with current use of specific glucose-lowering drugs, and not to make inferences about causal mechanisms. Finally, inclusion of prevalent cases of Type 2 DM might have biased our results, however our estimates from sensitivity analyses did not change even after restricting the results among patients who were recently diagnosed.

Large database studies that examine the prognostic effect of Type 2 DM or glucose-lowering therapy will often be based on historical data and include a mixture of prevalent and incident Type 2 DM and drug users [36,37]. Thus, we believe our data are useful and important to evaluate confounding in such studies, in which lifestyle factors are often not available.

Conclusions

In conclusion, among participants in a large Danish population survey, patients with Type 2 DM were substantially more obese than other individuals, but otherwise reported a similar or healthier lifestyle after controlling for age and gender differences. Patients treated with metformin generally presented high BMI and tended to have less physical exercise and increased alcohol intake, whereas insulin users reported the lowest BMI and highest physical exercise. Patients on sulfonylureas tended to smoke more than other drug users. These estimates may be useful in external adjustment for unmeasured confounding in future database studies [10].

Supporting Information

Appendix S1 World Health Organization International Classification of Diseases 8th Edition (ICD-8) and 10th Edition (ICD-10) codes, and Anatomical Therapeutical Chemical classification system (ATC) codes used in this study.

Acknowledgments

We would like to thank all the participants of "*Hvordan har du det?*"/ "How are you?" survey who helped us in conducting this study by completing the questionnaires.

Author Contributions

Conceived and designed the experiments: SPU FBL AM ES RWT. Performed the experiments: SPU. Analyzed the data: SPU AM ES RWT. Wrote the paper: SPU AM ES FBL RWT.

References

1. Shaw JE, Sicree RA, Zimmet PZ (2010) Global estimates of the prevalence of diabetes for 2010 and 2030. Diabetes Res Clin Pract 87(1): 4–14.
2. Thomsen R, Mor A (2012) Diabetes and risk of community-acquired respiratory tract infection, urinary tract infections, and bacteraemia: A review. Open Infect Dis J 6(Suppl 1: M1): 27–39.
3. Emerging Risk Factors Collaboration, Seshasai SR, Kaptoge S, Thompson A, Di Angelantonio E, et al. (2011) Diabetes mellitus, fasting glucose, and risk of cause-specific death. N Engl J Med 364(9): 829–841.
4. Tabak A, Akbaraly T, Batty G, Kivimaki M (2014) Depression and type 2 diabetes: A causal association? Lancet Diabetes Endocrinol 2014; 2(3): 236–245.
5. Nwaneri C, Cooper H, Bowen-Jones D (2013) Mortality in type 2 diabetes mellitus: Magnitude of the evidence from a systematic review and meta-analysis. The British Journal of Diabetes & Vascular Disease 13(4): 192–207.
6. Carstensen B, Witte DR, Friis S (2012) Cancer occurrence in danish diabetic patients: Duration and insulin effects. Diabetologia 55(4): 948–958.
7. Leegaard A, Riis A, Kornum JB, Prahl JB, Thomsen VØ, et al. (2011) Diabetes, glycemic control, and risk of tuberculosis: A population-based case-control study. Diabetes care 34(12): 2530–2535.
8. Garg SK, Maurer H, Reed K, Selagamsetty R (2013) Diabetes and cancer: Two diseases with obesity as a common risk factor. Diabetes Obes Metab [Epub ahead of print]; doi: 10.1111/dom.12124.
9. Horsdal HT, Mehnert F, Rungby J, Johnsen SP (2012) Type of preadmission antidiabetic treatment and outcome among patients with ischemic stroke: A nationwide follow-up study. J Stroke Cerebrovasc Dis 21(8): 717–725.
10. Schneeweiss S (2006) Sensitivity analysis and external adjustment for unmeasured confounders in epidemiologic database studies of therapeutics. Pharmacoepidemiol Drug Saf May; 15(5): 291–303.
11. Laugesen K, Telen Andersen AB, Norgaard M, Nielsen RB, Thomsen RW, et al. (2013) Use of selective serotonin reuptake inhibitors and lifestyle among women of childbearing age: A danish cross-sectional survey. BMJ Open 3(7): 10.1136/bmjopen,2013-003024.
12. Schmidt M, Pedersen L, Sorensen HT (2014) The Danish Civil Registration System as a tool in epidemiology. Eur J Epidemiol 29(8): 541–49.
13. Edwards P, Roberts I, Clarke M, DiGuiseppi C, Pratap S, et al. (2002) Increasing response rates to postal questionnaires: systematic review. BMJ 324(7347): 1183.
14. Larsen F, Nordvig L (2008) Hvordan har du det. Sundhedsprofil for region og kommuner. Accessed on 15.08.2014 from: http://www.cfk.rm.dk/udgivelser/befolkningsundersøgelser.
15. WHO Expert Consultation (2004) Appropriate body-mass index for asian populations and its implications for policy and intervention strategies. Lancet 363(9403): 157–163.
16. Toft U, Kristoffersen LH, Lau C, Borch-Johnsen K, Jorgensen T (2007) The dietary quality score: Validation and association with cardiovascular risk factors: The Inter99 study. Eur J Clin Nutr 61(2): 270–278.
17. Lynge E, Sandegaard JL, Rebolj M (2011) The danish national patient register. Scand J Public Health 39(7 Suppl): 30–33.
18. Ehrenstein V, Antonsen S, Pedersen L (2010) Existing data sources for clinical epidemiology: Aarhus university prescription database. Clin Epidemiol 2: 273–279.
19. Charlson ME, Pompei P, Ales KL, MacKenzie CR (1987) A new method of classifying prognostic comorbidity in longitudinal studies: Development and validation. J Chronic Dis 40(5): 373–383.
20. Thygesen SK, Christiansen CF, Christensen S, Lash TL, Sørensen HT (2011) The predictive value of ICD-10 diagnostic coding used to assess charlson comorbidity index conditions in the population-based danish national registry of patients. BMC Med Res Methodol 11: 83.
21. Cichosz SL, Fleischer J, Hoeyem P, Laugesen E, Poulsen PL, et al. (2013) Objective measurements of activity patterns in people with newly diagnosed type 2 diabetes demonstrate a sedentary lifestyle. Diabet Med 30(9): 1063–1066.

22. Thomsen RW, Nielsen JS, Ulrichsen SP, Pedersen L, Hansen AM, et al. (2012) The danish centre for strategic research in type 2 diabetes (DD2) study: Collection of baseline data from the first 580 patients. Clin Epidemiol 4: 43–48.
23. Magas S, Poljicanin T, Sekerija M, Ajdukovic D, Metelko Z, et al. (2009) Lifestyle habits of croatian diabetic population: Observations from the croatian adult health survey. Coll Antropol 33 Suppl 1: 115–159.
24. Murray AE, McMorrow AM, O'Connor E, Kiely C, Mac Ananey O, et al. (2013) Dietary quality in a sample of adults with type 2 diabetes mellitus in ireland; a cross-sectional case control study. Nutr J 12: 110.
25. Nichols M, Townsend N, Luengo-Fernandez R, Leal J, Gray A, et al. (2012) European Cardiovascular Disease Statistics 2012 edition. European Heart Network, Brussels, European Society of Cardiology, Sophia Antipolis.
26. Inzucchi SE, Bergenstal RM, Buse JB, Diamant M, Ferrannini E, et al. (2012) Management of hyperglycaemia in type 2 diabetes: A patient-centered approach. Position statement of the american diabetes association (ADA) and the european association for the study of diabetes (EASD). Diabetologia 55(6): 1577–1596.
27. UK Prospective Diabetes Study (UKPDS) Group (1998) Effect of intensive blood-glucose control with metformin on complications in overweight patients with type 2 diabetes (UKPDS 34). Lancet 352(9131): 854–865.
28. Mor A, Berencsi K, Svensson E, Rungby J, Nielsen JS, et al. (2014) Abstracts of the 50th EASD Annual Meeting. Diabetologia 57(Suppl 1): S-139, poster no. 321.
29. Ekstrom N, Schioler L, Svensson AM, Eeg-Olofsson K, Miao Jonasson J, et al. (2012) Effectiveness and safety of metformin in 51 675 patients with type 2 diabetes and different levels of renal function: A cohort study from the swedish national diabetes register. BMJ Open 2(4): doi: 10.1136/bmjopen-2012-001076.
30. Bo S, Ciccone G, Rosato R, Villois P, Appendino G, et al. (2012) Cancer mortality reduction and metformin: A retrospective cohort study in type 2 diabetic patients. Diabetes Obes Metab 14(1): 23–29.
31. Carstensen B, Kristensen JK, Ottosen P, Borch-Johnsen K, Steering Group of the National Diabetes Register (2008) The Danish National Diabetes Register: trends in incidence, prevalence and mortality. Diabetologia 51(12): 2187–96.
32. Christensen AI, Ekholm O, Glümer C, Andreasen AH, Hvidberg MF, et al. (2012) The Danish National Health Survey 2010. Study design and respondent characteristics. Scand J Public Health 40(4): 391–97.
33. Samuel-Hodge CD, Fernandez LM, Henriquez-Roldan CF, Johnston LF, Keyserling TC (2004) A comparison of self-reported energy intake with total energy expenditure estimated by accelerometer and basal metabolic rate in african-american women with type 2 diabetes. Diabetes Care 27(3): 663–669.
34. Yannakoulia M (2006) Eating behavior among type 2 diabetic patients: A poorly recognized aspect in a poorly controlled disease. Rev Diabet Stud 3(1): 11–16.
35. de Leeuw E, Hox J, Dillmann D (2008) International handbook of survey methodology. New York: Taylor & Francis Group.
36. Thomsen RW, Riis A, Christensen S, Norgaard M, Sørensen HT (2006) Diabetes and 30-day mortality from peptic ulcer bleeding and perforation: A danish population-based cohort study. Diabetes Care 29(4): 805–810.
37. Christiansen CF, Johansen MB, Christensen S, O'Brien JM, Tonnesen E, et al. (2013) Preadmission metformin use and mortality among intensive care patients with diabetes: A cohort study. Crit Care 17(5): R192.

Impaired Glucose Metabolism in Response to High Fat Diet in Female Mice Conceived by *In Vitro* Fertilization (IVF) or Ovarian Stimulation Alone

Miaoxin Chen[1,2,3], Linda Wu[1], Fang Wu[3,4], Gary A. Wittert[3], Robert J. Norman[1], Rebecca L. Robker[1], Leonie K. Heilbronn[1,3]*

1 Robinson Research Institute, School of Paediatrics and Reproductive Health, The University of Adelaide, Adelaide, Australia, 5005, **2** Department of Obstetrics and Gynaecology, The Affiliated Hospital of Guiyang Medical College, Guiyang, China, 550004, **3** Discipline of Medicine, The University of Adelaide, Adelaide, Australia, 5005, **4** Department of Emergency, The Affiliated Hospital of Guiyang Medical College, Guiyang, China, 550004

Abstract

Individuals conceived by *in vitro* fertilization (IVF) may be at increased risk of cardio-metabolic disorders. We recently reported that IVF conceived male mice displayed impaired glucose metabolism at normal and high body weights. In this study, we examined glucose metabolism in mature female C57BL/6J mice that were conceived by natural conception (NC), by ovarian stimulation (OS) or by IVF following chow or high-fat diet (HFD) for 8 weeks. By design, litter size was comparable between groups, but interestingly the birth weight of IVF and OS females was lower than NC females ($p \leq 0.001$). Mature IVF female mice displayed increased fasting glucose as compared to NC and OS mice, irrespective of diet. Mature IVF and OS mice were also more susceptible to the metabolic consequences of high fat diet as compared with NC females, with impaired glucose tolerance ($p \leq 0.01$), whereas peripheral insulin resistance and increased hepatic expression of gluconeogenic genes *Ppargc1α, Pck1* and *G6pc* was observed in IVF mice only ($p < 0.05$). This study suggests that ovarian stimulation alone and IVF program distinct metabolic effects in females, but that high fat diet may be required to unmask these effects. This study adds to the growing body of literature that assisted reproduction procedures may increase the risk of developing type 2 diabetes in an obesity prone environment.

Editor: Martin Young, University of Alabama at Birmingham, United States of America

Funding: This work and LH was supported by ARC Future Fellowship FT120100027. The funders had no role in study design, data collection and analysis, decision to publish, or preparation of the manuscript.

Competing Interests: The authors have declared that no competing interests exist.

* Email: leonie.heilbronn@adelaide.edu.au

Introduction

Adverse prenatal environments are linked to the development of cardiovascular disease and type 2 diabetes in adult human, rodent and sheep offspring [1–4]. In particular, maternal low protein diets fed exclusively during the preimplantation period, resulted in hypertension in mature rats [5,6] and mice [7], as well as cardiovascular dysfunction in mature sheep [8]. *In vitro* fertilization (IVF) exposes the preimplantation embryo to a non-physiological environment during embryo culture, and has been associated with changes in embryo growth and development in animal models and humans [9,10]. An increased risk of metabolic and cardiovascular disease has also been shown in some cohorts of IVF children [11–14] and is documented in mouse models [15–17]. We have recently demonstrated insulin resistance in a small cohort of IVF-conceived young adult men and women, and also showed that these individuals were more susceptible to adverse outcomes of short-term high fat overfeeding versus naturally conceived controls [18]. Similarly, we observed that mature IVF male mice displayed impaired glucose tolerance, under chow and high fat fed conditions [18].

Evidence from humans and animal models shows that male embryos grow faster than female embryos [19], and metabolic differences are generally more profound in male than female offspring in response to an adverse periconceptional maternal environment [4,20]. However, a previous mouse study [16] reported that IVF female offspring were glucose intolerant, but males maintained normal glucose tolerance, although both sexes displayed evidence of insulin resistance.

The process of IVF generally involves not only embryo culture, but ovarian hyperstimulation (OS), which itself has been associated with poorer perinatal outcomes, including low birth weight and preterm birth [21–23]. One study showed that 4-year-old children conceived following stimulated IVF had higher systolic blood pressure versus 4 year IVF children conceived following unstimulated or 'natural IVF' [24]. This study suggests the process of ovarian stimulation may be responsible for at least some of the phenotypes, however these differences may also have been related to the genetics or subfertility of the parent/s. In mature male mice, we recently showed that poor fetal growth could be attributed to ovarian stimulation since birth weight was lower in both OS and

IVF groups, but that differences in glucose metabolism were evident solely in mice generated by IVF and not OS alone [18].

The aim of the current study was to examine whether mature female C57BL/6J mice conceived by IVF or by ovarian stimulation alone have differences in birth weights or glucose metabolism as compared with naturally conceived female mice following chow or high fat diet (HFD) for 8 weeks.

Materials and Methods

Mice

C57BL/6J male and female mice were obtained at 6 weeks of age, and vasectomized (CBA X C57BL/6) F1 male mice were obtained at 8 weeks of age from the Animal Resource Centre (Perth, Western Australia). (CBA X C57BL/6) F1 female mice were obtained at 6 weeks of age from the University of Adelaide Laboratory Animal Services (Adelaide, South Australia). All mice were maintained at 24°C on a 12 h light, 12 h dark cycle, with standard rodent chow diet with 20% of calories from fat, 16% of calories from protein, and 64% of calories from carbohydrate (SF06-105, Specialty Feeds, Glen Forrest, Australia) and water available ad libitum. All mice were acclimatised for 2 weeks on chow before experimentation. All experiments were approved by the University of Adelaide Animal Ethics Committee (Permit Number: M-2011-248) and were conducted in accordance with the Australian Code of Practice for the Care and Use of Animals for Scientific Purposes. All surgeries were performed under Avertin anesthesia, and all efforts were made to minimize suffering.

Generating blastocysts

Mouse blastocysts were generated by natural conception (NC group), or by ovarian hormonal stimulation followed by either mating (OS group) or by IVF and embryo culture (IVF group) as reported [18]. For the NC group, female C57BL/6J mice were placed with male C57BL/6J mice overnight. For the OS group, female C57BL/6J mice were superovulated with intraperitoneal injections of 7.5 IU equine chorionic gonadotropin (Calbiochem, San Diego, CA) followed by 7.5 IU human chorionic gonadotropin (hCG; Calbiochem) 48 h later. Hormone dosages for hyperovulation in mouse strains range from 2.5 to 10 IU [25], and7.5 IU was selected in this study following testing for the optimal dose and as reported previously [26]. After injection with hCG, these females were placed with male C57BL/6J mice overnight. The following morning, female mice (NC and OS groups) with the presence of vaginal plugs were considered pregnant and were humanely sacrificed by cervical dislocation 3 days later. Blastocysts were collected by flushing dissected uteri with pre-warmed HEPES-buffered minimal essential medium (Invitrogen Australia Pty. Ltd.) supplemented with 5 mg/ml human serum albumin (SAGE Media ART-3001, CooperSurgical, USA). Blastocysts from the NC and the OS group were placed in Research Vitro Cleave Media (Cook Medical; QLD, Australia) for no more than 1 hour prior to being transferred to uteri of pseudopregnant mice (see below).

For the IVF group, the ovarian stimulation protocol was the same as for the OS group. *In vitro* fertilization was performed using a modified version of that described previously [27]. At 13 hours after injection with hCG, female C57BL/6J mice were humanely killed by cervical dislocation. Cumulus-oocyte complexes were placed in Research Vitro Fertilization Media (Cook Medical; QLD, Australia) under paraffin oil (Calbiochem) and incubated in a modular incubator chamber at 37°C in 6% CO_2, 5% O_2, 89% N_2 for 5–6 hours with sperm, collected from the cauda epidydimis of male C57BL/6J mice, that had been previously incubated for 1 hour in Research Vitro Fertilization Media (Cook Medical; QLD, Australia) for capacitation. Putative zygotes were placed in Research Vitro Cleave Media (10 zygotes/ 20 µl drop; Cook Medical; QLD, Australia) and checked for fertilization/cleavage the next morning. Embryos (2-cell) were then transferred to a new drop of Research Vitro Cleave Media (Cook Medical; QLD, Australia) and cultured in the modular incubator chamber at 37°C in 6% CO_2, 5% O_2, 89% N_2 for a further 2 days to the blastocyst stage (90–96 hours post-hCG injection).

Blastocysts transfer

Sterility of vasectomized (CBA X C57BL/6) F1 males was confirmed by mating them three times with superovulated (CBA X C57BL/6) F1 females and verifying the absence of embryos in the reproductive tract three days later. To generate pseudopregnant recipient females for embryo transfer, unstimulated (CBA X C57BL/6) F1 female mice were mated with vasectomized (CBA X C57BL/6) F1 male mice and those with copulatory plugs the next morning were considered as day 0.5 of pseudopregnancy. At day 2.5 of pseudopregnancy, totally 7 to 10 blastocysts were transferred to uteri (3–5 blastocysts/horn) of each pseudopregnant mouse anesthetized by i.p. injection of Avertin (0.5 mg/g body weight, Sigma-Aldrich, St. Louis, MO). Analgesia Carprofen (5 mg/kg) (Rimadyl Pfizer) was injected subcutaneously once after the surgery.

Pups and diets

Pups were born on day 19.5 of pregnancy and birth weights measured the next morning. Body weights of pups were measured weekly. Growth rate was calculated as described previously [28]. Pups were weaned at 3 weeks of age onto chow diet or high-fat diet (HFD) for 8 weeks. High-fat diet was made in house using the same recipe as D12492 of Research Diets (New Brunswick, NJ); 60% energy from fat with 91% lard and 9% soybean oil, 20% energy from protein, and 20% energy from carbohydrate. Only one or two female offspring were taken from each litter and were examined for separate tests below in this study.

Glucose and insulin tolerance tests

At 11 weeks of age, mice (n = 6–8) were fasted for 6 hours (from 8 am to 2 pm) and were then challenged with either an intraperitoneal injection of glucose (2 g/kg) or insulin (Actrapid, 0.75 U/kg, Novo Nordisk Australasia) for glucose or insulin tolerance tests respectively. Blood samples were obtained from the tail tip for assessment of glucose at 0, 15, 30, 60, 120 minutes with a glucometer (AccuChek Performa Monitor, Roche Diagnostics, Indianapolis, USA), and for insulin assays at 0, 30, 60, 120 minutes during glucose tests only by ultra-sensitive ELISA kits (Millipore). At 12 weeks of age, mice were sacrificed by cervical dislocation; inguinal fat, parametrial fat, quadriceps and liver were immediately excised and snap-frozen. Tissue samples were frozen at −80°C for later assessment.

Quantitative real-time PCR

Total RNA (n = 6) was extracted from liver and quadriceps using Trizol (Invitrogen, USA) following manufacturer's instructions. The concentration and purity of RNA were determined by Nanodrop (Thermo Fisher Scientific, California, USA). cDNA was synthesized from 1 µg of each RNA sample in 20 µl reactions using the QuantiTect reverse transcription kit (Qiagen, Valencia, CA). Standard control samples (25 ng/µl) pooled from each cDNA sample were diluted to create a standard curve as described previously [29].

Quantitative real-time PCR was performed as described previously [29] in duplicate with the ABI 7500 sequence detection system (Applied Biosystems, Foster City, CA) using TaqMan Fast Universal Master Mix and TaqMan primers and probes listed in Table S1. These genes are key regulators of mitochondrial biogenesis *Ppargc1α* (peroxisome proliferator-activated receptor gamma, coactivator 1 alpha), *Ndufb5* (NADH dehydrogenase (ubiquinone) 1 beta subcomplex, 5) and *Tfam* (Mitochondrial transcription factor A), lipid metabolism *Srebf1* (Sterol regulatory element-binding transcription factor 1) and *Cpt1a* (carnitine palmitoyltransferase 1A), and glucose metabolism *Gck* (Glucokinase), *G6pc* (Glucose-6-phosphatase catalytic subunit) and *Pck1* (phosphoenolpyruvate carboxykinase 1, cytosolic). The NormFinder program was used as described previously [30] and *Hprt* (Hypoxanthine phosphoribosyltransferase) and *Ppia* (Cyclophilin-A) out of 7 potential reference genes were identified as the best combination of reference genes. Data were analyzed using the $2^{-(\Delta\Delta CT)}$ method and expressed as the fold change relative to a control sample, which was selected from the NC group fed on chow and was included in each run.

Western immunoblotting

Liver and quadriceps (n = 4) were lysed and protein concentration was determined by bicinchoninic acid assay (Pierce BCA Protein Assay Kit, Thermo Scientific). Lysates (20 µg protein) were resolved by SDS-PAGE (Criterion XT 10% Bis Tris precast gels, Bio-Rad, Australia) and transferred onto PVDF membranes (criterion gel blotting sandwiches, Bio-Rad, Australia). Membranes were blocked in Tris-buffered saline with Tween 20 (TBST) [10 mM Tris, 150 Mm NaCl, and 0.1% Tween 20 (pH 7.5)] containing 5% (wt/vol) Amersham ECL blocking agent (GE Healthcare Australia Pty. Ltd., NSW, Australia) for 1 hour at room temperature. Membranes were then incubated with primary antibodies overnight at 4°C in 5% bovine serum albumin/TBST. Primary antibodies used were PPARGC1A antibody at 1:1000 (Abcam, MA, USA, Cat. No ab54481) and Total OXPHOS (oxidative phosphorylation) antibody cocktail at 1:1000 (Abcam, Cat. No ab110413). Beta-tubulin antibody at 1:1000 (Cell Signaling, Cat. No 2146) was used as reference protein. Membranes were then washed in TBST and incubated with sheep anti-rabbit IgG alkaline phosphatase conjugated secondary antibody at 1:2500 (Millipore, Temecula, CA) or goat anti-mouse IgG alkaline phosphatase conjugated secondary antibody at 1:2000 (Millipore, Temecula, CA) for 1 hour. ECF substrate (GE Healthcare) was prepared and applied to the blots and then all blots were scanned for fluorescence by the Typhoon Trio$^+$ (GE Healthcare) following the manufacturer's instructions. The band intensity was measured using Image J software (The National Institutes of Health, USA).

Mitochondrial DNA (mtDNA) copy number quantification

DNA were extracted from quadriceps (10 mg) using a QIAamp DNA Micro Kit (Qiagen) following manufacturer's instructions. The concentration and purity of DNA were determined by Nanodrop (Thermo Fisher Scientific). DNA was then used to estimate average mtDNA copy number/cell as described in [31]. The primers for amplification of the mitochondrial gene (12S rRNA) were 5′-CGT TAG GTC AAG GTG TAG CC-3′ and 5′-CCA GAC ACA CTT TCC AGT ATG-3′. The primers for amplification of the nuclear gene (β-actin) were 5′-GGAAAA-GAGCCTCAGGGCAT-3′ and 5′-CTGCCTGACGGCCAGG-3′. PCR amplification of mitochondrial DNA and nuclear DNA was performed simultaneously in each sample in triplicate using SYBR Green PCR Master Mix (Applied Biosystems) and a Rotor-Gene 6000 (Corbett, Valencia, CA) real-time rotary analyzer. The Ct value for β-actin was subtracted from that for 12S rRNA to give the ΔCt value and mtDNA copy number per nuclear genome (two actin gene copies) is calculated as $2\times2^{-(\Delta Ct)}$.

Statistical analysis

Data are shown as mean ± the standard error of the mean, unless otherwise stated. Data were analyzed statistically with SPSS 20 (SPSS, Chicago, IL, USA) and log-transformed for analysis if not normally distributed. Area under the curve(AUC) for glucose and insulin was calculated using the trapezoidal rule [32]. Total OXPHOS protein levels were calculated as the mean of OXPHOS complexes I–V and the relative density of PPARGC1A and total OXPHOS was normalized by beta-tubulin. Single comparisons were performed with one-way ANOVA for treatment effect or two-way ANOVA with diet and treatment as between group factors, whereas time-courses were analyzed by repeated-measures ANOVA and Bonferroni post hoc analysis. Insulin sensitivity assessed by insulin tolerance test is represented by delta glucose levels between baseline (0 minute) and 15 minutes and analyzed by two-way ANOVA, adjusting for baseline glucose levels which were significantly different between groups and were related to the change in glucose. Nonparametric tests (Mann-Whitney U test or Kruskal-Wallis test) were used when required. Chi square tests were used for nominal data. Differences were considered statistically significant at $P<0.05$.

Results

Reduced fetal growth and postnatal catch-up growth in OS and IVF mice

Litter size and sex ratio were not different between groups (Both $P = 0.5$, Table 1). Despite this, birth weight was significantly lower in the IVF and OS versus the NC female pups ($P\leq0.001$, Table 1). This difference in body weight was maintained in the IVF female pups until weaning ($P = 0.04$, Figure 1A), whereas the OS pups displayed rapid catch-up growth as shown by increased growth rate as compared with the NC pups at 1 week ($P = 0.004$; Figure 1 A,B). After weaning, a significantly increased growth rate was observed at 4 weeks of age in IVF vs NC females fed a chow diet and at 8 weeks of age in IVF vs NC and OS females fed a HFD ($P<0.04$, Figure1 D,F). OS mice weighed significantly less than IVF and NC mice from 4 weeks after exposure to HFD ($P<0.01$, Figure 1E). In a subset of animals (n = 4/group), liver weight and adipose tissue fat pads were weighed. As expected, the liver weight ratio was decreased and adipose tissue weight ratio increased in mice that were fed a HFD ($P<0.001$, Figure S1). However, a significantly higher percentage of body weight was in the inguinal and parametrial fat pads in OS and IVF versus NC mice fed HFD ($P\leq0.001$, Figure S1).

Impaired glucose metabolism in OS and IVF female mice following HFD

Fasting glucose was significantly higher in IVF versus NC and OS mice, independently of diet ($P<0.05$, Figure 2A). However, no other different phenotypes were noted in IVF or OS females versus NC females fed a chow diet. HFD increased fasting glucose, fasting insulin, glucose area under curve (AUC), insulin AUC and reduced insulin sensitivity (diet effect, $P<0.05$, Figure 2) and OS and IVF mice were more susceptible to adverse effects of HFD as evidenced by impaired glucose tolerance versus NC mice ($P\leq0.01$, Figure 2E). Insulin sensitivity as assessed by insulin tolerance test was also significantly lower in IVF mice versus NC mice only at

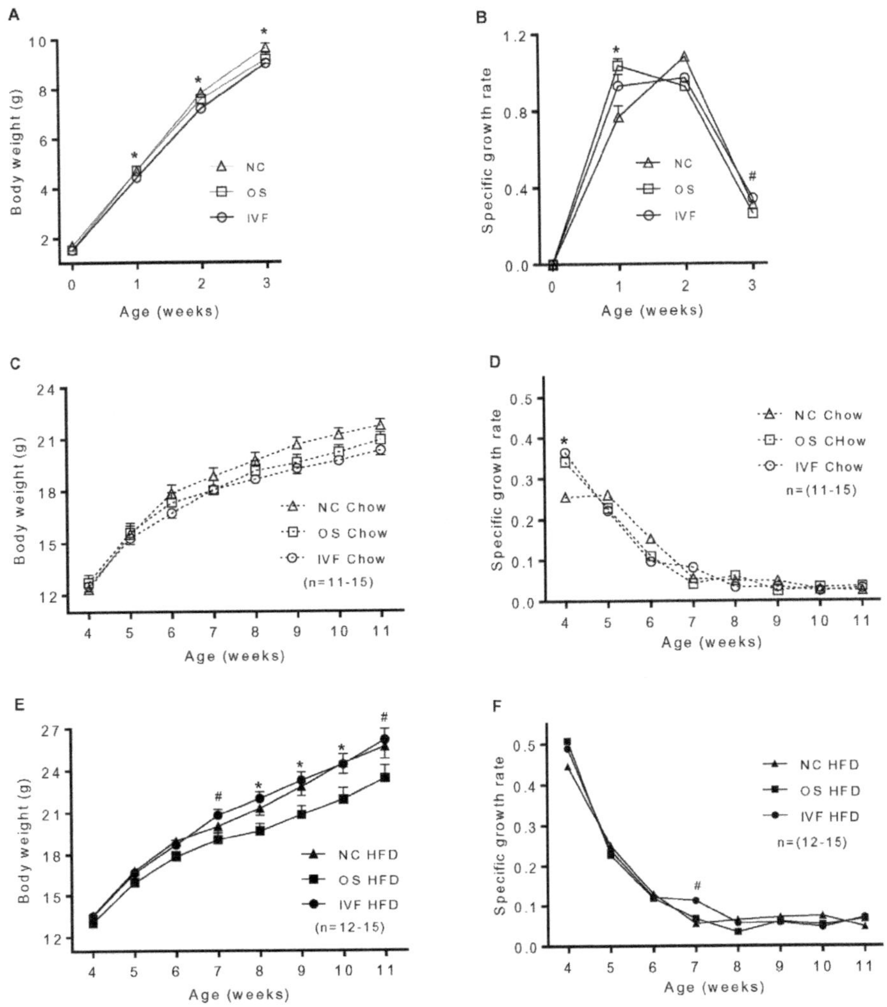

Figure 1. Body weight and growth rate in female mice offspring. Specific growth rate was calculated as follow: (Wn−W(n−1)/W(n−1). W is body weight, and n is age in weeks. (A), *IVF vs NC, P = 0.04; (n = 21–26). (B), *OS vs NC, P = 0.004; #IVF vs OS, P = 0.006. (n = 21–26). (D), Chow: *IVF vs NC, P = 0.03. (E), HFD: #IVF vs OS, P<0.001; *IVF & NC vs OS; P<0.01. (F), HFD: #IVF vs OS & NC, P<0.01.

15 minutes (P<0.001, Figure 2K). Lower fasting insulin (P = 0.03, Figure 2B) and lower insulin AUC was observed in OS mice as compared with NC and IVF mice in response to glucose tolerance test (P<0.05, Figure 2H).

We also examined the mRNA expression of genes involved in glucose and lipid metabolism in liver. HFD increased the expression of the genes *Srebf1, Cpt1a, Ppargc1α, Tfam,* and *Gck*, but not gluconeogenic genes *Pck1* and *G6pc* (Figure 3). Significant differences were also noted between groups, with increased hepatic expression of *Ppargc1α* and *Pck1* in IVF mice and decreased expression of *Cpt1a* in OS mice, independently of diet. The expression of *G6pc* and *Tfam* was also higher in IVF versus NC or OS mice respectively (Figure 3). However, no difference was observed in protein levels of mitochondrial biogenesis markers PPARGC1A and total OXPHOS in liver (Figure 4). These genes were also assessed in quadriceps muscle from animals fed HFD. No difference was observed in either gene expression or mitochondrial DNA copy number or protein levels of these makers in quadriceps muscle (data not shown).

Discussion

Children conceived by IVF have some evidence of altered cardio-metabolic outcomes [14,33]. We recently showed that IVF young adult humans displayed peripheral insulin resistance [18], an early risk factor in the development of type 2 diabetes [34,35], and significantly greater increases in systolic blood pressure when exposed to a high fat overfeeding diet for 3 days [18]. Furthermore, we showed that male C57BL6/J mice conceived by IVF displayed hyperglycemia and impaired glucose tolerance when fed chow or HFD [18]. In this study, we now report that female mice conceived by IVF also exhibited higher fasting glucose levels, independently of diet. However, IVF female mice fed a chow diet did not display any other adverse risk factors, whereas impaired glucose tolerance was unmasked by HFD, but this was apparent in both IVF and OS females. This study suggests that manipulation of the preimplantation embryo may predispose mature female mice to increased risk of developing type 2 diabetes, in an obesogenic environment.

In this study, birth weight was lower in female mice conceived either by ovarian stimulation alone or by IVF. This is consistent with the results we have recently reported in male mice [18].

Table 1. Litter characteristics and birth weight of female pups.

Group	Pups	Litters	Litter size	Range of litter size	Sex ratio(M/F)	Females	Birth weight(g)
NC	49	8	6.2± 0.6	4–8	1:1.33	28	1.69 ± 0.04
OS	51	7	7.4± 0.7	5–10	1:0.82	23	1.54 ± 0.03$^{\Delta}$
IVF	54	8	6.9± 0.5	5–9	1:1.08	28	1.52 ± 0.03*

NC: natural conception; OS: ovarian stimulation; IVF: in vitro fertilization. Data presented as mean ± SEM; Litter size (P = 0.5); M/F: male/female (P = 0.5); The litter is used for comparisons of birth weight;
$^{\Delta}$OS vs NC, P = 0.001,
*IVF vs NC, P<0.001.

Lower fetal weights have also been reported in mice conceived following ovarian stimulation at day 14 and day 18 of gestation [36,37]. Lower birth weights are also reported in human infants conceived by ovarian stimulation alone or by IVF after either fresh or frozen embryo transfer as compared with naturally conceived infants [21,22,38–43], although fresh embryo transfer further increases the risk of low birth weight and preterm birth in human infants as compared with frozen-thaw embryo transfer cycles [40,42,43]. In this study, while female donor mice for both the IVF and OS groups underwent ovarian hyperstimulation, the blastocysts for the OS group were developed in a hormonally stimulated reproductive tract prior to transfer, whereas the IVF blastocysts were developed *in vitro* in culture media prior to transfer. Previous studies have shown that both stimulated oviductal and *in vitro* culture environments are suboptimal and can impair embryo and fetal development in mice [44,45].The mechanism underlying the association between ovarian stimulation and low birth weight was not a focus of this study. However, since the embryos were transferred to unstimulated recipients in this study, this suggests that differences may be due to impaired oocyte quality and/or subsequent embryonic and fetal development, rather than changes in endometrial receptivity [36,37,44,46]. Further study is needed to determine if lower doses of gonadotropin result in less severe phenotypes in C57BL/6J mice and whether the OS phenotype is altered if kept in the stimulated uterine environment rather than undergoing embryo transfer.

Accelerated postnatal catch-up growth in infancy and early childhood are independent risk factors for cardiovascular disease and type 2 diabetes in humans [1,2,47–51] and rodents [52–54]. Accelerated weight gain in late infancy has been reported in IVF children as compared with spontaneously conceived children born to subfertile parents, and early childhood growth was also related to increased blood pressure in IVF children [55]. In this study, both OS and IVF female pups displayed catch-up growth. Of note, catch-up growth was observed in OS females soon after birth but occurred much later in IVF females after weaning, and OS mice on HFD failed to maintain this increase after 4 weeks on HFD. Sequential assessments of growth axis factors such as growth hormone, IGF, and ghrelin are needed during the early growth phase to tease out potential mechanisms underlying these differences in weight gain. Interestingly, and unlike our findings in males [18], both OS and IVF females fed on HFD displayed relatively higher adiposity, although this was only examined in 4 animals per group and thus should be confirmed with greater numbers and by other assessments of body composition. Further, assessments of food intake and energy metabolism should also be included in future studies to determine mechanisms underlying this difference in energy needs between groups. In this study, we also observed that IVF and OS mice displayed impaired glucose tolerance following HFD. Scott et al. also reported impaired glucose tolerance, and a compensatory insulin response to glucose in IVF versus naturally conceived B6C3F1 female mice at 8 weeks of age, even in response to chow diet [16]. Two more recent studies reported no differences in glucose tolerance between chow fed CF1xB6D2F1 or chow and HFD fed C57BL/6J female mice conceived by ovarian stimulation alone versus IVF [56,57], whereas glucose intolerance was observed in IVF females when embryos were cultured in more stressful conditions as compared with OS females, but notably these studies did not test relative to an unstimulated naturally conceived control mouse, as was performed in this study by including the NC group.

Interestingly, the pathways underlying these differences in glucose tolerance may be distinct between OS and IVF groups. In OS females, impaired glucose tolerance was observed in

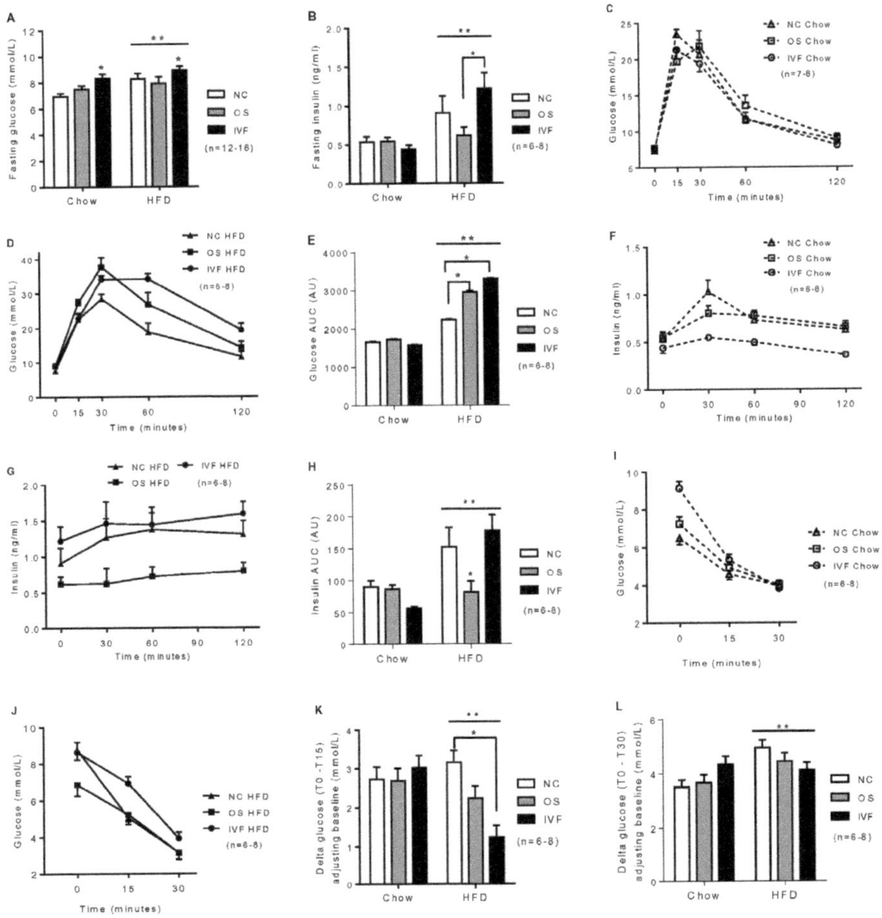

Figure 2. Fasting glucose, fasting insulin, glucose (C–E) and insulin (F–H) response to intraperitoneal glucose tolerance tests, and insulin tolerance tests (I–K) in female mice offspring. AU, arbitrary unit. (A), *IVF vs NC, P = 0.01; IVF vs OS, P = 0.03; **Diet effect, P = 0.01. (B), *IVF vs OS, P = 0.03; **Diet effect, P = 0.002. (E), *OS vs NC, P = 0.01; IVF vs NC, P<0.001; **Diet effect, P<0.001. (H), *OS vs IVF, P = 0.001,OS vs NC, P = 0.04; **Diet effect, P<0.001. (I–J), The glucose levels at T0 and T30 following insulin i.p. (K), Insulin sensitivity is represented by delta glucose adjusting baseline (T0–T15);*IVF vs NC, P<0.001; **Diet effect, P = 0.02. (L), Insulin sensitivity is represented by delta glucose adjusting baseline (T0–T30); **Diet effect, P = 0.01.

conjunction with lower insulin, possibly indicating impaired β-cell function. However, we did not collect the pancreas, and thus cannot assess islet numbers or size, nor investigate the insulin response to IV or oral GTT. In IVF females fed a HFD, peripheral insulin resistance as assessed by insulin tolerance test was noted and likely responsible for the impaired glucose tolerance. These data supports our previous findings of peripheral insulin resistance in IVF young adults, of whom 70% were women, and in this group we did not detect any differences in β-cell secretory capacity in response to intravenous injection of glucose [18].

We recently showed that only IVF, and not OS, conceived male mice displayed impaired glucose intolerance versus NC, and that this was observed following either chow or HFD [18]. This difference between sexes indicates that sexual dimorphism may exist in offspring conceived by IVF. Sex differences in phenotypes have been identified in several developmental programming models of adult diseases both in humans and animals [4,20]. Some of these differences may be because males grow faster than females in utero and thus are more vulnerable to malnutrition [58]. Furthermore, marked differences in the gene expression patterns are noted in male and female preimplantation embryos [59].

Uniquely, higher fasting blood glucose was observed in IVF females on chow and high fat diet, which we also observed in IVF males generated from the same litters [18]. We speculate this may be due to increased hepatic gluconeogenesis, since we observed increased expression of key gluconeogenic genes including *Ppargc1α*, *Pck1* and *G6pc* in the livers of IVF females. *Ppargc1α* is a key regulator of hepatic gluconeogenesis that contributes to circulating hyperglycemia [60], and liver-specific *Ppargc1α*-deficient mice have reduced *Pck1* and *G6pc* expression and mild hypoglycaemia [61]. IVF male mice displayed increased hepatic expression of key lipogenic gene *Srebf1* and impaired hepatic insulin sensitivity as evidenced by reduced AKT phosphorylation in liver following an insulin stimulation test [18]. Thus, whilst male and female IVF offspring both display hyperglycemia, this may be due to alternative activation of *Ppargc1α* or *Srebf1* pathway[62]. However, this result requires further testing. Importantly, our findings support previous results in humans that have shown higher fasting glucose levels in pubertal IVF children that could not be explained by environmental factors, including parental subfertility [12]. Taken together, the data suggests that *in vitro* culture induces profound alterations of metabolic regulatory pathways compared to the in vivo hormonally stimulated tract environment.

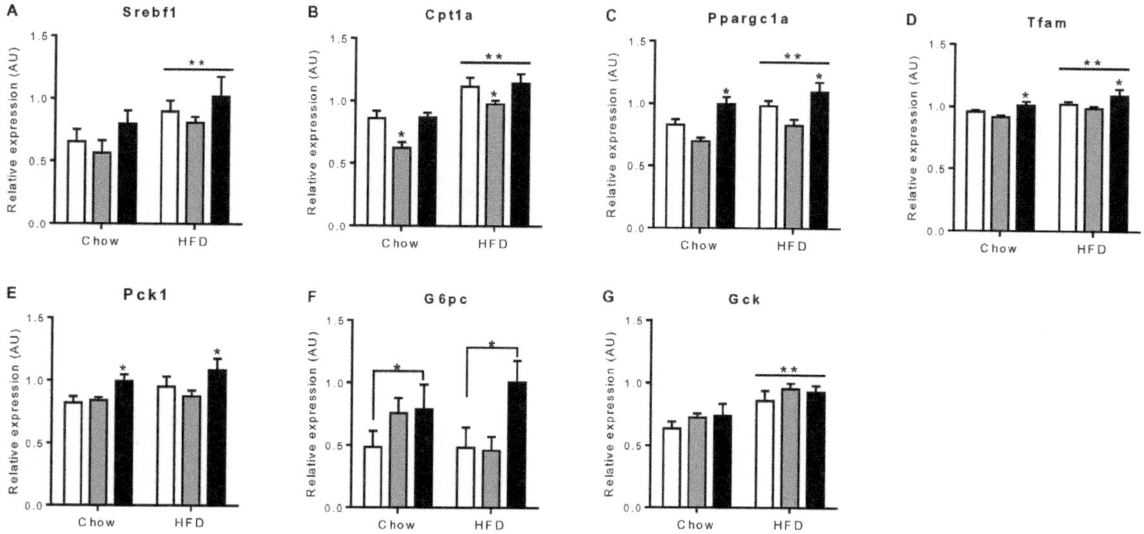

Figure 3. Hepatic gene expression of female mice offspring. White bars represent the NC group, grey bars represent the OS group and black bars represent the IVF group (n = 6). (A), **Diet effect, P = 0.009. (B), *OS vs IVF & NC, P<0.01; **Diet effect: P<0.001. (C), *IVF vs NC, P = 0.03; IVF vs OS, P<0.001; **Diet effect, P = 0.005. (D), *IVF vs OS, P = 0.003; **Diet effect, P = 0.003. (E), *IVF vs NC, P = 0.05; IVF vs OS, P = 0.02. (F), *IVF vs NC, P = 0.03. (G), **Diet effect, P<0.001.

To our knowledge, only three studies have examined the long term effects of IVF on glucose metabolism in mouse models to date [16,56,57]. However, one group did not control for litter size or genetics between IVF and control groups, which may have impacted the outcomes. Two more recent studies compared IVF to models of ovarian stimulation alone [56,57], which we and others have shown impairs fetal growth, and may also alter metabolic outcomes [36,37,44,46], and one study utilized outbred mice, which are less suited for metabolic studies [57]. In this study, we performed blastocyst transfer in all three groups so that we could control for any effects of embryo transfer, and more importantly enabled matching of litter size, as well as maternal environment across all three groups.

In conclusion, ovarian stimulation reduced fetal growth in utero, and when coupled with accelerated catch up growth and HFD, results in adiposity and impaired glucose tolerance. Further, *in vitro* culture of embryos uniquely increased fasting glucose and markers of hepatic gluconeogenesis, suggesting that IVF in particular, may increase the risk of developing type 2 diabetes in adulthood.

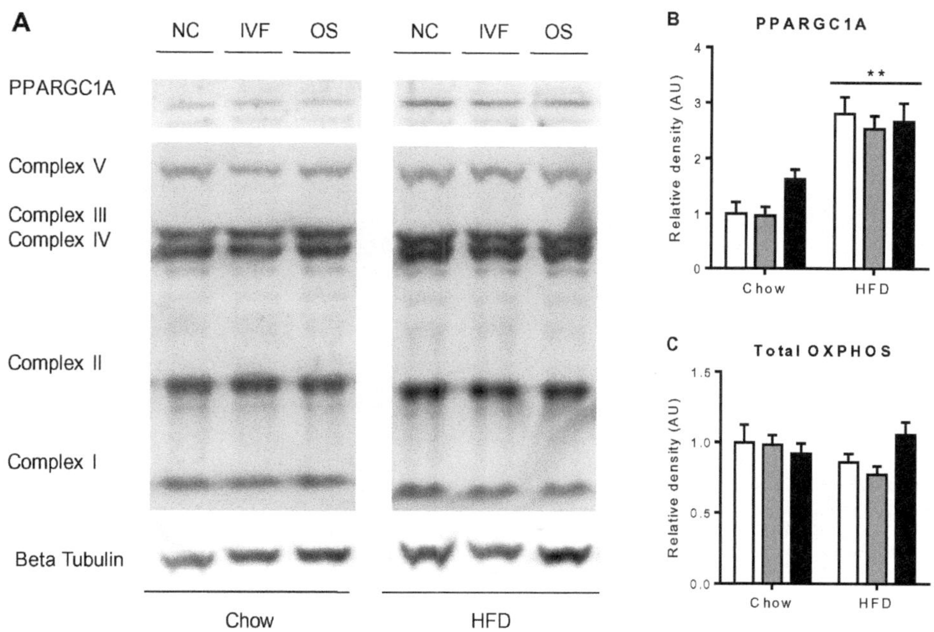

Figure 4. Protein levels of mitochondrial biogenesis markers PPARGC1A and total oxidative phosphorylation (OXPHOS) in liver of female mice offspring. White bars represent NC group, grey bars represent OS group and black bars represent IVF group (n = 4). (A), representative blots of PPARGC1A, OXPHOS complexes I–V and beta-tubulin. (B), **Diet effect, P<0.001.

Supporting Information

Figure S1 Tissue weight ratio (normalized to body weight) in female mice offspring. **Diet effect, P<0.001. (A) Liver; (B), Inguinal fat, *OS vs NC, P = 0.02; IVF vs NC, P = 0.001; (C), Parametrial fat, *OS vs NC, P = 0.01; IVF vs NC, P<0.001.

Table S1 TaqMan primers and probes used for gene expression analysis.

Acknowledgments

The authors thank Kylie Lange, Centre of Research Excellence in Translating Nutritional Science to Good Health, The University of Adelaide, for her expert statistical advice; Anita Peura, Discipline of Obstetrics & Gynaecology, The University of Adelaide, and George Hatzinikolas, Discipline of Medicine, The University of Adelaide, for their technical assistance in the study; and Julie Owens, School of Paediatrics and Reproductive Health, The University of Adelaide, for her critical comments in the study.

Author Contributions

Conceived and designed the experiments: RR LH. Performed the experiments: MC LW FW. Analyzed the data: MC GW RN RR LH. Contributed reagents/materials/analysis tools: MC LW FW. Contributed to the writing of the manuscript: MC GW RN RR LH.

References

1. Barker DJ, Hales CN, Fall CH, Osmond C, Phipps K, et al. (1993) Type 2 (non-insulin-dependent) diabetes mellitus, hypertension and hyperlipidaemia (syndrome X): relation to reduced fetal growth. Diabetologia 36: 62–67.
2. Barker DJ, Winter PD, Osmond C, Margetts B, Simmonds SJ (1989) Weight in infancy and death from ischaemic heart disease. Lancet 2: 577–580.
3. Edwards LJ, McMillen IC (2002) Periconceptional nutrition programs development of the cardiovascular system in the fetal sheep. Am J Physiol Regul Integr Comp Physiol 283: R669–679.
4. Aiken CE, Ozanne SE (2013) Sex differences in developmental programming models. Reproduction 145: R1–13.
5. Kwong WY, Wild AE, Roberts P, Willis AC, Fleming TP (2000) Maternal undernutrition during the preimplantation period of rat development causes blastocyst abnormalities and programming of postnatal hypertension. Development 127: 4195–4202.
6. Kwong WY, Miller DJ, Wilkins AP, Dear MS, Wright JN, et al. (2007) Maternal low protein diet restricted to the preimplantation period induces a gender-specific change on hepatic gene expression in rat fetuses. Mol Reprod Dev 74: 48–56.
7. Watkins AJ, Ursell E, Panton R, Papenbrock T, Hollis L, et al. (2008) Adaptive responses by mouse early embryos to maternal diet protect fetal growth but predispose to adult onset disease. Biol Reprod 78: 299–306.
8. Gardner DS, Pearce S, Dandrea J, Walker R, Ramsay MM, et al. (2004) Peri-implantation undernutrition programs blunted angiotensin II evoked baroreflex responses in young adult sheep. Hypertension 43: 1290–1296.
9. Fleming TP, Kwong WY, Porter R, Ursell E, Fesenko I, et al. (2004) The embryo and its future. Biol Reprod 71: 1046–1054.
10. Santos MA, Kuijk EW, Macklon NS (2010) The impact of ovarian stimulation for IVF on the developing embryo. Reproduction 139: 23–34.
11. Ceelen M, van Weissenbruch MM, Roos JC, Vermeiden JP, van Leeuwen FE, et al. (2007) Body composition in children and adolescents born after in vitro fertilization or spontaneous conception. J Clin Endocrinol Metab 92: 3417–3423.
12. Ceelen M, van Weissenbruch MM, Vermeiden JP, van Leeuwen FE, Delemarre-van de Waal HA (2008) Cardiometabolic differences in children born after in vitro fertilization: follow-up study. J Clin Endocrinol Metab 93: 1682–1688.
13. Sakka SD, Loutradis D, Kanaka-Gantenbein C, Margeli A, Papastamataki M, et al. (2010) Absence of insulin resistance and low-grade inflammation despite early metabolic syndrome manifestations in children born after in vitro fertilization. Fertil Steril 94: 1693–1699.
14. Scherrer U, Rimoldi SF, Rexhaj E, Stuber T, Duplain H, et al. (2012) Systemic and pulmonary vascular dysfunction in children conceived by assisted reproductive technologies. Circulation 125: 1890–1896.
15. Rexhaj E, Paoloni-Giacobino A, Rimoldi SF, Fuster DG, Anderegg M, et al. (2013) Mice generated by in vitro fertilization exhibit vascular dysfunction and shortened life span. J Clin Invest 123: 5052–5060.
16. Scott KA, Yamazaki Y, Yamamoto M, Lin Y, Melhorn SJ, et al. (2010) Glucose parameters are altered in mouse offspring produced by assisted reproductive technologies and somatic cell nuclear transfer. Biol Reprod 83: 220–227.
17. Watkins AJ, Platt D, Papenbrock T, Wilkins A, Eckert JJ, et al. (2007) Mouse embryo culture induces changes in postnatal phenotype including raised systolic blood pressure. Proc Natl Acad Sci U S A 104: 5449–5454.
18. Chen M, Wu L, Zhao J, Wu F, Davies MJ, et al. (2014) Altered glucose metabolism in mouse and humans conceived by in-vitro fertilization (IVF). Diabetes doi:10.2337/db14-0103.
19. Mittwoch U (1993) Blastocysts Prepare for the Race to Be Male. Hum Reprod 8: 1550–1555.
20. Grigore D, Ojeda NB, Alexander BT (2008) Sex differences in the fetal programming of hypertension. Gend Med 5 Suppl A: S121–132.
21. Klemetti R, Sevon T, Gissler M, Hemminki E (2010) Health of children born after ovulation induction. Fertil Steril 93: 1157–1168.
22. Pelinck MJ, Hadders-Algra M, Haadsma ML, Nijhuis WL, Kiewiet SM, et al. (2010) Is the birthweight of singletons born after IVF reduced by ovarian stimulation or by IVF laboratory procedures? Reprod Biomed Online 21: 245–251.
23. Ombelet W, Martens G, De Sutter P, Gerris J, Bosmans E, et al. (2006) Perinatal outcome of 12,021 singleton and 3108 twin births after non-IVF-assisted reproduction: a cohort study. Hum Reprod 21: 1025–1032.
24. La Bastide-Van Gemert S, Seggers J, Haadsma ML, Heineman MJ, Middelburg KJ, et al. (2014) Is ovarian hyperstimulation associated with higher blood pressure in 4-year-old IVF offspring? Part II: an explorative causal inference approach. Hum Reprod 29: 510–517.
25. Nagy A, Gersenstein M, Behringer R (2003) Manipulating the Mouse Embryo: A Laboratory Manual 3rd edition. Cold Spring Harbor Laboratory Press, New York, USA.
26. Le F, Wang LY, Wang N, Li L, Li le J, et al. (2013) In vitro fertilization alters growth and expression of Igf2/H19 and their epigenetic mechanisms in the liver and skeletal muscle of newborn and elder mice. Biol Reprod 88: 75.
27. Wu LL, Russell DL, Norman RJ, Robker RL (2012) Endoplasmic reticulum (ER) stress in cumulus-oocyte complexes impairs pentraxin-3 secretion, mitochondrial membrane potential (DeltaPsi m), and embryo development. Mol Endocrinol 26: 562–573.
28. Wander PL, Boyko EJ, Leonetti DL, McNeely MJ, Kahn SE, et al. (2013) Change in visceral adiposity independently predicts a greater risk of developing type 2 diabetes over 10 years in Japanese Americans. Diabetes Care 36: 289–293.
29. Chen M, Macpherson AM, Owens JA, Wittert GA, Heilbronn LK (2012) Obesity alone or with type 2 diabetes is associated with tissue specific alterations in DNA methylation and gene expression of PPARGC1A and IGF2. J Diab Res Clin Met 1: 16.
30. Andersen CL, Jensen JL, Orntoft TF (2004) Normalization of real-time quantitative reverse transcription-PCR data: a model-based variance estimation approach to identify genes suited for normalization, applied to bladder and colon cancer data sets. Cancer Res 64: 5245–5250.
31. Aiken CE, Cindrova-Davies T, Johnson MH (2008) Variations in mouse mitochondrial DNA copy number from fertilization to birth are associated with oxidative stress. Reprod Biomed Online 17: 806–813.
32. Matthews JN, Altman DG, Campbell MJ, Royston P (1990) Analysis of serial measurements in medical research. BMJ 300: 230–235.
33. Chen M, Norman RJ, Heilbronn LK (2011) Does in vitro fertilisation increase type 2 diabetes and cardiovascular risk? Curr Diabetes Rev 7: 426–432.
34. Warram JH, Martin BC, Krolewski AS, Soeldner JS, Kahn CR (1990) Slow glucose removal rate and hyperinsulinemia precede the development of type II diabetes in the offspring of diabetic parents. Ann Intern Med 113: 909–915.
35. Lillioja S, Mott DM, Spraul M, Ferraro R, Foley JE, et al. (1993) Insulin resistance and insulin secretory dysfunction as precursors of non-insulin-dependent diabetes mellitus. Prospective studies of Pima Indians. N Engl J Med 329: 1988–1992.
36. Ertzeid G, Storeng R (2001) The impact of ovarian stimulation on implantation and fetal development in mice. Hum Reprod 16: 221–225.
37. Van der Auwera I, D'Hooghe T (2001) Superovulation of female mice delays embryonic and fetal development. Hum Reprod 16: 1237–1243.
38. D'Angelo DV, Whitehead N, Helms K, Barfield W, Ahluwalia IB (2011) Birth outcomes of intended pregnancies among women who used assisted reproductive technology, ovulation stimulation, or no treatment. Fertil Steril 96: 314–320 e312.
39. Pandey S, Shetty A, Hamilton M, Bhattacharya S, Maheshwari A (2012) Obstetric and perinatal outcomes in singleton pregnancies resulting from IVF/ICSI: a systematic review and meta-analysis. Hum Reprod Update 18: 485–503.

40. Pinborg A, Wennerholm UB, Romundstad LB, Loft A, Aittomaki K, et al. (2013) Why do singletons conceived after assisted reproduction technology have adverse perinatal outcome? Systematic review and meta-analysis. Hum Reprod Update 19: 87–104.
41. Gaudoin M, Dobbie R, Finlayson A, Chalmers J, Cameron IT, et al. (2003) Ovulation induction/intrauterine insemination in infertile couples is associated with low-birth-weight infants. Am J Obstet Gynecol 188: 611–616.
42. Pelkonen S, Koivunen R, Gissler M, Nuojua-Huttunen S, Suikkari AM, et al. (2010) Perinatal outcome of children born after frozen and fresh embryo transfer: the Finnish cohort study 1995–2006. Hum Reprod 25: 914–923.
43. Pinborg A, Loft A, Aaris Henningsen AK, Rasmussen S, Andersen AN (2010) Infant outcome of 957 singletons born after frozen embryo replacement: the Danish National Cohort Study 1995–2006. Fertil Steril 94: 1320–1327.
44. Van der Auwera I, Pijnenborg R, Koninckx PR (1999) The influence of in-vitro culture versus stimulated and untreated oviductal environment on mouse embryo development and implantation. Hum Reprod 14: 2570–2574.
45. Kelley RL, Kind KL, Lane M, Robker RL, Thompson JG, et al. (2006) Recombinant human follicle-stimulating hormone alters maternal ovarian hormone concentrations and the uterus and perturbs fetal development in mice. Am J Physiol Endocrinol Metab 291: E761–770.
46. Ertzeid G, Storeng R (1992) Adverse effects of gonadotrophin treatment on pre- and postimplantation development in mice. J Reprod Fertil 96: 649–655.
47. Hales CN, Barker DJ, Clark PM, Cox LJ, Fall C, et al. (1991) Fetal and infant growth and impaired glucose tolerance at age 64. BMJ 303: 1019–1022.
48. Eriksson JG, Forsen T, Tuomilehto J, Osmond C, Barker DJ (2001) Early growth and coronary heart disease in later life: longitudinal study. BMJ 322: 949–953.
49. Bhargava SK, Sachdev HS, Fall CH, Osmond C, Lakshmy R, et al. (2004) Relation of serial changes in childhood body-mass index to impaired glucose tolerance in young adulthood. N Engl J Med 350: 865–875.
50. Ong KK, Dunger DB (2004) Birth weight, infant growth and insulin resistance. Eur J Endocrinol 151 Suppl 3: U131–139.
51. Ong KKL, Ahmed ML, Emmett PM, Preece MA, Dunger DB (2000) Association between postnatal catch-up growth and obesity in childhood: prospective cohort study. BMJ 320: 967–971.
52. Crescenzo R, Samec S, Antic V, Rohner-Jeanrenaud F, Seydoux J, et al. (2003) A role for suppressed thermogenesis favoring catch-up fat in the pathophysiology of catch-up growth. Diabetes 52: 1090–1097.
53. Jimenez-Chillaron JC, Hernandez-Valencia M, Reamer C, Fisher S, Joszi A, et al. (2005) beta-cell secretory dysfunction in the pathogenesis of low birth weight-associated diabetes - A murine model. Diabetes 54: 702–711.
54. Jimenez-Chillaron JC, Hernandez-Valencia M, Lightner A, Faucette RR, Reamer C, et al. (2006) Reductions in caloric intake and early postnatal growth prevent glucose intolerance and obesity associated with low birthweight. Diabetologia 49: 1974–1984.
55. Ceelen M, van Weissenbruch MM, Prein J, Smit JJ, Vermeiden JP, et al. (2009) Growth during infancy and early childhood in relation to blood pressure and body fat measures at age 8–18 years of IVF children and spontaneously conceived controls born to subfertile parents. Hum Reprod 24: 2788–2795.
56. Feuer SK, Liu X, Donjacour A, Lin W, Simbulan RK, et al. (2014) Use of a mouse in vitro fertilization model to understand the developmental origins of health and disease hypothesis. Endocrinology 155: 1956–1969.
57. Donjacour A, Liu X, Lin W, Simbulan R, Rinaudo PF (2014) In vitro fertilization affects growth and glucose metabolism in a sex-specific manner in an outbred mouse model. Biol Reprod 90: 80.
58. Eriksson JG, Kajantie E, Osmond C, Thornburg K, Barker DJ (2010) Boys live dangerously in the womb. Am J Hum Biol 22: 330–335.
59. Bermejo-Alvarez P, Rizos D, Lonergan P, Gutierrez-Adan A (2011) Transcriptional sexual dimorphism during preimplantation embryo development and its consequences for developmental competence and adult health and disease. Reproduction 141: 563–570.
60. Yoon JC, Puigserver P, Chen GX, Donovan J, Wu ZD, et al. (2001) Control of hepatic gluconeogenesis through the transcriptional coactivator PGC-1. Nature 413: 131–138.
61. Lin J, Wu PH, Tarr PT, Lindenberg KS, St-Pierre J, et al. (2004) Defects in adaptive energy metabolism with CNS-linked hyperactivity in PGC-1alpha null mice. Cell 119: 121–135.
62. Finck BN, Kelly DP (2006) PGC-1 coactivators: inducible regulators of energy metabolism in health and disease. J Clin Invest 116: 615–622.

10

Assessment of CD4+ T Cell Responses to Glutamic Acid Decarboxylase 65 Using DQ8 Tetramers Reveals a Pathogenic Role of GAD65 121–140 and GAD65 250–266 in T1D Development

I-Ting Chow[1], Junbao Yang[1], Theresa J. Gates[1], Eddie A. James[1], Duy T. Mai[1], Carla Greenbaum[1], William W. Kwok[1,2]*

1 Benaroya Research Institute at Virginia Mason, Seattle, WA, United States of America, **2** Department of Medicine, University of Washington, Seattle, WA, United States of America

Abstract

Susceptibility to type 1 diabetes (T1D) is strongly associated with MHC class II molecules, particularly HLA-DQ8 (DQ8: DQA1*03:01/DQB1*03:02). Monitoring T1D-specific T cell responses to DQ8-restricted epitopes may be key to understanding the immunopathology of the disease. In this study, we examined DQ8-restricted T cell responses to glutamic acid decarboxylase 65 (GAD65) using DQ8 tetramers. We demonstrated that $GAD65_{121-140}$ and $GAD65_{250-266}$ elicited responses from DQ8+ subjects. Circulating CD4+ T cells specific for these epitopes were detected significantly more often in T1D patients than in healthy individuals after in vitro expansion. T cell clones specific for $GAD65_{121-140}$ and $GAD65_{250-266}$ carried a Th1-dominant phenotype, with some of the $GAD65_{121-140}$-specific T cell clones producing IL-17. $GAD65_{250-266}$-specific CD4+ T cells could also be detected by direct ex vivo staining. Analysis of unmanipulated peripheral blood mononuclear cells (PBMCs) revealed that $GAD65_{250-266}$-specific T cells could be found in both healthy and diabetic individuals but the frequencies of specific T cells were higher in subjects with type 1 diabetes. Taken together, our results suggest a proinflammatory role for T cells specific for DQ8-restricted $GAD65_{121-140}$ and $GAD65_{250-266}$ epitopes and implicate their possible contribution to the progression of T1D.

Editor: Matthias G. von Herrath, La Jolla Institute for Allergy and Immunology, United States of America

Funding: This work was supported by JDRF center funding for Translational Research at BRI and DP3 DK097653 grant from National Institutes of Health. The funders had no role in study design, data collection and analysis, decision to publish, or preparation of the manuscript.

Competing Interests: The authors have declared that no competing interests exist.

* Email: bkwok@benaroyaresearch.org

Introduction

Type 1 diabetes (T1D) results from destruction of the insulin-producing beta cells of the pancreas. A number of genes have been implicated in T1D development, but genes within the HLA class II region confer most of the disease risk [1]; in particular, it is estimated that 90% of T1D subjects have either an HLA-DQ8 or DQ2 allele [2]. Subjects with the DRB1*04:01 (DR0401)-DQ8 haplotype have an odds ratio of 8.4 for T1D [3], and the predisposing effect of this haplotype is supported by meta-analysis of data sets from different geographic regions [4]. In accordance with the importance of MHC class II molecules in antigen presentation, DQ8-restricted CD4+ T cells are likely to have an essential and pathogenic role in the progression of T1D.

A special feature of DQ8 is the absence of an aspartic acid residue at position 57 of the beta chain [5]. Lack of this Asp residue at beta 57 leads to reduced affinity for antigenic peptides, giving rise to diabetic pathology as a result of ineffective tolerance induction in the thymus [6,7]. Identification and characterization of DQ8-restricted self-epitopes may be key to comprehending DQ8-mediated autoimmunity. A number of DQ8-restriced self-epitopes have been identified using DQ8 transgenic mice (for a recent review see [8]). Some of the reported peptides also elicit responses in HLA-DQ8+ individuals. However, monitoring of specific CD4+ T cells during the progression of diabetes, especially direct assessment of responses in the periphery, has been hampered by low frequencies of effector cells [9] and heterogeneity of the disease.

Autoantibodies against insulin (IA), glutamic acid decarboxylase 65 (GAD65), islet tyrosine phosphatase (IA-2), and zinc transporter 8 (ZnT8) have been used as predictive markers for T1D [10–13]. The appearance of autoantibodies is clear indication of beta cell autoimmunity and the combined measurement of insulin, GAD65, IA-2, and ZnT8 autoantibodies raise the detection rate to 98% at disease onset [12]. Despite their predictive value, some people with autoantibodies never develop diabetes [14]. In addition, the presence of autoantibodies does not necessarily indicate insulitis, the histopathologic hallmark of T1D that is mainly mediated by T-lymphocytes [15,16]. Therefore, identification of T cell biomarkers correlated with pathogenesis of T1D, together with the presence of autoantibodies, will facilitate disease prediction and prevention.

In this study, we investigated DQ8-restricted CD4+ T cell responses to GAD65. Responses of CD4+ T lymphocytes from T1D subjects to $GAD65_{121-140}$ and $GAD65_{250-266}$ were visualized using DQ8 tetramers after in vitro expansion of antigen-specific cells with the relevant peptides. In vitro responses and intracellular cytokine staining suggested a strong association of $GAD65_{121-140}$ and $GAD65_{250-266}$ to the disease. Direct ex vivo staining of peripheral blood mononuclear cells (PBMCs) for $GAD65_{250-266}$ revealed higher frequencies of CD4+ and CD4+CD45RO+ T cells in the T1D group. Collectively, our work indicates that T cells specific for $GAD65_{121-140}$ and $GAD65_{250-266}$ may contribute to the pathogenesis of T1D, and suggests $GAD65_{250-266}$-specific T cells as a potential biomarker for T1D.

Results

CD4+ T cell responses to $GAD65_{121-140}$ and $GAD65_{250-266}$ are detected more often in subjects with type 1 diabetes after in vitro expansion

Seven peptides derived from GAD65 were selected in this study to evaluate their relevance to the progression of autoimmune diabetes. All seven peptides are immunogenic in DQ8 transgenic mice [17–19], but DQ8-restricted responses in human subjects were not well demonstrated. Among the seven peptides, $GAD65_{121-140}$, $GAD65_{206-220}$, $GAD65_{250-266}$ bound to DQ8 with strong affinities (Table 1). The IC_{50} values of $GAD65_{121-140}$, $GAD65_{206-220}$, and $GAD65_{250-266}$ were comparable to that of influenza A/Puerto Rico/8/34 Matrix Protein M1 ($H1MP_{185-204}$) epitope.

The three strong DQ8 binders were used to stimulate CD4+ T cells from DQ8+ T1D subjects. After two-week stimulation, $GAD65_{121-140}$ and $GAD65_{250-266}$ elicited CD4+ T cell responses in multiple subjects. Examples of positive tetramer staining for the two epitopes that elicited responses are shown in Fig. 1. Responses to $GAD65_{206-220}$ were negative in five T1D subjects examined and were not further investigated. The association of $GAD65_{121-140}$ and $GAD65_{250-266}$ with T1D was next examined by comparing the prevalence of specific CD4+ T cell responses in T1D patients and healthy controls. $GAD65_{121-140}$- and $GAD65_{250-266}$-specific CD4+ T cell responses were detected more often in T1D subjects than controls ($GAD65_{121-140}$: 6/10 T1D and 0/9 controls ($p = 0.0108$); $GAD65_{250-266}$: 9/17 T1D and 1/11 controls (Table 2, $p = 0.0407$); p value evaluated by two-tailed Fisher's exact tests), demonstrating a clear association of DQ8-restricted GAD65 T cell responses with disease.

DQ8-restricted self-epitopes elicit pathogenic responses

Self-peptides can modulate autoimmunity by induction of pathogenic (Th1/Th17) or suppressive (Th2/Treg) responses. To examine functional properties of DQ8-restricted self epitopes, $GAD65_{121-140}$- and $GAD65_{250-266}$-specific CD4+ T cells were cloned from in vitro expanded cultures of multiple subjects with type 1 diabetes. Representative tetramer staining for a $GAD65_{121-140}$ and a $GAD65_{250-266}$ clone is shown in Fig. 2A. These DQ8 tetramer-sorted clones were antigen-specific and the responses could be blocked by anti-DQ (SPVL3) antibodies (Fig. 2B). The GAD65-specific cells were assayed for cytokine production by intracellular cytokine staining (ICS) (Fig. S1A). All $GAD65_{250-266}$-specific clones produced Th1-type cytokine IFN- γ (Fig. 2C). One $GAD65_{250-266}$-specific clone also produced IL-4, but production of IFN- γ was still dominant in these cells (Fig. S1B). IL-17 was not detected in $GAD65_{250-266}$ cells. The ICS data were in agreement with the cytokine ELISA results as IFN- γ was the main cytokine secreted from $GAD65_{250-266}$ clones after peptide specific stimulation (Fig. 2D). Conversely, the cytokine profile for the four $GAD65_{121-140}$-specific T clones was more diversified. Two $GAD65_{121-140}$-specific clones isolated from different patients produced IL-17 (Fig. 2C). One of the IL-17-producing cells exhibited a Th1/Th17 double positive phenotype by co-expressing IFN- γ. Production of IL-17 was not a result of in vitro priming of naïve cells, as cells isolated from the memory population (CD45RA-CD4+) maintained the Th17-like phenotype (data not shown). The two IL-17-negative $GAD65_{121-140}$-specific clones were positive for IFN- γ, IL-4, and IL-10. However, these two clones might have distinct functionality as suggested by the ratio of IFN- γ to IL-4 producing cells (Fig. S1B) and the cytokine ELISA results (Fig. 2D). Although multiple clones isolated from one donor might be the same T cell captured at different stages of differentiation, our T cell clone data from different patients suggest that DQ8-restricted GAD65-specific epitopes could induce proinflammatory responses in T1D subjects.

Higher frequencies of $GAD65_{250-266}$-specific T cells are observed in subjects with type 1 diabetes

In vitro responses can be affected by numbers and activity of monocytes and lymphocytes in the blood samples. To confirm the disease association of DQ8/GAD65-specific cells in an unmanipulated state, ex vivo tetramer staining was performed for DQ8-specific T cells in DQ8+ patients and DQ8+ controls (average age for patients: 28.8, and for controls: 34.6, $p = 0.2809$). Direct ex vivo analysis was able to detect $GAD65_{250-266}$-specific CD4+ T cells in DQ8+ subjects, but not for $GAD65_{121-140}$-specific cells

Table 1. List of DQ8-restricted GAD65 peptides used in this study.

Peptide	IC_{50} (μM)	Sequence
GAD65 121–140	1.6	YVVKS**FDRSTKVID**FHYPNE
GAD65 176–190	>50	PRY**FNQLSTGLD**MVG
GAD65 206–220	1.5	TYE**IAPVFVLLE**YVT
GAD65 250–266	2.3	AMMI**ARFKMFPE**VKEKG
GAD65 427–441	>50	FQQDKH**YDLSYDTGD**
GAD65 461–475	>50	AKG**TTGFEAHVD**KCL
GAD65 508–521	>50	YIPPS**LRTLEDNEE**

*IC_{50} value for the control $H1MP_{185-204}$ peptide was 1.4 μM.
*Predicted binding registers are indicated in boldface.

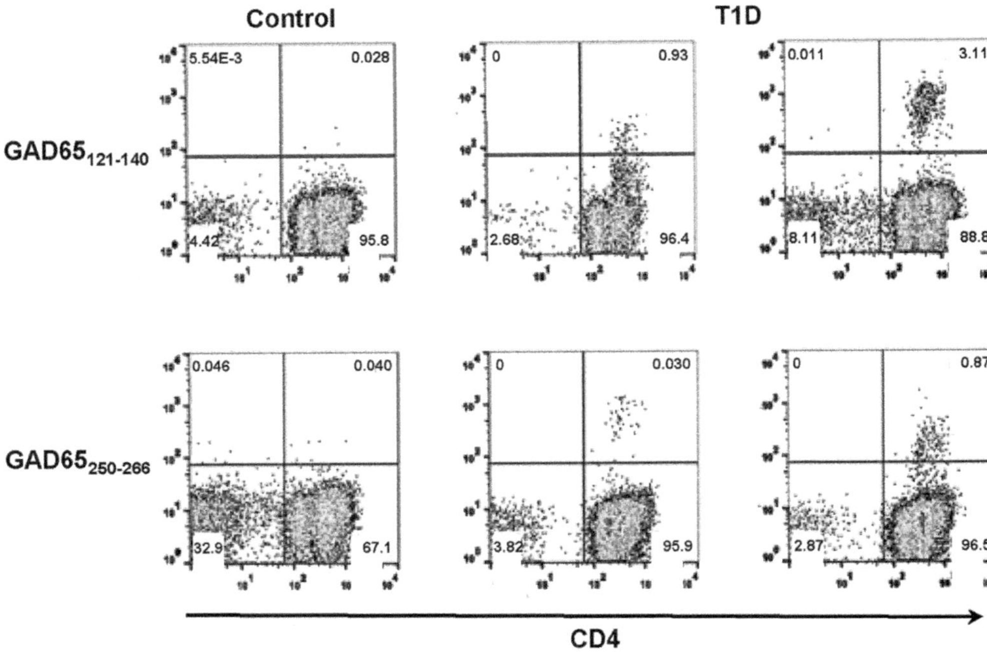

Figure 1. Detection of DQ8-specific self-reactive T cells in T1D patients. CD4+ T cells from T1D patients were stimulated with self-peptides derived from GAD65. The cells were cultured for two weeks and stained with PE-tetramers. CD4+ T cell responses to $GAD65_{121-140}$ and $GAD65_{250-266}$ were detected in multiple subjects. Representative tetramer staining of DQ8-specific self-reactive T cells was shown. Left column: negative staining from a healthy control. Middle and right columns: positive staining from two different T1D patients. Subjects were considered tetramer-positive if a distinct population that was more than three-fold above background in the same experiment was labeled.

(Fig. S2A and S2B). The unsuccessful detection might be due to low avidity or low frequencies of T cells specific for DQ8/$GAD65_{121-140}$. A representative ex vivo staining for DQ8/$GAD65_{250-266}$ from one T1D and one healthy subject is shown in Fig. 3A. The ex vivo staining for DQ8/$GAD65_{250-266}$ is specific as these cells can be co-stained by DQ8/$GAD65_{250-266}$ tetramers labeled with two different fluorochromes (PE or APC) (Fig. 3B).

Results of the ex vivo experiments are summarized in Table 3. The average frequencies of $GAD65_{250-266}$-specific cells and $GAD65_{250-266}$-specific CD45RO+ cells were found to be higher in the T1D group compared to the healthy control (Fig. 3C). There was no correlation between frequencies of $GAD65_{250-266}$-specific CD45RO+ cells and disease duration ($r^2 = 0.0218$).

Discussion

DQ8 possesses a predisposing non-aspartic acid residue at beta 57 and confers the highest risk to T1D. Substantial efforts have been made to identify DQ8-restricted responses which can closely monitor the progression of diabetes in human. However, detection of disease-related reactions from the rare islet-specific T cell populations is extremely challenging. In this study, we demonstrated DQ8 tetramers as a tool to study islet-specific T cell reactivity and identified two disease-associated peptides, $GAD65_{121-140}$ and $GAD65_{250-266}$ (Table 2, Fig. 2). In addition, T cells specific for $GAD65_{250-266}$ possessed several attributes that render these cells a potential biomarker for T1D. $GAD65_{250-266}$-

Table 2. Prevalence of GAD65-specific T cells in T1D and healthy subjects.

	Responses			
	+	-	Total	*P*
GAD65 121–140				
T1D	6	4	10	0.0108
Control	0	9	9	
Total	6	13	19	
GAD65 250–266				
T1D	9	8	17	0.0407
Control	1	10	11	
Total	10	18	28	

Not all peptides were tested on each subject.
Statistical analysis was performed using two-tailed Fisher's exact tests.

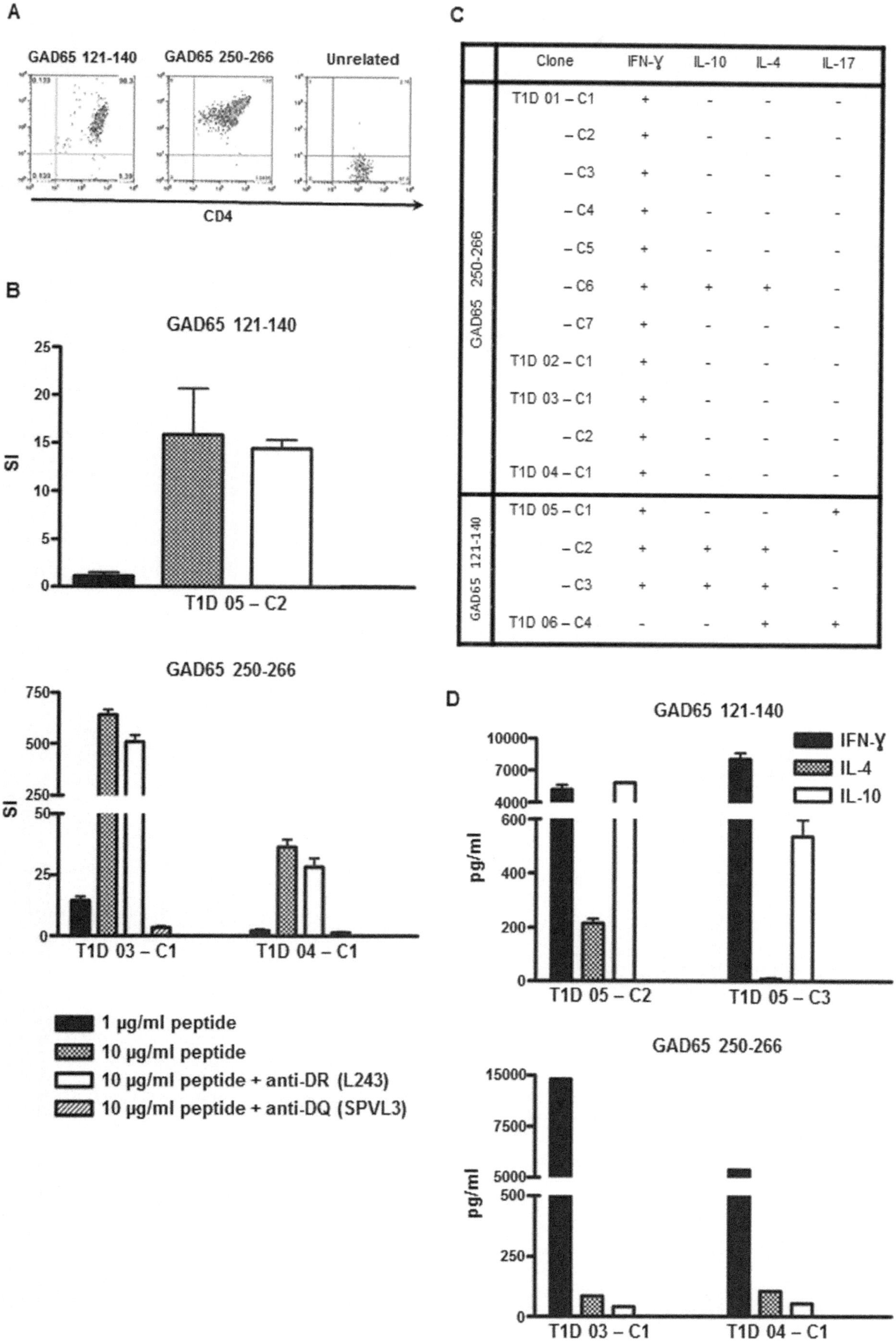

	Clone	IFN-Ɣ	IL-10	IL-4	IL-17
GAD65 250-266	T1D 01 – C1	+	-	-	-
	– C2	+	-	-	-
	– C3	+	-	-	-
	– C4	+	-	-	-
	– C5	+	-	-	-
	– C6	+	+	+	-
	– C7	+	-	-	-
	T1D 02 – C1	+	-	-	-
	T1D 03 – C1	+	-	-	-
	– C2	+	-	-	-
	T1D 04 – C1	+	-	-	-
GAD65 121-140	T1D 05 – C1	+	-	-	+
	– C2	+	+	+	-
	– C3	+	+	+	-
	T1D 06 – C4	-	-	+	+

Figure 2. Functional analysis of DQ8-specific self-reactive T cells. T cell clones isolated by DQ8 tetramers were assayed for specificity and functionality. (**A**) Tetramer staining for $GAD65_{121-140}$-specific (clone T1D05-C2), $GAD65_{250-266}$-specific (clone T1D04-C1) and unrelated T cell clones. (**B**) Representative proliferation results of one $GAD65_{121-140}$- and two $GAD65_{250-266}$-specific T cell clones using APCs from a DR0401/DQ8 homozygous individual. Cells were stimulated with specific or irrelevant control peptide in the absence or presence of 20 μg/ml of L243 (HLA-DR blocking antibody) or SPVL3 (HLA-DQ blocking antibody). SI: stimulation index; cpm of specific peptide divided by cpm of irrelevant peptide. (**C**) Summary of cytokine-positive clones (for definition see Materials and methods) for $GAD65_{121-140}$ and $GAD65_{250-266}$. T cell clones were stimulated with 50 ng/mL phorbol 12-myristate 13-acetate and 1 μg/mL ionomycin in the presence of 10 μg/mL Brefeldin A in 1 mL of T cell medium for 4 hours at 37°C. Cells were fixed, permeabilized, stained with antibodies for IFN-γ, IL-10, IL-4, and IL-17, and analyzed on a LSRII multicolor flow cytometer. (**D**) Secretion of IFN-γ, IL-4, and IL-10 from two $GAD65_{121-140}$-specific and two $GAD65_{250-266}$-specific T cell clones. Clones were stimulated in the presence of 10 μg/ml of specific peptide with DQ8 antigen presenting cells.

specific cells exhibited robust responses upon peptide stimulation (Fig. 1), and could be detected directly in unmanipulated PBMCs (Fig. 3A). Most importantly, differences between patients and healthy subjects in frequencies of CD4+ and CD4+CD45RO+ cells specific for $GAD65_{250-266}$ could readily be seen by ex vivo analysis (Fig. 3C). Monitoring of $GAD65_{250-266}$-specific T cells can potentially provide new insights into the etiology and treatment of the disease, although further longitudinal studies to link specific responses to the beta cell function are essential to confirm its suitability as a biomarker.

Schneider et al. suggest that self-reactive T effector cells are less resistant to peripheral regulation in T1D patients [20]. The current $GAD65_{121-140}$- and $GAD65_{250-266}$-reactive T cell data support this model as responses to both peptides were more prevalent in T1D patients compared to controls (Fig. 1). Higher numbers of total antigen specific cells and CD4+CD45RO+ cells for $GAD65_{250-266}$ (Fig. 3C) were also found in the periphery of subjects with T1D by ex vivo tetramer staining. Other studies show that DRB1*04:01 (DR0401)-restricted GAD65-reactive T cells of certain specificities are preferentially activated in T1D patients while other specificities are not [21–24]. The discrepancy in GAD65 responses to peripheral regulation might reflect that self-reactive T cells for different specificities are subjected to various degree of regulation. Further study in examining whether discrepancy in regulation of DR0401 and DQ8 restricted responses will be of interest. Previous studies show some islet-reactive T cells exhibit protective phenotype in healthy subjects [25,26]. The presence of multiple effector properties for $GAD65_{121-140}$ (Fig. 2C, Fig. 2D, and Fig. S1B) implies the potential of $GAD65_{121-140}$-specific cells to modulate the immune balance between tolerance and autoimmunity. Future studies to compare the dynamics of T cell responses for each HLA haplotype during disease development will help to shed more insight into the immunopathology of T1D.

The presence of self-reactive T cells in healthy individuals highlights the importance of peripheral regulation as a checkpoint in the progression of T1D. The higher frequencies of $GAD65_{250-266}$-specific total and memory CD4+ T cells in subjects with type 1 diabetes (Fig. 3C) suggest that quantity and phenotypic changes for self-reactive T cells might be an indicator for loss of tolerance. DQ8 tetramers can therefore be a useful tool for the identification of disease-related self-reactive T cells as reliable biomarkers. Monitoring of these cells could assist with early-detection of risk or progression to T1D. In conclusion, DQ8-restricted CD4+ T cells specific for $GAD65_{121-140}$ and $GAD65_{250-266}$ were detected in multiple T1D subjects. $GAD65_{121-140}$- and $GAD65_{250-266}$-reactive T cells were more prevalent in T1D patients. Further evaluation of T cell responses for beta cell autoantigens should facilitate our understanding of the role of autoreactive DQ8 T cells in type 1 diabetes and selection of autoreactive DQ8 T cells as T1D biomarkers.

Materials and Methods

Subjects

The studies were approved by the Institutional Review Board of Benaroya Research Institute (BRI, Seattle, WA). All DQ8+ subjects were volunteers of Caucasian descent and were recruited with written consent from participating individuals or their guardians. HLA typing was conducted by BRI sequencing and genotyping core facilities. Samples from DQ8-positive T1D (n = 33, age from 9 to 56, days of disease duration from 281 to 7507) or DQ8-positive individuals without T1D or other autoimmune disease (healthy controls, n = 23, age from 18 to 56) were obtained under the auspices of the BRI JDRF Center for Translational Research at Benaroya Research Institute and Seattle Children's.

DQ8 protein and tetramers

Recombinant DQ8 protein was produced as previously described [27]. Briefly, soluble DQ8 was purified from insect cell culture supernatants by affinity chromatography and dialyzed against citric/phosphate storage buffer, pH 5.4. For the preparation of HLA class II tetramers, DQ8 protein was in vivo biotinylated in Drosophila S2 cells [28] prior to harvest and dialyzed into citric/phosphate buffer. The biotinylated monomer was loaded with 0.2 mg/ml of peptide by incubating at 37°C for 72 h in the presence of 0.2 mg/ml n-Dodecyl-β-maltoside and 1 mM Pefabloc SC (Sigma–Aldrich, St. Louis, MO). Peptide loaded monomers were subsequently conjugated into tetramers using R-PE streptavidin (Biosource International, Camarillo, CA) at a molar ratio of 8:1.

Peptides

Peptides derived from GAD65 (Table 1) were synthesized by Mimotopes (Clayton, Australia). The biotinylated reference peptide $GAD65_{250-266}$ (AMMIARFKMFPEVKEKG) was synthesized by Genscript with one 6-aminohexanoic acid spacer added between the N-terminal biotin label and the remainder of the peptide sequence.

Peptide binding competition

$GAD65_{250-266}$ is a good binder for DQ8 [29] and was used as the index peptide in the competition study. Various concentrations of each test peptide were incubated in competition with 0.04 μM biotinylated $GAD65_{250-266}$ peptide in wells coated with DQ8 protein. After washing, the remaining biotin-$GAD65_{250-266}$ peptide was labeled using europium-conjugated streptavidin (Perkin Elmer) and quantified using a Victor2 D time resolved fluorometer (Perkin Elmer). Peptide binding curves were simulated by non-linear regression with Prism software (Version 5, GraphPad Software Inc.) using a sigmoidal dose–response curve. IC_{50} binding values were calculated from the resulting curves as

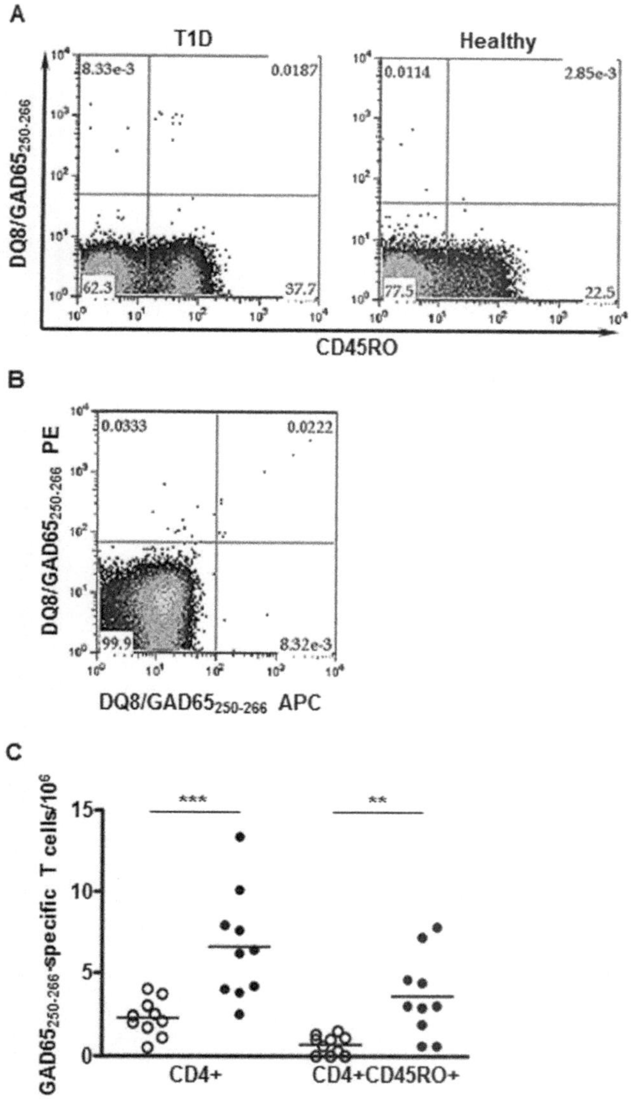

Figure 3. Direct ex vivo analysis of GAD65-specific T cells. Unmanipulated PBMCs were stained with DQ8/GAD65$_{250-266}$ PE-tetramer. Antigen-specific CD4+ T cells were enriched, stained with antibodies against surface markers of interest, and analyzed on a Calibur multi-color flow cytometer. (**A**) Representative ex vivo analysis of the surface memory marker CD45RO for GAD65$_{250-266}$. The frequency of GAD65$_{250-266}$-specific CD45RO+CD4+ T cells was 4.4 per million CD4+ T cells for the T1D patient (left panel) and 0.6 per million for the healthy subject (right panel). (**B**) Ex vivo co-staining of GAD65$_{250-266}$-specific cells with DQ8/GAD65$_{250-266}$ PE- and DQ8/GAD65$_{250-266}$ APC-tetramers. Cells were stained with PE-labeled DQ8/GAD65$_{250-266}$ tetramers first. After enrichment, tetramer-positive cells were stained again with APC-labeled DQ8/GAD65$_{250-266}$ tetramers at 37°C for 1 h. (**C**) Cumulative total CD4+ and CD45RO+CD4+ T cell frequencies for GAD65$_{250-266}$ in controls (open circles, n = 10) and T1D patients (closed circles, n = 10). *** $P<0.001$, ** $P<0.01$, as evaluated by Mann-Whitney U-test.

the peptide concentration needed for 50% inhibition of reference peptide binding.

Self-reactive T cell identification

PBMCs were prepared from the blood of T1D or healthy DQ8 subjects by Ficoll underlay. CD4+ T cells were isolated using the Miltenyi CD4+ T cell isolation kit, plated in 48-well plates with APCs, and stimulated with 20 µg/ml peptides from the selected peptide set. The cells were cultured for two weeks in the presence of T cell medium (RPMI-1640 (Gibso) +10% pooled human serum +1% penicillin-streptomycin) and IL-2 (Hemagen Diagnostics, Inc.) at 37°C, stained with PE-tetramers and antibodies of interest, and analyzed by flow cytometry. 20000 total events were collected for each staining. Lymphoid cells were gated based on forward and side scatter profile. The negative threshold for gating for Fig. 1 was set based on the staining of samples with empty tetramers. Our criterion for positivity was distinct staining that labeled a compact tetramer positive CD4+ population, and was more than three-fold above background (cells from an unstimulated well) in the same experiment.

Ex vivo analysis of self-reactive T cells

Ex vivo tetramer staining was performed as previously described [30]. Briefly, 30 million PBMCs in culture medium at a concentration of 150 million/mL were incubated with 50 nM dasatinib (LC Laboratories, dissolved in DMSO) for 10 min at 37°C. The cells were next stained with 20 µg/mL phycoerythrin (PE)–labeled tetramers at room temperature for 120 minutes, followed by antibody staining for 20 minutes at 4°C with CD4 APC (clone RPA-T4, eBioscience), CD45RO FITC (clone UCHC1, eBioscience), and a combination of CD14 PerCP (clone MφP9, BD PharMingen) and CD19 PerCP (clone SJ25C1, BD PharMingen) to exclude B cells and monocytes from the analysis. Cells were washed twice with FACS running buffer (0.5% BSA and 2mM EDTA in PBS) and incubated with anti-PE magnetic beads (Miltenyi Biotec, Bergisch Gladbach, Germany) at 4°C for another 20 minutes. The cells were washed again and enriched with a Miltenyi MS magnetic column. Samples were labeled with ViaProbe (BD Biosciences) and analyzed on a BD FACS Calibur flow cytometer. Frequencies were calculated by dividing the number of tetramer positive cells in the bound fraction by the number of total CD4+ T cells in the sample.

Statistical analysis

Statistical analysis was performed with Prism software (Version 5.03, GraphPad Software Inc.). The Mann-Whitney U-test was used to preform two group comparisons of T cell frequency. Fisher's exact test was used to compare the prevalence of T cell responses in T1D and healthy subjects.

T cell clone isolation

T cell clones were generated by staining cultured T cells with tetramers, sorting gated tetramer-positive CD4+ cells using a FACS Aria (at single-cell purity, applying a singlet gate to the lymphocyte population) and expanding in a 96-well plate in the presence of 1.0×10^5 irradiated PBMCs and 2 µg/ml phytohemagglutinin (Remel Inc. Lenexa, KS). After expansion of each T cell clone to a single 48 well, clones were stained again with tetramer and also stimulated in parallel with the corresponding peptides (10 µg/mL), adding HLA-DQ-matched irradiated PBMCs as antigen presenting cell and measuring thymidine uptake to verify epitope specificity.

Intracellular cytokine staining

Autoreactive-T cell clones isolated from T1D patients were resuspended in 200 µl of T cell medium (RPMI-1640 (Gibco) + 10% pooled human serum +1% penicillin-streptomycin), and stimulated with 50 ng/mL phorbol 12-myristate 13-acetate and 1 µg/mL ionomycin in the presence of 10 µg/mL Brefeldin A for 4 hours at 37°C. After incubation cells were stained with surface

Table 3. Summary of ex vivo results for $GAD65_{250-266}$.

T1D

Age	Duration (Days)	Frequency per 10^6 cells		% Memory	IAA	GADA	IA-2A	ZnT8A
		CD4+	CD4+CD45RO+					
14	1632	2.5	0.6	24.0	-	-	-	-
14	2439	3.8	0.6	15.8	+	-	-	-
17	1190	13.4	7.8	58.2	N/A	-	+	N/A
24	1379	6.2	2.9	46.8	+	+	+	+
25	292	7.9	3.0	38.0	-	+	+	+
25	1247	7.6	4.6	60.5	+	+	-	+
30	6564	4.2	1.9	45.2	-	-	+	+
41	1094	4.0	3.0	75.0	-	+	-	-
42	281	6.4	4.4	68.8	-	+	+	+
56	7507	10.1	7.2	71.0	+	+	-	-

Healthy

Age	Frequency per 10^6 cells		% Memory	IAA	GADA	IA-2A	ZnT8A
	CD4+	CD4+CD45RO+					
21	3.7	1.5	40.5	-	-	-	-
29	2.5	1.3	52.0	-	-	-	-
29	2.1	0.0	0.0	-	+	-	-
33	2.0	1.0	50.0	-	-	-	-
33	3.0	0.6	20.0	-	-	-	-
33	2.4	0.0	0.0	-	-	-	-
35	1.7	1.1	64.7	-	-	-	-
35	4.0	1.0	25.0	-	-	-	-
42	1.1	0.0	0.0	-	-	-	-
56	0.5	0.3	60.0	-	-	-	-

N/A: not available.

antibodies including CD3 PE-Cy5 (clone HIT3a, BioLegend) and CD4 v500 (clone RPA-T4, BD Biosciences) as well as Fixable Viability Stain 450 (BD Horizon). Cells were then fixed and permeabilized as per the manufacturer's instructions (eBioscience). Cells were next stained with antibodies against IFN-γ AF700 (clone 4S.B3, BioLegend), IL-10 PE Cy7 (clone MQ1-17H12, BioLegend), IL-17A APC Cy7 (clone BL168, BioLegend), and IL-4 FITC (clone 8D4-8, eBioscience) for 20 minutes at 4°C. Cells were then washed in PBS and immediately analyzed by flow cytometry on a BD LSRII multi-color flow cytometer. Clones were considered cytokine positive if more than 10% of the cells produced that particular cytokine.

Supporting Information

Figure S1 Intracellular cytokine staining for DQ8-specific T cell clones. T cell clones specific for $GAD65_{121-140}$ and $GAD65_{250-266}$ were stimulated with 50 ng/mL phorbol 12-myristate 13-acetate and 1 mg/mL ionomycin in the presence of 10 mg/mL Brefeldin A in 1 mL of T cell medium for 4 hours at 37°C. Cells were fixed, permeabilized, stained with antibodies for IFN- γ, IL-10, IL-4, and IL-17, and analyzed on a LSRII multicolor flow cytometer. (**A**) Representative intracellular cytokine staining analysis for the $GAD65_{250-266}$ T cell clone T1D01-C6. Staining results (open histograms) were compared to cells incubated with nonspecific isotype matched IgG control antibodies (gray histograms). Numbers indicate the percentage of cytokine-producing cells. (**B**) The ratio of IFN- γ producing cells to IL-4 producing cells in IFN- γ^+ IL-4^+ clones for $GAD65_{121-140}$ and $GAD65_{250-266}$. Each dot represents one IFN- γ^+IL-4^+ clone from Fig 2(C) (T1D05-C2 and T1D05-C3 for $GAD65_{121-140}$, and T1D01-C6 for $GAD65_{250-266}$, respectively).

Figure S2 Direct ex vivo flow cytometric analysis of DQ8/GAD65-specific T cells. (**A**) Gating strategy for Tetramer+ cells. Lymphoid cells were selected based on forward and side scatter profile. A dump channel was used to exclude monocytes (CD14+), B cells (CD19+), and dead cells (ViaProbe) from lymphocytes. Viable Tetramer+CD4+CD45RO+ T cells were gated based on the staining of unenriched cells, and the gating was applied to enriched populations. Numbers indicate the percentage of cells in the gated regions or each quadrant. (**B**) Representative ex vivo analysis of the surface memory marker CD45RO for $GAD65_{121-140}$-specific cells in a T1D subject. The frequency of these cells is below the threshold of detection.

Acknowledgments

We thank Dr Catherine Pihoker, Seattle Children's, and coordinators from BRI and Seattle Children's for help with subject recruitment. The administrative support of Diana Sorus is greatly appreciated.

Author Contributions

Conceived and designed the experiments: IC JY WWK. Performed the experiments: IC JY TJG EAJ DTM. Analyzed the data: IC. Contributed reagents/materials/analysis tools: IC. Wrote the paper: IC CG WWK.

References

1. Todd JA, Walker NM, Cooper JD, Smyth DJ, Downes K, et al. (2007) Robust associations of four new chromosome regions from genome-wide analyses of type 1 diabetes. Nat Genet 39: 857–864.
2. Ide A, Eisenbarth GS (2003) Genetic susceptibility in type 1 diabetes and its associated autoimmune disorders. Rev Endocr Metab Disord 4: 243–253.
3. Erlich H, Valdes AM, Noble J, Carlson JA, Varney M, et al. (2008) HLA DR-DQ haplotypes and genotypes and type 1 diabetes risk: analysis of the type 1 diabetes genetics consortium families. Diabetes 57: 1084–1092.
4. Thomson G, Valdes AM, Noble JA, Kockum I, Grote MN, et al. (2007) Relative predispositional effects of HLA class II DRB1-DQB1 haplotypes and genotypes on type 1 diabetes: a meta-analysis. Tissue Antigens 70: 110–127.
5. Todd JA, Bell JI, McDevitt HO (1987) HLA-DQ beta gene contributes to susceptibility and resistance to insulin-dependent diabetes mellitus. Nature 329: 599–604.
6. Corper AL, Stratmann T, Apostolopoulos V, Scott CA, Garcia KC, et al. (2000) A structural framework for deciphering the link between I-Ag7 and autoimmune diabetes. Science 288: 505–511.
7. Yoshida K, Corper AL, Herro R, Jabri B, Wilson IA, et al. (2010) The diabetogenic mouse MHC class II molecule I-Ag7 is endowed with a switch that modulates TCR affinity. J Clin Invest 120: 1578–1590.
8. Di Lorenzo TP, Peakman M, Roep BO (2007) Translational mini-review series on type 1 diabetes: Systematic analysis of T cell epitopes in autoimmune diabetes. Clin Exp Immunol 148: 1–16.
9. Oling V, Marttila J, Ilonen J, Kwok WW, Nepom G, et al. (2005) GAD65- and proinsulin-specific CD4+ T-cells detected by MHC class II tetramers in peripheral blood of type 1 diabetes patients and at-risk subjects. J Autoimmun 25: 235–243.
10. Achenbach P, Warncke K, Reiter J, Naserke HE, Williams AJ, et al. (2004) Stratification of type 1 diabetes risk on the basis of islet autoantibody characteristics. Diabetes 53: 384–392.
11. Bingley PJ (2010) Clinical applications of diabetes antibody testing. J Clin Endocrinol Metab 95: 25–33.
12. Wenzlau JM, Juhl K, Yu L, Moua O, Sarkar SA, et al. (2007) The cation efflux transporter ZnT8 (Slc30A8) is a major autoantigen in human type 1 diabetes. Proc Natl Acad Sci U S A 104: 17040–17045.
13. Achenbach P, Lampasona V, Landherr U, Koczwara K, Krause S, et al. (2009) Autoantibodies to zinc transporter 8 and SLC30A8 genotype stratify type 1 diabetes risk. Diabetologia 52: 1881–1888.
14. Narendran P, Estella E, Fourlanos S (2005) Immunology of type 1 diabetes. QJM 98: 547–556.
15. Willcox A, Richardson SJ, Bone AJ, Foulis AK, Morgan NG (2009) Analysis of islet inflammation in human type 1 diabetes. Clin Exp Immunol 155: 173–181.
16. Gianani R, Campbell-Thompson M, Sarkar SA, Wasserfall C, Pugliese A, et al. (2010) Dimorphic histopathology of long-standing childhood-onset diabetes. Diabetologia 53: 690–698.
17. Wen L, Wong FS, Burkly L, Altieri M, Mamalaki C, et al. (1998) Induction of insulitis by glutamic acid decarboxylase peptide-specific and HLA-DQ8-restricted CD4(+) T cells from human DQ transgenic mice. J Clin Invest 102: 947–957.
18. Herman AE, Tisch RM, Patel SD, Parry SL, Olson J, et al. (1999) Determination of glutamic acid decarboxylase 65 peptides presented by the type I diabetes-associated HLA-DQ8 class II molecule identifies an immunogenic peptide motif. J Immunol 163: 6275–6282.
19. Liu J, Purdy LE, Rabinovitch S, Jevnikar AM, Elliott JF (1999) Major DQ8-restricted T-cell epitopes for human GAD65 mapped using human CD4, DQA1*0301, DQB1*0302 transgenic IA(null) NOD mice. Diabetes 48: 469–477.
20. Schneider A, Rieck M, Sanda S, Pihoker C, Greenbaum C, et al. (2008) The effector T cells of diabetic subjects are resistant to regulation via CD4+ FOXP3+ regulatory T cells. J Immunol 181: 7350–7355.
21. Danke NA, Yang J, Greenbaum C, Kwok WW (2005) Comparative study of GAD65-specific CD4+ T cells in healthy and type 1 diabetic subjects. J Autoimmun 25: 303–311.
22. Yang J, James EA, Sanda S, Greenbaum C, Kwok WW (2013) CD4+ T cells recognize diverse epitopes within GAD65: implications for repertoire development and diabetes monitoring. Immunology 138: 269–279.
23. Monti P, Scirpoli M, Rigamonti A, Mayr A, Jaeger A, et al. (2007) Evidence for in vivo primed and expanded autoreactive T cells as a specific feature of patients with type 1 diabetes. J Immunol 179: 5785–5792.
24. Oling V, Reijonen H, Simell O, Knip M, Ilonen J (2012) Autoantigen-specific memory CD4+ T cells are prevalent early in progression to Type 1 diabetes. Cell Immunol 273: 133–139.
25. Arif S, Tree TI, Astill TP, Tremble JM, Bishop AJ, et al. (2004) Autoreactive T cell responses show proinflammatory polarization in diabetes but a regulatory phenotype in health. J Clin Invest 113: 451–463.
26. van Lummel M, Duinkerken G, van Veelen PA, de Ru A, Cordfunke R, et al. (2014) Posttranslational modification of HLA-DQ binding islet autoantigens in type 1 diabetes. Diabetes 63: 237–247.
27. Novak EJ, Liu AW, Gebe JA, Falk BA, Nepom GT, et al. (2001) Tetramer-guided epitope mapping: rapid identification and characterization of immunodominant CD4+ T cell epitopes from complex antigens. J Immunol 166: 6665–6670.
28. Yang J, Jaramillo A, Shi R, Kwok WW, Mohanakumar T (2004) In vivo biotinylation of the major histocompatibility complex (MHC) class II/peptide

complex by coexpression of BirA enzyme for the generation of MHC class II/ tetramers. Hum Immunol 65: 692–699.
29. Kwok WW, Domeier ML, Raymond FC, Byers P, Nepom GT (1996) Allele-specific motifs characterize HLA-DQ interactions with a diabetes-associated peptide derived from glutamic acid decarboxylase. J Immunol 156: 2171–2177.
30. Scriba TJ, Purbhoo M, Day CL, Robinson N, Fidler S, et al. (2005) Ultrasensitive detection and phenotyping of CD4+ T cells with optimized HLA class II tetramer staining. J Immunol 175: 6334–6343.

11

Foreign Body Response to Subcutaneous Implants in Diabetic Rats

Teresa Oviedo Socarrás[1,2], Anilton C. Vasconcelos[1], Paula P. Campos[1]*, Nubia B. Pereira[1], Jessica P. C. Souza[1], Silvia P. Andrade[3]

1 Department of General Pathology, Institute of Biological Sciences, Federal University of Minas Gerais, Belo Horizonte, Minas Gerais, Brazil, 2 Department of Livestock Sciences, University of Córdoba, Montería, Córdoba, Colombia, 3 Department of Physiology and Biophysics, Institute of Biological Sciences, Federal University of Minas Gerais, Belo Horizonte, Minas Gerais, Brazil

Abstract

Implantation of synthetic matrices and biomedical devices in diabetic individuals has become a common procedure to repair and/or replace biological tissues. However, an adverse foreign body reaction that invariably occurs adjacent to implant devices impairing their function is poorly characterized in the diabetic environment. We investigated the influence of this condition on the abnormal tissue healing response in implants placed subcutaneously in normoglycemic and streptozotocin-induced diabetes in rats. In polyether-polyurethane sponge discs removed 10 days after implantation, the components of the fibrovascular tissue (angiogenesis, inflammation, fibrogenesis, and apoptosis) were assessed. Intra-implant levels of hemoglobin and vascular endothelial growth factor were not different after diabetes when compared with normoglycemic counterparts. However, there were a lower number of vessels in the fibrovascular tissue from diabetic rats when compared with vessel numbers in implants from non-diabetic animals. Overall, the inflammatory parameters (neutrophil accumulation - myeloperoxidase activity, tumor necrosis factor alpha, and monocyte chemotactic protein-1 levels and mast cell counting) increased in subcutaneous implants after diabetes induction. However, macrophage activation (N-acetyl-β-D-glucosaminidase activity) was lower in implants from diabetic rats when compared with those from normoglycemic animals. All fibrogenic markers (transforming growth factor beta 1 levels, collagen deposition, fibrous capsule thickness, and foreign body giant cells) decreased after diabetes, whereas apoptosis (TUNEL) increased. Our results showing that hyperglycemia down regulates the main features of the foreign body reaction induced by subcutaneous implants in rats may be relevant in understanding biomaterial integration and performance in diabetes.

Editor: Mário A. Barbosa, Instituto de Engenharia Biomédica, University of Porto, Portugal

Funding: The work was supported by Conselho Nacional de Desenvolvimento Científico e Tecnológico CNPq- processo n°481659/2012-9 http://www.cnpq.br/. The funders had no role in study design, data collection and analysis, decision to publish, or preparation of the manuscript.

Competing Interests: The authors have declared that no competing interests exist.

* Email: paulapc@icb.ufmg.br

Introduction

The foreign body response refers to the non-specific immune response to implanted foreign materials [1–2]. It results from persistent inflammatory stimuli, such as the presence of implant devices in which a series of cellular alterations such as continuous inflammation are mediated by the various cell lineages. In this inflamed environment, macrophages, lymphocytes, mast cells, and their granular products contribute to the formation of foreign body giant cells (multinucleated fused macrophages) and the development of a dense of layer of fibrotic connective tissue which is detrimental to the implants' function, safety, and biocompatibility [1–4]. In an experimental model of foreign body reaction induced by polyether-polyurethane sponge implants in normoglycemic animals, we have characterized a series of overlapping events, such as leukocyte/mast cell recruitment, angiogenesis, fibrogenesis, apoptosis, and the formation of foreign body giant cells [5–6]. All these features that vary in intensity and severity depending on the nature of the implanted material, characterize the host response to foreign materials in a number of different studies [4,7]. Thus, while much is known about the foreign body reaction to indwelling medical devices in normoglycemic experimental animals, there is little information on the diabetic body's response to injury inflicted by internal implants [8]. This is despite the fact that complications associated with the diabetes often require implantable devices such as glucose sensors, orthopedic implants, catheter, vascular grafts, drug-eluting stents, artificial organs, biosensors, scaffolds for tissue engineering, heart valves, and others [9]. In one study involving diabetic baboons bearing polystyrene subcutaneous implants, the inflammatory cell response, granulation tissue, and connective tissue ingrowth were shown to be reduced [10]. Similarly, delayed in matrix maturation and angiogenesis and higher numbers of inflammatory cells in titanium fiber mesh were seen around percutaneous implants in diabetic rabbits [11]. However, the prevalence of diabetes and the potential number of individuals that will need indwelling medical devices warrant further investigation to determine to what extent the diabetes state modifies the features of foreign body reaction. Therefore, we investigated the influence of hyperglycemia in the inflammatory cells recruitment/activation, neovascularization, apoptosis, foreign body giant cell, and fibrous capsule induced by synthetic matrix implanted subcutaneously in rats. We have shown that the pattern of the reaction to the synthetic polyether-polyurethane matrix differs in important ways between diabetic and non-diabetic rats.

Materials and Methods

Ethics Statement

The use of animals and procedures for this study was approved by the Ethics Committee of Animal Experimentation (CETEA) of Federal University of Minas Gerais, (protocol number 176/11). All surgery was performed under ketamine and xylazine anesthesia, and all efforts were made to minimize suffering.

Animals

We used male Wistar laboratory rats weighing 300–350 g provided by Centro de Bioterismo (CEBIO) of Universidade Federal de Minas Gerais (UFMG). The animals were housed in polypropylene cages inside a well-ventilated room, provided with chow pellets and water *ad libitum* and maintained under a 12-hour light/dark cycle. All animal procedures were in accordance with the standards set forth in the guidelines for the care and use of experimental animals by our local Institutional Animal Welfare Committee.

Induction of Diabetes Mellitus

Streptozotocin (STZ) was obtained from Sigma – Aldrich, St. Louis, MO, USA. STZ was dissolved in 10 mM citrate buffer (pH 4.5) and always prepared for immediate use within 5 to 10 min. STZ doses were determined according to the animals' body weight and were administered intravenously in a single 60-mg/kg injection. The blood glucose level was measured before injection and subsequently every 4 days with On Call Plus Blood Glucose Meter (ACON Laboratories, Inc. San Diego CA, USA). Animals whose blood glucose level exceeded 200 mg/dl after treatment were considered diabetic.

Preparation of sponge discs and implantation

Polyether–polyurethane sponge discs, 5 mm thick×12 mm diameter (Vitafoam Ltd, Manchester, U.K.) were used as the matrix for fibrovascular tissue growth. The sponge discs were soaked overnight in 70% ethanol and sterilized by boiling in distilled water for 30 min prior to the implantation surgery.

Thirteen days after STZ injection in the diabetic groups, all animals were anesthetized with a mixture of ketamine and xylazine (60 mg/kg and 10 mg/kg, respectively). The dorsal hair was shaved and the exposed skin wiped with 70% ethanol. Two sponges discs per animal (11 non diabetic and 12 diabetic) were aseptically implanted into a subcutaneous pouch through a 1 cm long dorsal mid-line incision. The incisions were closed with a silk braided nonabsorbable suture.

At 10 days post implantation (23 days after diabetes induction), the animals were anesthetized with ketamine and xylazine and later killed by cervical dislocation. The sponge discs were carefully dissected from the adherent tissue, removed, and weighed. They were then processed as described below and subjected to several assays.

Tissue extraction and hemoglobin (Hb) measurement

Sponge implant vascularization was evaluated indirectly by the amount of Hb in the tissue detected by the Drabkin method. This method has been modified and used to determine angiogenesis in various experimental models and tissues, including the sponge implant model [6,12–13]. All implants were individually homogenized (Tekmar TR-10, Cincinnati, OH) in 5 mL of Drabkin reagent (Labtest, São Paulo, Brazil) and centrifuged at 12.000 rpm for 20 min. The supernatants were filtered through a 0.22 mm filter (Millipore, São Paulo, Brazil). Hb concentration in the samples was determined spectrophotometrically by measuring absorbance at 540 nm using an enzyme linked immunosorbent assay (ELISA) plate reader and compared against a standard Hb curve. The Hb content in the implant sponge was expressed as µg Hb/mg of wet tissue.

Determination of myeloperoxidase (MPO) activity

Neutrophil infiltration in the implants was measured indirectly by assaying MPO activity as previously described [14]. After using the sponge implant for Hb measurement, a part of the pellet was weighed and homogenized in 2 mL of pH 4.7 phosphate buffer (0.1 M NaCl, 0.02 M Na_3PO_4, 0.015 M NaEDTA, pH 4.7), and centrifuged at 12,000×g for 15 min. The pellet was resuspended in 0.05 M sodium phosphate buffer (pH 5.4) containing 0.5% hexa-1,6-bisdecyltrimethylammonium bromide (HTAB, Sigma Chemical Co., USA). Afterwards, the suspensions were freeze–thawed three times using liquid nitrogen and centrifuged at 10,000×g for 10 min. MPO activity in the supernatant samples was evaluated by quantifying the change in absorbance (optical density, OD) at 450 nm using tetramethylbenzidine (1.6 mM) and H_2O_2 (0.3 mM). The reaction was ended by adding 50 µl of H_2SO_4 (4 M). Results were expressed as a change in OD/mg of wet tissue.

Determination of N-acetyl-β-D-glucosaminidase (NAG) activity

The extent of mononuclear cells in the sponge implants was quantitated by measuring the levels of the lysosomal enzyme, N-acetyl-glucosaminidase (NAG), present in high levels in activated macrophages [12,15–16]. The implants were homogenized in 2 mL NaCl solution (0.9% w/v) containing 0.1% v/v Triton X-

Table 1. Blood glucose level and animal weight in non-diabetic and diabetic rats during the study.

		Non-diabetic (n = 11)	Diabetic (n = 12)	ANOVA
Blood glucose level (mg/dL) (mean ± SEM)	0th day	86.64±3.4	78.67±1.7	-
	23th days	99.45±3.4	462.6±22.1	<0,0001
Animal weight (g) (mean ± SEM)	0th day	219.8±6.5	237.7±4.9	-
	23th days	325.4±7.2	267.3±8.3	<0,0001

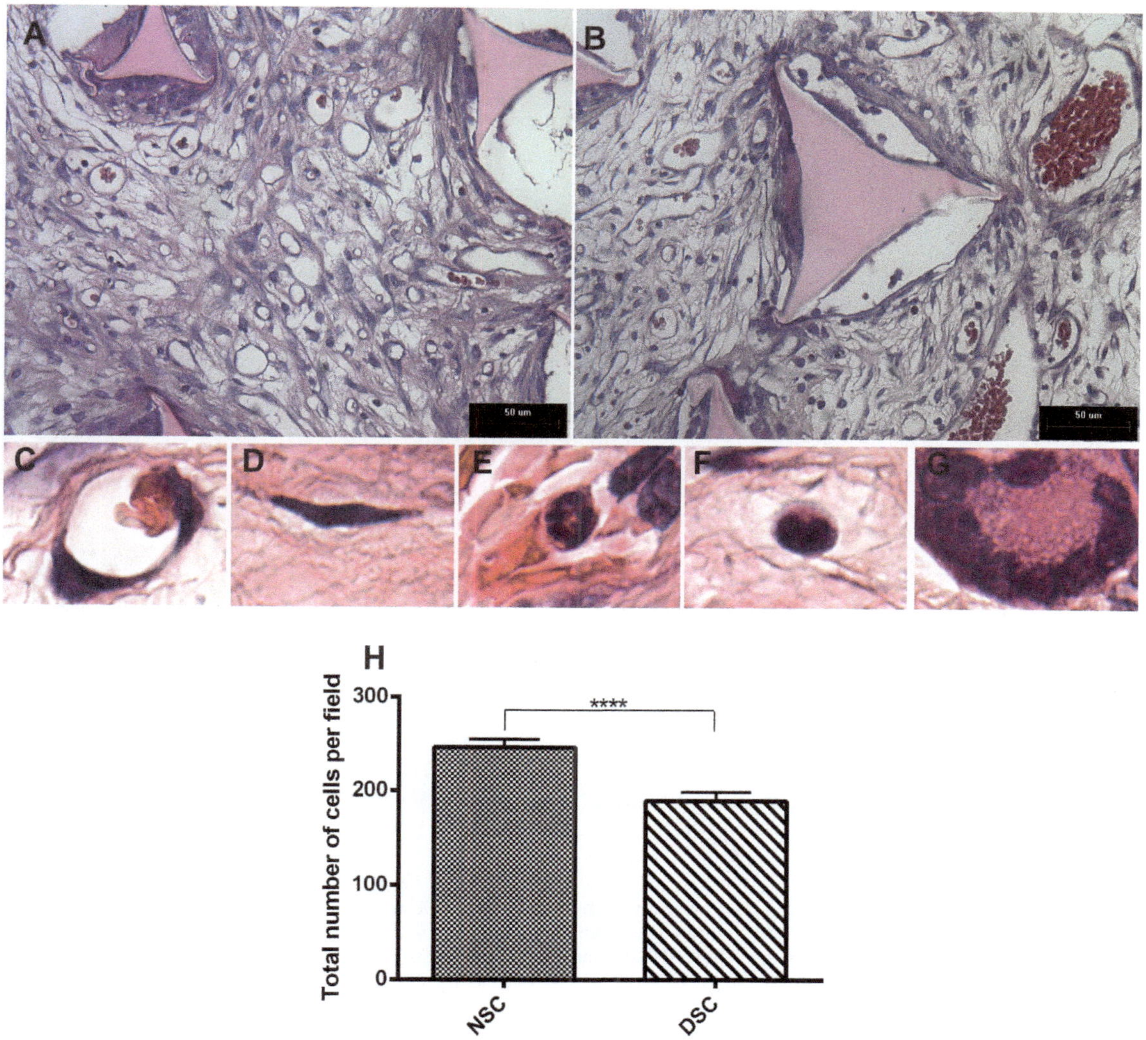

Figure 1. Histological analysis of 10-day old implants from non-diabetic and diabetic rats. Representative histological sections stained with H&E of fibrovascular tissue from diabetic (A) and non diabetic (B) rats. The pores of the sponge matrix, seen as triangular shapes, is composed of microvessels (C), spindle-shaped fibroblasts (D) and inflammatory infiltrate consisting of neutrophils (E), macrophages (F), and foreign body giant cells (G). Dilated microvessels and low cellularity were characteristics of implants from diabetic rats (H). Data are expressed as means ± SEM. *Significant difference between non-diabetic and diabetic; $p<0.05$; Mann-Whitney test. NSC, non-diabetic implant; DSC, diabetic implant; scale bar, 50 μm.

100 (Promega, Madison, WI) and centrifuged at 3000 rpm; 10 min at 4°C. One hundred μl of the supernatant was incubated for 10 min with 100 mL of pnitrophenyl-N-acetyl-b-D-glucosaminide (Sigma, Saint Louis, MO) prepared in citrate/phosphate buffer (0.1 M citric acid, 0.1 M Na_2HPO_4; pH 4.5) with a final concentration of 2.24 mM. The reaction was terminated by the adding 100 μl of 0.2 M glycine buffer (pH 10.6). Hydrolysis of the substrate was determined by the color absorption at 400 nm. A standard curve was constructed with *p*-nitrophenol (0–500 nmol/ml) and NAG activity was expressed as a change in nmol/mg of wet tissue.

Measurement of VEGF, TNF-α, MCP-1, and TGF- β1 content of the sponge implants

Implants were homogenized in PBS pH 7.4 containing 0.05% Tween and centrifuged at 10,000×*g* for 30 min. The cytokines vascular endothelial growth factor (VEGF), tumor necrosis factor alpha (TNF-α), monocyte chemotactic protein-1 (MCP-1), and Transforming growth factor beta (TGF- β1) were measured in 100 μl of the supernatant using Immunoassay Kits (R and D Systems, USA) and following the manufacturer's protocol. Dilutions of cell-free supernatants were added to ELISA plates coated with a specific murine monoclonal antibody against cytokine, followed by adding a second horseradish peroxidase-conjugated polyclonal antibody against cytokine. After washing to remove any unbound antibody-enzyme reagent, a substrate solution (50 μL of a 1:1 solution of hydrogen peroxide and tetramethylbenzidine 10 mg/ml in DMSO) was added to the wells. Color development was stopped after 20 min incubation with 2N sulphuric acid (50 μL) and color intensity was measured at 540 nm on a spectrophotometer (E max – Molecular Devices). Standards were 0.5-log10 dilutions of recombinant murine cytokines from 7.5 pg/ml to 1000 pg/ml (100 μl). The results were expressed as picogram of cytokine/mg of wet tissue.

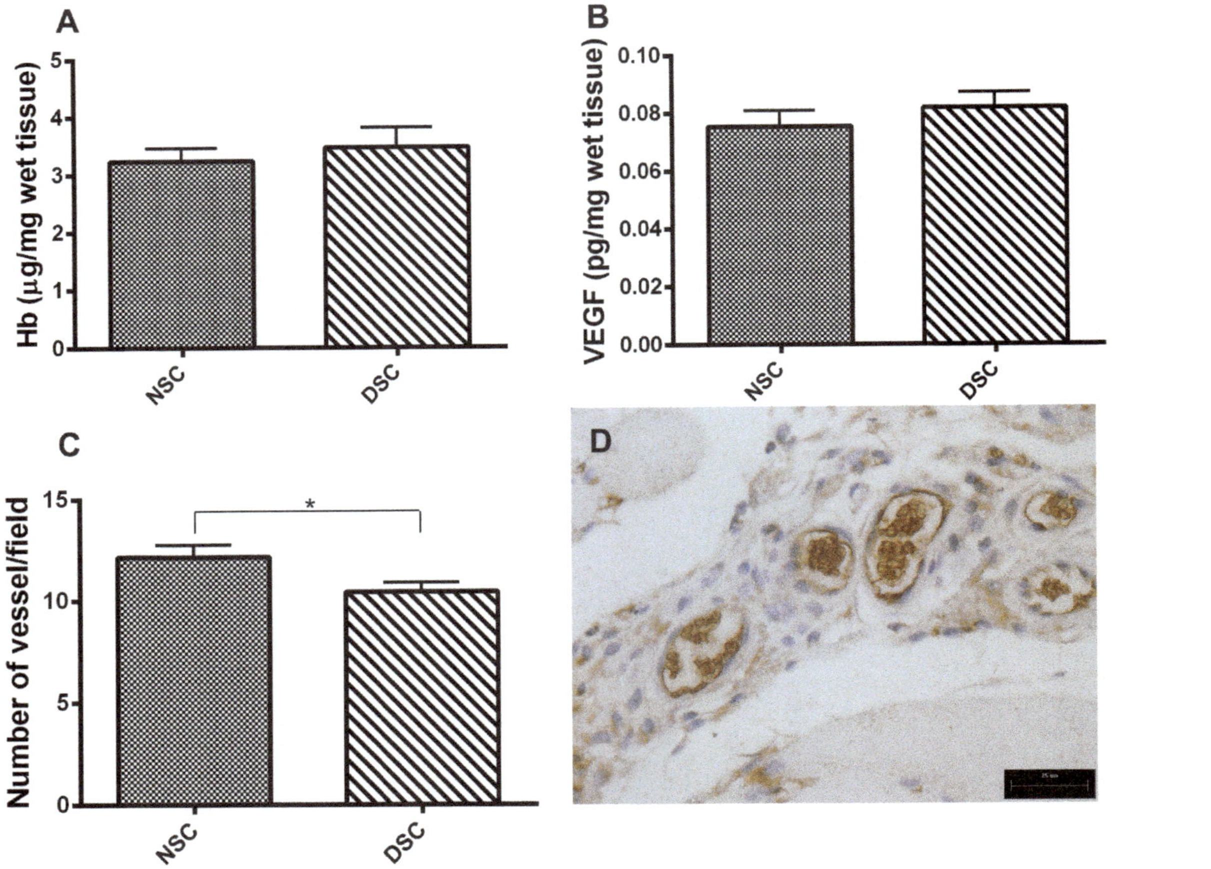

Figure 2. Vascularization in 10-day old implants from non-diabetic and diabetic rats. Hemoglobin content (A) and VEGF levels (B), both angiogenic markers, were not altered after diabetes induction. Morphometric analysis showed a decreased number of blood vessels in implants from diabetic as compared with non-diabetic rats (C). Representative CD31-immunostained section shows the newly formed vascular structures (D). Values shown are expressed as mean±SEM. *Significant difference between non-diabetic and diabetic; $p<0.05$. Student's t-test. NSC, non-diabetic implant; DSC, diabetic implant; scale bar, 25 μm.

Histological staining, immunohistochemistry, and morphometric analysis

The sponge implants from both groups (non-diabetic and diabetic) were fixed in 10% buffered formalin, pH 7.4, and processed for paraffin embedding. Sections with a thickness of 5 mm were stained with hematoxylin/eosin (H&E) and Dominici for light microscopic studies. Picrossirius-red staining followed by polarized-light microscopy was used to visualize and identify collagen fibers. The presence of apoptosis was investigated by TUNEL (TdT mediated dUTP nick end labeling) in histological sections, with a thickness pf 5 μm, using a commercial kit (TdT-FragEL DNA Fragmentation Detection Kit, Cat QIA33; Calbiochem, San Diego, CA, USA) to identify cells in apoptosis in marked terminal fragments of DNA (portion 3′-OH), associated with the characteristically fragmented nuclear DNA, allowing the morphological identification of cells undergoing apoptosis. The method was applied according to the manufacturer's instructions.

Immunohistochemistry (IHC) reactions for the detection of endothelial cells/blood vessels were performed using the monoclonal antibody clone CD 31, (Fitzgerald MA, USA). Tissue sections (5 μm) were dewaxed and antigens retrieved from the citrate buffer (pH 6). The slides were boiled in the citrate buffer for 25 minutes at 95°C and then cooled for 1 hour in the same buffer. Sections were incubated for 5 min in 3% hydrogen peroxide to quench endogenous tissue peroxidase. Nonspecific binding was blocked by using normal goat serum for 10 minutes (1:10 in phosphate-buffered saline) with 1% bovine serum albumin (in phosphate-buffered saline). The sections were then immunostained with monoclonal antibody to CD31 (1:40 dilution, DAKO Corporation, Carpinteria, CA, USA) for 60 min at room temperature. After washing in Tris–HCl buffer, sections were incubated for 30 min at room temperature with byotinylated Link Universal Streptavidin- HRP (Dako; Carpinteria, CA, USA). The reactions were revealed by applying 3,3′-diaminobenzidine in chromogen solution (DAB) (Dako; Carpinteria, CA, USA). The sections were counterstained with hematoxylin and mounted in Permount (Fisher Scientific; NJ, USA). Immunostaining was performed manually, and the spleen was used as a positive control. Negative controls were carried out by omitting the primary antibody, resulting in no detectable staining. The expression of these proteins was evaluated on the basis of the extent of cytoplasmic immunolabeling in endothelial cells forming lumen in six high-power fields, regardless of staining intensity (×400).

The number of blood vessels and giant cells, area of total collagen, capsule thickness, and number of mast cells and apoptotic cells were evaluated morphometrically. To perform the morphometric analysis, images of sequential cross sections from each implant were obtained from 25 fields for total number of cells, 35 fields for the number of blood vessels, and 20 fields for

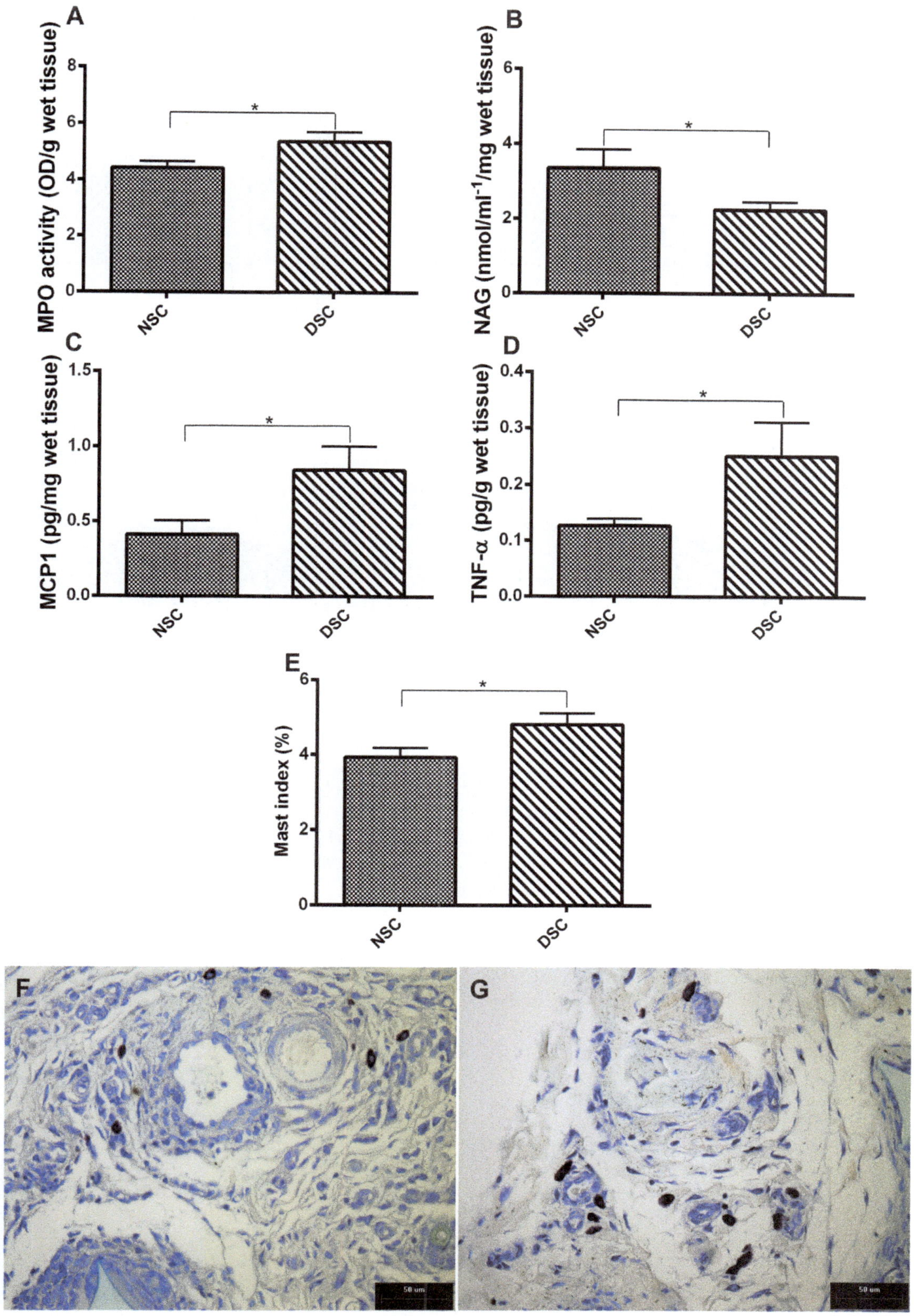

Figure 3. Markers of inflammation in 10-day old implants from non-diabetic and diabetic rats. Neutrophils and macrophages recruited to the implant were determined through MPO and NAG activities, respectively. An increase in MPO activity (A) and decreased in NAG activity (B) were observed after diabetes induction, indicating a persistence of acute inflammatory response and delay in the chronic response. An increase in other inflammatory indicators MCP-1 (C), TNF-α (D), and mast cell index (E) was observed. Representative histological images stained with Dominicci show mast cells in implants from non-diabetic (F) and diabetic rats (G). Values shown are expressed as mean±SEM. *Significant difference between non-diabetic and diabetic; $p<0.05$. Student's t-test and Mann-Whitney test. NSC, non-diabetic implant; DSC, diabetic implant; scale bar, 50 μm.

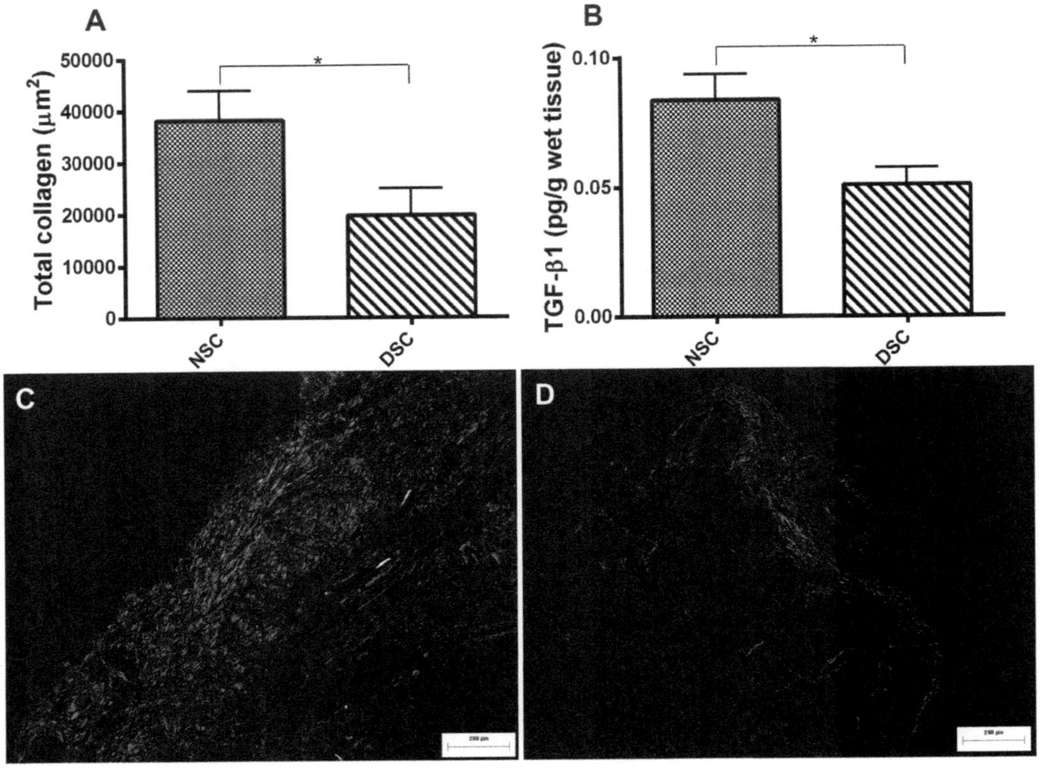

Figure 4. Markers of fibrogenesis in 10-day old implants from non-diabetic and diabetic rats. The amount of collagen (A) and levels of TGFβ1 (B) were increased in implants of non-diabetic rats as compared with that of diabetic rats. Representative histological sections (Picrossiurus-red staining) of implants from both groups of animals show distinct types of collagen in the implants (C) and (D). Values shown are expressed as mean±SEM. *Significant difference between non-diabetic and diabetic; $p<0.05$. Student's t-test. NSC, non-diabetic implant; DSC, diabetic implant; scale bar, 200 μm.

the number of mast cells, apoptotic cells, and giant cells. The images were captured with a planapochromatic objective (40x) in light microscopy (final magnification = 400x). For collagen analysis and wall thickness, images were obtained from three representative fields at 20x (final magnification = 200x). The images were digitized through a JVC TK-1270/JCB microcamera and transferred to an analyzer (software Image-Pro Plus 4.5, Media Cybernetics, Inc. Silver Spring, MD, USA). A countable vessel was defined as a structure with a lumen whether or not it contained red blood cells.

Statistics

Results are presented as mean±SEM. The assumptions of normality and homoscedasticity were determined for subsequent statistical analysis. Comparisons between the two groups (non-diabetic and diabetic groups) were made using Student's t-test or Mann-Whitney for unpaired groups. $P<0.05$ was considered significant. Analysis of the data was carried out using the GraphPad Prism program 6.0 version (La Jolla, CA, USA).

Results

A single intravenous injection of streptozotocin (STZ) (60 mg/kg) rendered the rats diabetic with blood glucose levels at 425.8±12 mg/dl five days after the treatment, which remained unaltered for the entire experimental period (23 days). The body weight of diabetic animals was affected by the diabetogenic treatment. At the beginning of the experiment, the mean weight of the animals was 229±4.4 g. Twenty-three days after the diabetogenic treatment, the animals weighed 267±8.3 g and the control animals gained 96.3 g (325±7) (Table 1). Macroscopically, no signs of rejection were observed at the implantation site in diabetic and non-diabetic rats.

Histological examination of sponge implants

In histological sections of the implants (H&E), the synthetic matrix induced the formation of a fibrovascular tissue that differed in important ways between implants from diabetic and non-diabetic rats. In normoglycemic rats, the granulation tissue that filled the subcutaneous matrix was composed of spindle-shaped fibroblasts, microvessels, and a dense inflammatory infiltrate containing macrophages, neutrophils, and foreign body giant cells embedded in an extracellular matrix. However, in implants from diabetic rats, the connective tissue was immature with little matrix deposition. A lower number of blood vessels and cellularity was observed when compared with implants from non-diabetic animals. One striking difference between both implants was the vasodilation observed in the microvasculature in the hyperglycemic environment when compared with that in normoglycemic rats (Fig. 1A–H).

Measurement of angiogenesis

The diabetogenic treatment did not alter the amount of Hb intraimplant or the levels of VEGF (a potent proangiogenic factor). However, the number of vessels, as determined in H&E stained sections and confirmed by CD31- immunostained sections, were lower in implants from diabetic rats (Fig. 2A–D).

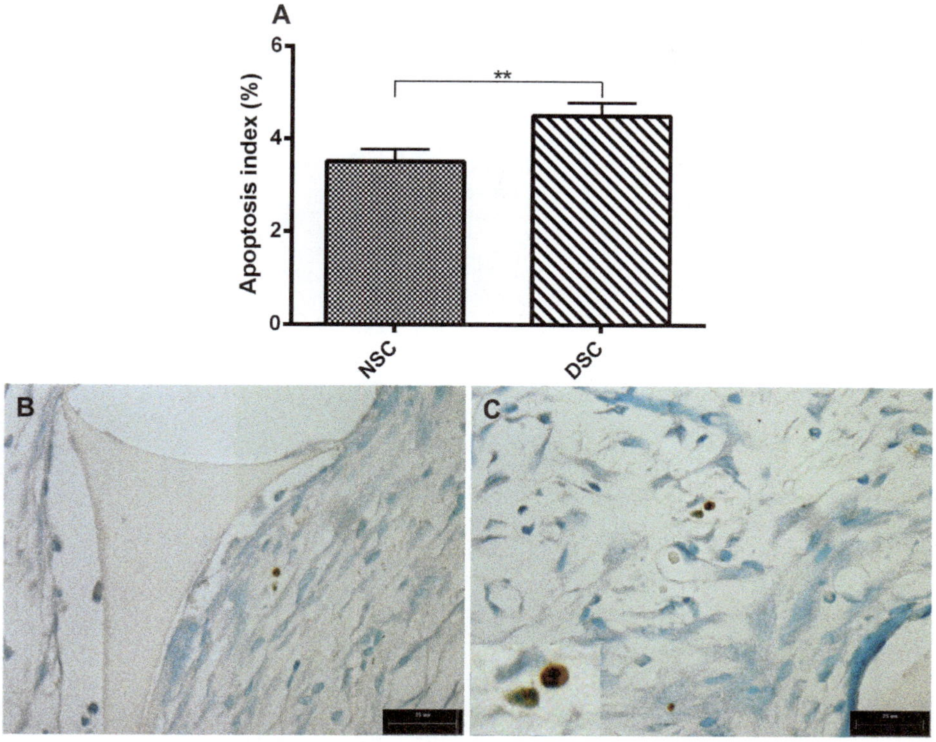

Figure 5. Pattern of apoptosis in 10-day old implants from non-diabetic and diabetic rats. Apoptotic index was increased in implants from diabetic rats as compared with non-diabetic rats (A). Values shown are expressed as mean±SEM. *Significant difference between non-diabetic and diabetic rats; $p<0.05$. Mann-Whitney test. NSC, non-diabetic implant; DSC, diabetic implant; scale bar, 25 μm. Representative histological sections (TUNEL staining) of the fibrovascular tissue induced by sponge implants at 10 post implantation show apoptotic cells in non-diabetic (B) and diabetic rats (C).

Inflammation in sponge implants

Several measurements of the inflammatory component of the implants (inflammatory enzyme activities and pro-inflammatory cytokines and mast cell index) were made. As shown in Fig. 3A–D, there were diabetes-related differences in leukocyte recruitment/ activation in these parameters in 10-day old implants. In subcutaneous implants from non-diabetic rats, MPO activity, TNF-α, and MCP-1 levels were lower when compared with the values in implants from diabetic animals. NAG activity was higher in implants from non-diabetic animals than in diabetic rats. An increased number of mast cells (Dominici staining) was detected in implants from diabetic rats when compared with the number in implants from normoglycemic animals (Fig. 3E). Representative photomicrographs of mast cells in both groups are shown in Fig. 3F and 3G.

Measurement of TGFβ1 levels and total collagen deposition

Fibrogenesis as an important wound healing and repair mechanism was measured by the cytokine TGF-β1 levels and total area of collagen (μm^2) in the sponge implants (Picrossirius staining). A significant decrease in both parameters was observed in implants from diabetic when compared with that from non-diabetic rats (Fig. 4A–D).

Apoptosis in sponge implants

In sponge sections stained with TUNEL, the number of positive cells was clearly higher in implants from diabetic rats than it was in normoglycemic rats (Fig. 5A). Representative photomicrograph of apoptotic cells are presented in Fig. 5B and 5C. Dark-brown TUNEL positive nuclei with other morphological features of cellular death (apoptotic bodies, cellular shrinkage, and condensed chromatin) are clearly marked.

Histological examination of the implant fibrous capsule and foreign body giant cells

One of the most striking differences between the implants from normoglycemic and hyperglycemic animals was the thickness of the capsule. In implants from non-diabetic rats, the thickness was 294.5±18.5 μm versus 169.4±10.8 μm in implants from diabetic animals (Fig. 6A–C). Similarly, a decrease in the number of foreign body giant cells in implants from diabetic animals was observed when compared with those from non-diabetic animals (Fig. 6D–F).

Discussion

Implantation of devices or biomaterials triggers a series of host reactions at the injury site that include interactions material/tissue, provisional matrix formation, acute and chronic inflammation, granulation tissue development, foreign body reaction, and fibrosis and fibrous capsule development [2,7]. Invariably, this foreign body reaction affects the implanted material's efficiency, leading to device failure [4,8,17]. Much of the knowledge on this adverse healing following biomaterial implantation has come from normoglycemic individuals, despite the fact that complications associated with diabetes often requires implantable devices such as glucose sensors, orthopedic implants, catheter, vascular grafts, drug-eluting stents, artificial organs, biosensors, scaffolds for tissue

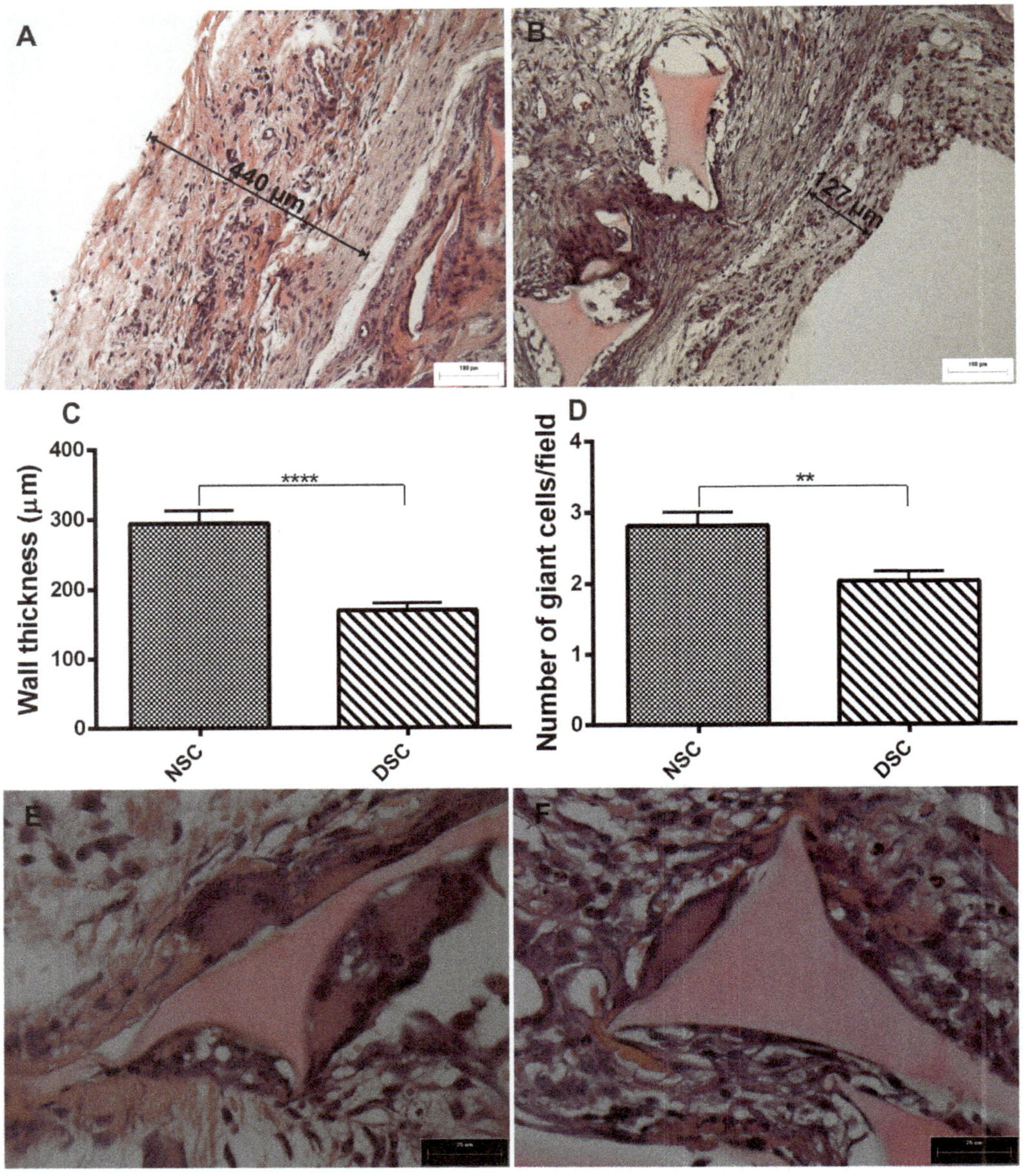

Figure 6. Histological characteristics of implant fibrous capsule. Representative histological sections of fibrous capsule in 10-day old implants from non-diabetic (A) and diabetic rats (B) (H&E staining) scale bar, 100 µm. Wall thickness was decreased after diabetes induction (C). Values shown are expressed as mean±SEM. *Significant difference between non-diabetic and diabetic; $p<0.05$. Student's t-test. Furthermore, the number foreign body giant cells was equally reduced in implants from diabetic rats (D). Values shown are expressed as mean±SEM. *Significant difference between non-diabetic and diabetic; $p<0.05$. Mann-Whitney test. Representative histological sections of foreign body giant cells in 10-day old implants from non-diabetic (E) and diabetic rats (F) (H&E staining); scale bar, 25 µm. NSC, non-diabetic implant; DSC, diabetic implant.

engineering, and heart valves in diabetic individuals [9]. By studying the inflammatory, angiogenic, apoptotic, and fibrogenic components of the foreign body response induced by subcutaneous polyether-polyurethane implants in rats, we have been able to identify a number of diabetes-related alterations of this reaction within and around the synthetic matrix.

In the descriptive histologic analysis of the implants from diabetic animals, a less mature and less dense extracellular matrix with fewer, but more dilated blood vessels (H&E stained sections and in CD31-immunostained sections) was observed in contrast with implants from non-diabetic rats. This result is consistent with reduced amounts of collagen and impaired angiogenesis in cutaneous wound healing and soft-tissue around implanted devices in diabetes [10–11,18–19]. However, Hb content and VEGF levels (angiogenic markers) in implants from diabetic rats were not altered in our experiments. This apparent discrepancy between a decreased number of vessels in implants from diabetic animals and no change in hemoglobin content may be explained by the increased vasodilatation observed in the histological sections of implants from the same group. Vascular dysfunctions, such as increased permeability, vasodilatation, and structural changes, are well established abnormalities in the diabetic state in experimental animal and human microvasculature [10,20–21]. Because we have shown an increased number of mast cells in implants from diabetic animals when compared with that from normoglycemic rats, it is possible that the histamine's well-known vasodilator effect may have contributed to maintaining the Hb content in both implants, despite the smaller number of blood vessels in implants from diabetic rats.

The inflammatory components of the skin wound's microenvironment in diabetes is altered in several aspects, including abnormal cellular infiltration, cytokine production, and protease release [2,22–23]. However, less is known about the inflammatory component of internal injury following device implantation in diabetes [8]. We measured four inflammation markers (MPO and NAG activities and two cytokines, TNF-α and MCP-1levels), in 10-day old implants from both groups of animals. We have also determined the number of mast cells within the fibrovascular tissue in the implants. All parameters, except for NAG activity (macrophage activation), were higher in implants from diabetic rats when compared with those from non-diabetic animals. We did not expect to find that, in implants from diabetic rats, the levels of MCP-1 (relevant chemoattractant chemokine) did not parallel NAG activity as previously demonstrated [24]. One possible explanation for this discrepancy is that, in the hyperglycemic environment, macrophages may be defective in their response to the chemoattractant stimulus. Alternatively, MCP-1 production and macrophage recruitment in the foreign body reaction may differ between internal and skin injuries. Apart from this, our findings are in accordance with the notion of an altered inflammatory microenvironment in diabetic skin wounds and this concept is extended to the foreign body reaction in rats. To same extent, our results are also in agreement with the studies performed in subcutaneous and percutaneous implants from diabetic baboons and rabbits, in which persistent infiltration of neutrophils and a reduced number of macrophages were observed in internal wounds [10–11]. These changes have occurred together with changes in chemokine and growth factor expression (increase levels of MCP-1 and TNF-α). An increased production of the same inflammatory cytokines was observed in the wounds of type-1 diabetic patients [25]. In the excisional skin wound mice model of type 1 and 2 diabetes, increased TNF-α levels were reported and proposed to account for fibroblast apoptosis, which, in turn, resulted in a failure to produce sufficient matrix deposition at the injury site [26]. In our findings, TNF-α levels and the apoptotic index were also higher in the internal fibrovascular tissue in diabetes. These may be one possible explanation for the decreased levels of TGB-β1 production, collagen deposition, fibrous capsule formation and number of foreign body giant cells found in implants from diabetic rats compared with that from normoglycemic animals. In fact, it has been proposed that processes that interfere with sufficient number of cells involved in the various phases of repair, such as fibroblast apoptosis, impair wound healing [26–28].

Numerous reports indicate that encapsulation is influenced by several factors, including properties of the biomaterial, biomaterial porosity, surface texture, and implantation site [29]. In fact, our observation of the events following intraperitoneal (i.p.) implantation of sponge discs in diabetic rats showed increased levels of angiogenic (VEGF) and fibrogenic (TGF-β1) cytokines and an increase in macrophage accumulation [30] which are in contrast with the findings from subcutaneous implants in the hyperglycemic environment. Nevertheless, the outcome of our experiments was an attenuated fibrogenic response in both intraperitoneal and subcutaneous implants in diabetic animals.

The main findings that have emerged from our work were that the changes observed in the foreign body reaction induced by synthetic implants in diabetic rats shared similarities with those seen in cutaneous tissue reported in the literature (decreased collagen deposition, disturbed inflammatory infiltrate, decreased angiogenesis, and increased apoptosis) in diabetic animals. More importantly, fibrous capsule formation and presence of foreign body giant cells, the typical features of the foreign body reaction, were attenuated in the hyperglycemic environment. These findings may be critical in developing strategies that may improve the performance and function of implanted biomaterials in diabetes.

Supporting Information

Data S1 Analyses of implants from normoglycemic and hyperglycemic animals.

Author Contributions

Conceived and designed the experiments: TOS SPA ACV PPC. Performed the experiments: TOS PPC NBP JPCS. Analyzed the data: TOS SPA PPC. Contributed reagents/materials/analysis tools: TOS SPA PPC ACV. Contributed to the writing of the manuscript: TOS SSP.

References

1. Anderson JM, McNally AK (2011) Biocompatibility of implants: lymphocyte/macrophage interactions. Semin Immunopathol 33: 221–233. http://www.ncbi.nlm.nih.gov/pubmed/21271251.
2. Luttikhuizen DT, Harmsen MC, Van Luyn MJ (2006) Cellular and molecular dynamics in the foreign body reaction. Tissue Eng 12: 1955–1970. http://www.ncbi.nlm.nih.gov/pubmed/16889525.
3. Wynn TA (2007) Common and unique mechanisms regulate fibrosis in various fibroproliferative diseases. J Clin Invest 117: 524–529. http://www.ncbi.nlm.nih.gov/pubmed/17332879.
4. Morais JM, Papadimitrakopoulos F, Burgess DJ (2010) Biomaterials/tissue interactions: Possible solutions to overcome foreign body response. The AAPS Journal 12: 188–196. http://www.ncbi.nlm.nih.gov/pubmed/20143194.
5. Campos PP, Andrade SP, Moro L, Ferreira MA, Vasconcelos AC (2006) Cellular proliferation, differentiation and apoptosis in polyether-polyurethane sponge implant model in mice. Histol Histopathol 21: 1263–1270. http://www.ncbi.nlm.nih.gov/pubmed/16977576.
6. Mendes JB, Rocha MA, Araújo FA, Moura SA, Ferreira MA, et al. (2009) Differential effects of rolipram on chronic subcutaneous inflammatory angiogenesis and on peritoneal adhesion in mice. Microvascular Research 78: 265–271. http://www.ncbi.nlm.nih.gov/pubmed/19732781.
7. Anderson JM, Rodriguez A, Chang DT (2008) Foreign body reaction to biomaterials. Semin Immunol 20: 86–100. http://www.ncbi.nlm.nih.gov/pubmed/18162407.
8. Le NN, Rose MB, Levinson H, Klitzman B (2011) Implant healing in experimental animal models of diabetes. J Diabetes Sci Technol 5: 605–618. http://www.ncbi.nlm.nih.gov/pubmed/21722576.
9. Onuki Y, Bhardwaj U, Papadimitrakopoulos F, Burgess DJ (2008) A review of the biocompatibility of implantable devices: current challenges to overcome foreign body response. J Diabetes Sci Technol 2: 1003–1015. http://www.ncbi.nlm.nih.gov/pubmed/19885290.
10. Thomson SE, McLennan SV, Hennessy A, Boughton P, Bonner J, et al. (2010) A novel primate model of delayed wound healing in diabetes: dysregulation of connective tissue growth factor. Diabetologia 53: 572–583. http://www.ncbi.nlm.nih.gov/pubmed/20091023.
11. Gerritsen M, Lutterman JA, Jansen JA (2000) A percutaneous device to study glucose kinetics in subcutaneous tissue fluid. J Mater Sci Mater Med 11: 499–503. http://www.ncbi.nlm.nih.gov/pubmed/15348000.
12. Campos PP, Bakhle YS, Andrade SP (2008) Mechanisms of wound healing responses in lupus-prone New Zealand White mouse strain. Wound Repair Regen 16: 416–424. http://www.ncbi.nlm.nih.gov/pubmed/18471260.
13. Araújo FA, Rocha MA, Ferreira MA, Campos PP, Capettini LS, et al. (2011) Implant-induced intraperitoneal inflammatory angiogenesis is attenuated by fluvastatin. Clin Exp Pharmacol Physiol 38: 262–268. http://www.ncbi.nlm.nih.gov/pubmed/21309808.
14. Bailey PJ (1988) Sponge implants as models. Methods Enzymol. 162: 327–334. http://www.ncbi.nlm.nih.gov/pubmed/3226313.
15. Ferreira MA, Barcelos LS, Campos PP, Vasconcelos AC, Teixeira MM, et al. (2004) Sponge-induced angiogenesis and inflammation in PAF receptor-deficient mice (PAFR-KO). Br J Pharmacol 141: 1185–1192. http://www.ncbi.nlm.nih.gov/pubmed/15023865.
16. Mendes JB, Campos PP, Ferreira MA, Bakhle YS, Andrade SP. (2007) Host response to sponge implants differs between subcutaneous and intraperitoneal

sites in mice. J Biomed Mater Res B Appl Biomater 83: 408–415. http://www.ncbi.nlm.nih.gov/pubmed/17415768.
17. Kyriakides TR, Bornstein P (2003) Matricellular proteins as modulators of wound healing and the foreign body response. Thromb Haemost 90: 986–992. http://www.ncbi.nlm.nih.gov/pubmed/14652628.
18. Altavilla D, Saitta A, Cucinotta D, Galeano M, Deodato B, et al. (2001) Inhibition of lipid peroxidation restores impaired vascular endothelial growth factor expression and stimulates wound healing and angiogenesis in the genetically diabetic mouse. Diabetes 50: 667–674. http://www.ncbi.nlm.nih.gov/pubmed/11246889.
19. Brem H, Tomic-Canic M (2007) Cellular and molecular basis of wound healing in diabetes. J Clin Invest 117: 1219–1222. http://www.ncbi.nlm.nih.gov/pubmed/17476353.
20. Kilzer P, Chang K, Marvel J, Rowold E, Jaudes P (1985) Albumin permeation of new vessels is increased in diabetic rats. Diabetes 34: 333–6. http://www.ncbi.nlm.nih.gov/pubmed/2579004.
21. Kahn AM, Seidel CL, Allen JC, O'Neil RG, Shelat H, et al. (1993) Insulin reduces contraction and intracellular calcium concentration in vascular smooth muscle. Hypertension 22: 735–742. http://www.ncbi.nlm.nih.gov/pubmed/8225533.
22. Blakytny R, Jude E (2006) The molecular biology of chronic wounds and delayed healing in diabetes. Diabet Med 23: 594–608. http://www.ncbi.nlm.nih.gov/pubmed/16759300.
23. Falanga V. Wound healing and its impairment in the diabetic foot (2005) Lancet 366: 1736–1743. http://www.ncbi.nlm.nih.gov/pubmed/16291068.
24. Engelhardt E, Toksoy A, Goebeler M, Debus S, Bröcker EB, et al. (1998) Chemokines IL-8, GROalpha, MCP-1, IP-10, and Mig are sequentially and differentially expressed during phase-specific infiltration of leukocyte subsets in human wound healing. Am J Pathol 153: 1849–1860. http://www.ncbi.nlm.nih.gov/pubmed/9846975.
25. Chatzigeorgiou A, Harokopos V, Mylona-Karagianni C, Tsouvalas E, Aidinis V, et al. (2010) The pattern of inflammatory/anti-inflammatory cytokines and chemokines in type 1 diabetic patients over time. Ann Med 42: 426–438. http://www.ncbi.nlm.nih.gov/pubmed/20568978.
26. Siqueira MF, Li J, Chehab L, Desta T, Chino T, et al. (2010) Impaired wound healing in mouse models of diabetes is mediated by TNF-α dysregulation and associated with enhanced activation of forkhead box O1 (FOXO1). Diabetologia 53: 378–388. http://www.ncbi.nlm.nih.gov/pubmed/19902175.
27. Darby IA, Bisucci T, Hewitson TD, MacLellan DG (1997) Apoptosis is increased in a model of diabetes-impaired wound healing in genetically diabetic mice. Int J Biochem Cell Biol 29: 191–200. http://www.ncbi.nlm.nih.gov/pubmed/9076954.
28. Rai NK, Suryabhan, Ansari M, Kumar M, Shukla VK, et al. (2005) Effect of glycaemic control on apoptosis in diabetic wounds. J Wound Care 14: 277–281. http://www.ncbi.nlm.nih.gov/pubmed/15974415.
29. Mikos AG, McIntire LV, Anderson JM, Babensee JE (1998) Host response to tissue engineered devices. Adv Drug Deliv Rev; 33: 111–139. http://www.ncbi.nlm.nih.gov/pubmed/10837656.
30. Oviedo-Socarrás T, Vasconcelos AC, Barbosa IX, Pereira NB, Campos PP, et al. (2014) Diabetes alters inflammation, angiogenesis, and fibrogenesis in intraperitoneal implants in rats. Microvasc Res 93: 23–29. http://www.ncbi.nlm.nih.gov/pubmed/24594441.

12

Hypoxia in Vascular Networks: A Complex System Approach to Unravel the Diabetic Paradox

Yérali Gandica[1], Tobias Schwarz[1,2], Orlando Oliveira[1], Rui D. M. Travasso[1,3]*

1 Center for Computational Physics, Department of Physics, University of Coimbra, Coimbra, Portugal, 2 Heinz-Brandt-Schule, Berlin, Germany, 3 Center of Ophthalmology and Vision Sciences(COCV), Institute for Biomedical Imaging and Life Sciences (IBILI), Faculty of Medicine, University of Coimbra, Coimbra, Portugal

Abstract

In this work we model the extent of hypoxia in the diabetic retina as a function of the area affected by vessel disruption. We find two regimes that differ on the ratio between the area of disrupted vasculature and the area of tissue in hypoxia. In the first regime the hypoxia is *localized* in the vicinity of the vascular disruption, while in the second regime there is a *generalized* hypoxia in the affected tissue. The transition between these two regimes occurs when the tissue area affected by individual sites of vessel damage is on the order of the square of the characteristic irrigation length in the tissue (the maximum distance that an irrigated point in the tissue is from an existing vessel). We observe that very high levels of hypoxia are correlated with the rupture of larger vessels in the retina, and with smaller radii of individual sites of vessel damage. Based on this property of vascular networks, we propose a novel mechanism for the transition between the nonproliferative and the proliferative stages in diabetic retinopathy.

Editor: Timothy W. Secomb, University of Arizona, United States of America

Funding: Y.G., T.S. and R.D.M.T. acknowledge financial support from Fundos FEDER through Programa Operacional Factores de Competitividade – COMPETE and by Fundação para a Ciência e Tecnologia, through project FCOMP-01-0124-FEDER-015708. The authors acknowledge support from Fundação para a Ciência e Tecnologia through project PEst-OE/FIS/UI0405/2014. R.D.M.T. acknowledges financial support from Fundação para a Ciência e Tecnologia through the Investigador FCT program. The funders had no role in study design, data collection and analysis, decision to publish, or preparation of the manuscript.

Competing Interests: The authors have declared that no competing interests exist.

* Email: rui@teor.fis.uc.pt

Introduction

Diabetes occurs when the pancreas does not secrete enough insulin or the body is unable to process it properly [1]. High levels (and/or wide fluctuations) of glucose concentration in the blood can lead to a number of complications, including an increased risk of cardio-vascular disease, kidney disease (nephropathy), neural damage (neuropathy), and retinal disease (diabetic retinopathy, DR) [2]. The number of deaths attributed to diabetes is about 9% of the global total of deaths [3].

Diabetic retinas suffer extensive blood vessel disruption (e.g. the formation of defects such as micro-aneurisms, and dramatic vessel proliferation increase, leading to the formation of small blood lakes and to loss of vessel function) [4] which stems from the inflammatory environment that is associated with high levels of methilglyoxal [5], and lead to the production of several proteins that have a vascular destabilization action. An example is the angiopoietin-2 (Ang-2) [6] that binds the receptors Tie-2 at the membrane of the vessels' endothelial cells, thus preventing the mediation of angiopoietin-1 in the maturation of the capillaries. Therefore, in the absence of pro-angiogenic factors, high levels of Ang-2 induce an increase of vessel permeability, with the consequence of a deficient tissue irrigation [7] (note, however, that the loosening of the Tie-2 junctions between endothelial cells is also an important step of the angiogenic process, and therefore, Ang-2 is able to promote angiogenesis depending on the presence of pro-angiogenic factors). It has been shown experimentally in mice that retinal vascular network damage is able to drive neo-vascularization characteristic of the later stages of DR [8,9].

A large body of work has been done to understand the pathogenesis of diabetic microvasculopathy [10,11]. Most of these efforts have been centered in the mechanisms related to specific signaling pathways [12,13]. Nevertheless, we argue in the present work that the spatial distribution of areas with deficient irrigation, i.e. in hypoxia, also play an important role in the determining the progression of the disease. In these regions, the lack of oxygen leads to higher levels of angiogenic factors that promote the remodeling of the vasculature as well as the growth of neo-vessels, both hallmarks of DR [14]. In consequence, the study of how the distribution of hypoxic regions depends on vascular damage is essential for the understanding of DR's progression. In this work we will focus on the changes in irrigation after events of vessel blockage, inspired by the effect of factors such as Ang-2, that are present in high levels in a DR setting, and that have the potential to drive extensive vessel damage rendering the smaller vessels non-functional. This study is closely related with the analysis of resilience in spatial complex networks, where is investigated the effect of a particular amount of damage in the nodes and/or links on the integrity of the complex network.

The resilience of complex networks to damage has attracted a great deal of attention in the past years [15–23]. Most of the studies on this topic link the random or selected removal of nodes to the alteration in the structural properties of networks and have important applications. For example, the study of the percolation properties of a network of social relations upon node removal can be applied directly to viral epidemics. In this case, random node removal gives information about the amount of agents to immunize in order to prevent the propagation of the epidemics

[24]. Also, the consequences of the breakdown of power lines resultant from a natural hazard, for example, is a problem that can be formulated in terms of the failure of interconnected networks, see e.g. [25,26].

Networks are studied by defining the nodes of the system and the connectivity between them by means of edges or bonds. Other specific characteristics can be added according to the system that is modeled, such as bond weights, directionality, etc [15–17]. Typically, when structural and dynamic characteristics of a network are determined solely by their connectivity, it can be considered to be embedded in an abstract "network space" [27]. However, when networks have the role of delivering energy, water or nutrients, the physical space constraints are important. In these networks, resilience after the rupture of bonds at a particular location is connected to the lack of goods, energy, water or nutrients in spatial regions, and not to the number of nodes and bonds affected per se [28]. Not surprisingly, the applications of the study of the resilience in spatial networks are vast, however most previous studies in resilience of complex networks have not considered spatial constraints [27].

Vascular networks are a particular type of spatial network constituted by two different topologies of connections that fulfill different functions [29]. Larger vessels, arterioles and venules form *specific* fractal tree-like networks [30–33] that are responsible for blood transport [34]. In these structures, alterations in the branching pattern [35], branching lengths [36,37], fractal dimension [32,38] among others, are often an indication of a pathology. On the other hand, nutrient and oxygen diffusion is carried out mainly by capillaries which are laid down in space approximately in a lattice-like structure [29,39,40]. Vascular networks are dynamic, since they can adapt to the nutrient requirements of the tissue they irrigate [41]. Therefore, spatial constraints, such as the nutrient and protein diffusion, affect not only the tissue cells survival, but also the structure of the vascular network itself.

Earlier studies on the hypoxia in damaged vascular networks showed a localized decrease in irrigation after specific targeting of blood vessels. Blinder et al. [30] studying robustness of distribution of blood in rodent neocortex to occlusion experiments found that removing 15% of the connections in the backbone isolates 5% of the cortex from perfusion. More recently, the same authors investigated experimentally the volume of micro-infarctions in the rat brain, resultant of the occlusion of specific arterioles [42], demonstrating that even small volumes of low irrigation have important cognitive consequences.

Our aim is to relate the different stages of DR with the distribution of tissue irrigation decrease after a total loss of vascular function in localised regions in the retina. This article is organized as follows. In the next section the retina vessel network is described, together with the details of calculation of the tissue irrigation. In the Simulation and Results section we investigate how the affected irrigation changes with the damaged vasculature. In the Discussion section the results are analyzed and its physio-pathological implications to the development of DR are discussed. Finally, in the last section we summarize and conclude.

Materials and Methods

The aim of this work is to propose a mechanism relating the evolution of the proliferative stage of DR with the patterns of hypoxia in the retinal tissue after damage of its vascular network. Therefore, we start with a vascular network that mimics the retinal vasculature. The top layer of the vasculature at the retina is almost two dimensional [43], so that its approximate structure can be obtained from the digitalization of an angiography. In this work we used an angiography of a human retina (with 1684×1192 lattice units, equivalent to 9.4×6.6 mm; each lattice unit corresponds to 5.6 μm), obtained from a patient in the early stages of diabetic retinopathy (left panel in Fig. 1). Patients at Coimbra's University Hospitals routinely perform angiographies to assess the progress of different diseases (normally DR or age related macular degeneracy). This results in an image where the deficiencies of the retinal vascular network can be clearly visualized. The hospital stores several of these images obtained from anonymous patients as example of the different stages of relevant pathologies. We chose one image from that set corresponding to a very early stage of DR, where the pathology-driven vasculature alteration was the least perceptible. No human tissues or cells were used in this study.

A closed vascular network is obtained extending manually the thinner arterial vessels to intercept the thinner veins (see Fig. 1 center). Taking into account the thickness and contrast in the original angiography, we are able to manually identify the sites where the vessels overlap without establishing bifurcations. Even missing the thinnest capillaries, this network provides the basic structure of in-vivo retinal networks. The measured number of bifurcations between the main vessel (artery or vein) and the furthermost capillary is 35. This number is of the same order of magnitude as the number of successive vessel bifurcations observed in higher organisms [44].

The blood flow in the network (right panel in Fig. 1) is approximated by assuming Poiseuille flow in all vessels, i.e., that they have cylindrical symmetry and that the blood viscosity is high enough to neglect turbulence and inertial effects [44]. For the human body, this is a good approximation, except for the larger arteries and veins [44]. At every bifurcation in the vessel network we apply blood flow conservation, i.e. the sum of incoming flows to a node matches the sum of the outgoing flows. In all calculations we also disregard the alterations in blood viscosity due to the Fahreus-Lindqvist effect and the viscoelasticity of the blood (in the Text S1 we demonstrate that the inclusion of the Fahreus-Lindqvist effect does not affect in a significant way our results).

Our analysis is based on a steady state study, and therefore we do not take into account the pressure and radii variation at the larger vessels due to the heart beat. Also, given that most of the flow in the retinal vessels is laminar, solving the full Navier-Stokes equation can only change the pressure at the vessels for a small amount, leaving essentially unchanged the calculated hypoxia regions after vessel suppression.

Very high levels of Ang-2 increase the vessel permeability, and, in the limit, render them incapable of irrigating the tissue. In this work we take this limit, and consider the total loss of function of individual thin vessels in the regions affected by vessel damage. We use a simplified method to estimate the effects of vascular disruptions on tissue oxygen levels. In reality, the oxygen level declines nonlinearly with the distance along each vessel, depending on the flow rate, the oxygen consumption rate, and on the nonlinear oxygen binding characteristics of hemoglobin. For simplicity, we here use intravascular hydrostatic pressure as an index of position along each flow pathway, and assume a linear dependence of the oxygen concentration on pressure, setting the levels of oxygen at the retinal artery equal to 1 and the concentration at the veins equal to 0. Since the model used is linear in the levels of oxygen in the tissue, the profile of hypoxia observed is independent of the values of the oxygen levels at the arteries and veins, if the critical oxygen concentration for hypoxia in the tissue is altered accordingly. In fact, we expect that the observed hypoxic regions after vessel suppression will depend

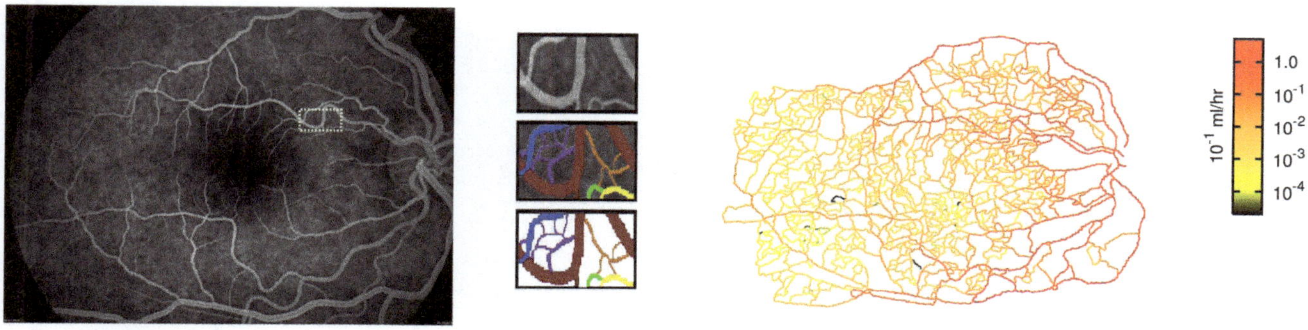

Figure 1. Characterization of the vascular network. Left panel: The original angiography of the retina that was digitalized. Identified with a small rectangle is the area that is amplified in the central panel. Center panel: Zoom of detail in angiography: original detail (top); manual identification of vessels with different colors indicating joined vessels of similar caliber (center); geometry that is digitalized to obtain the reconstructed network (bottom). Right panel: The blood flow in the reconstructed network. The color gradient indicates the flow intensity.

mainly on the diffusion of oxygen in the tissue (and in particular on the characteristic irrigation length, i.e. the maximum distance that an irrigated point in the tissue is from a vessel, function of the oxygen diffusion length, the oxygen consumption rate and the critical oxygen concentration for hypoxia), and not on the details of how the oxygen levels at the vessels are calculated (see below and Text S1).

The transport of oxygen to the tissues occurs via a diffusive process. We consider that the oxygen consumption rate in the tissue is constant and, therefore, the time-independent concentration of oxygen c_O can be obtained from the Poisson equation

$$L^2\nabla^2 c_O = c_O, \quad (1)$$

where L is the tissue oxygen diffusion length. In this equation, we linearize the Michaelis-Menten kinetics normally used for the consumption of oxygen by the tissue [45,46], since the regions of hypoxia that are analyzed in this work are determined by the characteristic irrigation length (see below and Text S1), i.e. by the levels of oxygen far from the immediate vicinity of the capillaries, which is where the non-linear behavior of the Michaelis-Menten is relevant.

Equation (1) is solved in a large rectangular domain that includes the totality of vessel network. We use the successive over-relaxation method setting the concentration of oxygen to zero at the borders of the domain, and having as boundary condition the concentration of oxygen at the vessels that are able to irrigate. The capillary endothelium is highly specialized to permit the exchange of oxygen between the blood and the tissue. In contrast, main arteries and veins have the function of transporting the blood to and from the capillaries [34] and have thick walls that often require their proper irrigation to be oxygenated. For this reason, we consider that only the thinner vessels (venules, arterioles and capillaries) with flow larger than zero can irrigate (in the model we assign this function to vessels with diameter smaller than 24 μm so that most of the vessels in the simulation participate actively in irrigation of the tissue). Therefore, when equation (1) is solved for every point in the tissue, the concentration of oxygen is fixed as boundary condition at the smaller vessels (with diameter smaller than 24 μm) if their flow is larger than zero.

If c_O falls below a critical value, C_m, the tissue cells will enter in hypoxia. In Fig. 2 we show the maximum value for C_m such that all the tissue region highlighted in the inset (inside the turquoise dashed rectangle) is in normoxia as a function of L (since a site is in normoxia if $c_O > C_m$, the plot corresponds to the minimum value of c_O inside the highlighted region as a function of L). In order to avoid the irregular boundary of the network, we will focus on the rectangular region highlighted in the inset of Fig. 2 in the rest of the work. The lower the value L, the faster equation (1) is solved numerically. We chose $L=20$ lattice units (112μm) and $C_m=0.06$ (corresponding to a point on the beginning of the rising part of the curve in Fig. 2) for faster run times and we have found that our results are independent of this particular choice for L (see also Text S1).

Results

To simulate the effect of localized vascular loss of function of the thinner vessels, we consider small circular regions of radius R in the vascular network where the vessel damage occurs. Inside these regions, we block all vessels with diameter smaller than a cutoff, Λ. These circular regions are distributed randomly within the highlighted area in the inset of Fig. 2. The area fraction covered by these blocking regions will be deemed A_{blk}. In what follows we will take $\Lambda=4.35$ lattice units, i.e. 24 μm, the average of the

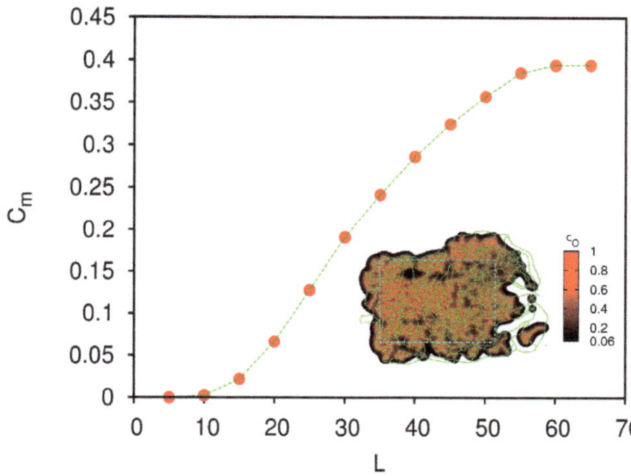

Figure 2. Plot of the C_m required for the normoxia of all tissue inside the rectangle (inset) as a function of the diffusion length of oxygen, L. Inset: In this diagram we represent the vascular network analyzed (in green), the c_O in the retina (in the gradient black-red) for $L=20$ lattice units and $C_m=0.06$, and the boundary of the region of the retina analyzed in this work (in turquoise).

diameters of the vessels in our network. The results will be compared to those using a larger cutoff $\Lambda=8$ lattice units, i.e. 45 μm. Physiologically, taking larger values of Λ means considering also the suppression of thicker vessels.

Once the vessels are blocked, the blood flow will be altered (i.e. we re-calculate the flow, now in the altered vessel network), the irrigation of the retina will be lower and this may lead to new regions in hypoxia. We measure how the total area in hypoxia changes with A_{blk}, the area where the thin vessels are blocked.

Fig. 3 depicts the average area in hypoxia, A_H, for only one blocking circular area of radius R. The data in the plot are the average over 500 random realisations of the blocking sites. The picture shows the results for different values of diffusion length L and two different cutoffs Λ. Interestingly, for all these different parameters there is a single critical value of the radius ($R_c \approx 50$) below which only one blocking circle does not induce an appreciable change in the irrigation of the network. It is therefore necessary a minimal size of the blocking target to produce an area in hypoxia. We observe that this characteristic distance in the system does not depend on the value of L or Λ, but on the maximum distance that a point is from a capillary vessel in the analyzed network (see Text S1). Hence, R_c will be designated by the characteristic irrigation length.

We proceed by increasing the number of damaged circular neighborhoods, which are distributed randomly (they may overlap). We calculate the fraction of area in hypoxia, A_H, as a function of the area fraction of retina affected by the vessel disrupting proteins, A_{blk}, see Fig. 4. Each curve corresponds to vessel damaged regions built with blocking circles with the same radius R. The radii are indicated in lattice units. For equal blocked areas the hypoxia can be considerably different, depending on the radii of the blocking regions.

We observe a monotonic increase of A_H with A_{blk} for all the values of R. In general, for large blocked areas, a larger R corresponds to a smaller area in hypoxia. However, for small values of A_{blk} we found a different behavior depending if R is larger or lower than the characteristic irrigation length, $R_c \approx 50$. Above this radius (Fig. 4 left), at blocking areas below a critical area $A_c \approx 0.47$, and contrary to what happens for $A_{blk} > A_c$, a larger R corresponds to a larger area in hypoxia. On the other hand, for $R < R_c$ (Fig. 4 right) the area in hypoxia is independent of the radius for very low A_{blk}, i.e. all the curves collapse into a single curve at low A_{blk} (the section of the curve where this collapse occurs depends on the value of R, with a larger overlap region for larger values of R). Besides, for $R < R_c$, the value of A_{blk} at which the transition to the large area regime occurs is lower than $A_c \approx 0.47$ and strongly dependent on the radius, in opposition to the situation where $R > R_c$. This transition for $R < R_c$ is associated with a very steep increase in A_H. The slope of this increase is larger for smaller values of R.

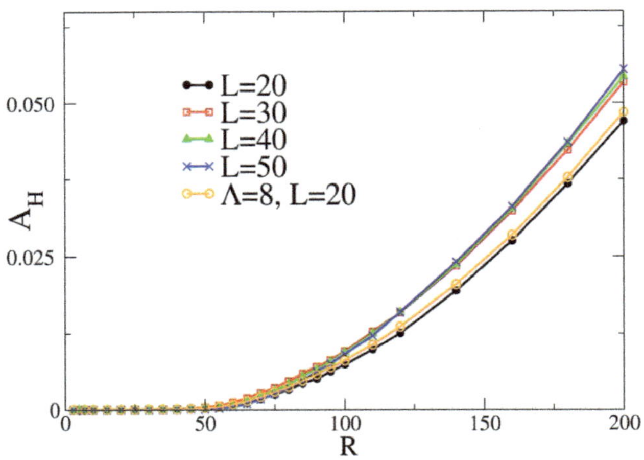

Figure 3. Resulting area in hypoxia for one blocking spot of radius *R*. Each curve has a different diffusion length, $L=20$, 30, 40 and 50 (each point in the graphic represents the average of 500 runs). Also shown are the results for $L=20$ with $\Lambda=8$. The curves for different Λ and $L=20$ are, essentially, undistinguishable. In all cases the radius of the circle necessary for an average hypoxia region larger than zero is $R_c \approx 50$.

Discussion

Damage and Hypoxia

To understand the dependence of the A_H on A_{blk} and R, we will start by analyzing how hypoxia regions are formed after vessel blockage in this system.

The blockage induced by a single circular region with radius larger than the characteristic irrigation length produces an area in hypoxia which is smaller than the blocked region (Fig. 5a). Points inside the blocking region that are at a distance larger than the characteristic irrigation length R_c from the circumference of the region, are in hypoxia. Hence, for blocking circles with $R > R_c$, the area that is still irrigated is approximately equal to $2\pi R R_c$, i.e. it grows linearly with R and not with R^2. Therefore, for larger blocking circles, the areas inside each circle that are still irrigated are proportionally smaller. Consequently, for $R > R_c$, for a small number of these regions and for the same covered area, we observe that higher values of R will correspond to a higher hypoxic area (see Fig. 4 left).

As the number of blocked areas gets larger, A_{blk} increases until the system reaches a regime in which regions are not irrigated, in spite of not having their vessels blocked. This is the consequence of being surrounded by the circular blocking areas (Fig. 5b)). In this regime, the number of such oxygen deprived regions will be larger if R is smaller, since for smaller R the number of circular blocking areas is higher, for the same A_{blk}. With a higher number of circular regions becomes easier to surround not affected areas, blocking the required vessels to deprive those regions of irrigation. Therefore, if $A_{blk} > A_c$, smaller R will correspond to larger A_H, in opposition to what is observed for $A_{blk} < A_c$.

A completely different scenerio occurs for $R < R_c$, i.e. when we are covering the network with targets smaller than its characteristic irrigation length. In this regime the effect of covering areas loses its local nature, because a single blocking region can not create hypoxia (as seen in Fig. 3). Hypoxia can only be reached with the cooperating effect of many blocking regions. This can be clearly seen in Fig. 5c, where the few hypoxic areas are the result of the particular disposition of various neighboring blocking spots.

As the number of blocking spots increases, there will be a density at which these spots have a high probability for blocking vessels separated by R_c. Above this density, that corresponds to a critical area A^*_{blk}, hypoxia will occur everywhere in the tissue. An example of such a situation is in Fig. 5d. We expect a sharp transition between $A_H \approx 0$ and almost total hypoxia at this particular density of blocking sites. For A^*_{blk} the area in hypoxia will be dramatically larger than A_{blk}. This effect can be clearly seen in the steep slope of the curves in right panel of Fig. 4.

It is possible to obtain the dependence of the critical area A^*_{blk} on R for very small R, disregarding overlap between the circles. Consider a blocking region of radius R much smaller than R_c. To have hypoxia, circles have to block vessels that are located at least at a distance $2R_c$. One of these circles blocks a given vessel, if its

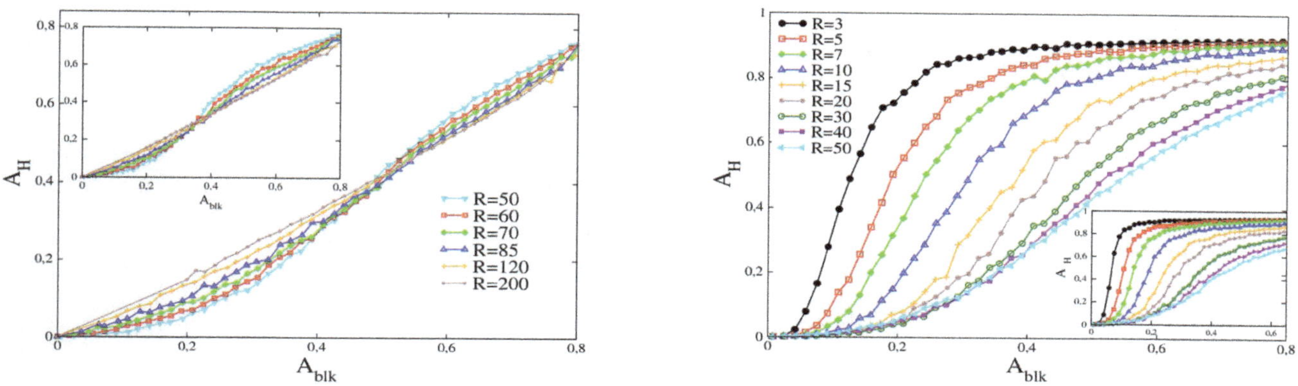

Figure 4. Fraction of area in hypoxia (A_H) versus fraction of area vessel disruption in the retina (A_{blk}). Left panel: Plots for $\Lambda=4.35$ and radii of each blocking circular neighborhood larger than 50 lattice units. The inset corresponds to $\Lambda=8$, i.e. when vessels with diameter smaller than 8 lattice units are compromised. Right panel: Same as in the left panel, but for radii smaller than 50.

center is closer to the vessel than a distance R. The associated probability for cutting the vessel is then of the order $p\sim\frac{R}{R_c}$. On the other hand, in 2D the number of blocking regions in a square of side $2R_c$ will be $4\rho R_c^2$, where ρ is the number of blocking circles per unit area. In order to have hypoxia everywhere, the critical A^*_{blk} should be such that is able to block the vessels, i.e. the probability of blocking a vessel is on the order of unity. Hence, the minimum density of points required, ρ^* obeys

$$4\rho^* R_c^2\frac{R}{R_c}=4\rho^* R_c R\sim 1\ .$$

We approximate $\rho^*\approx\frac{A^*_{blk}}{\pi R^2}$, obtaining finally that $A^*_{blk}\sim\frac{\pi R}{4R_c}\sim R$, i.e. the blocking area at the steepest slope in the right panel of Fig. 4 has a linear dependence with R.

For $R>R_c$ to have a large hypoxic region, the distance between the blocked centers should be on the order of the blocking circles radius, i.e. $\sqrt{1/\rho^*}\sim 2R$. Then, $\frac{\pi R^2}{A^*_{blk}}\sim 4R^2$ and for $R>R_c$, $A^*_{blk}\equiv A_c\sim O(1)$ is independent of R.

In Fig. 6 we show the log-log graph of the inflexion points for the curves plotted in Fig. 4. The inflexion points are obtained through a fit of the curves to an hyperbolic tangent function superimposed on a linear function. The error bars correspond to the statistical error of the non-linear fit. We associate the inflexion points to the transition values for A^*_{blk}. We can see that the dependence of A^*_{blk} is linear for R much smaller than R_c, becoming independent of R for $R>R_c$, in good agreement with the predictions discussed above.

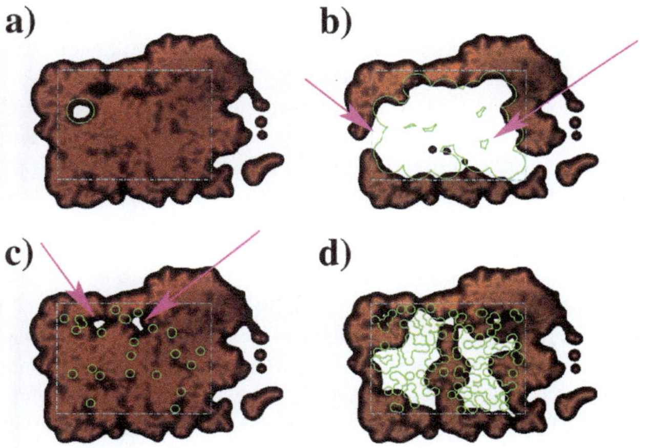

Figure 5. Irrigation, i.e. the density plot of c_O, in different scenarios. a) one blocking circle with $R=80$, b) 50 blocking circles with $R=80$ (arrows signal sites with no irrigation or vessel damage), c) 24 blocking circles with $R=25$ (arrows signal areas in hypoxia resultant from the combined action of several blocking sites) and d) 153 blocking circles with $R=25$. For each plot, the blocked regions are in green, the local irrigation are represented by the color gradient, from black (lower) to red (higher) and the areas in white inside rectangle of interest have $c_O<C_m$, and are in hypoxia.

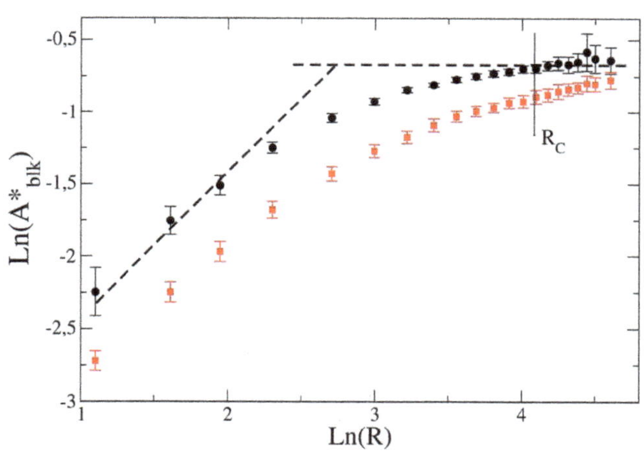

Figure 6. In black circles, the logarithm of inflexion points, from curves showed in Fig. 4, versus the logarithm of R. We compare to two straight dashed lines with slope 1 and 0. We observe that the transition points follow $A^*_{blk}\sim R$ for R much smaller than R_c and $A^*_{blk}\sim O(1)$ for $R>R_c$. In red squares the same for $\Lambda=8$ lattice units.

For $R > R_c$ the size of the blocking circles are larger than any characteristic scale in the underlining network, and the irrigation of the tissue will be blocked only when the blocking circles percolate the system. We also verify the non-dependence of A^*_{blk} on R which is characteristic of the circular blocking neighborhoods percolation (see Text S1). Therefore in this regime the transition does not depend on the underlining network.

Consequences for DR progression

We observed that the complex effects of covering areas with targets smaller than the lattice parameter produces hypoxic regions that can grow easily larger than the affected area for $R < R_c$. This regime can have important consequences in the progression of the disease.

It is a known fact that DR can be divided in two main stages with different phenotypes. The earliest stage of DR is nonproliferative diabetic retinopathy (NPDR). Though this stage can be itself divided in different sub-stages [1,2], it is characterized by the presence of micro-aneurisms (swellings in capillaries and arterioles), a variable degree of vessel blockage and the consequent deprivation of irrigation in some regions of the retina. The most advanced stage of DR, the proliferative diabetic retinopathy, PDR, is characterized by neovascularization, the growth of abnormal (fragile and leaky) new blood vessels, which may lead to blindness through hemorrhage and scarring [47]. This pathological retinal angiogenesis generates randomly orientated and physiologically deficient vessels that do not conform to neuronal histology [14].

The creation of this abnormal and dense structures is rooted in the following paradox (often referred in the literature as the diabetic paradox [48,49]): if the prevalent action in DR is the regression, disruption and blockage of blood vessels, then how does the hallmark of the most advanced stage of the disease is a very high vascular density? Does the fact that the vascular disruption sites in DR are extremely small and localized [50,51] play an important role in the progression of the disease?

According to our study, the blockage of vessels, akin to what happens in DR, leads to a deficient irrigation of the tissue, and to an increase of hypoxia in the retina. However, a tissue in hypoxia leads to an increase in the production of the HIF-1 (Hypoxia Inducible Factor) transcription factor, which has angiogenic factors, such as VEGF, as targets. The consequence is the triggering of neovascularization in the tissue [52–54]. We expect that when this neovascularization occurs repeatedly in regions where vessel regression and blockage occurred, the increase in VEGF levels will occur locally, balancing the effects of the antiangiogenic factors that led to the vessel disruption. The result will be a vasculature with the same physiological density and caliber but with possible local malformations [55]. In these situations we expect to find a NPDR phenotype.

However, when the disruptions of the vasculature lead to hypoxia in regions with little or no vessel regression, the neovascularization resultant from the high VEGF levels in these regions will not counterbalance the original disruption. Therefore, the process of angiogenesis would lead to a denser vasculature. In these situations we expect to find a PDR phenotype.

As we mentioned, in the right panel of Fig. 4 we observe a regime where the area in hypoxia is larger than the affected area. In this regime, associated with low values of R and large A_{blk}, we clearly have areas that will be producing very high levels of VEGF, since they are in hypoxia, and still have functional vessels. This setting suggests a high vessel density as consequence, and we can associate this effect with a PDR phenotype.

Therefore, we predict that the PDR phenotype occurs when $R < R_c$ as the density of affected points increases, i.e. as the disease progresses. This will happen in sections where a fraction of the retina larger than A^*_{blk} is affected. Besides, the existence of very small and localized sites of vascular disruption in DR in vivo is in agreement with the hypothesis of $R < R_c$ being required for PDR to develop [50,51].

However, we found that there is a possibility to decrease A^*_{blk} and to obtain the PDR regime at lower affected areas. In the insets of Fig. 4 we show A_H as a function of A_{blk}, but now we change the cutoff of the system to $\Lambda = 8$ lattice units. In this case in each blocking region all vessels with radius smaller than 8 units will be compromised, i.e. thicker vessels may also be affected. In spite that, in this case the minimum radius R_c of a blocking circles that can induce hypoxia is still the same as it is shown in Fig. 3. Accordingly, we still observe in the inset of Fig. 4 left and in Fig. 6 the approximately constant value for A^*_{blk} for $R > R_c$. Of course that, as R grows, the value of A^*_{blk} should reach $A_c \approx 0.47$, the value associated with the percolation of the blocking circles in this system. However for $R > R_c$ the increase of A_{blk} is extremely slow (Fig. 6).

For all values of R we observe that the values of A^*_{blk} are much lower when the thick vessels are also affected. Even for the largest R in the left panel of Fig. 4 the value $A^*_{blk} \approx 0.4$ is lower than the case where only the capillaries are affected. This is consequence of the specific structure of the retina network. The largest vessels are few in number but have the important role of distributing the blood through all the network. Cutting these vessels lead to a larger loss in irrigation than cutting only the small capillaries. The consequence is a lower value for the critical A_{blk}.

In what concerns the progression of DR, we anticipate that the PDR phenotype can dominate in two scenarios: either the affected area increases, or the type of vessels affected is altered and larger vessels are also compromised. In both situations the phenotype is most severe when the radius of each focus of damage is smaller, for the same affected area.

Conclusion

We analyzed the effect of vessel damage in the retina irrigation, consequent of the high levels of vessel destabilizing proteins, such as Ang-2, in a diabetic environment. In this study we modelled blood flow and the oxygen concentration in the tissue. Although more exhaustive methods exist to describe oxygen pressure dynamics [45,56–59] and the flow in vascular networks [60], the present model captures the main ingredients of the processes involved. However, when more subtle vessel disruption events are considered, (e.g. increases in the permeability of the capillaries that do not compromise the vessel viability, partial blockage of vessels), a more complete description of oxygen transport needs to be implemented, including how the oxygen levels decline nonlinearly with distance along each vessel as a function of the flow rate, and how it is consumed in the tissue according to a Michaelis-Menten kinetics [45,58,59]. The study of oxygen levels in these situations complement the work presented, and will be the subject of a future study.

Having access to the basic topology of the vascular network of a human retina, we found two regimes delimited by a critical size of blocking spots radius. This critical radius corresponds to the characteristic irrigation length in the network. Furthermore, these results suggest that the prevalent phenotype of the pathology can be a direct consequence of the distribution of disrupted and hypoxic regions in the tissue. We associate the situation where the hypoxia occurs prevalently in the region of vessel disruption with the non-proliferative diabetic retinopathy phenotype. On the other hand, if the extensive regions of hypoxia occur outside the region of vessel disruption we expect a proliferative diabetic retinopathy phenotype.

Our results suggest that disrupting the vessels in the retina with targets of radius lower than the characteristic irrigation length in the tissue (typical in DR [50,51]), may lead to large hypoxia levels with relatively low values of vessel destabilizing areas. These areas will be even lower if the vessel destabilizing environment is able to rupture thicker vessels. These results convey a new way of thinking about the diabetic paradox [48,49]: allowing the possibility that localized vessel disruption points lead to the formation of large regions in hypoxia, which have the ability to drive neovascularization [52,53], excessive angiogenesis is able to occur in pathologies that are driven by regression and blockage of blood vessels.

These conclusions on the mechanisms for the early development of the two phenotypes of DR may be of high importance in the definition of prevention strategies for the development of DR is risk patients.

Supporting Information

Text S1 In this text we discuss several details of our model. We focus on the relation between the characteristic irrigation length and the geometry of the network, on the relevance of modeling the Fahreus-Lindqvist effect, and on the relation between the percolation transition and the transition from the non proliferative phenotype to the proliferative phenotype.

Acknowledgments

The authors thank fruitful discussions with João Carvalho, Jaime Silva, Rui Bernardes, Conceição Lobo, Rosa Fernandes and the Henrique Girão's group. The authors would also like to thank the editor and the anonymous referees for their comments and helpful discussions which contributed to improve the final version of the text.

Author Contributions

Conceived and designed the experiments: TS OO RDMT. Performed the experiments: YG TS RDMT. Analyzed the data: YG TS RDMT. Contributed reagents/materials/analysis tools: TS RDMT. Wrote the paper: YG OO RDMT.

References

1. Yun WL, Acharya R, Venkatesh YV, Chee C, Min L C, et al. (2008) Identification of different stages of diabetic retinopathy. Information Sciences 178: 106–121.
2. Bearse MA Jr, Adams AJ, Han Y, Schneck ME, Ng J, et al. (2006) A Multifocal Electroretinogram Model Predicting the Development of Diabetic Retinopathy. Prog Retin Eye Res 25: 425–448.
3. World Health Organization. Media Centre. Available: http://www.who.int/mediacentre/factsheets/fs236/en/. Accessed: 2014 October 28.
4. Barber AJ, Antonetti DA (2003) Mapping the blood vessels with paracellular permeability in the retinas of diabetic rats. Invest Ophthal & Vis Sci, 44: 5410–5416.
5. Bento CF, Fernandes R, Matafome P, Sena C, Seiça R, et al. (2010) Methylglyoxal-induced imbalance in the ratio VEGF/Ang-2 secreted by retinal pigment epithelial cells leads to endothelial dysfunction. Exp Physiol 95: 955–970.
6. Hammes HP, Lin J, Wagner P, Feng Y, Vom Hagen F, et al. (2004) Angiopoietin-2 causes pericyte dropout in the normal retina: evidence for involvement in diabetic retinopathy. Diabetes 53: 1104–1110.
7. Maisonpierre PC, Suri C, Jones PF, Bartunkova S, Wiegand SJ, et al. (1997) Angiopoietin-2, a natural antagonist for Tie2 that disrupts in-vivo angiogenesis. Science 277: 55–60.
8. Smith LE, Wesolowski E, McLellan A, Kostyk SK, D'amato R, et al. (1994) Oxygen-induced retinopathy in the mouse. Investigative Ophthalmology & Visual Science 35: 101–111.
9. Connor KM, Krah NM, Dennison RJ, Aderman CM, Chen J, et al. (2009) Quantification of oxygen-induced retinopathy in the mouse: a model of vessel loss, vessel regrowth and pathological angiogenesis. Nature Protocols 4:1565–1573.
10. Davis S, Gale NW, Rudge JS, Wiegand SJ, Holash J (2000) Vascular-specific growth factors and blood vessel formation. Nature 407: 242–248.
11. Acharya UR, Ng EYK, Tan JH, Sree SV, Ng KH (2012) An Integrated Index for the Identification of Diabetic Retinopathy Stages Using Texture Parameters. J Med Syst 36: 2011–2020.
12. Reiter C, Sandirasegarane L, Wu XH, Nakamura M, Barber AJ, et al. (2005) The retinal insulin receptor, signaling pathway is impaired by diabetes: A potential mechanism contributing to diabetic retinopathy. Diabetes 54: A222.
13. Jun JI, Lau LF (2011) Taking aim at the extracellular matrix: CCN proteins as emerging therapeutic targets. Nature Reviews Drug Discovery 10: 945–963.
14. Gariano RF, Gardner TW (2005) Retinal angiogenesis in development and disease. Nature 438: 960–6.
15. Newman M, Barabási A-L, Watts D (2006) Structure and Dynamics of Networks. Princeton, NJ: Princeton University Press.
16. Barrat A, Barthèlemy M, Vespignani A (2008) Dynamical Processes on Complex Networks. Cambridge: Cambridge University Press.
17. Paul G, Sreenivasan S, Stanley HE (2005) Resilience of complex networks to random breakdown, Phys Rev E 72: 056130.
18. Albert R, Jeong H, Barabási AL (2000) Error and attack tolerance of Complex Networks. Nature 406: 378–382.
19. Callaway DS, Newman MEJ, Strogatz SH, Watts DJ (2000) Network robustness and fragility: Percolation on random graphs. Phys Rev Lett 85: 5468–5471.
20. Cohen R, Erez K, Ben-Avraham D, Havlin S (2000) Resilience of the Internet to random breakdowns. Phys Rev Lett 85: 4626–4628.
21. Cohen R, Erez K, Ben-Avraham D, Havlin S (2001) Breakdown of the Internet under Intentional Attack. Phys Rev Lett 86: 3682–3685.
22. Dall'Asta L, Barrat A, Barthelemy M, Vespignani A (2006) Vulnerability of weighted networks. J Stat Mech P04006.
23. Paul G, Tanizawa T, Havlin S, Stanley HE (2004) Optimization of robustness of complex networks. The European Physical Journal B-Condensed Matter and Complex Systems 38: 187–191.
24. Pastor-Satorras R, Vespignani A (2002) Immunization of complex networks. Phys Rev E 65: 036104.
25. Vespignani A (2010) Complex networks: The fragility of interdependency. Nature 464: 984–985.
26. Buldyrev SV, Parshani R, Paul G, Stanley HE, Havlin S (2010) Catastrophic cascade of failures in interdependent networks. Nature 464: 1025–1028.
27. Gastner MT, Newman MEJ (2006) The spatial structure of networks. Eur. Phys. J. B 49:247–252.
28. Barthélemy M (2011) Spatial networks. Physics Reports 499: 1–101.
29. Secomb TW, Alberding JP, Hsu R, Dewhirst MW, Pries AR (2013) Angiogenesis: An Adaptive Dynamic Biological Patterning Problem. PLoS Computational Biology 9: e1002983.
30. Blinder P, Shih AY, Rafie C, Kleinfeld D (2010) Topological basis for the robust distribution of blood to rodent neocortex. Proc Natl Acad Sci USA 107: 12670–12675.
31. Guibert R, Fonta C, Plouraboué F (2010) A New Approach to Model Confined Suspensions Flows in Complex Networks: Application to Blood Flow. Transp Porous Med 83: 171–194.
32. Masters BR (2004) Fractal analysis of the vascular tree in the human retina. Annual Review of Biomedical Engineering 6: 427–552.
33. Avakian A, Kalina RE, Sage H, Rambhia AH, Elliott KE, et al. (2002) Fractal analysis of region-based vascular change in the normal and non-proliferative diabetic retina. Current Eye Research 24: 274–280.
34. Flores J, Corvera Poiré E, del Río JA, López de Haro M (2010) A plausible explanation for heart rates in mammals. J Theor Biol 265: 599–603.
35. Murray CD (1926) The Physiological Principle of Minimum Work: I. The Vascular System and the Cost of Blood Volume. Proc Natl Acad Sci USA 12: 207–214.
36. West GB (1999) The Origin of Universal Scaling Laws in Biology. Physica A 263: 104–113.
37. Herman AB, Savage VM, West GB (2011) A Quantitative Theory of Solid Tumor Growth, Metabolic Rate and Vascularization. Plos One 6: e22973.
38. Daxer A (1993) Characterisation of the neovascularisation process in diabetic refinopathy by means of fractal geometry: diagnostic implications. Graefe's Arch Clin Exp Ophthalmol 231: 681–686.
39. Blinder P, Tsai PS, Kaufhold JP, Knutsen PM, Suhl H, et al. (2013) The cortical angiome: an interconnected vascular network with noncolumnar patterns of blood flow. Nature Neuroscience 16: 889–897.
40. Owen MR, Alarcón T, Maini PK, Byrne HM (2009) Angiogenesis and vascular remodelling in normal and cancerous tissues. J Math Biol 58: 689–721.
41. Travasso RDM, Corvera Poiré E, Castro M, Rodríguez-Manzaneque JC, Hernández-Machado A (2011) Tumor angiogenesis and vascular patterning: a mathematical model. PLoS One 6: e19989.

42. Shih AY, Blinder P, Tsai PS, Friedman B, Stanley G, et al. (2012) The smallest stroke: occlusion of one penetrating vessel leads to infarction and a cognitive deficit. Nature Neuroscience 16: 55–63.
43. Milde F, Lauw S, Koumoutsakos P, Iruela-Arispe ML (2013) The mouse retina in 3D: quantification of vascular growth and remodeling. Integrative Biology 5: 1426–1438.
44. Flores J, Romero AM, Travasso RDM, Corvera Poiré EC (2013) Flow and anastomosis in vascular networks, J Theor Biol 317: 257–270.
45. Secomb TW, Hsu R, Park EY, Dewhirst MW (2004) Green's function methods for analysis of oxygen delivery to tissue by microvascular networks. Annals of Biomedical Engineering 32: 1519–1529.
46. Secomb TW, Alberding JP, Hsu R, Dewhirst MW, Pries AR (2013) Angiogenesis: An Adaptive Dynamic Biological Patterning Problem. PLoS Computational Biology 9: e1002983.
47. Sivakumar R, Ravindran G, Muthayya M, Lakshminarayanan S, Velmurughendran CU (2005) Diabetic Retinopathy Analysis. Journal of Biomedicine and Biotechnology 2005: 20–27.
48. Fadini GP, Sartore S, Baesso I, Lenzi M, Agostini C, et al. (2006) Endothelial progenitor cells and the diabetic paradox. Diabetes Care 29: 714–716.
49. Costa C (2011) Vasculogenesis in Diabetes-Associated Diseases: Unraveling the Diabetic Paradox. In: Simionescu DT, Simionescu A, editors. Vasculogenesis and Angiogenesis - from Embryonic Development to Regenerative Medicine. Rijeka: InTech open. pp 107–130.
50. Vinores SA, McGehee R, Lee A, Gadegbeku C, Campochiaro PA (1990) Ultrastructural localization of blood-retinal barrier breakdown in diabetic and galactosemic rats. Journal of Histochemistry & Cytochemistry 38: 1341–1352.
51. Vinores SA, Gadegbeku C, Campochiaro PA, Green WR (1989) Immunohistochemical localization of blood-retinal barrier breakdown in human diabetics. The American Journal of Pathology 134: 231–235.
52. Shweiki D, Itin A, Soffer D, Keshet E (1992) Vascular endothelial growth factor induced by hypoxia may mediate hypoxia-initiated angiogenesis. Nature 359: 843–845.
53. Pugh CW, Ratcliffe PJ (2003) Regulation of angiogenesis by hypoxia: role of the HIF system. Nature Medicine 9: 677–684.
54. Treins C, Giorgetti-Peraldi S, Murdaca J, Monthouël-Kartmann MN, Van Obberghen E (2005) Regulation of hypoxia-inducible factor (HIF)-1 activity and expression of HIF hydroxylases in response to insulin-like growth factor I. Molecular Endocrinology19: 1304–1317.
55. Jain RK (2005) Normalization of tumor vasculature: an emerging concept in antiangiogenic therapy. Science 307: 58–62.
56. Hellums JD, Nair PK, Huang NS, Ohshima N (1996) Simulation of intraluminal gas transport processes in the microcirculation. Ann Biomed Eng 24: 1–24.
57. Pittman RN (2011) Regulation of tissue oxygenation. Marston Gate: Morgan & Claypool Life Sciences.
58. Goldman D (2008) Theoretical models of microvascular oxygen transport to tissue. Microcirculation 15: 795–811.
59. Popel AS (1989) Theory of oxygen transport to tissue. Crit Rev Biomed Eng 17: 257–321.
60. Formaggia L, Lamponi D, Tuveri M, Veneziani A (2006) Numerical modeling of 1D arterial networks coupled with a lumped parameters description of the heart. Computer Methods in Biomechanics and Biomedical Engineering 9: 273–288.

13

Generation of Insulin-Producing Cells from the Mouse Liver Using β Cell-Related Gene Transfer Including *Mafa* and *Mafb*

Haruka Nagasaki[1]☯, Tokio Katsumata[1]☯, Hisashi Oishi[1,2]*, Pei-Han Tai[1], Yukari Sekiguchi[1], Ryusuke Koshida[1], Yunshin Jung[1], Takashi Kudo[1], Satoru Takahashi[1,2,3]*

1 Department of Anatomy and Embryology, Faculty of Medicine, University of Tsukuba, Tsukuba, Ibaraki, Japan, **2** Life Science Center, Tsukuba Advanced Research Alliance (TARA), University of Tsukuba, Tsukuba, Ibaraki, Japan, **3** International Institute for Integrative Sleep Medicine (WPI-IIIS), University of Tsukuba, Tsukuba, Ibaraki, Japan

Abstract

Recent studies on the large Maf transcription factors have shown that *Mafb* and *Mafa* have respective and distinctive roles in β-cell development and maturation. However, whether this difference in roles is due to the timing of the gene expression (roughly, expression of *Mafb* before birth and of *Mafa* after birth) or to the specific function of each gene is unclear. Our aim was to examine the functional differences between these genes that are closely related to β cells by using an *in vivo* model of β-like cell generation. We monitored insulin gene transcription by measuring bioluminescence emitted from the liver of insulin promoter-luciferase transgenic (MIP-Luc-VU) mice. Adenoviral gene transfers of *Pdx1/Neurod/Mafa* (PDA) and *Pdx1/Neurod/Mafb* (PDB) combinations generated intense luminescence from the liver that lasted for more than 1 week and peaked at 3 days after transduction. The peak signal intensities of PDA and PDB were comparable. However, PDA but not PDB transfer resulted in significant bioluminescence on day 10, suggesting that *Mafa* has a more sustainable role in insulin gene activation than does *Mafb*. Both PDA and PDB transfers ameliorated the glucose levels in a streptozotocin (STZ)-induced diabetic model for up to 21 days and 7 days, respectively. Furthermore, PDA transfer induced several gene expressions necessary for glucose sensing and insulin secretion in the liver on day 9. However, a glucose tolerance test and liver perfusion experiment did not show glucose-stimulated insulin secretion from intrahepatic β-like cells. These results demonstrate that bioluminescence imaging in MIP-Luc-VU mice provides a noninvasive means of detecting β-like cells in the liver. They also show that *Mafa* has a markedly intense and sustained role in β-like cell production in comparison with *Mafb*.

Editor: Bridget Wagner, Broad Institute of Harvard and MIT, United States of America

Funding: This work was supported by a Grant-in-Aid for Scientific Research (21220009) from the Japanese Ministry of Education, Culture, Sports, Science and Technology (MEXT). The funders had no role in study design, data collection and analysis, decision to publish, or preparation of the manuscript.

Competing Interests: The authors have declared that no competing interests exist.

* Email: hoishi@md.tsukuba.ac.jp (HO); satoruta@md.tsukuba.ac.jp (ST)

☯ These authors contributed equally to this work.

Introduction

The development of pancreatic β cells is a highly orchestrated process that involves many extracellular stimulants and intracellular signaling pathways. At embryonic day 9.5 (E9.5), the pancreas evolves from the dorsal and ventral buds of the foregut's endodermal epithelium [1]. After gut rotation and fusion of the dorsal and ventral rudiments at around E11.5, the pancreatic epithelium initiates branching by sending finger-like epithelial protrusions into the surrounding mesenchyme [2]. As a branching duct-like structure forms, endocrine progenitors expressing neurogenin 3 within the trunks delaminate from the developing epithelium. Subsequently, progenitor cells successively differentiate into each hormone-producing cell under the hierarchical control of a lineage-specific molecular cascade [2]. Among the 5 different types of endocrine cells in the Langerhans islets, the development of β cells has been the most intensively investigated in relation to future complementation therapy against diabetes.

The Maf family of transcription factors, which is a member of the basic leucine-zipper (bZip) transcription factor family, are homologs of v-Maf, the oncogenic component of the avian retrovirus AS42 originally identified in the genome of chicken musculoaponeurotic fibrosarcoma (MAF), and are subdivided into 2 groups, small and large MAF proteins, according to their structure, function, and molecular size [3–5]. Three small MAF proteins, MAFF, MAFG, and MAFK, lack a transactivation domain and regulate genes important in hematopoiesis and the stress response by forming a heterodimer with other bZIP factors such as cap'n'collar (CNC) family proteins. To date, abnormalities in pancreatic development and glucose homeostasis of small maf knockout mice have not been reported [6]. In contrast, the large MAF proteins comprise 4 distinct proteins,

MAFA, MAFB, c-MAF, and NRL, which are characterized by the presence of an N-terminal transactivation domain. In β-cell development, at E15.5, 50%, and 90% of insulin-positive cells express *Mafa* and *Mafb*, respectively; however, in adult mice, *Mafa* and *Mafb* are preferentially expressed in β cells and α cells, respectively [7]. Therefore, this switch from *Mafb* to *Mafa* expression in β cells probably has a crucial meaning for functional maturation in both mouse models and in human embryonic stem cell differentiation [7,8].

Bioluminescence imaging (BLI) in small animals is a versatile and cost-effective technology that has high sensitivity and efficiency [9]. In β-cell research, BLI has been employed for the quantification of β-cell mass, monitoring of islet graft survival after transplantation, and detection of reporter gene expression [10–12]. Recently, we have shown that BLI of luciferase reporter mice, which can express luciferase under the control of the *Ins1* gene, could also be useful for the detection of fetal β-cell genesis in utero and for intrahepatic insulin gene activity [13,14].

In this study, we aimed to examine the functional differences between *Mafa* and *Mafb* using an *in vivo* model of β-like cell conversion. Although these closely related genes each have their distinctive role in β-cell development (*Mafb*) and maturation (*Mafa*), whether the difference is due to the timing of the gene expression or to the characteristic features of each gene is unclear. Even though both *Mafa* and *Mafb* similarly activate insulin gene expression through the Maf recognition element (MARE) *in vitro*, the less-conserved N-terminal activation domain of the large Maf transcription factors raises the possibility of different activation potentials and/or downstream targets [7]. Here, we transduced β cell-related genes, including *Mafa* and *Mafb*, into the livers of insulin reporter mice and compared the transcriptional activities of insulin and glucose metabolism. Gene transfer including of *Mafb* could activate the insulin gene in the mouse liver. However, a combination gene transfer including *Mafa* demonstrated more efficient and sustainable insulin induction for most experiments when compared with *Mafb*. These findings provide insight into the reprogramming cell potency of the *Mafa* gene and the gene-specific functions of *Mafa* and *Mafb* in normal β-cell generation.

Materials and Methods

Animals

All experiments were performed in compliance with the relevant Japanese and institutional laws and guidelines and approved by the University of Tsukuba animal ethics committee (authorization number 13–072). Transgenic mice expressing luciferase under the control of the mouse *ins1* promoter [FVB/N-Tg(*Ins1-luc*)-VUPwrs/J; Stock number: 007800; MIP-Luc-VU] were purchased from the Jackson Laboratory (Bar Harbor, ME, USA). Jcl:ICR mice purchased from Clea (Clea Japan, Tokyo, Japan) were mated for the experiments. Mice were euthanized at the appropriate time points with carbon dioxide gas.

Preparation of recombinant adenovirus vectors

Recombinant adenoviruses expressing mouse *Pdx1*, *Neurod* (kindly gifted by Dr. S. Yoshida), *Mafa*, and *Mafb* were prepared using the ViraPower Adenoviral Gateway Expression kit (Life Technologies, Carlsbad, CA, USA). Each cDNA fragment was cloned into a pENTR4 entry vector. To create expression clones and produce recombinant adenoviruses, the pENTR4 inserts were transferred into pAd/CMV/V5-DEST destination vectors using the LR recombination reaction, and PacI-linearized plasmids were transfected into 293A cells (Life Technologies) by using Fugene 6 transfection reagent (Roche Diagnostics, Basel, Switzerland). The viruses were propagated in 293A cells and purified using $CsCl_2$ banding followed by dialysis against 10 mM Tris-HCl, pH 8.0 with 2 mM MgCl. The infectious titers were determined using the Adeno-X Rapid Titer kit (Takara, Shiga, Japan). The successful adenoviral gene transfer is shown in Figure S1A, in which 5×10^9 infectious units of the viruses were injected into wild-type mice, and immunohistochemistry using the target antibodies was performed 3 days after the infection. 39.6±3.9%, 26.4±5.8%, 46.5±3.2%, 57.3±5.8%, of liver cells reacted to PDX1, NEUROD, MAFA, and MAFB antibodies, respectively (n = 3) (Figure S1A).

Bioluminescence imaging

Adenoviral constructs (5×10^9 IFU) expressing GFP (Ad-GFP), PDX1, NEUROD, and MAFA (Ad-PDA) and PDX1, NEUROD, and MAFB (Ad-PDB) were intravenously injected into the MIP-Luc-VU mice. Serial BLI was performed before and after infection on the designated days. The day of injection was determined as day 0. To detect the bioluminescence signals emitted from the free-fed mice, D-luciferin (5 mg/kg body weight; Promega, Madison, WI, USA) was injected intraperitoneally, and bioluminescence images were taken using an IVIS spectrum 5 minutes later (Caliper Life Sciences, Hopkinton, MA, USA). Bioluminescence images were captured with an integration time of 1 minute, and isometric regions of interest (ROIs) were drawn over the location corresponding to the liver for the quantification using Living Image software (Xenogen Corporation, Alameda, CA, USA).

Quantitative RT-PCR

Total RNA was extracted from the liver using the NucleoSpin RNA II kit (Machery-Nagel, Düren, Germany), and 1 μg was used to prepare cDNA primed with random hexamers and reverse-transcribed with the QuantiTect Reverse Transcription kit (Qiagen, Hilden, Germany) according to the manufacturer's protocol. Gene expression levels were compared by real-time RT-PCR using the Thermal Cycler Dice Real Time system (Takara) with a SYBR Green PCR master mix (Takara). Values were normalized to expression levels of *Hprt* and shown in relative amount to the PDA group at day 3. All primer sequences are listed in Table 1 [15].

Measurement of insulin content

Hepatic insulin after adenovirus infection was extracted by the acid-ethanol method as described previously, and the content measured with an insulin enzyme-linked immunosorbent assay kit (Morinaga Bioscience, Yokohama, Japan) [16]. The insulin content was normalized to the total protein concentration measured by a Coomassie protein assay reagent (Thermo Scientific, Hudson, NH, USA).

Diabetes induction

Wild-type mice were rendered diabetic at 6 weeks of age by IP injection of streptozotocin (STZ, Sigma) at a dose of 200 mg/kg body weight in 0.1 M citrate buffer (pH 4.5). The serum glucose concentrations of the mice after they had been subjected to a 12-hour overnight fast were measured using a Dry-chem 3500 automated analyzer for routine laboratory tests (Fujifilm, Tokyo, Japan). The serum insulin levels were measured with an ultrasensitive insulin enzyme-linked immunosorbent assay kit (Morinaga).

Table 1. Primer sequences used in the study.

Gene symbol	Forward primer sequences	Reverse primer sequences
Ins1	5′-CCAGCTATAATCAGAGACCA-3′	5′-GGGCCTTAGTTGCAGTAGTT-3′
Ins2	5′-AGGAAGCCTATCTTCCAGGT-3′	5′-ATTCATTGCAGAGGGGTAGG-3′
Slc2a2	5′-TGGGATGAAGAGGAGACTGAA-3′	5′-CATCCGTGAAGAGCTGGATCA-3′
Pcsk2	5′-AATGACCCCTAACCCATACCC-3′	5′-GAGGAGGGTTCGATGATGTC-3′
islet Gck	5′-TGGATGACAGAGCCAGGATGG-3′	5′-ACTTCTGAGCCTTCTGGGGTG-3′
Sur1	5′-CTGGTCCTCAGCAGCACAT-3′	5′-GGAACTCTTGGGACGAGACA-3′
Kcnj11 (Kir6.2)	5′-GTAGGGGACCTCGGAAAGAG-3′	5′-TGGAGTCGATGACGTGGTAG-3′
Sytl4	5′-CCAGCACACAAAGGCGAGT-3′	5′-GAAGGAGGTATCCCTTGACAAAG-3′
Hprt	5′-GGCTTCCTCCTCAGACCGCTTT-3′	5′-AGGCTTTGTATTTGGCTTTTCC-3′

Immunostaining

The MIP-Luc-VU mice were euthanized at 8 weeks of age, and the livers removed. Tissues were fixed in 10% formalin and embedded in paraffin. The tissue sections were incubated with anti-insulin antibody (Abcam, Cambridge, UK) for 8 hours at 4°C. The antigens were visualized using appropriate secondary antibody conjugated with Alexa 596 with nuclear staining using 4′,6-diamidino-2-phenylindole (DAPI) (Invitrogen). Images of the sections were scanned and analyzed using a Biorevo BZ-9000 microscope (Keyence, Osaka, Japan) and BZ-II Analyzer software (Keyence).

In situ liver perfusion

The experiment was performed according to a previous report by Yechoor et al [17]. Briefly, anesthetized mice were cannulated via the portal vein for infusion and via the inferior vena cava (IVC) through the right atrium for collection of the effusate. After the initial washout, a peristaltic pump was used to perfuse the isolated liver with KRB buffer (119 mM NaCl, 4.7 mM KCl, 25 mM $NaHCO_3$, 2.5 mM $CaCl_2$, 1.2 mM $MgSO_4$, 1.2 mM KH_2PO_4, and 0.25% BSA) containing different concentrations of glucose. Finally, after another washout, glibenclamide (10 nM; Sigma) and KCl (25 mM) were added. The insulin concentration of the effusate was measured 10 minutes after each perfusion of glucose.

Statistical analysis

Data were expressed as the means ± standard errors of the means and compared using an unpaired t test, unless otherwise stated. Probability values of less than 0.05 were considered significant.

Results

To screen the transcriptional activity of the intrahepatic insulin gene in a noninvasive manner, we monitored the bioluminescence emissions from MIP-Luc-VU mice after adenovirus-mediated gene transfer (Figure 1A). We transferred a 3-gene combination of *Pdx1*, *Neurod*, and *Mafa* into the MIP-Luc-VU mice with different infectious titers to detect the bioluminescence signal 3 days after infection, according to a previous study (Figure 1B) [18]. After luciferin injection (5 mg/kg body weight, IP) into the gene-transferred mouse, within minutes the emission from the liver rose quickly and then gradually attenuated (Figure S1B). The 3-gene transfer resulted in a dose-dependent bioluminescence emission in the hepatic region, which was identified as originating from the liver by imaging of the extracted tissues and by immunohistochemistry using anti-luciferase antibody (Figure 1B, C, D). Most hepatic cells exhibit reporter expression, whereas immunohistochemistry using anti-insulin antibody showed very few luciferase-positive cells expressing insulin protein, indicating the existence of some regulatory mechanisms of the transcription and the protein levels of insulin, such as mRNA and protein degradation and leakage of produced insulin into the blood circulation (Figure S1C).

To compare the effects of *Mafa* and *Mafb* on the transcriptional activity of the insulin gene through measurement of the bioluminescence emission, we examined 3 different gene combinations – *Pdx1/Neurod* (PD); *Pdx1*, *Neurod*, and *Mafa* (PDA); and *Pdx1*, *Neurod*, and *Mafb* (PDB) – in MIP-Luc-VU mice (Figure 2A). The bioluminescence signals induced by the 3 different combinations peaked at day 3 and gradually disappeared over 14 days in the same way. The PDA ($1.81\pm0.34\times10^9$/photons/sec/cm^2/steradian; n = 7) and PDB ($1.70\pm0.33\times10^9$/photons/sec/cm^2/steradian; n = 8) transductions induced comparable but significantly higher signal intensities than the peak emission of PD ($4.49\pm2.6\times10^7$/photons/sec/cm^2/steradian; n = 4) at day 3 (Figure 2B). In contrast, only the PDA-transferred mice continued to emit substantial bioluminescence, even at day 10, suggesting that *Mafa* is capable of inducing a peak emission similar to but a more sustainable insulin gene activity than that of *Mafb* (PD: $1.28\pm0.1\times10^5$/photons/sec/cm^2/steradian; n = 4, PDA: $2.46\pm0.8\times10^7$/photons/sec/cm^2/steradian; n = 7, PDB: $1.96\pm0.4\times10^5$/photons/sec/cm^2/steradian; n = 8) (Figure 2C). Furthermore, immunohistochemistry using anti-insulin antibody revealed that some PDA- and PDB-transferred liver cells reacted to the antibody at days 3 and 9 after infection (Figure 2D). To confirm the presence of insulin-positive cells in PDB-transferred liver, DAB (3, 3′-diaminobenzidine) visualization is also shown in Figure S2A. We next examined the insulin content of the gene-transferred livers at days 3 and 9 after infection (Figure 3). Consistent with the bioluminescence results, we found no difference among the groups at day 3 (GFP: 0.31±0.2 ng/mg; n = 4; PDA: 1.26±0.5 ng/mg; n = 7; PDB: 2.6±0.3 ng/mg; n = 5), but the PDA-transferred liver at day 9 (6.23±1.3 ng/mg, n = 4) contained fairly abundant amounts of insulin protein when compared with the other groups. Interestingly, the insulin content of the PDA-transferred liver at day 9 was increased 5-fold over that of day 3, suggesting that newly synthesized insulin protein is gradually stored in the liver.

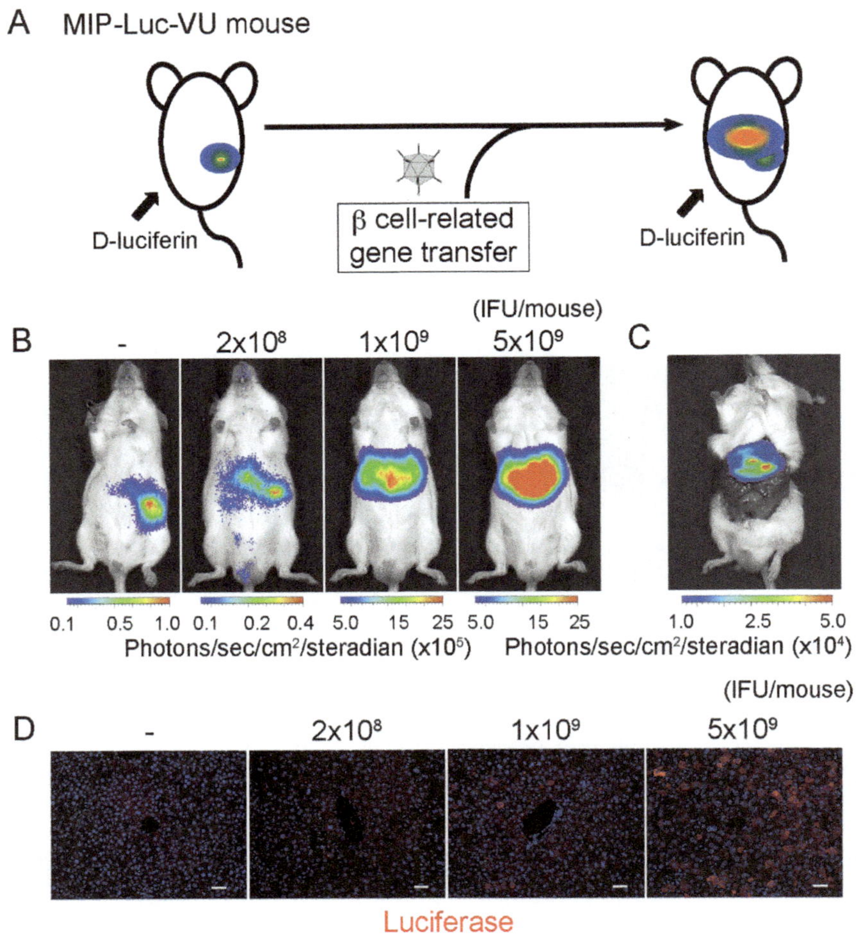

Figure 1. Bioluminescence emission from the hepatic region of MIP-Luc-VU mice after β cell-related gene transfer. (A) Diagrammatic representation of bioluminescence monitoring of insulin transcriptional activity. (B) Representative example of dose-dependent bioluminescence emission from the hepatic region. (C) Bioluminescence images of the abdominal section of MIP-Luc-VU mice 3 days after infection. (D) Tissue sections of MIP-Luc-VU liver stained with anti-luciferase antibody with 4′,6-diamidino-2-phenylindole (DAPI) 3 days after gene transfer. Scale bar indicates 100 μm.

To examine the gene expression profiles related to β-cell function, we performed quantitative RT-PCR analysis using RNAs recovered from whole liver cells (GFP, n = 6) (Figure 4). The expressions of *Pdx*1, *Neurod*, *Mafa*, and *Mafb* are shown in Figure S2B. Both Ad-PDA (n = 7) and Ad-PDB (n = 7) treatment induced comparable expression levels of β cell-related genes, including *Slc2a2* and *Pcsk2*, 3 days after infection, but only in the PDA-transfer group were the expressions sustained for longer than 1 week. In contrast to this significant β cell-related gene induction, immunohistochemistry showed that other hormones including glucagon, pancreatic polypeptide (PP), and somatostatin were not induced by the Ad-PDA and Ad-PDB treatments (data not shown). Furthermore, other β cell-specific transcription factors, such as *Nkx2.2*, *Nkx6.2*, and *Pax4* that are detected in normal β-cell development, were neither induced nor increased by PDA-gene transfer, suggesting that transient β-like cell induction does not occur in the similar molecular cascade to that of the regular developmental process of β cells.

Next, to examine whether hepatic insulin production induced by PDA can ameliorate blood glucose levels in the diabetic model, we injected 200 mg/kg STZ into ICR mice, followed by control Ad-GFP (n = 8) or Ad-PDA (n = 5) treatment on day 7 after diabetes induction. As shown in Figure 5A, fasting blood glucose levels were recovered by Ad-PDA treatment for up to 21 days, which was more pronounced and persistent than the effects of Ad-PDB treatment (n = 7) (Figure 5A). Consistent with this result, serum insulin levels after 12 hours of fasting in the mice treated with Ad-PDA (3.87±1.2 ng/ml, n = 4) were significantly higher than those in the mice treated with Ad-GFP (0.088±0.02 ng/ml, n = 5) or Ad-PDB (0.18±0.07 ng/ml, n = 4) (Figure 5B). Furthermore, we also performed an intraperitoneal glucose tolerance test 7 and 14 days after the adenovirus injection. As shown in Figure 5C (7 days) and 5D (14 days), the Ad-PDA-treated mice showed lower glucose levels at each time point after the glucose stimulation; however, the reduction in blood glucose levels in the Ad-PDA-treated mice (n = 4) was very consistent at all time points – about 150 mg/dL (day 7) and 50 mg/dL (day 14) – when compared with those in the Ad-GFP-treated mice (n = 6). These results raise the possibility that Ad-PDA treatment could not give rise to mature insulin-producing cells capable of secreting insulin in response to glucose levels despite the significant improvement in fasting blood glucose levels in the STZ diabetic model.

Finally, to examine directly whether PDA-transferred liver cells are capable of secreting insulin in respond to glucose stimulation, we performed an *in situ* liver perfusion experiment (Figure 6A, B).

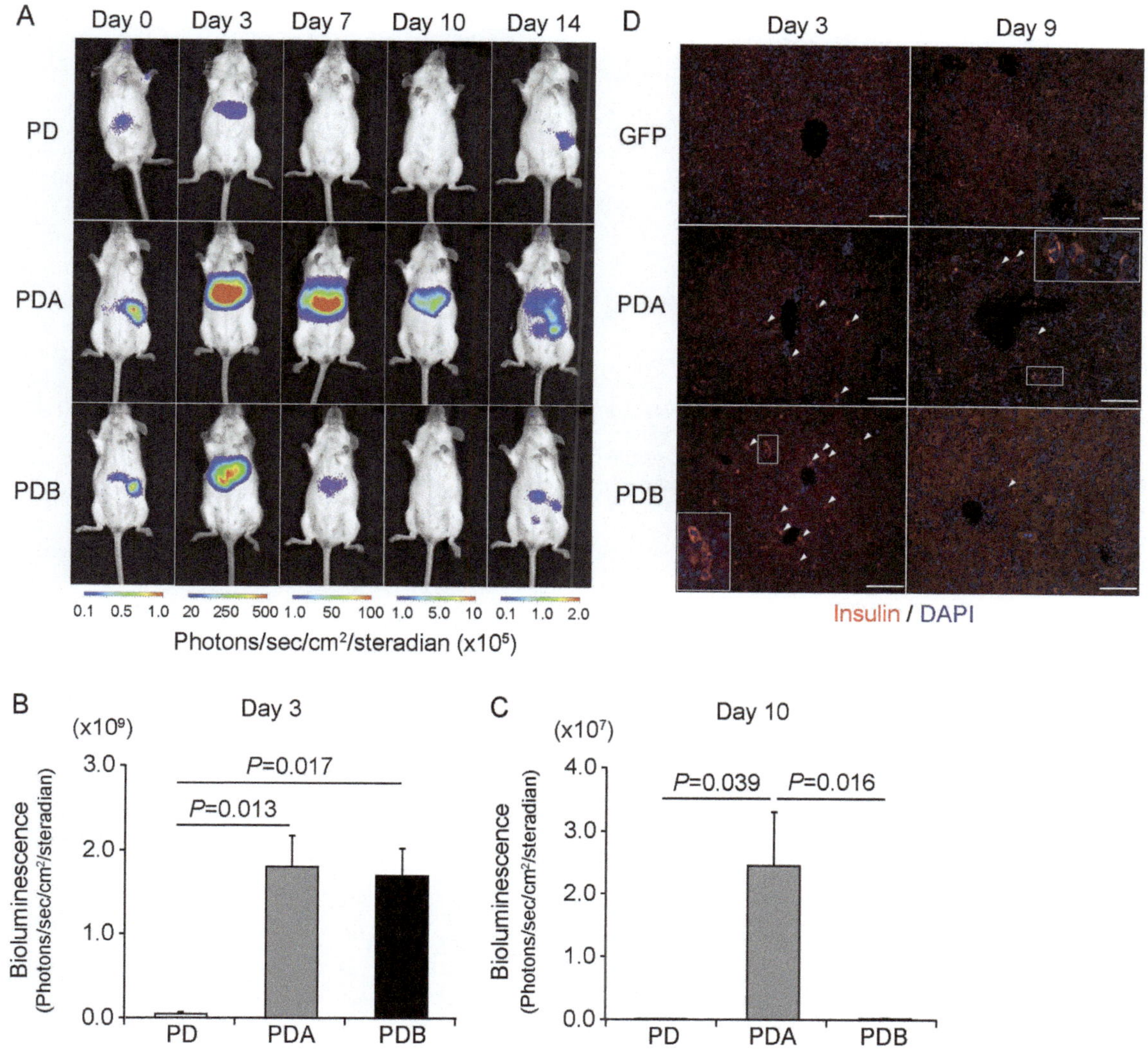

Figure 2. Comparison of the transcription of insulin in the liver by use of bioluminescence imaging. (A) Representative bioluminescence imaging of MIP-Luc-VU mice after *Pdx1/Neurod* (PD), *Pdx1/Neurod/Mafa* (PDA), and *Pdx1/Neurod/Mafb* (PDB) gene transfer. (B, C) Quantification of signal intensity after PD (n = 6), PDA (n = 7), and PDB (n = 7) gene transfer at days 3 (B) and 10 (C). (D) Tissue sections of wild-type mouse liver stained with anti-insulin antibody (red) and 4′6-diamidino-2-phenylindole (DAPI) (blue) after GFP-, PDA-, and PDB-gene transfer. Arrowheads indicate insulin-positive cells. Scale bars indicate 100 μm.

Solutions containing different glucose concentrations were infused via the portal vein, and the liver effusion was collected for the measurement of insulin and glucose concentrations. In contrast to the Ad-GFP treatment, the Ad-PDA and Ad-PDB treatments led to high insulin secretion at all time points; however, stepwise increase in insulin secretion did not occur during glucose stimulation in the infusate from 2.8 to 11.1 and 25 mM. Consistent with the result of the intraperitoneal glucose tolerance test, this result indicates that liver cells after PDA-gene transfer secrete insulin independent of glucose concentration, similar to basal insulin secretion.

Discussion

In this study, we used β-like cell induction in the mouse liver to examine the functional differences between 2 large Maf transcription factor genes that are expressed in the pancreatic islets. Although no reports have been published on the successful generation of β-like cells by overexpression of gene combination including *Mafb* by other types of cells, we transiently but successfully induced insulin-producing cells by overexpression of *Mafb* in combination with *Pdx1* and *Neurod* [19]. However, hepatic insulin-producing cells induced by Ad-PDB treatment demonstrated defective expressions of *Pcsk2* and *islet Gck* (Figure 4) and insulin release in a glucose-independent manner (Figures 5, 6), suggesting that *Mafb* is capable of stimulating β-cell conversion to the immature and transitional states [20]. Meanwhile, the possibility remained that PDB and PDA transfer induced a few mature β cells, the phenotype of which is masked by the majority of immature β cells. Notably, $MAFB^+$ $insulin^+$ cells are generated during the normal β-cell differentiation process before the emergence of $MAFA^+$ $insulin^+$ cells, implying that the transition from *Mafb* to *Mafa* is critical to β-cell maturation [5,7]. Meanwhile, β cells acquire the capability of glucose-stimulated insulin secretion during postnatal days 0 to 10, when downregulation of *Mafb* expression takes place in β cells [21,22]. Therefore, alteration of gene expression profiles after birth might also be

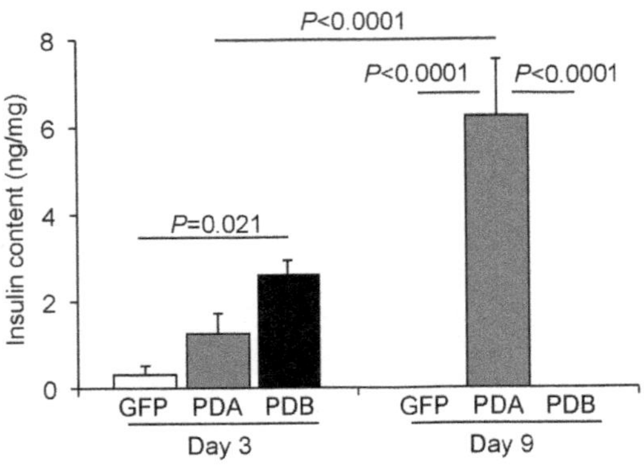

Figure 3. Insulin content in mouse liver after β-like cell-related gene transfer. Insulin content of wild-type mouse liver at days 3 and 9 after GFP (n = 7), *Pdx1/Neurod/Mafa* (PDA, n = 8), and *Pdx1/Neurod/Mafb* (PDB, n = 5) gene transfer. Data were expressed as the means ± standard errors of the means and analyzed by one-way ANOVA followed by the Tukey-Kramer honestly significant difference (HSD) test.

considered for deeper understanding of the molecular mechanism of β-cell maturation [23].

Large Maf transcription family proteins show relatively high levels of amino acid similarity in each domain. In mice, MAFB shares 57%, 86%, and 72% amino acid sequence identities with the individual acidic, basic, and leucine zipper moieties of MAFA, respectively [24]. Although we have not determined which amino acids or regions in MAFA are dominant for the generation of β-like cells from liver cells, the C-terminal DNA-binding region of MAFA has been shown to be critical for insulin induction [19]. In addition, the difference in activity between MAFA and MAFB might also be related to posttranslational modifications, including phosphorylation, ubiquitination, and sumoylation [25–30]. Recent studies using gene knockout mice revealed that *Mafa* and *Mafb* regulate different genes critical for glucose-stimulated insulin secretion and β-cell development, respectively, supporting our results indicating the different conversion capabilities of these 2 genes [31].

We demonstrated that bioluminescence monitoring using an apparatus equipped with a sensitive CCD camera capable of detecting slight bioluminescence from reporter mice could be useful for noninvasive monitoring of intrahepatic insulin gene activity *in vivo*. Indeed, it has been demonstrated that hepatocytes or hepatocyte precursors could be converted to insulin-producing cells using different gene combinations [17,18,32–34]. However, a comprehensive method for comparing these protocols and determining the optimal conditions for β-cell generation has not been established [14]. Our simple and repetitive monitoring described here provides readily quantifiable data to examine the efficiency of β-cell induction under different protocols.

In this study, we transduced the same PDA gene combination as that of a previous report by Kaneto et al [18]. In contrast to ours, their results demonstrated fairly good insulin secretion in response to glucose stimulation. This discrepancy is probably due to the different mouse strains and PDX1 used. They injected adenovirus expressing a constitutively active form of PDX1, PDX1-VP16 fusion protein, into C57BL/6 mice, whereas we used wild-type PDX1 and ICR mice. Especially, the PDX1-VP16 form, of which VP16 is the activation domain from the herpes simplex virus, has been demonstrated to show potent transdifferentiation activity when compared with wild-type PDX1 [35,36].

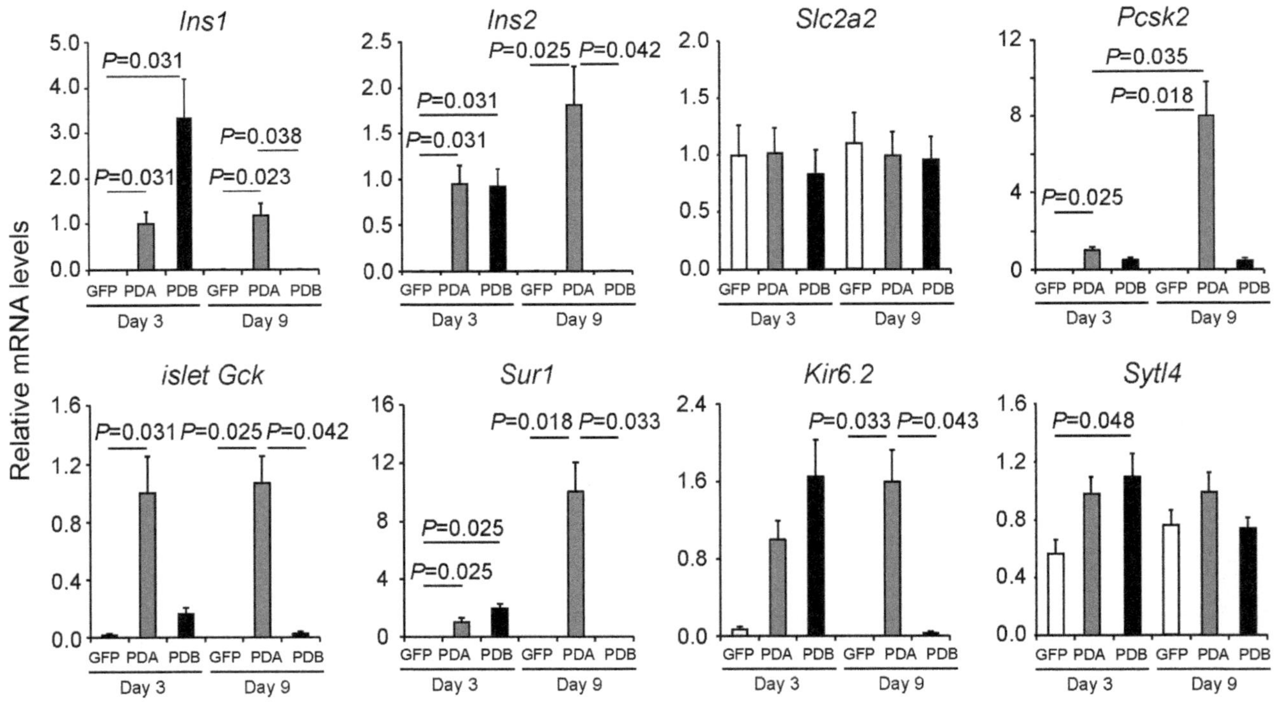

Figure 4. Expression of β cell-related genes in mouse liver after *Pdx1/Neurod* in combination with *Mafa* (PDA) or *Mafb* (PDB) gene transfer. Wild-type mouse liver treated with Ad-PDA (PDA, n = 7) displayed a significant increase in β cell-related mRNAs at day 9 (*Ins1*, *Ins2*, *PC2*, *i-GK*, *Sur1*, *Kir6.2*) on Q-PCR analysis. In contrast, the Ad-PDB treated group of mice (PDB, n = 7) displayed a significant increase in *Ins1*, *Ins2*, *Sur1*, and *Kir6.2* only at day 3. Data were normalized to *Hprt* mRNA abundance and shown as relative expression levels to that of the Ad-PDA-treated group at day 3. Data were expressed as the means ± standard errors of the means and analyzed using the Steel-Dwass multiple comparison test.

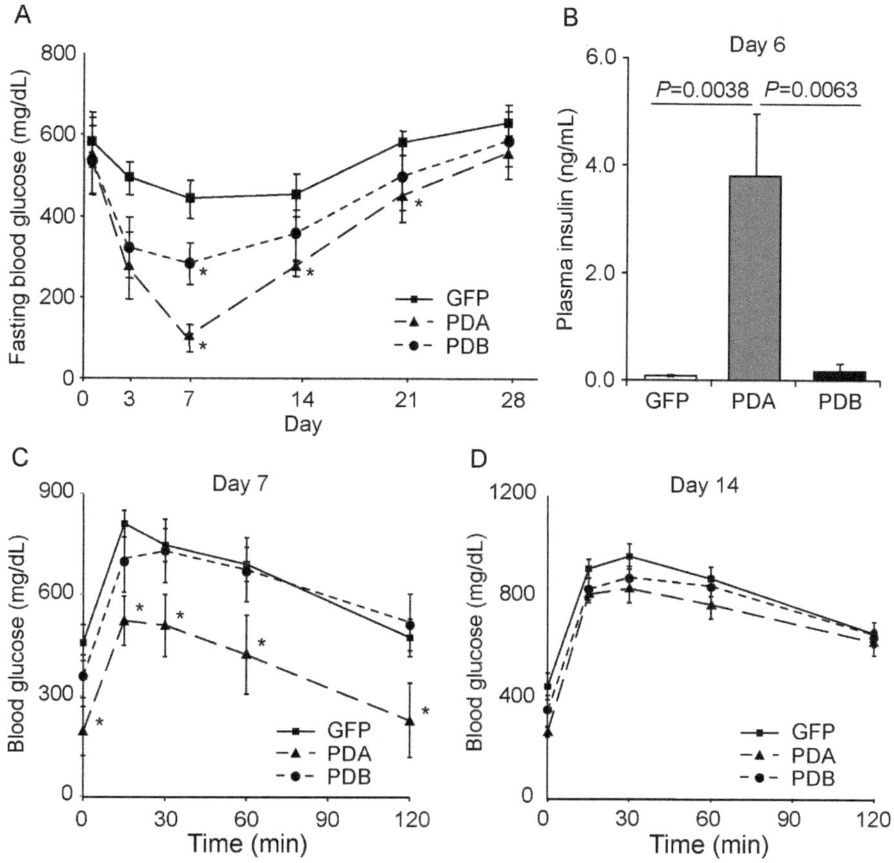

Figure 5. *Pdx1*, *Neurod*, and *Mafa* gene transfer in the liver significantly improved blood glucose levels in a streptozotocin-induced diabetic model in comparison with *Pdx1*, *Neurod*, and *Mafb* gene transfer. (A) ICR mice were rendered diabetic by intraperitoneal injection of streptozotocin (STZ; 200 mg/kg) followed by treatment with Ad-GFP, Ad-PDA, or Ad-PDB (2.5×10^9 IFU). Fasting blood glucose levels were measured 0 to 28 days after the treatment. Data were expressed as the means ± standard errors of the means and analyzed using the Steel-Dwass multiple comparison test. (B) Plasma insulin levels in the fasting state 6 days after the treatment. Data were expressed as the means ± standard errors of the means, and *P* values calculated using the Tukey-Kramer honestly significant difference (HSD) test. (C–D) Intraperitoneal glucose tolerance tests 7 (C) and 14 (D) days after the treatment. After an overnight fast, the STZ-induced diabetic mice were injected intraperitoneally with 2.0 g/kg body weight of glucose. Blood samples collected at the designated times after glucose challenge were used to measure blood glucose levels. Data were expressed as the means ± standard errors of the means, and *P* values calculated using the Tukey-Kramer HSD test. *$P<0.05$.

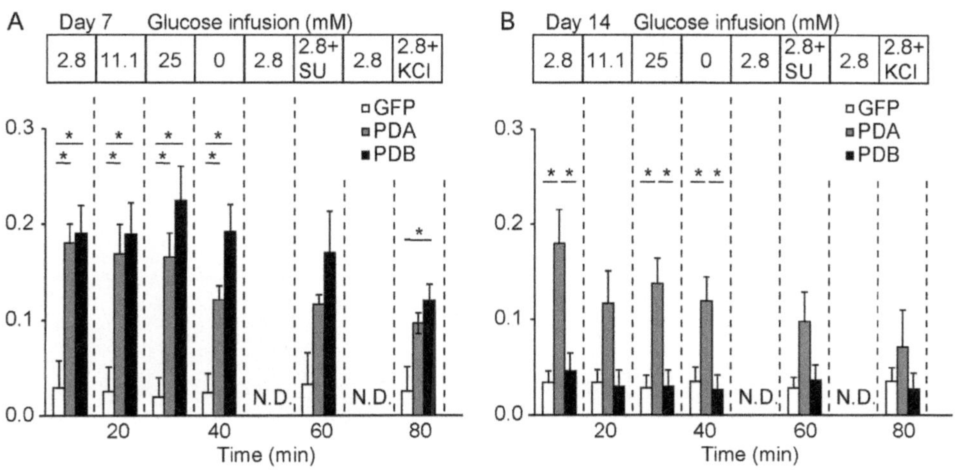

Figure 6. Glucose-independent insulin release from the mouse liver after β-like cell-related gene transfer. (A–B) Glucose-stimulated insulin release from the livers of Ad-GFP- (n = 6), Ad-PDA- (n = 6), and Ad-PDB- (n = 7) treated mice 7 days (A) and 14 days (B) after treatment by *in situ* liver perfusion. Data were expressed as the means ± standard errors of the means, and *P* values calculated using the Tukey-Kramer honestly significant difference (HSD) test. *$P<0.05$. N.D. indicates no data.

In summary, we have demonstrated that bioluminescence imaging in MIP-Luc-VU mice provides a noninvasive means of monitoring insulin transcriptional activity and the presence of β-like cells in the liver, and *Mafa* has a markedly sustainable role in β-like cell induction in comparison with *Mafb*.

Supporting Information

Figure S1 (A) Immunohistochemistry of wild-type mouse liver infected with the indicated viruses 3 days after induction. Liver tissues were fixed in 4% paraformaldehyde overnight and embedded in OCT compound (Sakura, Tokyo, Japan). The tissue sections were incubated with anti-PDX1 (Abcam, ab47267), NEUROD (Santa Cruz, sc-1084), MAFA (Bethyl, BL1069) and MAFB (Bethyl, IHC-00351) antibodies and visualized using appropriate secondary antibodies conjugated with Alexa 596 with nuclear staining using 4′,6-diamidino-2-phenylindole (DAPI) (Invitrogen). Lower panels indicate negative control sections. Scale bars indicate 50 μm. (B) Bioluminescence emission from the liver of PDA-transferred MIP-Luc-VU mice following intraperitoneal injection of luciferin. (C) Tissue sections of MIP-Luc-VU liver stained with anti-luciferase (Promega, G475A) and anti-insulin (Abcam, ab7842) antibodies with 4′,6-diamidino-2-phenylindole (DAPI) 3 days after PDA gene transfer. Scale bar indicates 100 μm.

Figure S2 (A) Immunohistochemistry for anti-insulin antibody in the livers treated with Ad-GFP (Left), Ad-PDB (Center) and islets treated with Ad-PDB (Right). Scale bars indicate 50 μm. (B) Expression of genes delivered in mouse liver treated with Ad-GFP, Ad-PDA, and Ad-PDB. Primer sequences: 5′-TTCCCGAATGGAACCGAGC-3′ and 5′-GTAGGCAGTACGGGTCCTCT-3′ for *Pdx1*; 5′-ACAGACGCTCTGCAAAGGTTT-3′ and 5′-GGACTGGTAGGAGTAGGGATG-3′ for *Neurod*; 5′-CACTGGCCATCGAGTAGTCA-3′ and 5′-CTTCACCTCGAACTTCATCAGGTC-3′ for *Mafa*; 5′-TGAGCATGGGGCAAGAGCTG-3′ and 5′-CCATCCAGTACAGGTCCTCG-3′ for *Mafb*; and 5′-GCTATGTGAGCACTCCACAG-3′ and 5′-CCATCCAGTACAGGTCCTCG-3′ for exogenous specific *Mafb*.

Acknowledgments

The authors thank Masami Ojima for technical assistance and Flaminia Miyamasu for grammatical revision of the manuscript.

Author Contributions

Conceived and designed the experiments: ST HO. Performed the experiments: T. Katsumata HO PT YS YJ HN. Analyzed the data: T. Katsumata HO RK. Contributed reagents/materials/analysis tools: HO ST T. Kudo. Wrote the paper: HO ST.

References

1. Zhou Q, Law AC, Rajagopal J, Anderson WJ, Gray PA, et al. (2007) A multipotent progenitor domain guides pancreatic organogenesis. Dev Cell 13: 103–114.
2. Puri S, Hebrok M (2010) Cellular plasticity within the pancreas – lessons learned from development. Dev Cell 18: 342–356.
3. Nishizawa M, Kataoka K, Goto N, Fujiwara KT, Kawai S (1989) v-maf, a viral oncogene that encodes a "leucine zipper" motif. Proc Natl Acad Sci U S A 86: 7711–7715.
4. Kataoka K (2007) Multiple mechanisms and functions of maf transcription factors in the regulation of tissue-specific genes. J Biochem 141: 775–781.
5. Hang Y, Stein R (2011) MafA and MafB activity in pancreatic β cells. Trends Endocrinol Metab 22: 364–373.
6. Yamazaki H, Katsuoka F, Motohashi H, Engel JD, Yamamoto M (2012) Embryonic lethality and fetal liver apoptosis in mice lacking all three small Maf proteins. Mol Cell Biol 32: 808–816.
7. Nishimura W, Kondo T, Salameh T, El Khattabi I, Dodge R, et al. (2006) A switch from MafB to MafA expression accompanies differentiation to pancreatic beta-cells. Dev Biol 293: 526–539.
8. Kroon E, Martinson LA, Kadoya K, Bang AG, Kelly OG, et al. (2008) Pancreatic endoderm derived from human embryonic stem cells generates glucose-responsive insulin-secreting cells in vivo. Nat Biotechnol 26: 443–452.
9. Zinn KR, Chaudhuri TR, Szafran AA, O'Quinn D, Weaver C, et al. (2008) Noninvasive bioluminescence imaging in small animals. ILAR J 49: 103–115.
10. Virostko J, Radhika A, Poffenberger G, Chen Z, Brissova M, et al. (2010) Bioluminescence imaging in mouse models quantifies beta cell mass in the pancreas and after islet transplantation. Mol Imaging Biol 12: 42–53.
11. Lu Y, Dang H, Middleton B, Zhang Z, Washburn L, et al. (2004) Bioluminescent monitoring of islet graft survival after transplantation. Mol Ther 9: 428–435.
12. Sadikot RT, Blackwell TS (2008) Bioluminescence: imaging modality for in vitro and in vivo gene expression. Methods Mol Biol 477: 383–394.
13. Sekiguchi Y, Owada J, Oishi H, Katsumata T, Ikeda K, et al. (2012) Noninvasive monitoring of β-cell mass and fetal β-cell genesis in mice using bioluminescence imaging. Exp Anim 61: 445–451.
14. Katsumata T, Oishi H, Sekiguchi Y, Nagasaki H, Daassi D, et al. (2013) Bioluminescence imaging of β cells and intrahepatic insulin gene activity under normal and pathological conditions. PLoS One 8: e60411.
15. Palumbo MO, Levi D, Chentoufi AA, Polychronakos C (2006) Isolation and characterization of proinsulin-producing medullary thymic epithelial cell clones. Diabetes 55: 2595–2601.
16. im Walde SS, Dohle C, Schott-Ohly P, Gleichmann H (2002) Molecular target structures in alloxan-induced diabetes in mice. Life Sci 71: 1681–1694.
17. Yechoor V, Liu V, Espiritu C, Paul A, Oka K, et al. (2009) Neurogenin3 is sufficient for transdetermination of hepatic progenitor cells into neo-islets in vivo but not transdifferentiation of hepatocytes. Dev Cell 16: 358–373.
18. Kaneto H, Matsuoka TA, Nakatani Y, Miyatsuka T, Matsuhisa M, et al. (2005) A crucial role of MafA as a novel therapeutic target for diabetes. J Biol Chem 280: 15047–15052.
19. Artner I, Hang Y, Guo M, Gu G, Stein R (2008) MafA is a dedicated activator of the insulin gene in vivo. J Endocrinol 198: 271–279.
20. Minami K, Okuno M, Miyawaki K, Okumachi A, Ishizaki K, et al. (2005) Lineage tracing and characterization of insulin-secreting cells generated from adult pancreatic acinar cells. Proc Natl Acad Sci U S A 102: 15116–15121.
21. Blum B, Hrvatin SS, Schuetz C, Bonal C, Rezania A, et al. (2012) Functional beta-cell maturation is marked by an increased glucose threshold and by expression of urocortin 3. Nat Biotechnol 30: 261–264.
22. Aguayo-Mazzucato C, Zavacki AM, Marinelarena A, Hollister-Lock J, El Khattabi I, et al. (2013) Thyroid hormone promotes postnatal rat pancreatic β-cell development and glucose-responsive insulin secretion through MAFA. Diabetes 62: 1569–1580.
23. Szabat M, Lynn FC, Hoffman BG, Kieffer TJ, Allan DW, et al. (2012) Maintenance of β-cell maturity and plasticity in the adult pancreas: developmental biology concepts in adult physiology. Diabetes 61: 1365–1371.
24. Kajihara M, Sone H, Amemiya M, Katoh Y, Isogai M, et al. (2003) Mouse MafA, homologue of zebrafish somite Maf 1, contributes to the specific transcriptional activity through the insulin promoter. Biochem Biophys Res Commun 312: 831–842.
25. Benkhelifa S, Provot S, Nabais E, Eychene A, Calothy G, et al. (2001) Phosphorylation of MafA is essential for its transcriptional and biological properties. Mol Cell Biol 21: 4441–4452.
26. Rocques N, Abou Zeid N, Sii-Felice K, Lecoin L, Felder-Schmittbuhl MP, et al. (2007) GSK-3-mediated phosphorylation enhances Maf-transforming activity. Mol Cell 28: 584–597.
27. Han SI, Aramata S, Yasuda K, Kataoka K (2007) MafA stability in pancreatic beta cells is regulated by glucose and is dependent on its constitutive phosphorylation at multiple sites by glycogen synthase kinase 3. Mol Cell Biol 27: 6593–6605.
28. Shao C, Cobb MH (2009) Sumoylation regulates the transcriptional activity of MafA in pancreatic beta cells. J Biol Chem 284: 3117–3124.
29. Guo S, Burnette R, Zhao L, Vanderford NL, Poitout V, et al. (2009) The stability and transactivation potential of the mammalian MafA transcription factor are regulated by serine 65 phosphorylation. J Biol Chem 284: 759–765.
30. Guo S, Vanderford NL, Stein R (2010) Phosphorylation within the MafA N terminus regulates C-terminal dimerization and DNA binding. J Biol Chem 285: 12655–12661.
31. Artner I, Hang Y, Mazur M, Yamamoto T, Guo M, et al. (2010) MafA and MafB regulate genes critical to beta-cells in a unique temporal manner. Diabetes 59: 2530–2539.
32. Ferber S, Halkin A, Cohen H, Ber I, Einav Y, et al. (2000) Pancreatic and duodenal homeobox gene 1 induces expression of insulin genes in liver and ameliorates streptozotocin-induced hyperglycemia. Nat Med 6: 568–572.

33. Kojima H, Fujimiya M, Matsumura K, Younan P, Imaeda H, et al. (2003) NeuroD-betacellulin gene therapy induces islet neogenesis in the liver and reverses diabetes in mice. Nat Med 9: 596–603.
34. Banga A, Akinci E, Greder LV, Dutton JR, Slack JM (2012) In vivo reprogramming of Sox9+ cells in the liver to insulin-secreting ducts. Proc Natl Acad Sci U S A 109: 15336–15341.
35. Horb ME, Shen CN, Tosh D, Slack JM (2003) Experimental conversion of liver to pancreas. Curr Biol 13: 105–115.
36. Ham DS, Shin J, Kim JW, Park HS, Cho JH, et al. (2013) Generation of functional insulin-producing cells from neonatal porcine liver-derived cells by PDX1/VP16, BETA2/NeuroD and MafA. PLoS One 8: e79076.

14

Relationship of Dickkopf1 (DKK1) with Cardiovascular Disease and Bone Metabolism in Caucasian Type 2 Diabetes Mellitus

Antonia Garcia-Martín[1,2], Rebeca Reyes-Garcia[1,3], Beatriz García-Fontana[1], Sonia Morales-Santana[1,4], Ana Coto-Montes[5], Manuel Muñoz-Garach[6], Pedro Rozas-Moreno[7], Manuel Muñoz-Torres[1]*

1 Bone Metabolic Unit (RETICEF), Endocrinology Division, Hospital Universitario San Cecilio, Instituto de Investigación Biosanitaria de Granada, Granada, Spain, **2** Endocrinology, Hospital Comarcal del Noroeste, Caravaca de la Cruz, Murcia, Spain, **3** Endocrinology Unit, Hospital General Universitario Rafael Mendez, Lorca, Murcia, Spain, **4** Proteomic Research Service, Fundación para la Investigación Biosanitaria de Andalucía Oriental -Alejandro Otero- (FIBAO), Granada, Spain, **5** Department of Morphology and Cellular Biology (RETICEF), Faculty of Medicine, University of Oviedo, Oviedo, Spain, **6** Critical Care and Emergencies Unit, Hospital Universitario San Cecilio, Granada, Spain, **7** Endocrinology Division, Hospital General de Ciudad Real, Ciudad Real, Spain

Abstract

Objectives: Dickkopf-1 (DKK1) is a potent inhibitor of Wnt signalling, which exerts anabolic effects on bone and also takes part in the regulation of vascular cells. Our aims were to evaluate serum DKK1 in type 2 diabetes (T2DM) patients and to analyze its relationships with cardiovascular disease (CVD). We also evaluated the relationship between DKK1 and bone metabolism.

Design: We conducted a cross-sectional study in which we measured serum DKK1 (ELISA, Biomedica) in 126 subjects: 72 patients with T2DM and 54 non-diabetic subjects. We analysed its relationship with clinical CVD, preclinical CVD expressed as carotid intima media thickness (IMT), and bone metabolism.

Results: T2DM patients with CVD ($P=0{,}026$) and abnormal carotid IMT ($P=0{,}038$) had higher DKK1 concentrations. DKK1 was related to the presence of CVD in T2DM, independently of the presence of risk factors for atherosclerosis. Therefore, for each increase of 28 pg/ml of serum DKK1 there was a 6,2% increase in the risk of CVD in T2DM patients. The ROC curve analysis to evaluate the usefulness of DKK1 as a marker for high risk of CVD showed an area under the curve of 0,667 (95% CI: 0,538–0,795; $P=0{,}016$). In addition, there was a positive correlation between serum DKK1 and spine bone mineral density in the total sample ($r=0{,}183$; $P=0{,}048$).

Conclusion: In summary, circulating DKK1 levels are higher in T2DM with CVD and are associated with an abnormal carotid IMT in this cross-sectional study. DKK1 may be involved in vascular disease of T2DM patients.

Editor: Rudolf Kirchmair, Medical University Innsbruck, Austria

Funding: This work was supported in part by Consejería de Salud y Bienestar Social, Junta de Andalucia (PI-0514-2012) and Red de Investigación Colaborativa en Envejecimiento y Fragilidad (RETICEF) (RD06/0013/1014-RD12/0043/0014). The funders had no role in study design, data collection and analysis, decision to publish, or preparation of the manuscript.

Competing Interests: The authors have declared that no competing interests exist.

* Email: mmt@mamuto.es

Introduction

Patients with type 2 diabetes mellitus (T2DM) have a higher risk of cardiovascular disease (CVD). This association has serious consequences on the morbidity and the mortality in this population. Atherosclerosis is the main pathological mechanism in macrovascular disease in T2DM, which causes the development of atheroma plaques and the major life-threatening events in atherosclerosis, including myocardial infarction and stroke [1].

Patients with osteoporosis have a higher prevalence of cardiovascular disease, and it has been proposed that both pathologies share common pathophysiologic pathways [2]. In T2DM there is an increased risk of fractures at any skeletal site even with greater bone mineral density (BMD) [3,4], and there are data from epidemiological studies supporting a relationship between low bone mineral density (BMD) and atherosclerosis in T2DM [5,6]. Thus, a better characterization of the pathways that could be involved in both processes is of interest, and may help in the development of new therapeutic tools.

The Wnt signalling pathways are involved in several developmental and physiological processes, including the cell differentiation and tissue/organ morphogenesis [7]. The discovery of the Wnt signaling pathway and its relevance in bone homeostasis has contributed to a better knowledge of the cellular and molecular mechanisms of bone biology [8]. The activation of this pathway results in an expansion of osteoprogenitor cells and also determines a reduction in the apoptosis of osteoblasts, which leads to anabolic effects on bone [8]. The canonical Wnt pathway is regulated by several families of secreted antagonists, such as the soluble frizzled-related receptors, dickkopf-1 (DKK1) and sclerostin. DKK1 regulates the Wnt signaling by binding to the Wnt co-receptor, the low-density lipoprotein-related receptor (LRP) 5/6. In addition to its binding to LRP 5/6, DKK1 binds to other trans-membrane molecules as proteins Kremen, which increases their inhibitory activity on the Wnt signaling pathway [9].

The role of Wnt signaling pathways in atherosclerosis it is a matter of growing interest. In preclinical studies the Wnt signaling pathways are involved in atherosclerosis-related processes as vascular calcification [10], inflammation [11], and the monocyte adhesion and its trans-endothelial migration [12]. In a recent study conducted in bovine aortic endothelial cells (ECs) [13], the authors found that Msx2 and Wnt7 family members stabilize the aortic ECs phenotype, whereas DKK1 promotes an endothelial–mesenchymal transition in cultured bovine aortic ECs, a process associated to the pathogenesis of myocardial fibrosis with ischemia [14] and valve calcification [15]. In addition, in animal models of CKD-MBD (chronic kidney disease-mineral bone disease) [16] there is an increased renal production of Wnt inhibitor family members and higher levels of circulating DKK1, sclerostin, and secreted klotho. In this model, the neutralization of DKK1 by administration of a monoclonal antibody after renal injury stimulated bone formation rates, corrected the osteodystrophy, and prevented CKD-stimulated vascular calcification. Besides, the neutralization of DKK1 suppressed aortic expression of the osteoblastic transcription factor Runx2, increased expression of vascular smooth muscle protein 22-α, and restored aortic expression of klotho"

There is also recent data showing a relationship between serum DKK1 and atherosclerosis in humans [17,18]. In a previous study from Register and colleagues, DKK1 concentrations were inversely related to coronary artery disease and aortic calcification. However, as the authors point, this study has been conducted in Afro-Americans (AAs) with T2DM, which has a different prevalence of atherosclerotic disease and osteoporosis compared to European populations. These differences make it interesting to explore this relationship in Caucasian type 2 diabetes. Besides, the relationship between DKK1 concentrations and bone mass has been explored with conflicting data [19–21], so its evaluation in a population with a high risk of bone fragility such as T2DM is of interest.

In this context, the objectives of our study were to evaluate serum DKK1 levels in a cohort of T2DM patients and to analyze its relationships with CVD and bone metabolism. In addition, we compared serum DKK1 concentrations between T2DM and non-diabetic subjects. Thus, our hypothesis was that DKK1 concentrations may be related to CVD and bone metabolism in T2DM patients.

Materials and Methods

Study population

Our study was a cross-sectional one that included 126 subjects. The estimated size of the sample considering an error of 5% and a statistical power of 80% was 84 subjects. The T2DM group included 72 patients with a diagnosis of diabetes according to the American Diabetes Association criteria (ADA, 2005). From January 2006 to December 2007 we consecutively recruited patients who had been referred to our outpatient clinic from community clinics for treatment of diabetes. The control group included 54 non-diabetic subjects who were consecutively recruited from the general community in the same period of time.

All participants were recruited according to the following criteria: Caucasian, free-living, aged 35 to 65 years and normal values for blood count, renal creatinine, hepatic function, calcium and phosphorus. We considered as exclusion criteria the presence of chronic diseases apart from T2DM in the non-diabetic group, the presence of diseases affecting bone (Paget's disease, rheumatoid arthritis, hyperparathyroidism, hypercortisolism, malignant tumors, renal bone disease, chronic liver disease and post-transplantation bone disease) and also previous or current treatment with drugs affecting bone metabolism (calcium supplements, vitamin D preparations, selective estrogen receptor modulators, calcitonin, estrogens therapy, antiresorptive therapy, thiazides, steroids, glucocorticoids or anticonvulsants). Patients treated with thiazolidinediones were also excluded.

The presence of cardiovascular disease was recorded by the medical history and after that it was checked in medical records. T2DM patients were classified into two groups according to the presence of clinical CVD: CVD group and non-CVD group. Inclusion criteria for patients with CVD were cerebrovascular disease (ischemic stroke or transient ischemic attack); coronary heart disease (previous myocardial infarction, diagnosed stable or unstable angina, or coronary revascularization surgery) or ischemic peripheral arterial disease (diagnosed by a positive Doppler ultrasound or arteriogram, or by a previous revascularization surgery).

The study was approved by the ethical review board of the Hospital Universitario San Cecilio and it was done conformed to the ethical guidelines for research in humans. All the participants in the study provided written informed consent after a full explanation of the purpose of the study and the nature of all the procedures that will be used in the study. Written informed consent was approved for the ethical review board of our hospital, and after that it was filed in the medical record of each patient.

Clinical evaluation

Height, weight, and waist circumference were measured at baseline according to standard procedures. Weight was measured to the nearest 100 grams using digital electronic scales. Height and waist circumference were measured to the nearest 1 mm using a stadiometer and a metal anthropometric tape, respectively. Body mass index (BMI) in Kg/m^2 was calculated as weight divided by the square of height in meters.

Blood pressure was measured in a standardized manner. The subjects remained at rest for at least 5 minutes, and after that blood pressure was measured twice using a standard mercury sphygmomanometer (12 centimeters long, 35 cm wide). The mean of the two values was used for analysis. We defined hypertension when blood pressure values were higher than 140/90 mmHg and/or where subjects were on antihypertensive treatment.

The participants reported their alcohol use, smoking status and their level of physical activity with a specific health questionnaire. Patients were classified as having a significant alcohol intake if it was higher than 40 grams/day in males and 24 grams/day in women; smoking status was categorized as no tobacco use or current tobacco use. Physical activity was collected through a specific questionnaire in which study subjects scored their physical activity on a scale from 0 (none) to 10 (sport more than one hour four times per week). Based on the results, the study sample was divided into two groups: sedentary (<5 on the scale) and no sedentary (≥5 on the scale).

Serum measurements

Samples of venous blood were taken in the morning after a fasting overnight. The sera were stored at −80°C until examina-

Table 1. Characteristics of the study population.

	Total Group (n=126)	T2DM Group (n=72)	Non-diabetic Group (n=54)	P Value
Age (years)	57±6	58±6	55±7	0,018
Male/female (n)	62/64	39/33	25/29	0,472
Medical history				
Duration of diabetes (years)	-	13,7±7,6	-	
Hypertension (%)	53,2	80,6	46,3	<0,001
Dyslipidaemia (%)	65,9	94,4	70,4	<0,001
Albuminuria (%)	20,5	35,0	4,0	0,006
Chronic kidney disease (KDOQI stages) (%)				
Stage 1	51	52	52	0,938
Stage 2	46	44	48	0,815
Stage 3	3	4	0	0,155
Smoker or ex-smoker (%)	15,1	16,7	13	0,623
Alcohol (%)	8,7	6,9	11,1	0,104
Sedentarism (%)	47,6	55,6	37,0	0,048
Clinical evaluation:				
BMI (kg/m^2)	102,6±12,4	31,4±5,7	29,3±5,9	0,043
Waist circumference (cm)	130±20	106,4±11,4	97,4±11,9	<0,001
SBP (mm Hg)	80±13	134±97	124±17	0,002
DBP (mm Hg)	30,5±5,9	80±12	79±15	0,705
Serum parameters:				
FPG (mg/dL)	137,2±61,9	173±60,1	89,4±10,4	<0,001
HbA1$_c$ (%)	6,7±2,2	8±1,9	4,8±0,4	<0,001
GFR (MDR/CKD-EPI)(ml/min/1,73 m^2)	92±23	92±23	93±22	0,745
Calcium (mg/dL)	9,5±0,5	9,6±0,5	9,3±0,4	0,001
Phosphorus (mg/dL)	3,6±0,5	3,7±0,5	3,5±0,5	0,01
PTH (pg/mL)	43,6±19,5	38,5±18,4	50,4±19,1	<0,001
25(OH) D (ng/mL)	19,5±11,3	17,8±11,5	21,6±10,9	0,06
Triglyceride (mg/dl)	142±121	169,9±149,8	104,9±47,7	<0,001
HDL-c (mg/dl)	53,5±15,5	49±16	59,5±12,5	<0,001
LDL-c (mg/dl)	111,7±35,5	96,9±34,1	130,8±27,4	<0,001
DKK1 (pg/ml)	629±374	669±395	575±340	0,163
DXA parameters and VF:				
BMD LS (g/cm^2)	0,977±0,148	0,954±0,146	1±0,148	0,068
BMD FN (g/cm^2)	0,820±0,124	0,817±0,132	0,823±0,117	0,792
BMD TH (g/cm^2)	0,906±0,135	0,903±0,145	0,911±0,125	0,772
T-score LS	−1,08±1,36	−1,3±1,3	0,82±1,3	0,058
T-score FN	−0,55±1,01	−0,6±1,04	−0,49±0,99	0,565
T-score TH	−0,55±0,98	−0,62±1	−0,51±0,92	0,557
Osteoporosis (%)	15,9	24,6	9,4	0,047
Morphometric VF (%)	23,0	30,3	20,0	0,274
Cardiovascular disease:	35,7	58,3	5,6	<0,001
Cerebrovascular disease (%)	11,9	19,4	1,9	0,002
Coronary heart disease (%)	23,8	38,9	3,7	<0,001
Peripheral artery disease (%)	7,9	13,9	0	0,005
Abnormal intima-media thickness (%)	35,7	54,2	11,1	<0,001
Carotid plaques (%)	15,9	29,4	0	<0,001

Data for continuous variables are presented as mean ±SD. Data for categorical variables are presented as numbers and/or percentages. The comparison between groups was done by Student's t test (continuous variables) or Chi-square test (categorical variables).

T2DM: type 2 diabetes mellitus; BMI: body mass index; SBP: sistolic blood pressure; DBP: diastolic blood pressure; FPG: fasting plasma glucose; HbA1c: glycated hemoglobin; GFR: glomerular filtration rate; MDR/CKD-EPI: Chronic Kidney Disease Epidemiology Collaboration; PTH: parathormone; 25(OH) D: 25-hydroxyvitamin D; HDL-c: High-density lipoprotein; LDL-c: Low-density lipoprotein; BMD: bone mineral density; LS: lumbar spine; FN: femoral neck; TH: total hip; VF: vertebral fractures.

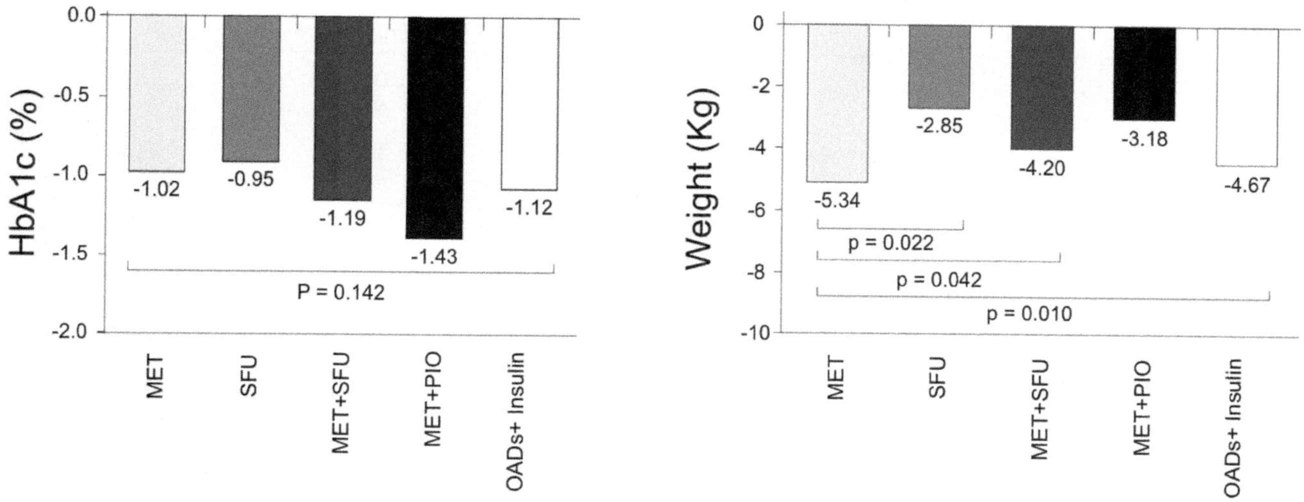

Figure 1. DKK1 serum levels in T2DM patients according to the presence of cardiovascular disease and abnormal intima-media thickness. Between groups differences are indicated through a bar with the P-value given above.

tion. Fasting plasma glucose (FPG), glycated hemoglobin (HbA1c), calcium, phosphorus and creatinine were measured using standard automated laboratory techniques. Glomerular filtration rate (GFR) was calculated by MDRD/CKD-EPI formula [22]. High-density lipoprotein (HDL), low-density lipoprotein (LDL) cholesterol and triglycerides (TGs) were measured by standard biochemical methods. Dyslipidemia was defined according to third report of the expert panel on detection, evaluation, and treatment of high blood cholesterol in adults (ATP-III) criteria or current treatment with statins.

Calciotropic hormones measurement included serum intact parathormone (Two-site immunoassay for iPTH, Roche Diagnostics SL, Barcelona, Spain; intra and interassay variability of 3%) and 25-hydroxyvitamin D (25-OH-D, radioimmunoassay, DiaSorin, Stillwater, Minnesota USA. Serum DKK1 was measured using quantitative sandwich enzyme-linked immunosorbent assay (ELISA) developed by Biomedica (Biomedica Medizinprodukte GmbH and Co. KG, Wien, Austria) according to the manufacturer's instructions. The Biomedica DKK-1 ELISA (BI-20412) detects free DKK-1. Intra-assay and interassay variability were of 7% and 9%, respectively. DKK1 measurements are reported throughout in pg/ml after conversion from pMol/L. 1 pMol/l is equivalent to 28,68 pg/ml.

Bone density measurement and vertebral fractures assessment

Bone mineral density at lumbar spine (LS) L2–L4, femoral neck (FN) and total hip (TH) was performed in all patients by dual-energy X-ray absorptiometry (DXA) using Hologic QDR 4500 densitometer (Whatman, MA; variation coefficient <1%). All the BMD measurements were done by the same experienced operator. We used the World Health Organization criteria for osteoporosis (Kanis JA, 1994).

Standardized spinal X-rays were taken for morphometric analysis of all participants of the study and they were interpreted according to the algorithm developed by McCloskey and colleagues [23].

Carotid intima-media thickness Ultrasonographic examination of the carotid arteries was performed with patients in supine position using Doppler ultrasonography (Toshiba PowerVision 6000). The maximum intima-media thickness (IMT) at the carotid bifurcation (BIF) was determined between the near and far walls of the carotid bifurcation on the right and left sides. Each part was measured from views of both longitudinal and vertical sections at the bifurcation. If a discrepancy was observed in the measured values between longitudinal and vertical sections, the smaller value was selected to avoid overestimation. BIF–IMT was defined as the mean of the measurements from the right and left sides. The value for each side was obtained from the mean of 10 wall measurements. The BIF–IMT, measured in millimeters (mm), was considered pathological if it was ≥0.9 mm, and was considered to be carotid atherosclerosis if the BIF–IMT was ≥ 1.2 mm or 50% greater than the BIF–IMT in the adjacent area [24]. Plaques were identified as calcified by findings of bright white echoes on sonography. A single trained sonographer performed the study in all subjects.

Statistical analysis

Data for continuous variables are presented as mean ± standard deviation (SD). Data for categorical variables are presented as numbers and/or percentages. Kolmogorov–Smirnov test was used to test the normality of distribution of continuous variables. The association between continuous variables was described by Pearson's or Spearman's correlation coefficients. The comparison of categorical variables among groups was performed using Chi-square test or Fisher test. The comparison of continuous variables among groups was performed using unpaired Student's t test or Mann-Whitney test. To determine the independent variables which correlated with DKK1 (dependent variable), the parameters that correlate significantly in univariate analysis and other which are biologically linked to DKK1 were tested in multiple backward model linear regression analysis. Multiple backward model of logistic regression analysis was performed to identify DKK1 as independent predictor for CVD (dependent variable) in T2DM patients. The model included established atherosclerotic risk factors (age, gender, body mass index, hypertension, dislipidaemia, smoking, sedentarism, HbA1c, GFR and intima-media thickness). CVD-defining parameters (cerebrovascular disease, coronary heart disease or ischemic peripheral arterial disease) were not included in the multiple logistic regression model. The usefulness of serum DKK1 as a marker of high risk of atherosclerotic disease in T2DM was

Table 2. DKK1 concentrations according to the presence of cardiovascular disease in the T2DM group.

	Yes	No	P value
Cardiovascular disease	757±416	547±333	0,026
Cerebrovascular disease	854±480	625±363	0,045
Coronary heart disease	694±379	654±408	0,677
Peripheral artery disease	634±247	675±415	0,762
Abnormal intima-media thickness	756±433	567±322	0,042
Carotid plaque	730±422	661±395	0,522

The comparison between groups was done by Student's t test.

analyzed using a receiver operating characteristic curve (ROC Curve). A p value of less than 0,05 was considered to be significant (two-tailed). Data were recorded and analyzed using SPSS version 18.0 software (SPSS Inc, Chicago, IL, USA).

Results

The clinical characteristics of the study population are summarized in Table 1. Serum DKK1 was significantly higher ($P = 0{,}026$) in T2DM patients with CVD (757±416 pg/ml) compared with those without CVD (547±333 pg/ml). (Figure 1 and Table 2). T2DM patients with abnormal IMT (756±433 pg/ml *vs* 563±322 pg/ml; $P = 0{,}042$) and cerebrovascular disease (854±480 pg/ml *vs* 625±363; $P = 0{,}045$) had higher DKK1 concentrations. (Figure 1 and Table 2). However, we did not find differences in DKK1 concentrations according to the presence of carotid plaque ($P = 0{,}522$), coronary heart disease ($P = 0{,}677$) or ischemic peripheral artery disease ($P = 0{,}762$).

A model of logistic regression analysis was performed using the presence of CVD as a dependent variable. Independent variables were serum DKK1 levels and risk factors for atherosclerosis (age, gender, body mass index, hypertension, dislipidaemia, smoking, sedentarism, HbA1c, GFR, and IMT). DKK1 levels were independently associated with the presence of CVD in T2DM (odds ratio: 1,062, 95% confidence interval: 1,003–1,125; $P = 0{,}04$). Therefore, for each increase of 28 pg/ml of serum DKK1 there was a 6,2% increased risk of CVD in T2DM patients.

In the ROC curve analysis to evaluate the usefulness of DKK1 as a marker for high risk of CVD, the area under the curve was 0,667 (95% confidence interval: 0,538–0,795; $P = 0{,}016$) (Figure 2). A concentration of 494 pg/ml or higher showed a sensitivity of 71,4% and a specificity of 60% to identify an increased risk of CVD.

We found no differences in DKK1 between study groups: T2DM 669±395 vs non-diabetic 575±340 pg/ml, $P = 0{,}163$. Serum DKK1 concentrations were significantly higher in females than in males in total sample (697±434 vs 563±293 pg/ml, $P = 0{,}046$) and in T2DM group (788±493 vs 569±255 pg/ml, $P = 0{,}025$) but were not significantly increased in control females (593±335 vs 553±349 pg/ml, $P = 0{,}682$).

Linear regression analysis was performed to determine the influence of independent factors identified in univariate correlation analysis, including group, gender, age, HbA1c, CVD and IMT as independent variables that explain serum DKK1 levels. The analysis demonstrated that gender ($\beta = -0{,}299$, $P = 0{,}002$) and CVD ($\beta = 0{,}292$, $P = 0{,}007$) were positively associated with serum DKK1.

Regarding bone metabolism, lumbar spine BMD was positively related to serum DKK1 in total sample ($r = 0{,}183$, $P = 0{,}048$). In contrast, we did not found a significant relationship with bone remodelling markers osteoporosis diagnosis or morphometric vertebral fractures (data not shown), in the total sample or in the study groups separately.

Discussion

To our knowledge, there is no previous study evaluating DKK1 concentrations and its relationship with CVD in Caucasian T2DM patients. There is also scarce data concerning the relationship between DKK1 and bone metabolism in T2DM. Our results show that higher levels of DKK1 are associated with clinical CVD and abnormal IMT in T2DM patients. These findings suggest that serum DKK1 are related to the presence of CVD in this population. However, our data showed no differences in serum DKK1 between T2DM patients and non-diabetic patients. Regarding bone metabolism, we found a significant relationship with bone mineral density.

In our study, higher DKK1 levels were positively related to cardiovascular disease in T2DM patients independently of the presence of others risk factors for atherosclerosis, and high concentrations of DKK1 were related to abnormal IMT in these patients. Our results are in accordance with previous reports showing the relationship between vascular disease and DKK1 in other populations. Patients with cerebrovascular disease have higher serum DKK1 levels compared with control subjects [25], and serum DKK1 correlated with coronary artery calcification and atherosclerotic plaques evaluated by coronary computed tomography and coronary artery calcium scoring [17]. Previously, Ueland and colleagues [26] demonstrated that DKK1 expression is enhanced in advanced carotid plaques and that DKK1 is a novel mediator in platelet-mediated endothelial cell activation, which could occur within the atherosclerotic lesions. Moreover, current data clearly demonstrate a novel role for Wnt proteins in the proliferation, migration, and survival of smooth muscle cells (SMCs) [27]. Regarding this, higher levels of DKK1 are present in advanced carotid plaques and DKK1 promotes platelet-mediated activation of endothelial cells. Thus, it has been proposed that this could lead to enhanced inflammation in the atherosclerotic lesion; however, it may also lead to a reduced survival, proliferation, and migration of SMCs, thereby reinforcing the potential complexity of the participation of Wnt proteins in atherosclerosis [27].

In contrast to our findings, DKK1 concentrations were negatively associated with atherosclerotic calcified plaque in African-Americans (AAs) patients with T2DM [18]. There are several reasons that might contribute to this discrepancy. As the authors point, AAs have lower rates of vascular calcification. It has

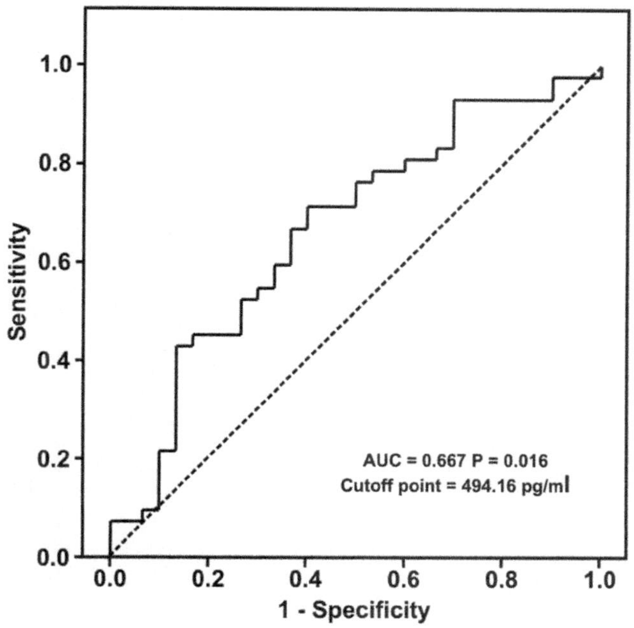

Figure 2. DKK1 ROC curve for cardiovascular disease.

been reported lower levels of coronary artery calcified plaque relative to European Americans (EAs) despite similar or more detrimental cardiovascular risk factor profiles [28,29]. This observation is consistent both in T2DM and subjects without diabetes [30,31], and suggests a differential impact of CV risk factors on atherosclerosis based on ethnicity although the underlying causes of ethnic differences in vascular calcification are not well established [32]. Reinforcing these ethnic differences, AAs are at lower risk for myocardial infarction based on less coronary artery calcification, and they have significantly lower rates of myocardial infarction than EAs, provided equal access to healthcare [33,34]. It has been suggested that AAs may be less susceptible than whites to hyperglycaemia–induced macrovascular disease [35]. Thus, these findings may explain the differences observed in the relationship between vascular disease and DKK1 between our study and the data from Register and colleagues.

Recent data suggest that the association between vascular calcification and osteoporosis is not simply a consequence of age, stressing that the co-incidence of vascular calcification with low bone activity and osteoporosis could be biologically linked. During the development of vascular calcification, there is a transition of vascular SMCs towards an osteoblast- like phenotype, which promotes the mineralization within these structures. In this process there are several players, including those related to mineral metabolism, like phosphorus, calcium or parathyroid hormone, which influences the expression of osteogenic factors [36]. There is emerging evidence suggesting that some inhibitors of the Wnt pathway, such as secreted frizzled Proteins 2 and 4 and DKK-1, may play a role linking vascular calcification and bone loss [26,27]. AAs manifest a skeletal resistance to the effects of parathyroid hormone [37,38] and exhibit opposite relationships between arterial calcification and serum vitamin D concentrations compared with Europeans [39]. In our opinion, these ethnic differences in the effects of calciotropic hormones on bone and vessels may indicate that differences in other pathways, as Wnt pathway, may be expected according to race. However, this hypothesis must be confirmed.

There are other differences between the study from Register and colleagues and ours, which may explain the discrepancy of results. First, the prevalence of cardiovascular disease is lower, 27%, compared to our study where a 58% of patients had previous cardiovascular disease. Second, in the study from Register and colleagues 28,3% of subjects were taking hormonal therapy while no women were on hormonal therapy in our study. Estradiol and progesterone has shown to regulate Wnt pathways in endometrial tissue [40] and brain [41], so an influence of hormonal therapy in DKK1 concentrations can not be excluded. Finally, despite the low expected incidence of arterial calcification in AAs, in the study from Register and colleagues there is a high prevalence of aortic calcification. Thus, differences between study populations apart from the ethnicity may influence the discrepancy of results.

There are no previous studies evaluating differences in serum DKK1 concentrations according to the presence of diabetes. We did not find differences in DKK1 between T2DM patients and subjects without diabetes. These results contrast with our previous data showing higher sclerostin concentrations in the same group of type 2 diabetes patients [42]. However, serum DKK1 and sclerostin have shown to be barely correlated [43], as we found in our sample (data not shown). In addition, the effects of DKK1 and sclerostin may differ due to differences in Kremen binding. While DKK1 is always an inhibitor of Wnt signaling, the effect of sclerostin is variable depending on context [44]. Unlike our previous results about sclerostin, women had higher DKK1 concentrations both in the total sample and in the T2DM group. Estradiol and progesterone have shown to take part in the regulation of the Wnt pathways in endometrial tissue [40] and brain [41], so a sex steroid-induced effect may explain gender differences in DKK1 although this hypothesis must be confirmed.

Regarding the relationship between bone metabolism and DKK1 we only found a weak correlation with BMD at lumbar spine in the total sample, and no relationship with bone turnover markers, osteoporosis or morphometric vertebral fractures (data not shown). In addition, lumbar spine BMD may be affected by aortic calcification. Our findings confirm previous data showing no relationship between DKK1 and bone turnover markers in postmenopausal osteoporosis [20]. The relationship between DKK1 and BMD is not totally established. It has been reported no relationship with volumetric BMD in Afro-American T2DM patients [18]. However, is also been described and inverse relationship between DKK1 and BMD, and higher DKK1 concentrations in patients with osteoporosis [19]. Therefore, in our opinion the data about serum DKK1 and bone metabolism are controversial and thus no clear conclusions can be drawn.

Our study has some limitations. First, the cross-sectional design does not allow to establishing a cause-effect relationship. Second, the sample size is relatively small and might affect the statistic power. Our study has also several strengths, as the evaluation of circulating serum DKK1 in Caucasian patients with T2DM for the first time, the comparison to non-diabetic subjects and the evaluation both of bone metabolism and atherosclerotic disease.

In summary, serum levels of DKK1 are elevated in Caucasian patients with T2DM presenting CVD. These findings suggest that Wnt signaling pathway is involved in vascular disease in diabetic subjects. However, the relations of DKK1 with bone metabolism are inconsistent.

Author Contributions

None. Conceived and designed the experiments: AGM PRM RRG MMT. Performed the experiments: BGF SMS. Analyzed the data: AGM RRG MMT. Contributed reagents/materials/analysis tools: BGF SMS. Wrote the paper: AGM RRG MMT PRM ACM MMG.

References

1. Madonna R, De Caterina R (2011) Cellular and molecular mechanisms of vascular injury in diabetes–part I: Pathways of vascular disease in diabetes. Vascular Pharmacology 54: 68–74.
2. Magnus JH, Brussard DL (2005) Relationship between bone mineral density and myocardial infarction in US adults. Osteoporosis International 16: 2053–2062.
3. Hofbauer LC, Brueck CC, Singh SK, Dognig H (2007) Osteoporosis in patients with diabetes mellitus. Journal of Bone and Mineral Research 22: 1317–1328.
4. Epstein S, Leroith D (2008) Diabetes and fragility fractures — A burgeoning epidemic? Bone 43: 3–6.
5. Carr JJ, Register TC, Hsu FC, Lohman K, Lenchik L, et al. (2008) Calcified atherosclerotic plaque and bone mineral density in type 2 diabetes: the diabetes heart study. Bone 42: 43–52.
6. Divers J, Register TC, Langefeld CD, Wagenknecht LE, Bowden DW, et al. (2011) Relationships between calcified atherosclerotic plaque and bone mineral density in AAs with type 2 diabetes. Journal of Bone and Mineral Research 26: 1554–1560.
7. Gordon MD, Nusse R (2006) Wnt signalling: multiple pathways, multiple receptors and multiple transcription factors. Journal of Biology and Chemistry 281: 22429–22433.
8. Huang H, He X (2008) Wnt/beta-catenin signaling: new (and old) players and new insight. Current Opinion in Cell Biology 20: 119–125.
9. Mao B, Wu W, Davidson G, Marhold J, Li M, et al. (2002) Kremen proteins are Dickkopf receptors that regulate Wnt/-catenin signalling. Nature 417: 664–667.
10. Shao JS, Cheng SL, Pingsterhaus JM, Charlton-Kachigian N, Loewy AP, et al. (2005) Msx2 promotes cardiovascular calcification by activating paracrine Wnt signals. Journal of Clinical Investigation 115: 1210–1220.
11. Sen M, Ghosh G (2008) Transcriptional outcome of Wnt-Frizzled signal transduction in inflammation: evolving concepts. Journal of Immunology 181: 4441–4445.
12. Christman MA 2nd, Goetz DJ, Dickerson E, McCall KD, Lewis CJ, et al. (2008) Wnt5a is expressed in murine and human atherosclerotic lesions. American Journal of Physiology and Heart Circulation and Physiology 294: H2864–2870.
13. Cheng SL, Shao JS, Behrmann A, Krchma K, Towler DA (2013) Dkk1 and MSX2-Wnt7b signaling reciprocally regulate the endothelial-mesenchymal transition in aortic endothelial cells. Arterioscler Thromb Vasc Biol 33: 1679–89.
14. Krenning G, Zeisberg EM, Kalluri R (2010) The origin of fibroblasts and mechanism of cardiac fibrosis. J Cell Physiol 225: 631–637.
15. Wylie-Sears J, Aikawa E, Levine RA, Yang JH, Bischoff J (2011) Mitral valve endothelial cells with osteogenic differentiation potential. Arterioscler Thromb Vasc Biol 31: 598–607.
16. Fang Y, Ginsberg C, Seifert M, Agapova O, Sugatani T, et al. (2014) CKD-Induced Wingless/Integration1 Inhibitors and Phosphorus Cause the CKD-Mineral and Bone Disorder. J Am Soc Nephrol 25: 1760–73.
17. Kim KI, Park KU, Chun EJ, Choi SI, Cho YS, et al. (2011) A novel biomarker of coronary atheroesclerosis: serum DKK1 concentration correlates with coronary artery calcification and atherosclerotic plaques. Journal of Korean Medical Science 26: 1178–1184.
18. Register TC, Hruska KA, Divers J, Bowden DW, Palmer ND, et al. (2013) Plasma Dickkopf (DKK1) concentrations negatively associate with atherosclerotic calcified plaque in african-americans with type 2 diabetes. Journal of Clinical Endocrinology and Metabolism 98: 60–65.
19. Butler JS, Murray DW, Hurson CJ, O'Brien J, Doran PP, et al. (2011) The role of Dkk1 in bone mass regulation: correlating serum Dkk1 expression with bone mineral density. Journal of Orthopaedic Research 29: 414–418.
20. Polyzos SA, Anastasilakis AD, Bratengeier C, Woloszczuk W, Papatheodorou A, et al. (2012) Serum sclerostin levels positively correlate with lumbar spinal bone mineral density in postmenopausal women-the six-month effect of risedronate and teriparatide. Osteoporosis International 23: 1171–1176.
21. Cejka D, Jäger-Lansky A, Kieweg H, Weber M, Bieglmayer C, et al. (2012) Sclerostin serum levels correlate positively with bone mineral density and microarchitecture in haemodialysis patients. Nephrology Dialysis Transplantion 27: 226–230.
22. Levey AS, Stevens LA, Schmid CH, Zhang YL, Castro AF 3rd, et al. (2009) CKD-EPI (Chronic Kidney Disease Epidemiology Collaboration). A new equation to estimate glomerular filtration rate. Ann Intern Med 150: 604–612.
23. McCloskey EV, Spector TD, Eyres KS, Fern ED, O'Rourke N, et al. (1993) The assessment of vertebral deformity: a method for use in population studies and clinical trials. Osteoporosis International 3: 138–147.
24. Junyent M, Gilabert R, Nuñez I, Corbella E, Vela M, et al. (2005) Carotid ultrasound in the assessment of preclinical atherosclerosis. Distribution of intima-media thickness values and plaque frequency in a Spanish community cohort. Medicina Clinica 125: 770–774.
25. Seifert-Held T, Pekar T, Gattringer T, Simmet NE, Scharnagl H, et al. (2011) Circulating Dickkopf-1 in acute ischemic stroke and clinically stable cerebrovascular disease. Atherosclerosis 218: 233–237.
26. Ueland T, Otterdal K, Lekva T, Halvorsen B, Gabrielsen A, et al. (2009) Dickkopf-1 enhances inflammatory interaction between platelets and endothelial cells and shows increased expression in atherosclerosis. Arteriosclerosis Thrombosis and Vascular Biology 29: 1228–1234.
27. Mill C, George SJ (2012) Wnt signalling in smooth muscle cells and its role in cardiovascular disorders. Cardiovascular Research 95: 233–40.
28. Bild DE, Detrano R, Peterson D, Guerci A, Liu K, et al. (2005) Ethnic differences in coronary calcification: the Multi-Ethnic Study of Atherosclerosis (MESA). Circulation 111: 1313–20.
29. Lee TC, O'Malley PG, Feuerstein I, Taylor AJ (2003) The prevalence and severity of coronary artery calcification on coronary artery computed tomography in black and white subjects. J Am Coll Cardiol 41: 39–44.
30. Freedman BI, Hsu FC, Langefeld CD, Rich SS, Herrington DM, et al. (2005) The impact of ethnicity and sex on subclinical cardiovascular disease: the Diabetes Heart Study. Diabetologia 48: 2511–8.
31. Wade AN, Fedyna S, Mehta NN, St. Clair C, Ginwala N, et al. (2011) Type 2 diabetes does not attenuate racial differences in coronary calcification. Diabetes Res Clin Pract 91: 101–7.
32. Divers J, Palmer ND, Lu L, Register TC, Carr JJ, et al. (2013) Admixture mapping of coronary artery calcified plaque in African Americans with type 2 diabetes mellitus. Circ Cardiovasc Genet; 6: 97–105.
33. Karter AJ, Ferrara A, Liu JY, Moffet HH, Ackerson LM, et al. (2002) Ethnic disparities in diabetic complications in an insured population. JAMA 287: 2519–27.
34. Young BA, Maynard C, Boyko EJ (2003) Racial differences in diabetic nephropathy, cardiovascular disease, and mortality in a national population of veterans. Diabetes Care 26: 2392–9.
35. Freedman BI, Hsu FC, Langefeld CD, Rich SS, Herrington DM, et al. (2005) The impact of ethnicity and sex on subclinical cardiovascular disease: the Diabetes Heart Study. Diabetologia 48: 2511–8.
36. Cannata-Andia JB, Roman-Garcia P, Hruska K (2011) The connections between vascular calcification and bone health. Nephrol Dial Transplant 26: 3429–36.
37. Bell NH, Williamson B, Hollis B, Riggs BL (2001) Effects of race on diurnal patterns of renal conservation of calcium and bone resorption in premenopausal women. Osteoporos Int 12: 43–8.
38. Aloia J, Vaswani A, Yeh J, Flaster E (1996) Risk for osteoporosis in black women. Calcif Tissue Int 59: 415–23.
39. Freedman BI, Register TC (2012) Effect of race and genetics on vitamin D metabolism, bone and vascular health. Nature Review Nephrology 8: 459–466.
40. Wang Y, Hanifi-Moghaddam P, Hanekamp EE, Kloosterboer HJ, Franken P, et al. (2009) Progesterone inhibition of Wnt/beta-catenin signaling in normal endometrium and endometrial cancer. Clinical Cancer Research 15: 5784–5793.
41. Scott EL, Brann DW (2012) Estrogen regulation of Dkk1 and Wnt/β-Catenin signaling in neurodegenerative disease. Brain Research 1514: 63–74.
42. García-Martín A, Rozas-Moreno P, Reyes-García R, Morales-Santana S, García-Fontana B, et al. (2012) Circulating levels of sclerostin are increased in patients with type 2 diabetes mellitus. Journal of Clinical Endocrinology and Metabolism 97: 234–241.
43. Thambiah S, Roplekar R, Manghat P, Fogelman I, Fraser WD, et al. (2012) Circulating sclerostin and Dickkopf-1 (DKK1) in predialysis chronic kidney disease (CKD): relationship with bone density and arterial stiffness. Calcified Tissue International 90: 473–480.
44. Kawano Y, Kypta R (2003) Secreted antagonists of the Wnt signalling pathway. J Cell Sci 116: 2627–34.

Health Behaviour in Children and Adolescents with Type 1 Diabetes Compared to a Representative Reference Population

Sebastian Kummer[1*¶], Anna Stahl-Pehe[2¶], Katty Castillo[2], Christina Bächle[2], Christine Graf[3], Klaus Straßburger[2], Burak Salgin[4], Ertan Mayatepek[1], Guido Giani[2], Reinhard W. Holl[5], Thomas Meissner[1¶], Joachim Rosenbauer[2¶]

1 Department of General Pediatrics, Neonatology and Pediatric Cardiology, University Children's Hospital, Duesseldorf, Germany, **2** Institute for Biometrics and Epidemiology, German Diabetes Center (DDZ), Leibniz Institute for Diabetes Research at Heinrich Heine University, Duesseldorf, Germany, **3** Institute of Movement and Neurosciences, German Sport University, Cologne, Germany, **4** Department of Paediatrics, Cambridge University, Addenbrooke's Hospital, Cambridge, United Kingdom, **5** Institute for Epidemiology and Medical Biometry, University of Ulm, Ulm, Germany

Abstract

Objective: We provide a population-based overview of health behaviours of children and adolescents with type 1 diabetes in comparison to the general population, and analyse their relevance for glycaemic control and self-rated health status.

Methods: Data from questionnaires of 11- to 17-year-old children and adolescents with diabetes (n = 629) were compared to a representative sample (n = 6,813).

Results: Children and adolescents with type 1 diabetes had a significantly increased odds of infrequent physical activity (adjusted OR 1.56), short overall duration of physical activity per week (OR 1.55, difference -1.3 hours/week), and high daily computer use (OR 2.51). They had a lower odds of active and passive smoking (OR 0.31 and OR 0.29), and high daily television time (OR 0.68). The odds of an at least good and excellent self-rated health status was increased with intense physical activity, and decreased with active smoking and prolonged daily use of computer and television. Active smoking and prolonged daily use of computer were associated with higher HbA1c.

Conclusions: Children and adolescents with type 1 diabetes showed a different profile of health behaviour. Their overall health may improve if their education stresses specifically frequent physical activity with longer overall duration and less frequent television or computer use.

Editor: Jacobus van Wouwe, TNO, Netherlands

Funding: The study was supported by the Competence Network for Diabetes Mellitus funded by the Federal Ministry of Education and Research (support code 01GI0802, 01GI1109A, 01GI1106). The German Diabetes Center is institutionally funded by the German Ministry of Health and the Ministry of Innovation, Sciences and Research of the Federal State of North Rhine-Westphalia. The funders had no role in study design, data collection and analysis, decision to publish, or preparation of the manuscript.

Competing Interests: The authors have declared that no competing interests exist.

* Email: Sebastian.kummer@med.uni-duesseldorf.de

¶ These authors are shared first and senior authors on this work.

Introduction

Long-term prognosis in type 1 diabetes improves with good glycaemic control in childhood and adolescence [1]. This depends not only on adequate insulin substitution, but also on health-relevant behaviours such as physical activity, nutrition, smoking, and psychosocial parameters, which have a significant impact on the quality of glycaemic control. For example, physical activity has the potential to reduce cardiovascular risk, enhance quality of life and improve glucose control in patients with type 1 diabetes [2,3] as well as in healthy individuals [4]. Also on the tissue level, exercise results in beneficial effects, e.g. on pancreas, cardiovascular system, the kidneys, and skeletal muscle [5] Smoking negatively affects type 1 diabetes management and increases the risk especially for long-term sequelae of diabetes mellitus [6,7]. It was shown in a clinical sample of youths with type 1 diabetes that daily media consumption time is a significant risk factor for poor glycaemic control [8]. In healthy children and adolescents, computer use and watching television are associated with physical activity, eating behaviour and obesity [9,10]. However, the impact of these health-relevant activities has not been evaluated in detail for their relevance in patients with type 1 diabetes. To our knowledge, there is no population-based study to date that has compared these health behaviours between children and adolescents with type 1 diabetes and the general population.

Patients with early-onset type 1 diabetes are expected to be at increased risk of late complications compared with patients with later onset [11]. In addition, a doubling of new cases of type 1 diabetes in European children younger than 5 years of age between 2005 and 2020 has been predicted [12]. Associations between physical activity, smoking and media consumption on the one side and glycaemic control and health status on the other side are largely unexplored in this young patient group so far.

Our objective is to provide a population-based overview of health-relevant behaviours and their association with glycaemic control and self-rated health status in children and adolescents with early-onset and long-duration type 1 diabetes in comparison to peers from the general population in Germany.

Methods

Data source/study populations

Data sources have been described in detail elsewhere [13]. In brief, young patients with type 1 diabetes mellitus between 11 and 21 years of age and disease onset between age 0 and 4 years in the period from 1993 to 1999 were selected from the nationwide diabetes register (completeness of ascertainment 95%) maintained at the German Diabetes Center, Duesseldorf, Germany. Between September 2009 and December 2010, 2.241 patients and their parents received mailed/paper-based questionnaires, information about the study and a consent form. No financial incentives were paid for participation. Comprehensive questionnaires were obtained from 840 participants and their parents. Participants and non-participants did not differ significantly with respect to sex, but participants were 0.8 years younger, had 0.2 years earlier disease onset and 0.6 years shorter disease duration (each $p< 0.001$). For the analyses, all patients ≥18 years of age were excluded, leaving 629 children and adolescents between 11 and 17 years of age. The overall response rate was 43% in 11- to 13-year-olds and 42% in 14- to 17-year-olds.

As normative data, the Public Use File of the German Health Interview and Examination Survey for Children and Adolescents (KiGGS 2003–2006, Robert-Koch-Institute, Berlin, Germany) was used [14]. Data collection was performed between May 2003 and May 2006 from 17.641 children and adolescents aged between 0–17 years. 6,813 participants were in the age range 11 to 17 years. The response rate was 69% in 11- to 13-year-olds and 63% in 14- to 17-year-olds.

Both studies used identical extensive, standardized, self-administered questionnaires to obtain information from children and adolescents as well as from their parents. The study was approved by the commissioner responsible for data protection and the ethics committee of Düsseldorf University (study number 3254), and was conducted according to the principles expressed in the Declaration of Helsinki. Written and informed consent was obtained from all participating children and adolescents and all parents or respective legal guardians.

Variables

The children and adolescents answered questions concerning their health behaviour. They were asked how often (never, 1–2 times per month, 1–2 times per week, 3–5 times per week, approximately every day) and how many hours per week in total they were physically active in their leisure time in an intensity to cause sweating or hard breathing (e.g. by sports or bicycling). In addition, they were asked about their own smoking behaviour, and environmental smoking exposure (frequency of active and passive smoking: never, less than once per week, once per week, a number of times per week, every day), and about the average daily use of television and computers (never, about half an hour, about 1–2 hours, about 3–4 hours, more than 4 hours per day). To avoid small numbers of cases in subcategories for some analyses, the cut point for low and high frequency of physical activity was defined at 3 times per week instead of 7 times per week as recommended. For some analyses, duration of physical activity was dichotomized as low (<7 hours/week) and high (≥7 hours/week) according to international recommendations (at least 60 minutes of moderate to vigorous physical activity per day) [15]. The categorization for active and passive smoking was yes/no and >1 time/week/≤1 time/week, respectively. Time spent watching television and using the computer was categorized in ≥3 hours/day and <3 hours/day based on recent recommendations (limit entertainment screen time to <1 to 2 hours per day [16]).

Sociodemographic information was given by the parents. Participants were classified as having a migration background if they had emigrated from another country and at least one of their parents was not born in Germany or was of non-German nationality. Socioeconomic status was defined according to an established composite social status index, which integrated information obtained from the parents' questionnaires on parental level of education, parents' professional status, and household income. Each of the three components was rated with 1–7 points and summed up to a total score (range 3–21 points), which was categorized as low (3–8 points), intermediate (9–14) or high (15–21 points) socioeconomic status. The socioeconomic status is a statistical construct specifically recommended for epidemiological research in Germany [17,18]. Two regions of residence – East-Germany (former German Democratic Republic including Berlin), and West-Germany (former Federal Republic of Germany) – were differentiated. Weight status was classified as underweight, normal weight, and overweight including obesity using age- and sex-specific German reference data based on the body mass index [19]. Weight and height of the participants were self-reported in the diabetes study, but measured in a standardized way in the KiGGS.

Severe hypoglycaemic events were defined as hypoglycaemia with impaired consciousness and/or convulsion or glucagon treatment, according to 2009 International Society for Pediatric and Adolescent Diabetes (ISPAD) guidelines [20]. Glycaemic control derived from clinical records of a subgroup of 444 youths was classified for some analyses as optimal (HbA1c <7.5%), suboptimal (HbA1c 7.5%–9.0%), and poor (HbA1c >9.0%) according to the ISPAD Guidelines [21]. Self-rated health status had been assessed with the question "How would you describe your health in general?" with a 5-point Likert scale (excellent, good, moderate, poor, very poor).

Statistical analyses

Percentages or means and standard deviations (SD) are reported as descriptive statistics. A survey weighting factor was used for the KiGGS data to adjust for deviations of demographic characteristics between the sample and the general population in Germany related to age, sex, region and nationality [22]. This approach was necessary to compare data of the diabetes study with nationally representative data. For simple group comparisons of continuous and categorical variables t-test or Wilcoxon-test and χ^2-test were used, respectively.

Multivariable linear and logistic regression analysis was applied to identify differences between the patient group and the reference group adjusted for confounding factors. Dependent variables were frequency and duration of physical activity, active and passive smoking, time spent watching television, and time using the computer. For each outcome, study group, age, sex, socioeconomic status, migration background, region of residence, and weight status were included as independent variables. To explore differential effects of study groups on outcomes by age and sex, we added terms for study group by age and study group by sex interactions in the regression models. Adjusted differences (β) and odds ratios (OR) with 95% confidence intervals (95% CI) and respective p-values were obtained by applying the SAS SURVEYREG and SURVEYLOGISTIC procedures. Explorative analyses were performed for youths with type 1 diabetes to analyse associations between aspects of health behaviour and severe hypoglycaemic events, glycaemic control, and self-rated health status adjusted for confounders. We applied multivariable ordinal logistic regression (proportional odds model based on cumulative odds) [23] to severe hypoglycaemic events (0, 1≥2 events), glycaemic control (HbA1c <7.5%, 7.5–9.0%,>9.0%) and self-rated health status (ordinal: excellent, good, at most moderate) as ordinal outcomes. A Score test was used to test the proportional odds assumption (identical OR across different cut-offs of the outcome). As the Score test is anticonservative (i.e. the test rejects the proportional odds assumption too readily) [24], the test was performed at an α-level of 0.01. We applied multivariable linear regression to HbA1c as continuous outcome. Health behaviours were modelled as dichotomous and ordinal (linear score term for categories) independent variables. Odds ratios and adjusted differences with 95% confidence intervals (95% CI) and respective p-values were obtained by applying the SAS REG and LOGISTIC procedures. In case of the proportional odds model [23,24], ORs estimated for severe hypoglycaemic events as ordinal outcome refer to the odds of at least one versus no event and to the odds of at least 2 events versus at most 1 event, ORs estimated for ordinal HbA1c refer to the odds of HbA1c ≥7.5% versus HbA1c <7.5% and to the odds of HbA1c ≥9.0% versus HbA1c <9.0, ORs estimated for self-rated health status refer to the odds of at least good versus at most moderate health status and to the odds of excellent versus at most good health status. All tests were performed two-sided at a 5% significance level (with the exception of the Score test described above). SAS for Windows Version 9.3 (SAS Institute, Cary, North Carolina, USA) was used for all analyses.

Results

Description of study populations

A description of the two study populations is given in Table 1. Significant differences between both populations were found for age, socioeconomic status, migration background, region of residence, and weight status. All subsequent between-group analyses were adjusted for these variables. Children and adolescents with type 1 diabetes had a mean age at disease onset of 2.7 years (SD 1.1, range 0.6–4.9 years) and a mean diabetes duration of 12.5 years (SD 1.6, range 10.0–16.5 years). About half of them (48.8%) used continuous subcutaneous insulin infusion (CSII), 43.3% used multiple daily injections (≥4/day, MDI), and 7.9% used conventional therapy (1–3 injections/day, CT). Mean HbA1c among those with available data (n = 444) was 8.4% (SD 1.6); 24.5% of patients had optimal, 50.9% suboptimal, and 24.5% poor glycaemic control. A total of 19.8% of the patients reported excellent and 62.4% good general health. One or at least 2 severe hypoglycaemic events during the last 12 months were reported by 9.3% and 4.2%, respectively.

Health behaviour in children and adolescents with type 1 diabetes compared to the general population

Table 2 shows the descriptive statistics concerning physical activity, active/passive smoking, and television/computer use. Tables 3 and 4 show the results of the comparison of the two study populations by multivariable logistic and linear regression analyses. The frequency and duration of physical activity differed between the youths with diabetes and the reference group (Tables 2, 3, and 4). The adjusted odds of infrequent physical activity (≤2 times/week) was 56% higher in the total patient group than in the total reference group (adjusted OR 1.56, p<0.001). The crude mean duration of physical activity per week was 5.5 (SD 4.8) hours in the patient group and 7.0 (SD 7.1) hours in the reference group. Adjusted for confounders, children and adolescents with diabetes had on average a 1.26 hours (p<0.001) shorter weekly duration of physical activity than the reference group (Table 4). Concordantly, the adjusted odds for shorter physical activity (<7 hours/week) was increased in the physically active patient group compared to the physically active reference group (OR 1.55, p<0.001) (Table 3). Compared to the general population, children and adolescents with type 1 diabetes mellitus had a lower odds for active smoking (OR 0.31, p<0.001) and passive smoking (OR 0.29, p<0.001). Active smoking was virtually not reported in individuals 11 to 13 years of age. The odds of high daily television consumption (≥3 hours/day) was lower in the patient group than in the reference group (OR 0.68, p = 0.002). In contrast, the odds for youths with type 1 diabetes to have ≥ 3 hours of daily computer use was higher than in the reference group (OR 2.51, p<0.001).

Results of the regression models including terms for study group by sex and study group by age interactions showed that the adjusted ORs for health-related behaviours of children and adolescents with type 1 diabetes compared to KiGGS participants were similar among boys and girls (p>0.05 for testing study group by sex interaction) and independent of age (p>0.05 for testing study group by age interaction). Sex-specific differences between the patient group and the general population were only observed for computer use (OR significantly higher in girls than in boys: 3.89 vs. 1.51, p<0.001) (Table 3), and the adjusted difference in the duration of weekly physical activity (difference smaller in girls than in boys: −0.71 vs −1.78, p = 0.012) (Table 4).

Associations between health behaviours and hypoglycaemic events, glycaemic control, and self-rated general health status in children and adolescents with type 1 diabetes mellitus

The proportional odds assumption was not rejected in any of the ordinal logistic regression models (Score test p≥0.02), with the exception of the model with hypoglycaemic events as outcome and modelling active smoking as dichotomous independent variable (Score test p = 0.006) (Table 5).

Youths with a higher frequency of physical activity had an increased odds for 1 and ≥2 severe hypoglycaemic events per year according to dichotomous (OR = 1.75, p = 0.026) and ordinal modelling of physical activity (OR 1.29, p = 0.045) (Table 5). There was no statistically significant association between hypoglycaemic events and overall weekly duration of physical activity, the use of different media, and active smoking. Passive smoking as dichotomous factor was not associated with hypoglycaemic events in the proportional odds model. However, the proportional odds assumption was questionable in this model. When specifically modelling non-proportional odds passive smoking modelled as binary variable was significantly associated with ≥2 hypoglycaemic events (OR

Table 1. Description of the two study populations.

	Diabetes study [a]	KiGGS [b]	p-value [c]
Number of participants	629	6813	
Boys [%]	54.1	51.3	0.189
Age			
Mean (SD) [years]	15.3 (1.7)	14.6 (2.0)	<0.001
11–13 years [%]	24.0	39.6	<0.001
14–17 years [%]	76.0	60.4	
Socioeconomic status			
Low [%]	17.9	27.4	<0.001
Intermediate [%]	48.2	47.2	
High [%]	33.9	25.3	
Migration background [%]	1.8	17.5	<0.001
Region of residence			
West-Germany [%]	86.2	81.4	0.003
East-Germany [%]	13.8	18.6	
Family structure			
Biological parents [%]	79.2	74.6	0.070
Mother and partner/father and partner [%]	9.3	10.6	
Single mother/father [%]	10.4	13.6	
Other (relatives, foster parents, youth institutions) [%]	1.1	1.3	
Weight status			
Underweight [%]	3.3	7.5	<0.001
Normal weight [%]	80.7	74.8	
Overweight (incl. adiposity) [%]	16.0	17.7	

[a]Percentages and means (SD).
[b]Weighted percentages and weighted means (SD).
[c]χ^2-Test, t-Test.

3.16, p = 0.009) but not with ≥1 severe hypoglycaemic events (OR1.34, p = 0.340). In ordinal modelling, passive smoking was associated with a higher odds for severe hypoglycaemic events (OR 1.23, p = 0.034) (Table 5).

Frequency and weekly duration of physical activity and longer use of television were not significantly associated with the level of HbA1c irrespective of binary or ordinal modelling of variables and according to both the ordinal logistic and the linear regression models. However, active smoking (dichotomous/ordinal modelling: OR 2.65/1.54, p = 0.003/<0.001), passive smoking (OR 1.64/1.26, p = 0.040/0.004), and longer computer use (OR 1.62/1.23, p = 0.030/0.035) were associated with higher odds for moderate and poor glycaemic control in ordinal logistic regression independent of binary or ordinal modelling. Likewise, these behaviours were associated with higher HbA1c levels according to linear regression with the exception of dichotomous passive smoking (Table 5).

Higher frequency of physical activity (dichotomous/ordinal modelling OR = 1.70/1.30, p = 0.002/0.002) was associated with a higher odds for at least good and excellent self-rated health status. However, longer weekly duration of physical activity showed as significant association with health status only when modelled continuously (OR = 1.04, p = 0.049). Active smoking (OR = 0.29, p<0.001) and more than three hours daily use of television (OR = 0.58, p = 0.016) and computer (OR = 0.59, p = 0.008) were associated with decreased odds for at least good and excellent self-rated health status. The association of active smoking and duration of computer use was confirmed when modelled in ordinal approach (OR 0.66, p<0.001 and OR 0.78, p = 0.003). Passive smoking showed no significant association with self-rated health-status.

Additional adjustment for insulin therapy regimen, diabetes duration, region of residence, weight status and HbA1c (not for HbA1c outcome) affected estimates only little (data not shown).

Discussion

Children and adolescents with early disease onset and long diabetes duration are at particular risk for long term complications. Therefore, their health relevant behaviours have a high relevance. They differed from the peers of the general population in several aspects. A positive finding of our study is that children and adolescents with type 1 diabetes had a healthier profile with regard to smoking and time spent watching television compared to the general population in Germany. However, they were also characterized by less physical activity, and by spending more time at the computer.

The World Health Organization (WHO) recommends that youths should be physically active for at least one hour every day [15]. Only one third of children and adolescents of the KiGGS group was physically active as recommended. The children and adolescents of the diabetes study were physically active both less often and shorter than the reference group. An identical finding was reported very recently for youths with type 2 diabetes [25]. A

Table 2. Prevalence of health-related behaviours in children and adolescents with type 1 diabetes and KiGGS participants.

Health-related behaviour	Diabetes study [%] [a]	KiGGS [%] [b]	p-value [c]
Frequency of physical activity			
Never	6.4	10.2	<0.001
1–2 times/month	10.1	5.4	
1–2 times/week	39.6	29.9	
3–5 times/week	32.4	31.6	
Approximately every day	11.5	22.9	
Duration of physical activity in physically active youths			
Mean (SD) hours/week	5.5 (4.8)	7.0 (7.1)	<0.001
>0–<2 hours/week	11.1	7.0	<0.001
≥2–<5 hours/week	41.6	37.7	
≥5–<7 hours/week	19.3	18.6	
≥7–<10 hours/week	13.6	13.5	
≥10 hours/week	14.4	23.2	
Active smoking			
No	89.4	79.6	<0.001
Yes	10.6	20.4	
Passive smoking			
Never	26.8	14.0	<0.001
Once a week or less often	52.9	45.2	
Several times a week or daily	20.3	40.9	
Television			
0 hours/day	5.0	4.1	<0.001
0.5 hours/day	27.8	21.4	
1–2 hours/day	51.7	51.7	
3–4 hours/day	11.3	17.2	
≥4 hours/day	4.2	5.6	
Computer			
0 hours/day	6.6	24.0	<0.001
0.5 hours/day	27.9	35.4	
1–2 hours/day	39.5	28.9	
3–4 hours/day	16.0	7.6	
≥4 hours/day	10.0	4.1	

[a]Percentages and means (SD).
[b]Weighted percentages and weighted means (SD).
[c]χ^2-Test, Wilcoxon-Test.

reason may be the fear of hypoglycaemia associated with prolonged exercise [26]. Our explorative analyses support this hypothesis because frequency of physical activity was associated with a higher risk for severe hypoglycaemic events. Therefore, patient education should be intensified with regard to blood glucose awareness training, strategies to prevent activity-induced hypoglycaemia and behavioural therapy to manage the fear of hypoglycaemia.

Physical activity comes along with improved metabolic and cardiovascular parameters. There is an inverse association between physical activity performed regularly at least once a week for at least 30 minutes and HbA1c, and regular physical activity was not associated with a higher rate of severe hypoglycaemia based on a large patient database [2]. A review of 42 studies showed a significant relationship with insulin sensitivity in 78% of studies on physical activity, and 69% of studies on cardiorespiratory fitness [27]. Analysis of 23.251 patients from 209 centres in Germany and Austria revealed lower lipoprotein levels, diastolic blood pressure and HbA1c to be associated with increasing physical activity [28]. However, we could not confirm the beneficial effect of physical activity on HbA1c. Results indicated that longer overall physical activity per week was associated with a lower chance for optimal HbA1c and a higher risk for poor HbA1c. Also other authors raise questions about the beneficial effects of physical activity on metabolic control, using a similar measure for physical activity [29]. Perhaps, the used methods for assessing physical activity are not sensitive enough to detect an association.

A positive association was observed between physical activity and excellent self-rated health. This is in accordance with other studies, in which physical activity was positively correlated with nearly all markers of psychological health, including well-being,

Table 3. Odds ratios for health-related behaviours of children and adolescents with type 1 diabetes compared to KiGGS participants.

Health-related behaviour	Total groups	Girls	Boys		12 years	16 years	
	OR (95% CI) [a]	OR (95% CI) [b]	OR (95% CI) [b]	p [d]	OR (95% CI) [b]	OR (95% CI) [b]	ΔOR per year (95% CI) [b]
	p [c]	p [c]	p [c]		p [c]	p [c]	p [e]
Frequency of physical activity							
≤2 times/week vs. ≥3 times/week	1.56 (1.30; 1.88)	1.36 (1.04; 1.79)	1.75 (1.36; 2.25)	0.172	1.55 (1.07; 2.25)	1.54 (1.26; 1.88)	1.00 (0.90; 1.10)
	<0.001	0.026	<0.001		0.020	<0.001	0.959
Duration of physical activity [f]							
>0–<7 hours/week vs. ≥7 hours/week	1.55 (1.26; 1.91)	1.33 (0.94; 1.87)	1.57 (1.19; 2.05)	0.438	1.25 (0.83; 1.90)	1.59 (1.26; 2.01)	1.06 (0.95; 1.19)
	<0.001	0.105	0.001		0.283	<0.001	0.313
Active smoking							
Yes vs. no	0.31 (0.23; 0.42)	0.24 (0.14; 0.42)	0.33 (0.19; 0.55)	0.320	0.25 (0.11; 0.59)	0.30 (0.22; 0.41)	1.05 (0.87; 1.27)
	<0.001	<0.001	<0.001		0.002	<0.001	0.626
Passive smoking							
>1 time/week vs. ≤1 time/week	0.29 (0.23; 0.36)	0.37 (0.26; 0.52)	0.24 (0.17; 0.34)	0.061	0.32 (0.19; 0.55)	0.28 (0.22; 0.36)	0.97 (0.85; 1.11)
	<0.001	<0.001	<0.001		<0.001	<0.001	0.641
Television							
≥3 hours/day vs. ≤2 hours/day	0.68 (0.54; 0.87)	0.60 (0.42; 0.86)	0.71 (0.48; 1.04)	0.503	0.59 (0.34; 1.002)	0.70 (0.54; 0.90)	1.04 (0.91; 1.20)
	0.002	0.006	0.075		0.051	0.006	0.539
Computer							
≥3 hours/day vs. ≤2 hours/day	2.51 (2.01; 3.13)	3.89 (2.71; 5.59)	1.51 (1.09; 2.09)	<0.001	1.80 (1.09; 2.96)	2.93 (2.33; 3.69)	1.13 (0.998; 1.28)
	<0.001	<0.001	0.014		0.021	<0.001	0.055

[a]Estimated from separate logistic regression models including study group, age, sex, migration background, socio-economic status, region of residence, and weight status.
[b]Estimated from separate logistic regression model including study group, age, sex, terms for study group by sex and study group by age interactions, migration background, socio-economic status, region of residence, and weight status.
[c]P-value (Wald-χ^2-Test); [d] P-value (Wald-χ^2-Test) for comparison sex-specific odds ratios (corresponding to testing of study group by sex interaction).
[e]P-value (Wald-χ^2-Test) for testing ΔOR per year (relative change in OR per year, corresponding to testing of study group by age interaction).
[f]Physically inactive youths were excluded.

Table 4. Duration of weekly physical activity of children and adolescents with type 1 diabetes compared to KiGGS participants.

Health-related behaviour	Total groups	Girls	Boys		12 years	16 years	
	ß (95% CI) [a]	ß (95% CI) [b]	ß (95% CI) [b]	p [d]	ß (95% CI) [b]	ß (95% CI) [b]	Δß per year (95% CI) [b]
	p [c]	p [c]	p [c]		p [c]	p [c]	p [e]
Difference in duration of weekly physical activity [hours/week] [f]	1.26 (−1.70; −0.82)	−0.71 (−1.23; −0.20)	−1.78 (−2.43; −1.13)	0.012	−1.36 (−2.23; −0.50)	−1.17 (−1.72; −0.63)	0.05 (−0.24; 0.33)
	<0.001	0.007	<0.001		0.002	<0.001	0.740

[a] Estimated from linear regression model including study group, age, sex, migration background, socio-economic status, region of residence, and weight status.
[b] Estimated from linear regression model including study group, age, sex, terms for study group by sex and study group by age interactions, migration background, socio-economic status, region of residence, and weight status.
[c] p-value (Wald-χ^2-Test).
[d] p-value (Wald-χ^2-Test) for comparison sex-specific difference (corresponding to testing of study group by sex interaction).
[e] p-value (Wald-χ^2-Test) for testing Δß per year (change in ß per year, corresponding to testing of study group by age interaction).
[f] Physically inactive youths were excluded.

less worry, greater perception of health and general quality of life in patients with type 1 diabetes [29,30] as well as healthy peers [31]. However, most studies may not show the causal direction of the association between physical activity and self-rated health, as both influence each other.

In studies among older adolescents and emerging adults the observed prevalence of smoking was usually similar with and without diabetes [7,32,33]. In our study, the prevalence of regular active and passive smoking was only half as high as in the general population. This finding might be to some extend attributable to a cohort effect arising from the time span of 3-7 years between the data collection in both studies. Since the beginning of this millennium, a significant decrease in smoking prevalence was observed in the general population, as shown for adolescents in the USA [34] and Germany (decrease from 20.4% to 12.0 % between 2003-6 and 2009-12) [35]. However, children and adolescents with other chronic diseases, such as sickle cell anaemia and cystic fibrosis, reported less frequent use of tobacco than healthy controls as well [36]. This may indicate a generally better health awareness of the youths with type 1 diabetes – like for other chronic diseases - with regard to active smoking, because it is part of the education program for patients [37]. The reduced passive tobacco exposure might be caused by the youths' active avoidance of tobacco smoke or due to an improved health awareness of their family and friends. It was not explained by socioeconomic status or migration background, as analyses were adjusted for both variables. Smoking during adolescence increases the risk for developing chronic complications in patients with type 1 diabetes [38]. A more recent observation was that tobacco exposure is associated with worse glycaemic control and markers of higher cardiovascular risk already in children and adolescents with type 1 diabetes [39]. Our results confirm that active smoking is associated with an increased odds for poor glycaemic control in youths with early-onset type 1 diabetes. Moreover, smoking was associated with a decreased odds for excellent self-rated health status in our study population. This may be due to direct adverse effects of tobacco exposition or may reflect a generally lower health-promoting lifestyle in patients who smoke.

Patients showed increased computer use and decreased time spent watching television compared to KiGGS participants, which could at least in part be due to earlier data collection. During the past years, computers and internet became more available to youths. This cohort effect might explain why markedly less children and adolescents of the diabetes study than of the KiGGS reported to use a computer "not at all". The difference in time spent watching television is probably not due to time effects, because available literature suggests a minimal increase in daily television use over time [40]. Negative impact of media consumption on health is well documented in children and adolescents, as it increases the likelihood of overweight, unhealthy food preferences, and smoking [41]. Furthermore, it reduces beneficial activities such as reading or hobbies with physical activity [41]. In children and adolescents with type 1 diabetes, an increased daily time of media consumption is associated with higher HbA1c [42]. These findings are confirmed by our population-based study as both increased computer use and increased television consumption were associated with poor self-reported HbA1c. The association between less media consumption and optimal HbA1c was less pronounced. A new finding was that media consumption was negatively associated with self-rated health status. Possibly, children and adolescents with T1DM feeling more impaired have fewer joint activities with friends and prefer physically inactive leisure time activities. This behaviour

Table 5. Prevalence of outcomes in children and adolescents with type 1 diabetes dependent on health-related behaviours and respective odds ratios.

Health-related behaviour (independent variable)	Outcome: Severe hypoglycaemic events during past 12 months (ordinal: 0,1, ≥2)		HbA1c (ordinal: <7.5, 7.5–9.0,>9.0)		HbA1c (continuous)		Self-rated health status (ordinal: at most moderate, good, excellent)	
	[%] [a]	OR (95% CI) [c]	[%] [a]	OR (95% CI) [c]	Mean (SD) [e]	ß (95% CI) [g]	[%] [a]	OR (95% CI) [c]
	p [b]	p [d]	p [b]	p [d]	p [f]	p [h]	p [b]	p [d]
Frequency of physical activity		0.650 [i]		0.822 [i]				0.085 [i]
≤2 times/week	11.0	1	24.2	1	8.47 (1.60)	0	14.7	1
≥3 times/week	16.4	1.75 (1.07; 2.86)	26.8	1.20 (0.82; 1.74)	8.44 (1.51)	0.17 (−0.12; 0.46)	26.4	1.70 (1.21; 2.34)
	0.050	0.026	0.468	0.351	0.876	0.259	<0.001	0.002
Ordinal coding for categories (never, 1–2 times/month, 1–2 times/week, 3–5 times/week, approximately every day)		0.460 [i]		0.825 [i]		0.05 (−0.12; 0.21)		0.023 [i]
		1.29 (1.01; 1.66)		1.08 (0.89; 1.30)		0.583		1.30 (1.10; 1.53)
		0.045		0.441				0.002
Duration of physical activity [j]		0.577 [i]		0.651 [i]				0.076 [i]
>0–<7 hours/week	13.1	1	23.6	1	8.35 (1.45)	0	18.5	1
≥7 hours/week	15.0	1.25 (0.72; 2.16)	30.1	1.35 (0.89; 2.05)	8.61 (1.63)	0.34 (−0.01; 0.69)	26.1	1.37 (0.94; 2.01)
	0.561	0.423	0.114	0.162	0.122	0.059	0.044	0.102
Continuous hours/week		0.583 [i]		0.912 [i]		0.03 (−0.003; 0.06)		0.142 [i]
		1.00 (0.95; 1.06)		1.01 (0.98; 1.05)		0.078		1.04 (1.00; 1.08)
		0.874		0.550				0.049
Active smoking		0.121 [i]		0.836 [i]				0.030 [i]
No	13.3	1	22.4	1	8.33 (1.43)	0	21.6	1
Yes	14.1	1.19 (0.53; 2.67)	50.8	2.65 (1.41; 4.99)	9.54 (2.14)	1.07 (0.39; 1.75)	4.5	0.29 (0.17; 0.51)
	0.871	0.669	<0.001	0.003	<0.001	0.002	0.001	<0.001
Ordinal coding for categories (never, <1 time/week, 1 time/week, several times/week, every day)		0.486 [i]		0.864 [i]		0.44 (0.23; 0.64)		0.020 [i]
		1.04 (0.81; 1.34)		1.54 (1.24; 1.90)		<0.001		0.66 (0.56; 0.79)
		0.741		<0.001				<0.001
Passive smoking		0.006 [k]		0.801 [i]				0.175 [i]
≤1 time/week	12.1	1	23.4	1	8.40 (1.61)	0	21.2	1
>1 time/week	16.9	1.41 (0.78; 2.54)	34.2	1.64 (1.02; 2.63)	8.75 (1.35)	0.15 (−0.22; 0.52)	13.6	0.74 (0.49; 1.13)
	0.158	0.251	0.016	0.040	0.064	0.419	0.058	0.162
Ordinal coding for categories (never, <1 time/week, 1 time/week, several times/week, every day)		0.028 [i]		0.839 [i]		0.13 (0.02; 0.24)		167 [i]
		1.23 (1.02; 1.49)		1.26 (1.08; 1.47)		0.017		0.89 (0.78; 1.02)
		0.034		0.004				0.099

Table 5. Cont.

Health-related behaviour (independent variable)	Outcome: Severe hypoglycaemic events during past 12 months (ordinal: 0,1, ≥2) [%] [a]		HbA1c (ordinal: <7.5, 7.5–9.0,>9.0) [%] [a]		HbA1c (continuous) Mean (SD) [e]		Self-rated health status (ordinal: at most moderate, good, excellent) [%] [a]	
	[%] [a]	OR (95% CI) [c]	[%] [a]	OR (95% CI) [c]	Mean (SD) [e]	ß (95% CI) [g]	[%] [a]	OR (95% CI) [c]
	p [b]	p [d]	p [b]	p [d]	p [f]	p [h]	p [b]	p [d]
Television		0.205 [i]		0.878 [i]				0.078 [i]
≤2 hours/day	13.9	1	23.0	1	8.41 (1.53)	0	21.3	1
≥3 hours/day	11.5	0.89 (0.45; 1.74)	35.2	1.03 (0.63; 1.68)	8.58 (1.66)	0.07 (−0.34; 0.49)	10.5	0.58 (0.37; 0.90)
	0.521	0.725	0.014	0.917	0.386	0.735	0.015	0.016
Ordinal coding for categories (never, 0.5 hours/day, 1–2 hours/day, 3–4 hours/day, ≥4 hours/day)		0.365 [i]		0.822 [i]		−0.09 (−0.26; 0.09)		0.078 [i]
		0.97 (0.73; 1.29)		0.94 (0.76; 1.16)		0.325		0.94 (0.78; 1.13)
		0.833		0.545				0.505
Computer		0.558 [i]		0.781 [i]				0.063 [i]
≤2 hours/day	13.6	1	20.6	1	8.32 (1.47)	0	21.8	1
≥3 hours/day	13.3	1.11 (0.63; 1.95)	39.4	1.62 (1.05; 2.51)	8.86 (1.76)	0.38 (0.00; 0.75)	13.2	0.59 (0.40; 0.87)
	0.930	0.731	<0.001	0.030	0.005	0.050	0.018	0.008
Ordinal coding for categories (never, 0.5 hours/day, 1–2 hours/day, 3–4 hours/day, ≥4 hours/day)		0.399 [i]		0.455 [i]		0.19 (0.02; 0.36)		0.072 [i]
		1.10 (0.87; 1.40)		1.23 (1.02; 1.48)		0.026		0.78 (0.66; 0.92)
		0.420		0.035				0.003

[a]Percentage of patients with respective outcome.
[b]P-value (χ^2-Test).
[c]Odds ratio estimated from ordinal logistic regression (proportional odds model) adjusted for age, sex and socioeconomic status, separate model for each health related behaviour.
[d]P-value (Wald-χ^2-Test).
[e]Mean Hba1c by health-related behaviour.
[f]P-value (t-Test).
[g]Difference estimated from linear regression adjusted for age, sex and socioeconomic status, separate model for each health related behaviour, [d]p-value (t-Test).
[h]P-value (Wald-χ^2-Test).
[i]P-value (Score test for proportional odds assumption).
[j]Physically inactive youths were excluded.
[k]As in this model the proportional odds assumption was rejected, we also estimated ORs in a non-proportional odds model. The OR estimates for ≥1 and ≥2 severe hypoglycaemic events were 1.34 (95% CI 0.74; 2.44, p = 0.340) and 3.19 (95% CI 1.34; 7.44, p = 0.020), respectively.

might reduce their self-rated health and their motivation to be physically active (vicious circle).

A limitation of this study is that data, in particular on health-related behaviours, are based on self-administered questionnaires. These tend to over-estimate behaviours that participants believe to be socially desirable and underestimate behaviours that are undesirable. This limitation is unavoidable in population-based studies evaluating these factors, and can be assumed to be non-differential between both study groups. In addition, children and adolescents of the diabetes study were not as representative as the KiGGS participants were. However, as both groups were evaluated using identical questionnaires and confounding factors were considered in the analyses, it is unlikely that the observed between-group differences were artefacts due to differential reporting bias. The possible cohort effect with respect to computer use has already been mentioned. A limitation of the explorative analyses of the effects of health related behaviours on outcomes is the cross-sectional study design that hampers the differentiation between causes and consequences, e.g. it is possible that general health status has an impact on physical activity and vice versa. Further, HbA1c values from clinical records were available only for about 71% of patients limiting the analyses with respect to HbA1c to this subgroup.

In summary, we revealed that children and adolescents with early-onset and long-duration type 1 diabetes tended to smoke less, watch fewer TV, use the computer more often and be less physically active than the general population. Our study provides further evidence that less physical activity, more frequent media use and smoking are associated with worse glycaemic control and worse self-rated health in children and adolescents with type 1 diabetes. There is still the need for reduction of activity-related hypoglycaemia, while patients should be further encouraged to increase their overall physical activity and to decrease sedentary behaviours in order to achieve positive effects on health-status, glycaemic control and long-term sequelae of diabetes. In conclusion, besides physical activity and smoking, media consumption is an important factor contributing to the overall health and glycaemic control in children and adolescents with type 1 diabetes and should be intensely considered in diabetes education.

Author Contributions

Conceived and designed the experiments: SK ASP KC CB CG KS GG RWH TM JR. Analyzed the data: SK ASP KC CB CG KS BS EM GG RWH TM JR. Wrote the paper: SK ASP KC CB CG KS BS EM GG RWH TM JR.

References

1. DCCT Research Group (1994) Effect of intensive diabetes treatment on the development and progression of long-term complications in adolescents with insulin-dependent diabetes mellitus: Diabetes Control and Complications Trial. Diabetes Control and Complications Trial Research Group. J Pediatr 125: 177–188.
2. Herbst A, Bachran R, Kapellen T, Holl RW (2006) Effects of regular physical activity on control of glycemia in pediatric patients with type 1 diabetes mellitus. Arch Pediatr Adolesc Med 160: 573–577.
3. Heyman E, Berthon P, Youssef H, Delamarche A, Briard D, et al. (2012) Metabolic dysfunction in late-puberty adolescent girls with type 1 diabetes: Relationship to physical activity and dietary intakes. Diabetes Metab 38: 337–342.
4. Lindholm E, Brevinge H, Bergh CH, Korner U, Lundholm K (2003) Relationships between self-reported health related quality of life and measures of standardized exercise capacity and metabolic efficiency in a middle-aged and aged healthy population. Qual Life Res 12: 575–582.
5. Stehno-Bittel L (2012) Organ-based response to exercise in type 1 diabetes. ISRN endocrinology 2012: 318194.
6. Daneman D (2005) Early diabetes-related complications in adolescents: risk factors and screening. Hormone research 63: 75–85.
7. Mays D, Streisand R, Walker LR, Prokhorov AV, Tercyak KP (2012) Cigarette smoking among adolescents with type 1 diabetes: Strategies for behavioral prevention and intervention. Journal of Diabetes and its Complications 26: 148–153.
8. Galler A, Lindau M, Ernert A, Thalemann R, Raile K (2011) Associations between media consumption habits, physical activity, socioeconomic status, and glycaemic control in children, adolescents, and young adults with type 1 diabetes. Diabetes Care 34: 2356–2359.
9. Fulton JE, Wang X, Yore MM, Carlson SA, Galuska DA, et al. (2009) Television viewing, computer use, and BMI among U.S. children and adolescents. Journal of physical activity & health 6 Suppl 1: S28–35.
10. Marshall SJ, Biddle SJ, Gorely T, Cameron N, Murdey I (2004) Relationships between media use, body fatness and physical activity in children and youth: a meta-analysis. Int J Obes Relat Metab Disord 28: 1238–1246.
11. Salardi S, Porta M, Maltoni G, Rubbi F, Rovere S, et al. (2012) Infant and toddler type 1 diabetes: complications after 20 years' duration. Diabetes Care 35: 829–833.
12. Patterson CC, Dahlquist GG, Gyurus E, Green A, Soltesz G, et al. (2009) Incidence trends for childhood type 1 diabetes in Europe during 1989–2003 and predicted new cases 2005-20: a multicentre prospective registration study. Lancet 373: 2027–2033.
13. Stahl A, Strassburger K, Lange K, Bächle C, Holl RW, et al. (2012) Health-Related Quality of Life Among German Youths With Early-Onset and Long-Duration Type 1 Diabetes. Diabetes Care 35: 1736–1742.
14. Kurth BM, Kamtsiuris P, Holling H, Schlaud M, Dolle R, et al. (2008) The challenge of comprehensively mapping children's health in a nation-wide health survey: design of the German KiGGS-Study. BMC public health 8: 196.
15. WHO (2010) Global recommendations on physical activity for health. WHO Press, Switzerland.
16. Council On Communications And Media (2013) Children, Adolescents, and the Media. *Pediatrics* 132: 958–961.
17. Lange M, Kamtsiuris P, Lange C, Schaffrath Rosario A, Stolzenberg H, et al. (2007) Sociodemographic characteristics in the German Health Interview and Examination Survey for Children and Adolescents (KiGGS) - operationalisation and public health significance, taking as an example the assessment of general state of health. Bundesgesundheitsblatt, Gesundheitsforschung, Gesundheitsschutz 50: 578–589.
18. Lampert T, Kurth B-M (2007) Socioeconomic Status and Health in Children and Adolescents – Results of the German Health Interview and Examination Survey for Children and Adolescents (KiGGS). Dtsch Arztebl International, 104(43): 2944–2949.
19. Kromeyer-Hauschild K, Wabitsch M, Kunze D, Geller F, Geiß C, et al. (2001) Perzentile fuür den Body-mass-Index fuür das Kindes- und Jugendalter unter Heranziehung verschiedener deutscher Stichproben. Monatsschr Kinderheilkd 8: 807–818.
20. Clarke W, Jones T, Rewers M, Dunger D, Klingensmith GJ (2009) ISPAD Clinical Practice Consensus Guidelines 2009 Compendium. Assessment and management of hypoglycemia in children and adolescents with diabetes. Pediatric Diabetes 10 (Suppl 12): 134–144.
21. Rewers M, Pihoker C, Donaghue K, Hanas R, Swift P, et al. (2009) ISPAD Clinical Practice Consensus Guidelines 2009 Compendium. Assessment and monitoring of glycemic control in children and adolescents with diabetes. Pediatric Diabetes 10 (Suppl 12): 71–81.
22. Kamtsiuris P, Lange M, Schaffrath Rosario A (2007) The German Health Interview and Examination Survey for Children and Adolescents (KiGGS): sample design, response and nonresponse analysis. Bundesgesundheitsblatt, Gesundheitsforschung, Gesundheitsschutz 50: 547–556.
23. Agresti A (2010) Analysis of Ordinal Categorical Data, 2nd Edition. Hoboken, NJ: Wiley. 424 p.
24. Peterson B, Harrel FE (1990) Partial proportinal odss models for ordinal response variables. Appl. Statist 39: 205–217.
25. Kriska A, Delahanty L, Edelstein S, Amodei N, Chadwick J, et al. (2013) Sedentary behaviour and physical activity in youth with recent onset of type 2 diabetes. Pediatrics 131: e850–856.
26. Brazeau AS, Rabasa-Lhoret R, Strychar I, Mircescu H (2008) Barriers to physical activity among patients with type 1 diabetes. Diabetes Care 31: 2108–2109.
27. Berman LJ, Weigensberg MJ, Spruijt-Metz D (2012) Physical activity is related to insulin sensitivity in children and adolescents, independent of adiposity: a review of the literature. Diabetes Metab Res Rev 28: 395–408.
28. Herbst A, Kordonouri O, Schwab KO, Schmidt F, Holl RW (2007) Impact of physical activity on cardiovascular risk factors in children with type 1 diabetes: a multicenter study of 23,251 patients. Diabetes Care 30: 2098–2100.
29. Aman J, Skinner TC, de Beaufort CE, Swift PG, Aanstoot HJ, et al. (2009) Associations between physical activity, sedentary behaviour, and glycaemic control in a large cohort of adolescents with type 1 diabetes: the Hvidoere Study Group on Childhood Diabetes. Pediatr Diabetes 10: 234–239.

30. Li CL, Lai YC, Tseng CH, Lin JD, Chang HY (2010) A population study on the association between leisure time physical activity and self-rated health among diabetics in Taiwan. BMC public health 10: 277.
31. Aarnio M, Winter T, Kujala U, Kaprio J (2002) Associations of health related behaviour, social relationships, and health status with persistent physical activity and inactivity: a study of Finnish adolescent twins. Br J Sports Med 36: 360–364.
32. Palladino DK, Helgeson VS, Reynolds KA, Becker DJ, Siminerio LM, et al. (2013) Emerging adults with type 1 diabetes: a comparison to peers without diabetes. *J Pediatr Psychol* 38: 506–517.
33. Shah AS, Dabelea D, Talton JW, Urbina EM, Agostino J, et al. (2014) Smoking and Arterial Stiffness in Youth with Type 1 Diabetes: The SEARCH Cardiovascular Disease Study. The Journal of Pediatrics 165: 110–116.
34. Daniels SR, Pratt CA, Hayman LL (2011) Reduction of risk for cardiovascular disease in children and adolescents. Circulation 124: 1673–1686.
35. Lampert T, Kuntz B, KiGGS Study Group (2014) Tobacco and alcohol consumption among 11- to 17-year-old adolescents: results of the KiGGS study: first follow-up (KiGGS Wave 1). Bundesgesundheitsblatt Gesundheitsforschung Gesundheitsschutz 57: 830–839.
36. Britto MT, Garrett JM, Dugliss MA, Daeschner CW Jr, Johnson CA, et al. (1998) Risky behaviour in teens with cystic fibrosis or sickle cell disease: a multicenter study. Pediatrics 101: 250–256.
37. Swift PG (2009) Diabetes education in children and adolescents. Pediatr Diabetes 10 Suppl 12: 51–57.
38. Moy CS, LaPorte RE, Dorman JS, Songer TJ, Orchard TJ, et al. (1990) Insulin-dependent diabetes mellitus mortality. The risk of cigarette smoking. Circulation 82: 37–43.
39. Hofer SE, Rosenbauer J, Grulich-Henn J, Naeke A, Fröhlich-Reiterer E, et al. (2009) Smoking and metabolic control in adolescents with type 1 diabetes. J Pediatr 154: 20–23.
40. Marshall SJ, Gorely T, Biddle SJ (2006) A descriptive epidemiology of screen-based media use in youth: a review and critique. Journal of adolescence 29: 333–349.
41. Strasburger VC, Jordan AB, Donnerstein E (2010) Health effects of media on children and adolescents. Pediatrics 125: 756–767.
42. Margeirsdottir HD, Larsen JR, Brunborg C, Sandvik L, Dahl-Jorgensen K (2007) Strong association between time watching television and blood glucose control in children and adolescents with type 1 diabetes. Diabetes Care 30: 1567–1570.

Proximal Tubule Dysfunction Is Associated with Podocyte Damage Biomarkers Nephrin and Vascular Endothelial Growth Factor in Type 2 Diabetes Mellitus Patients

Ligia Petrica[1,5], Adrian Vlad[2,5]*, Gheorghe Gluhovschi[1,5], Florica Gadalean[1,5], Victor Dumitrascu[3,5], Cristina Gluhovschi[1,5], Silvia Velciov[1,5], Flaviu Bob[1,5], Daliborca Vlad[3,5], Roxana Popescu[4,5], Oana Milas[5], Sorin Ursoniu[6]

1 "Victor Babes" University of Medicine and Pharmacy, Dept. of Nephrology, Timisoara, Romania, 2 "Victor Babes" University of Medicine and Pharmacy, Dept. of Diabetes and Metabolic Diseases, Timisoara, Romania, 3 "Victor Babes" University of Medicine and Pharmacy, Department of Pharmacology, Timisoara, Romania, 4 "Victor Babes" University of Medicine and Pharmacy, Dept. of Cellular Biology, Timisoara, Romania, 5 County Emergency Hospital, Timisoara, Romania, 6 "Victor Babes" University of Medicine and Pharmacy, Dept. of Public Health Medicine, Timisoara, Romania

Abstract

Background: There is an ongoing debate as to whether early diabetic nephropathy in Type 2 diabetes mellitus may be attributed to the glomerulus or to the proximal tubule. Urinary excretion of nephrin and vascular endothelial growth factor may increase even in the normoalbuminuria stage. In the course of diabetic nephropathy, the proximal tubule may be involved in the uptake of urinary nephrin and vascular endothelial growth factor.

Materials and Methods: Two groups of consecutive Type 2 diabetes mellitus outpatients (38 normo-, 32 microalbuminuric) and 21 healthy subjects were enrolled in a cross-sectional study and evaluated concerning the relation of proximal tubule dysfunction with the podocyte biomarkers excretion, assessed by ELISA methods. The impact of advanced glycation end-products on this relation was also queried.

Results: Urinary alpha$_1$-microglobulin and kidney injury molecule-1 correlated with urinary albumin:creatinine ratio ($R^2=0.269$; $p<0.001$; $R^2=0.125$; $p<0.001$), nephrinuria ($R^2=0.529$; $p<0.001$; $R^2=0.203$; $p<0.001$), urinary vascular endothelial growth factor ($R^2=0.709$; $p<0.001$; $R^2=0.360$; $p<0.001$), urinary advanced glycation end-products ($R^2=0.578$; $p<0.001$; $R^2=0.405$; $p<0.001$), serum cystatin C ($R^2=0.130$; $p<0.001$; $R^2=0.128$; $p<0.001$), and glomerular filtration rate ($R^2=0.167$; $p<0.001$; $R^2=0.166$; $p<0.001$); nephrinuria and urinary vascular endothelial growth factor correlated with urinary albumin:creatinine ratio ($R^2=0.498$; $p<0.001$; $R^2=0.227$; $p<0.001$), urinary advanced glycation end-products ($R^2=0.251$; $p<0.001$; $R^2=0.308$; $p<0.001$), serum cystatin C ($R^2=0.157$; $p<0.001$; $R^2=0.226$; $p<0.001$), and glomerular filtration rate ($R^2=0.087$; $p=0.007$; $R^2=0.218$; $p<0.001$).

Conclusions: In Type 2 diabetes mellitus there is an association of proximal tubule dysfunction with podocyte damage biomarkers, even in the normoalbuminuria stage. This observation suggests a potential role of the proximal tubule in urinary nephrin and urinary vascular endothelial growth factor processing in early diabetic nephropathy, a fact which could be related to advanced glycation end-products intervention. Podocyte damage and proximal tubule dysfunction biomarkers could be validated as a practical approach to the diagnosis of early diabetic nephropathy by further studies on larger cohorts.

Editor: Effie C. Tsilibary, National Center for Scientific Research Demokritos, Greece

Funding: This research received funding from an internal grant of "Victor Babes" University of Medicine and Pharmacy Timisoara, PIII-C1-PCFI-2014/2015, www.umft.ro. LP received the funding. The funders had no role in study design, data collection and analysis, decision to publish, or preparation of the manuscript.

Competing Interests: The authors have declared that no competing interests exist.

* Email: vladrian@hotmail.com

Introduction

Due to the increasing epidemic of diabetes mellitus (DM) worldwide, diabetic kidney disease is now the leading cause of end-stage renal disease and may be attributed up to 40% of cases referred to renal replacement therapies, both in developed and emerging countries [1,2].

There is an ongoing debate as to whether early diabetic nephropathy (DN) in Type 2 DM may be attributed to the glomerulus or to the proximal tubule (PT). The interest for the PT involvement in the occurrence of early DN derives from the observation that patients with Type 2 DM may show a steady decline in renal function and may progress to more advanced stages of chronic kidney disease (CKD) despite the fact that they remain normoalbuminuric in the long term [3].

The classical concept concerning mechanisms of albuminuria in DN relies on defects in the glomerular filtration barrier [4,5]. According to this hypothesis, it is considered that albuminuria is determined by the severity of the glomerular lesions, but this correlation is not strict in preceding the onset of albuminuria, a fact demonstrated on iterated renal biopsies in patients with Type 2 DM [6].

Podocytes are onthogenetic terminally-differentiated cells, located on the outer aspect of the glomerular basement membrane. Nephrin, a transmembrane protein of the immunoglobulin superfamily, is an important component of the slit diaphragm located between the foot processes of the podocytes. Its alterations lead to the limitation of the size-selectivity of the slit diaphragm [4].

The importance of nephrin as a biomarker of early DN resides in the results provided by several studies which show that increased levels of nephrinuria may be found in Type 1 and Type 2 DM patients with normoalbuminuria, a fact which demonstrates that nephrinuria may precede microalbuminuria [7,8,9].

Vascular endothelial growth factor (VEGF) is a pro-angiogenic factor, produced mainly by the podocytes, which acts upon these cells through an autocrine mechanism. In the early stage of DN, VEGF expression is increased within the podocytes, leading to the increase in the endothelial permeability [10] and in the autocrine effects of VEGF upon the podocytes, with subsequent proteinuria [11]. Urinary excretion of VEGF may increase even in the normoalbuminuria stage, a fact which suggests that urinary VEGF may be used as a sensitive biomarker in the diagnosis of early DN [12].

The tubular theory concerning albuminuria in the course of DM states that albuminuria is caused primarily by impaired tubular uptake of intact albumin rather than by an increased leakiness of the glomerular filtration barrier [13,14]. In previous works performed by us in normoalbuminuric patients with Type 2 DM we demonstrated that PT dysfunction precedes the occurrence of albuminuria [15], a phenomenon which could be delayed by rosiglitazone [16] and pioglitazone [17].

Amongst other causative factors related to PT dysfunction, advanced glycation end- products (AGE) have been involved in the pathogenesis of diabetic tubulopathy, an emerging entity [18]. The aim of our study was to evaluate a potential relation of PT dysfunction with urinary nephrin and urinary VEGF excretion in normoalbuminuric patients with Type 2 DM as compared to microalbuminuric ones. Also, we queried if this association could be related to AGE intervention, which may impact both the PT and the podocytes. We found that in Type 2 DM there is an association of PT dysfunction with podocyte damage biomarkers, even in the normoalbuminuria stage. This observation suggests a potential role of the PT in urinary nephrin and urinary VEGF processing in early DN. Podocyte damage and PT dysfunction biomarkers could be validated as a practical approach to the diagnosis of early DN.

Materials and Methods

A total of 70 consecutive patients with Type 2 DM (38 patients with normoalbuminuria – group A – and 32 patients with microalbuminuria – group B) attending the Outpatient Department of Diabetes and Metabolic Diseases and 21 healthy control subjects (group C) were enrolled in a cross-sectional study. The inclusion criteria were duration of DM higher than 5 years, normoalbuminuria [urine albumin-to-creatinine ratio (UACR)< 30 mg/g] or microalbuminuria (UACR between 30 and 300 mg/g), therapy with oral antidiabetic drugs, angiotensin-converting enzyme inhibitors and/or angiotensin receptor blockers, and statins.

All patients were assessed concerning urinary alpha$_1$-microglobulin and urinary kidney injury molecule-1 (KIM-1) as biomarkers of PT dysfunction; urinary nephrin and urinary VEGF, as markers of podocyte damage; plasma and urinary AGE; UACR and serum cystatin C.

Serum and urinary biomarkers were determined in specimens frozen at −80°C and thawed before assay. CKD was defined according to the KDIGO Guideline for the Evaluation and Management of CKD (2009 CKD-EPI creatinine equation) [19].

Cystatin C was assessed in serum with N latex cystatin C kit (Siemens Healthcare Diagnostics, Marburg, Germany) through particle-enhanced immunonephelometry using the BNProSpec System. The reference interval was calculated nonparametrically and was determined to be 0.53–0.95 mg/l. The intra-assay precision was 2.5% coefficient of variation (CV) and inter-assay precision was 2.0% CV with a total of 2.8% CV. Analytical sensitivity was calculated as two standard deviations above the mean signal of 20 replicates of N diluent and was determined to be 0.005 mg/l. A typical detection for N latex cystatin C is 0.05 mg/l.

Alpha$_1$-microglobulin was evaluated in the second morning urine specimen with N α1-microglobulin kit (Siemens Healthcare Diagnostics, Marburg, Germany) through particle-enhanced immunonephelometry using the BNProSpec System. The reference interval was 12 mg/l or 0.07–5 mg/g creatinine. The intra-assay precision was 2.9–5.2% CV, while the inter-assay precision was 7.4–13.2% CV.

KIM-1 was assessed in the second morning urine specimen by KIM-1 ELISA test kit for the detection of KIM-1 in human urine, Cat No. H-RENA-E-001, Bio Assay Works, Ijamsville, MD, USA. A human KIM-1 antibody was utilised and the detection level was set at urinary KIM-1<0.150 ng/ml.

Albuminuria was measured in the second morning urine specimen through immunonephelometry on the BNProSpec System, with N Antiserum to Human Albumin (Siemens Healthcare Diagnostics, Marburg, Germany). Microalbuminuria was defined by UACR between 30 and 300 mg/g, and normoalbuminuria by UACR<30 mg/g. The N Antiserum to Human Albumin was evaluated for the assay of urine on a BN System and yielded a Within-Run CV of 2.2% and a total CV of 2.6% with a mean of 79 mg/l. The results (ten runs, four determinations per run) were evaluated by analysis of variance. Urine cultures were negative for bacteriuria in all patients.

Nephrin was assessed in the second morning urine specimen by human NPHN (Nephrin) ELISA kit, Cat No. E-EL-H1901 Elabscience Biotech Co. Ltd, Wuhan, Hubei Province, China. A human NPHN antibody was utilised. The sensitivity of the assessment showed that the minimum detectable dose of Human NPHN is 0.1 ng/ml. The detection range is 0.16–10 ng/ml. The repeatability of the test displayed a CV <10%.

VEGF was assessed in the second morning urine specimen by a VEGF human ELISA kit for the detection of urinary VEGF, Cat No. ab100663, Abcam, Cambridge, MA, USA. A human VEGF antibody was utilised and the minimum detectable dose of VEGF was typically less than 10 pg/ml. The intra-assay reproducibility was <10% CV, and the inter-assay reproducibility was <12% CV.

Plasma and urinary AGE peptides were assessed in two 24-hour urine samples by the ELISA method with human advanced glycosylation end-products ELISA kit (E01A0002), Shanghai Blue Gene Biotech Co., Shanghai, China. The sensitivity in this assay measured in two 24-hour urine samples was 1.0 pg/ml. This assay has high sensitivity and excellent specificity of AGE. This assay contains polyclonal antibodies which assess protein-bound AGE. The system utilized allows the assessment of both high and low molecular AGE species. No significant cross-reactivity or interference between AGE and analogues was observed.

Statistical analysis

Clinical and biological data are presented as medians and IQR, as for variables with skewed distribution. We used ANOVA test and the Bonferroni multiple-comparison test. We used simple and multiple linear regression analysis. Stata's regress command was applied for testing this. R-square and adjusted R-square are part of the output and the last one was reported in the results presented. The p values for all hypothesis tests were two-sided, and statistical significance was set at $p<0.00625$. All analyses were conducted with Stata 9.2 (Statacorp, Texas, USA).

Ethics statement

The County Emergency Hospital Timisoara Ethical Committee (Board of Human Studies) approved the protocol (approval number 3/5th January 2014), and every patient provided written informed consent before enrolment.

Results

All patients and controls were included in the analysis.

The demographic, clinical and laboratory data of the patients and control subjects are presented in Table 1. According to the study inclusion criteria, all patients were on ACEIs and/or ARBs, and statins. Therefore, these parameters were not entered in Table 1 and in uni/multivariate analyses.

Significant differences were found between groups A and B with regard to high sensitive C reactive protein (hsCRP) ($p<0.0001$), UACR ($p<0.0001$), serum cystatin C ($p = 0.020$), urinary alpha1-microglobulin ($p<0.0001$), urinary KIM-1 ($p = 0.003$), urinary nephrin ($p<0.0001$), urinary VEGF ($p<0.0001$), urinary AGE ($p<0.0001$), and plasma AGE ($p<0.0001$). Also, significant differences were found between groups A and C, and B and C, respectively, with regard to the same parameters, including cystatin C, as well (Table 1).

In *univariate regression analysis*, urinary alpha$_1$-microglobulin and urinary KIM-1 correlated directly with UACR, nephrinuria, urinary VEGF, urinary AGE, serum cystatin C, and inversely with the estimated Glomerular filtration rate (eGFR). Nephrinuria and urinary VEGF correlated directly with urinary alpha$_1$-microglobulin, urinary KIM-1, UACR, urinary AGE, serum cystatin C, and inversely with eGFR (Table 2). In *multivariate regression analysis*, urinary alpha$_1$-microglobulin correlated directly with urinary KIM-1, urinary AGE, nephrinuria, urinary VEGF, serum cystatin C, and inversely with eGFR; urinary KIM-1 correlated directly with urinary alpha$_1$-microglobulin, urinary AGE, nephrinuria, urinary VEGF, serum cystatin C, and inversely with eGFR; nephrinuria correlated directly with UACR, urinary AGE, and urinary VEGF, while urinary VEGF correlated directly with urinary AGE, serum cystatin C, urinary alpha$_1$-microglobulin, and inversely with eGFR. Due to the fact that inflammation increases VEGF expression and podocyte injury in the course of DN, hsCRP was also introduced in multivariate analysis. After adjustment for hsCRP in multivariate analysis, the association between PT dysfunction and podocyte damage biomarkers remained significant (Table 3).

Discussion

Podocyte damage biomarkers have been discussed in relation to PT dysfunction biomarkers and emphasis has been put on potential nephrin and VEGF uptake and processing by the PT in early DN. Subsequently, AGE involvement in this setting was also queried due to the fact that AGE may impact both the podocyte and the PT.

In patients with Type 2 DM we found an association between PT dysfunction and podocyte biomarkers, a phenomenon which was independent of the level of albuminuria and of renal function.

The biomarkers of PT dysfunction are increased in early DN and correlate with urinary AGE

The tubular theory concerning mechanisms of albuminuria in early DN states that there is a reduction in the retrieval pathway of albumin in the PT, and this impairment precedes glomerular damage [14]. AGE-modified peptides show tubulotoxic effects and lead to pathophysiologic responses described as diabetic tubulopathy [18].

Biomarkers of PT dysfunction are strongly associated to the levels of plasma and urinary AGE [20,21]. In our study we found a significant relation of plasma and urinary AGE with biomarkers of PT dysfunction, such as urinary alpha$_1$-microglobulin and urinary KIM-1.

Urinary alpha$_1$-microglobulin and urinary KIM-1 are sensitive biomarkers in detecting PT dysfunction in early DN, even in normoalbuminuric patients. Data provided by several studies performed in normoalbuminuric patients with Type 2 DM, who displayed increased levels of urinary alpha$_1$-microglobulin [15–17,22], and of urinary KIM-1 [23] show that tubular functional defects precede the onset of albuminuria. In a study performed in patients with Type 2 DM, urinary tubular markers were independently associated with albuminuria in the early stage of DN [23].

Higher levels of urinary KIM-1 were found in Type 2 DM patients with glomerular hyperfiltration, as compared to patients with normal eGFR, showing that this glomerular phenomenon is a trigger for PT dysfunction in early DN [24].

In our study, the levels of urinary KIM-1 were increased in both normo- and microalbuminuric patients, but significantly higher in the microalbuminuric group. These data are in keeping with the results shown in the study performed by Vaidya *et al.* in patients with Type 1 DM in who lower urinary KIM-1 and N-acetyl-beta-D glucosaminidase levels were associated with the regression of microalbuminuria to normoalbuminuria. Urinary levels of the two tubular injury biomarkers were significantly elevated in patients with microalbuminuria as compared to patients with normoalbuminuria and healthy controls [25].

In our patients urinary alpha$_1$-microglobulin and urinary KIM-1 correlated with UACR even at high-to-normal levels, thus raising the possibility that the PT injury may precede the onset of microalbuminuria. It is worth underlining that in our study, urinary alpha$_1$-microglobulin and urinary KIM-1 correlated with

Table 1. Clinical and biological data of the studied patients.

Parameter	Group A	Group B	Group C	p*	p**	p***	p
Number of subjects	38	32	21	–	–	–	–
Age (years)	56.5 (51–61)	58.5 (52–65)	57 (52–59)	0.417	0.899	0.479	0.635
DM duration (years)	9 (7–12)	9 (6–16)	–	0.893	–	–	0.545
BMI (kg/m^2)	31.6 (28.5–35.2)	31.7 (27.0–35.4)	23.9 (23.6–24.9)	0.969	<0.0001	<0.0001	<0.0001
SBP (mmHg)	130 (120–140)	130 (125–135)	120 (115–120)	0.693	0.003	0.0004	0.0036
DBP (mmHg)	75 (70–80)	75 (70–80)	70 (60–75)	0.646	0.002	0.020	0.0022
Hb (g/dl)	13 (12.3–14.2)	12.8 (12.4–13.5)	14.3 (13.6–14.7)	0.603	0.002	0.0006	0.0047
Serum creatinine (mg/dl)	0.98 (0.82–1.08)	0.99 (0.92–1.13)	0.82 (0.77–0.92)	0.254	0.015	0.003	0.034
eGFR (ml/min/1.73 m^2)	71.8 (60.9–86.9)	68.2 (58.1–83.0)	85.9 (82.6–95.3)	0.255	0.005	0.001	0.005
Glycaemia (mg/dl)	139 (117.5–196)	130.5 (105–210)	95 (85–100)	0.704	<0.0001	0.0004	0.001
HbA_{1c} (%)	7.0 (6.5–7.5)	7.2 (6.4–7.8)	5.1 (4.8–5.2)	0.889	<0.0001	<0.0001	0.0003
HbA_{1c} (mmol/mol)	53 (48–58)	55 (46–62)	32 (29–33)	0.889	<0.0001	<0.0001	0.0003
Serum cholesterol (mg/dl)	213 (182–253)	215 (191–268)	140 (135–170)	0.676	<0.0001	<0.0001	<0.0001
Triglycerides (mg/dl)	146 (108–190)	150 (121–183)	92 (85–107)	0.582	0.0004	0.0001	0.0014
hsCRP(mg/dl)	4.6 (3.3–11.5)	11.1 (9.3–16.7)	0.85 (0.8–1.2)	<0.0001	<0.0001	<0.0001	<0.0001
UACR (mg/g)	21.9 (16.2–28.1)	72.1 (42.9–103.0)	19.12 (17.82–24.45)	<0.0001	0.606	<0.0001	<0.0001
Serum cystatin C (mg/l)	0.87 (0.66–0.99)	0.92 (0.79–1.08)	0.63 (0.535–0.682)	0.061	0.0009	<0.0001	<0.0001
Urinary alpha1/creat (mg/g)	3.65 (3.39–6.18)	6.94 (4.56–9.08)	2.83 (2.75–3.21)	<0.0001	0.001	<0.0001	<0.0001
Urinary KIM-1/creat (ng/g)	71.26 (47.62–98.34)	107.58 (63.96–133.78)	43.2 (49.86–40.33)	0.004	0.003	0.0001	<0.0001
Urinary VEGF/creat (ng/g)	75.40 (41.75–110.55)	109.15 (84.70–200.80)	19.5 (7.4–35.4)	0.0009	<0.0001	<0.0001	<0.0001
Urinary nephrin/creat (mg/g)	0.11 (0.09–0.14)	0.89 (0.55–1.46)	0.036 (0.034–0.067)	<0.0001	<0.0001	<0.0001	<0.0001
Urinary AGE (pg/ml)	36.15 (32.81–56.25)	68.93 (35.21–108.20)	32.48 (30.36–34.10)	0.006	0.002	<0.0001	<0.0001
Plasma AGE (pg/ml)	373.41 (320.30–521.99)	649.88 (517.20–851.88)	280.62 (252.70–300.10)	<0.0001	0.0001	<0.0001	<0.0001

DM: diabetes mellitus; BMI: body mass index; SBP: systolic blood pressure; DBP: diastolic blood pressure; Hb: haemoglobin; eGFR: estimated glomerular filtration rate; HbA_{1c}: glycated haemoglobin; hsCRP: high sensitive C reactive protein; UACR: urine albumin to creatinine ratio; $alpha_1$/creat: $alpha_1$-microglobulin to creatinine ratio; KIM-1/creat: kidney injury molecule-1 to creatinine ratio; VEGF/creat: vascular endothelial growth factor to creatinine ratio; nephrin/creat: nephrin to creatinine ratio; AGE: advanced glycation end-products; group A: patients with normoalbuminuria; group B: patients with microalbuminuria; group C: healthy control subjects; parameters are expressed as medians and IQR, as for variables with skewed distribution; p*: Bonferroni's t-test for the differences between groups A and B; p**: Bonferroni's t-test for the differences between groups A and C; p***: Bonferroni's t-test for the differences between groups B and C; p: ANOVA analysis of variance for the differences between groups A, B, and C; statistical significance was set at 0.00625.

Table 2. Univariate regression analysis for the urinary biomarkers.

Variable	R-squared*	Coef β*	p*	R-squared#	Coef β#	p#	R-squared§	Coef β§	p§	R-squared∫	Coef β∫	p∫
eGFR	0.166	−0.953	<0.001	0.167	−0.053	<0.001	0.087	−0.008	0.007	0.218	−1.836	<0.001
Cystatin C	0.128	57.336	0.001	0.130	3.215	<0.001	0.157	0.809	<0.001	0.226	127.806	<0.001
Urinary AGE	0.405	0.825	<0.001	0.578	0.054	<0.001	0.251	0.008	<0.001	0.308	1.211	<0.001
UACR	0.125	0.427	<0.001	0.269	0.034	<0.001	0.498	0.010	<0.001	0.227	0.969	<0.001
KIM-1/creat	–	–	–	0.531	0.040	<0.001	0.203	0.005	<0.001	0.360	1.008	<0.001
Urinary alpha1/creat	0.531	13.107	<0.001	–	–	–	0.529	0.167	<0.001	0.709	25.469	<0.001
Nephrin/creat	0.203	35.316	<0.001	0.529	3.169	<0.001	–	–	–	0.527	95.648	<0.001
VEGF/creat	0.360	0.356	<0.001	0.709	0.027	<0.001	0.527	0.005	<0.001	–	–	–

KIM-1/creat: kidney injury molecule-1 to creatinine ratio; alpha1/creat: alpha$_1$-microglobulin to creatinine ratio; nephrin/creat: nephrin to creatinine ratio; VEGF/creat: vascular endothelial growth factor to creatinine ratio; eGFR: estimated glomerular filtration rate; AGE: advanced glycation end-products; UACR: urine albumin-to-creatinine ratio; *: data for KIM-1/creat; #: data for urinary alpha1/creat; §: data for nephrin/creat; ∫: data for VEGF/creat.

urinary AGE. In a recent experimental study it has been shown that diabetic mice had a greater renal burden of AGE, which correlated with UACR, hyperfiltration, and release of urinary KIM-1 [26]. It may be assumed that AGE may impact the PT in the early stages of DN, thus explaining increased levels of urinary alpha-1 microglobulin and urinary KIM-1 in normoalbuminuric patients with Type 2 DM.

Nephrinuria and urinary VEGF parallel PT dysfunction in patients with Type 2 DM

Nephrin is a podocyte-specific protein and its presence in the urine correlates with podocyte lesions in the course of DN. In a study conducted by Pätäri *et al.* in the urine of patients with Type 1 DM, nephrin was evidenced in 30% of normoalbuminuric patients, in 17% of those with microalbuminuria, in 28% of those with macroalbuminuria, and in 28% of those who were with recent onset albuminuria. The detection of nephrinuria in normoalbuminuric patients is highly predictive for the development of DN [7].

The results of our study substantiate the fact that nephrinuria is increased in patients with Type 2 DM, even in the normoalbuminuria stage. We found elevated levels of nephrinuria which correlated with the biomarkers of PT dysfunction, urinary AGE, UACR, cystatin C, and the eGFR. These correlations did not hold true for the healthy subjects studied, a fact which increases the predictive diagnostic power of nephrinuria in early DN.

Increased levels of nephrinuria, which paralleled the elevated levels of PT dysfunction markers, such as NGAL and heart-fatty acid binding protein, have been shown in a study conducted on an animal model in rats with streptozocin induced Type 1 DM and early DN [27].

In a study performed in patients with Type 2 DM, there has been evidenced an independent correlation between nephrinuria and UACR and eGFR, respectively. Nephrinuria was associated significantly with decreased levels of eGFR, even in normoalbuminuric patients, thus suggesting that nephrinuria may be potentially involved in the development of renal insufficiency in the stage of normoalbuminuria. Our results are in keeping with these data which point to the fact that patients with Type 2 DM and normoalbuminuria are very often perceived as a group of patients at low risk of developing CKD [8].

In another study performed in Type 2 DM patients, nephrinuria was detected in 54% of normoalbuminuric patients, suggesting its potential role as an early biomarker of DN. In this report, nephrinuria correlated significantly with albuminuria and showed a negative correlation with eGFR [9].

Although these data suggest that alterations of the glomerular filtration barrier may be present in the early stages of DN, nephrinuria is evidenced only in a reduced percentage of patients, a phenomenon which is expressed when PT dysfunction occurs. Retrieval of albumin by the PT through specific endocytotic mechanisms which utilize the megalin/cubilin receptor complex explains the delay in the occurrence of microalbuminuria even in patients with detectable nephrinuria. It has been assumed that the PT may be involved not only in albumin, but also in nephrin uptake in the course of DN, even in its early stages [8].

In our study, nephrinuria correlated with the biomarkers of PT dysfunction, a fact which forwards the hypothesis that the PT could have delayed the expression of glomerular involvement in early DN by coordinating nephrin uptake and processing.

In the study by Kim *et al.* urinary VEGF was increased in patients with Type 2 DM in the early stage of DN and correlated with albuminuria. Urinary VEGF excretion increased as DN

Table 3. Multivariate regression analysis for the urinary biomarkers.

Variable	Coef β	p	95% CI	F	Prob>F	R^2
Constant#	1.214	0.004	0.392 to 2.036	82.48##	<0.001##	0.887##
eGFR#	−1.666	0.006	−0.495 to −2.838			
Cystatin C#	1.866	<0.001	0.945 to 0.787			
Urinary AGE#	0.020	<0.001	0.013 to 0.028			
KIM-1/creat#	0.011	<0.001	0.005 to 0.018			
Nephrin/creat#	1.078	0.001	0.465 to 1.691			
VEGF/creat#	0.014	<0.001	0.009 to 0.019			
hsCRP#	−0.016	0.331	−0.050 to 0.017			
Constant*	1.513	0.002	0.211 to 3.098	86.31**	<0.001**	0.752**
eGFR*	−1.834	0.006	−0.204 to −3.116			
Cystatin C*	1.968	<0.001	1.098 to 3.689			
Urinary AGE*	0.063	<0.001	0.008 to 0.041			
Urinary alpha1/creat*	0.008	<0.001	0.029 to 0.018			
Nephrin/creat*	0.913	0.005	0.406 to 1.141			
VEGF/creat*	0.015	<0.001	0.012 to 0.027			
hsCRP*	−0.011	0.379	−0.039 to 0.006			
Constant^{f}	−38.012	0.025	−71.178 to −4.846	58.84^{ff}	<0.001^{ff}	0.796^{ff}
eGFR^{f}	− 61.423	0.008	−106.517 to −16.329			
Cystatin C^{f}	100.334	<0.001	60.706 to 139.962			
Urinary alpha1/creat^{f}	28.381	<0.001	23.483 to 33.279			
Urinary AGE^{f}	0.461	0.011	0.813 to 0.108			
hsCRP^{f}	−1.020	0.074	−2.140 to 0.100			
Constant§	−0.420	<0.001	−0.530 to −0.311	78.56§§	<0.001§§	0.775§§
UACR§	0.006	<0.001	0.004 to 0.008			
VEGF/creat§	0.003	<0.001	0.002 to 0.004			
Urinary AGE§	0.046	<0.001	0.011 to 0.063			
hsCRP§	−0.011	0.468	−0.133 to 0.046			

alpha1/creat: $alpha_1$-microglobulin to creatinine ratio; KIM-1/creat: kidney injury molecule-1 to creatinine ratio; VEGF/creat: vascular endothelial growth factor to creatinine ratio; nephrin/creat: nephrin to creatinine ratio; eGFR: estimated glomerular filtration rate; AGE: advanced glycation end-products; hsCRP-high sensitive C-reactive protein; UACR: urine albumin-to-creatinine ratio; #: variables correlated with urinary alpha1/creat; *: variables correlated with KIM-1/creat; ^{f}: variables correlated with VEGF/creat; §: variables correlated with nephrin/creat; ##: multivariate regression analysis for urinary alpha1/creat; **: multivariate regression analysis for KIM-1/creat; ^{ff}: multivariate regression analysis for VEGF/creat; §§: multivariate regression analysis for nephrin/creat.

advanced, thus suggesting that urinary VEGF is a sensitive biomarker of DN, predicting disease progression [12].

In our study, urinary VEGF correlated with nephrinuria and UACR, but also with the biomarkers of PT dysfunction, urinary AGE, cystatin C, and eGFR. As was the case with nephrinuria, these correlations were not found in the healthy controls.

We assume that this observation documents an association of PT with urinary VEGF uptake and processing, a fact substantiated by the strong correlation of the PT dysfunction biomarkers with urinary VEGF, even in normoalbuminuric patients. Most likely, as was the case with urinary nephrin, the PT interferes with the expression of podocyte damage markers in early DN.

The correlation of urinary VEGF with urinary AGE is in keeping with the observation that AGE induce increased VEGF expression by the podocytes in vivo and vitro [28]. In our patients, increased levels of urinary VEGF were present in both normo- and microalbuminuric patients, leading to the assumption that an increased AGE-induced VEGF expression by the podocytes may occur in the early stages of DN. Studies performed on kidney biopsies from diabetic mice [29] and Type 2 DM patients [30] show that increased levels of glycated albumin are associated with abnormal renal nephrin and VEGF expression, even in the early stages of DN.

Cystatin C is associated with biomarkers of PT dysfunction and of podocyte damage in patients with Type 2 DM

In our study, UACR, urinary $alpha_1$-microglobulin, urinary KIM-1, urinary nephrin, urinary VEGF, and plasma and urinary AGE correlated directly with serum cystatin C and negatively with eGFR. Other studies have also revealed that urinary PT damage biomarkers are associated with eGFR and cystatin C, independently of albuminuria [24,31]. Our data have also documented a correlation of urinary nephrin and urinary VEGF with cystatin C and eGFR, even in normoalbuminuric patients, thus suggesting that these podocyte damage biomarkers may be associated to renal function decline independently of albuminuria, but most likely related to PT dysfunction.

It has been shown that reduced eGFR may correlate with the degree of albuminuria within normal range [15-17,32]. Subtle changes in renal function in patients with Type 2 DM, as assessed by cystatin C, may parallel the degree of albuminuria, even in high-to- normal albuminuria [33–35], data which are similar to our findings. In our study, declined levels of eGFR were found in normoalbuminuric patients too, a fact that could have been attributed to PT dysfunction. These data are consistent with studies which provide evidence of a steady decline in renal function in normoalbuminuric patients with Type 2 DM [3,36].

Our study has several limitations. First, the small study cohort affects the statistical power of the study. Second, this is a cross-sectional study which requires validation by a longitudinal study in order to prove causality between urinary nephrin and urinary VEGF excretion and PT dysfunction in Type 2 DM patients. Third, despite significant correlations in multivariate analysis between the biomarkers studied, residual confounding factors could have interfered interpretation of data, such as the extent and intervention of tubulointerstitial injury. The differences between groups concerning hsCRP may be attributed to multiple comorbid inflammatory conditions recorded in microalbuminuric patients with Type 2 DM.

The strength of our study relies upon the documentation of an association between biomarkers of PT dysfunction and biomarkers of glomerular damage in patients with Type 2 DM, relation which was independent of the degree of albuminuria and level of renal function.

To sum up, in patients with Type 2 DM, there is an association of PT dysfunction and podocyte damage biomarkers, even in the normoalbuminuria stage. This observation raises the possibility of a putative role of the PT in urinary nephrin and urinary VEGF excretion in early DN. Moreover, it forwards the hypothesis according to which podocyte damage and PT dysfunction may precede the onset of microalbuminuria. AGE could impact both the PT and the glomerulus in the early stages of DN, thus explaining increased levels of urinary nephrin and urinary VEGF in normoalbuminuric patients with Type 2 DM.

It is possible that in early DN, sequentially, PT dysfunction biomarkers may be elevated before the increase in podocyte damage biomarkers in the normoalbuminuria stage.

Presumably, the PT interferes with the expression of glomerular injury in early DN by coordinating albumin, as well as nephrin and VEGF uptake and processing. These data point to the fact that podocyte damage and PT dysfunction biomarkers could be validated as a practical approach to the diagnosis of early DN by further prospective studies on larger cohorts.

Author Contributions

Conceived and designed the experiments: LP AV GG. Performed the experiments: FG CG SV DV RP. Analyzed the data: LP AV VD FB OM SU. Wrote the paper: LP AV FG VD. Revised the manuscript critically for important intellectual content: GG CG SV FB DV RP OM SU.

References

1. US Renal Data System (2008) USRDS 2008 Annual Data Report. Available: http://www.usrds.org. Accessed 11 February 2014.
2. Schernthaner G (2011) Kidney disease in diabetology: lessons from 2010. Nephrol Dial Transplant 26: 454–457.
3. MacIsaac RJ, Tsalamandris C, Panagiotopoulos S, Smith TJ, McNeil KJ, et al. (2004) Nonalbuminuric renal insufficiency in type 2 diabetes. Diabetes Care 27: 195–200.
4. Jefferson JA, Shankland SJ, Pichler RH (2008) Proteinuria in diabetic kidney disease: a mechanistic viewpoint. Kidney Int 74: 22–36.
5. Nakagawa T, Tanabe K, Croker BP, Johnson RJ, Grant MB, et al. (2011) Endothelial dysfunction as a potential contributor in diabetic nephropathy. Nat Rev Nephrol 7: 36–44.
6. Fioretto P, Mauer M (2007) Histopathology of diabetic nephropathy. Semin Nephrol 27: 195–207.
7. Pätäri A, Forsblom C, Havana M, Taipale H, Groop PH, et al. (2003) Nephrinuria in diabetic nephropathy of type 1 diabetes. Diabetes 52: 2969–2974.
8. Ng DPK, Tai BC, Tan E, Leong H, Nurbaya S, et al. (2011) Nephrinuria associates with multiple renal traits in type 2 diabetes. Nephrol Dial Transplant 26: 2508–2514.
9. Jim B, Ghanta M, Qipo A, Fan Y, Chuang PY, et al. (2012) Dysregulated nephrin in diabetic nephropathy of type 2 diabetes: a cross sectional study. PLoS One 7(5): e36041.
10. Ziyadeh FN, Wolf G (2008) Pathogenesis of the podocytopathy and proteinuria in diabetic glomerulopathy. Curr Diabetes Rev 4: 39–45.
11. Eremina V, Sood M, Haigh J, Nagy A, Lajoie G, et al. (2003) Glomerular-specific alterations of VEGF-A expression lead to distinct congenital and acquired renal diseases. J Clin Invest 111: 707–716.
12. Kim NH, Kim KB, Kim DL, Kim SG, Choi KM, et al. (2004) Plasma and urinary vascular endothelial growth factor and diabetic nephropathy in type 2 diabetes mellitus. Diabet Med 21: 545–551.
13. Comper WD, Haraldsson B, Deen WM (2008) Resolved: normal glomeruli filter nephrotic levels of albumin. J Am Soc Nephrol 19: 427–432.
14. Russo LM, Sandoval RM, Campos SB, Molitoris BA, Comper WD, et al. (2009) Impaired tubular uptake explains albuminuria in early diabetic nepropathy. J Am Soc Nephrol 20: 489–494.
15. Petrica L, Petrica M, Vlad A, Jianu DC, Gluhovschi G, et al. (2011) Proximal tubule dysfunction is dissociated from endothelial dysfunction in normoalbuminuric patients with type 2 diabetes mellitus: a cross-sectional study. Nephron Clin Pract 118: c155–c164.
16. Petrica L, Petrica M, Vlad A, Jianu DC, Gluhovschi G, et al. (2009) Nephro- and neuroprotective effects of rosiglitazone versus glimepiride in normoalbuminuric patients with type 2 diabetes mellitus: a randomized controlled trial. Wien Klin Wochenschr 121: 765–775.
17. Petrica L, Vlad A, Petrica M, Jianu CD, Gluhovschi G, et al. (2011) Pioglitazone delays proximal tubule dysfunction and improves cerebral vessels endothelial dysfunction in normoalbuminuric patients with type 2 diabetes mellitus. Diabetes Res Clin Pract 94: 22–32.
18. Tang SC, Leung JC, Lai KN (2011) Diabetic tubulopathy: an emerging entity. Contrib Nephrol 170: 124–134.
19. (2013) KDIGO clinical practice guideline for the evaluation and management of chronic kidney disease Kidney Int (Suppl) 3: 1–150.
20. Ozdemir AM, Hopfer U, Erhard P, Monnier VM, Weiss MF (2005) Processing advanced glycation end product-modified albumin by the renal proximal tubule and the early pathogenesis of diabetic nephropathy. Ann N Y Acad Sci 1043: 625–636.
21. Kern EF, Erhard P, Sun W, Gennth S, Weiss MF (2010) Early urinary markers of diabetic kidney disease: a nested case-control study from the Diabetes Control and Complications Trial (DCCT). Am J Kidney Dis 55: 824–834.
22. Hong CY, Hughes K, Chia KS, Ng V, Ling SL (2003) Urinary alpha$_1$-microglobulin as a marker of nephropathy in type 2 diabetic Asian subjects in Singapore. Diabetes Care 26: 338–342.
23. Kim SS, Song SH, Kim IJ, Yang JY, Lee JG, et al. (2012) Clinical implication of urinary tubular markers in the early stage of nephropathy with type 2 diabetic patients. Diabetes Res Clin Pract 97: 251–257.
24. Fu WJ, Li BL, Wang SB, Chen ML, Deng RT, et al. (2012) Changes of the tubular markers in type 2 diabetes mellitus with glomerular hyperfiltration. Diabetes Res Clin Pract 95: 105–109.
25. Vaidya VS, Niewczas MA, Ficociello LH, Johnson AC, Collings FB, et al. (2011) Regression of microalbuminuria in type 1 diabetes is associated with lower levels of urinary tubular injury biomarkers, kidney injury molecule-1, and N-acetyl-β-D-glucosaminidase. Kidney Int 79: 464–470.
26. Thallas-Bonke V, Coughlan MT, Tan AL, Harcourt BE, Morgan PE, et al. (2013) Targeting the AGE – RAGE axis improves renal function in the context of a healthy diet low in advanced glycation end-product content. Nephrology (Carlton) 18: 47–56.
27. Alter ML, Kretchmer A, von Websky K, Tsuprykov O, Reichetzeder C, et al. (2012) Early urinary and plasma biomarkers for experimental diabetic nephropathy. Clin Lab 58: 659–671.
28. Tsuchida K, Makita Z, Yamagishi S, Atsumi T, Mioshi H, et al. (1999) Suppression of transforming growth factor beta and vascular endothelial growth factor in diabetic nephropathy in rats by novel advanced glycation end product inhibitor, OPB – 9195. Diabetologia 42: 579–588.
29. Cohen MP, Chen S, Ziyadeh FN, Shea E, Hud EA, et al. (2005) Evidence linking glycated albumin to altered glomerular nephrin and VEGF expression, proteinuria, and diabetic nephropathy. Kidney Int 68: 1554–1561.
30. Doublier S, Salvidio G, Lupia E, Ruotsalainen V, Verzola D, et al. (2003) Nephrin expression is reduced in human diabetic nephropathy. Evidence for a distinct role for glycated albumin and angiotensin II. Diabetes 52: 1023–1030.
31. Nauta FL, Boertien WE, Bakker SJ, van Goor H, van Oeveren W, et al. (2011) Glomerular and tubular damage markers are elevated in patients with diabetes. Diabetes Care 34: 975–981.
32. Ritz E, Viberti GC, Ruilope LM, Rabelink AJ, Izzo JL Jr, et al. (2010) Determinants of urinary albumin excretion within the normal range in patients with type 2 diabetes: the Randomised Olmesartan and Diabetes Microalbuminuria Prevention (ROADMAP) study. Diabetologia 53: 49–57.

33. Kravaritou M, Thanopoulou A, Karamanos B, Kofinis A, Noutsou M, et al. (2009) Evidence that even "normal" albuminuria may denote incipient eGFR reduction in patients with type 2 diabetes mellitus. Diabetes Res Clin Pract 85: 317–321.
34. Borges RL, Hirota AH, Quinto BM, Ribeiro AB, Zanella MT, et al. (2010) Is cystatin C a useful marker in the detection of diabetic kidney disease? Nephron Clin Pract 114: c127–c134.
35. Jeon YK, Kim MR, Huh JE, Mok JY, Song SH, et al. (2011) Cystatin C as an early biomarker of nephropathy in patients with type 2 diabetes. J Korean Med Sci 26: 258–263.
36. Jerums G, Panagiotopoulos S, Premaratne E, MacIsaac RJ (2009) Integrating albuminuria and GFR in the assessment of diabetic nephropathy. Nat Rev Nephrol 5: 397–406.

17

Protective Effects of Astragaloside IV on db/db Mice with Diabetic Retinopathy

Yuzhi Ding[1⁹], Songtao Yuan[1⁹], Xiaoyi Liu[1⁹], Pingan Mao[2], Chen Zhao[1], Qiong Huang[3], Rihua Zhang[3], Yuan Fang[1], Qinglu Song[1], Dongqing Yuan[1], Ping Xie[1], Yun Liu[3]*, Qinghuai Liu[1]*

1 Department of Ophthalmology, The First Affiliated Hospital of Nanjing Medical University, Nanjing, China, **2** Department of Ophthalmology, No. 2 People's Hospital of Changzhou, Changzhou, China, **3** Department of Endocrinology, The First Affiliated Hospital of Nanjing Medical University, Nanjing, China

Abstract

Objectives: Diabetic retinopathy (DR) is a common diabetic eye disease which is well-known as the result of microvascular retinal changes. Although the potential biological functions of astragaloside IV (AS IV) have long been described in traditional system of medicine, its protective effect on DR remains unclear. This study aims to investigate the function and mechanism of AS IV on type 2 diabetic db/db mice.

Methods: Db/db mice were treated with AS IV (4.5 mg/kg or 9 mg/kg) or physiological saline by oral gavage for 20 weeks along with db/m mice. In each group, retinal ganglion cell (RGC) function was measured by pattern electroretinogram (ERG) and apoptosis was determined by Terminal deoxynucleotidyl transferase dUTP nick end labeling (TUNEL) staining. Blood and retina aldose reductase (AR) activity were quantified by chemiluminescence analysis. The expressions of phosporylated-ERK1/2, NF-κB were determined by Western blot analysis. Furthermore, the expression of related downstream proteins were quantified by Label-based Mouse Antibody Array.

Results: Administration of AS IV significantly improved the amplitude in pattern ERG and reduced the apoptosis of RGCs.in db/db mice. Furthermore, downregulation of AR activity, ERK1/2 phosphorylation, NF-κB and related cytokine were observed in AS IV treatment group.

Conclusions: Our study indicated that AS IV, as an inhibitor of AR, could prevent the activation of ERK1/2 phosporylation and NF-kB and further relieve the RGCs disfunction in db/db mice with DR. It has provided a basis for investigating the clinical efficacy of AR inhibitors in preventing DR.

Editor: Alfred S. Lewin, University of Florida, United States of America

Funding: This work was supported by grants from the National Basic Research Program of China (973 Program, No. 2013CB967500), the National Natural Science Foundation of China (Nos. 81270952, 81070684, 81170855, 81070743), the Jiangsu Province's Key Provincial Talents Program (BE 2011802), Jiangsu Science & Technology Pillar Program (BE 2011802), and Jiangsu Provincial Special Program of Medical Science (BL2014089). The funders had no role in study design, data collection and analysis, decision to publish, or preparation of the manuscript.

Competing Interests: The authors have declared that no competing interests exist.

* Email: liuqh@njmu.edu.cn (QL); liuyun@njmu.edu.cn (YL)

⁹ These authors contributed equally to this work.

Introduction

Diabetic retinopathy (DR) is known to be the most common microvascular complication of diabetes mellitus and is one of the most serious causes of visual impairment and blindness in developed countries [1–3]. Type 1 diabetic patients, along with approximately 80% of insulin-dependent type 2 diabetic patients and 50% of insulin-resistant type 2 diabetic patients, will suffer the retinopathy in the following 20 years since the first diagnosis [4]. Furthermore, DR accounts for 15 to 17% of total blindness [5]. Therefore, there is a pressing need for the development of novel and effective therapeutic approaches to halt the progression of DR. The prime-triggering factor for the progression of the disease is hyperglycemia [6,7]. However, the pathogenesis remains uncertain. Studies have shown this metabolic disorder can interfere with generation of neurotransmitters [8–10], inducing proapoptotic [11–14] and proinflammatory responses [15–17]. Accumulating evidence also suggested that immunologic and inflammatory mechanisms play important roles in its development and progression [18]. Recently, several vitro and vivo studies indicated that drugs with varying aldose reductase (AR) inhibiting efficacy show significant protection against diabetic complications, which provided evidences pointing to a significant role of AR in mediating hyperglycemic injury [19–23].

Astragaloside IV (AS IV), a novel saponin purified from Astragalus membranaceus (Fisch) Bunge, is one of the major and active components of the astragalus membranaceus. It has been reported of its hypoglycemic effect in diabetic mice by inhibiting of hepatic glycogen phosphorylase and glucose-6-phosphatase activities or the formation of advanced glycation end products [24,25].

Gui et al. suggested AS-IV prevents Glucose-Induced podocyte apoptosis as a novel antioxidant [26]. They also demonstrated significant efficacy against inflammation through inhibiting NF-κB in streptozotocin (STZ)-induced diabetic rats models in diabetic nephropathy (DN) [27]. In addition, AS IV showed its inhibitory effects on diabetic peripheral neuropathy in rats [28]. However, the inhibitory effect of this drug directly on DR has not been explored yet. Based on the observations described above, the aim of the present study was to investigate the protective effects and mechanism of AS IV on diabetic retinopathy in type 2 diabetic db/db mice.

Research Design and Methods

Materials

AS IV, extracted from Astragalus membranaceus (Fisch.) Bunge, was provided by the Institute of Botany, Jiangsu Province and Chinese Academy of Sciences (purity >98% using the HPLC method). The rabbit polyclonal antibodies against ERK/p-ERK, NF-κB were purchased from SANTA CRUZ, USA. Terminal Transferase dUTP Nick End Labeling (TUNEL) Assay kit was purchased from Roche, USA. Mouse Cytokine Array was purchased from RayBiotech, USA.

Experimental design

C57BLKsJ-db/db mice strain (db/db mice for short. Strain name BKS.Cg-Dock7^{m} +/+ Lepr^{db}/J and stock number 000642 in Jackson Laboratories) were purchased from Model Animal Research Center of Nanjing University. This study was carried out in strict accordance with the recommendations in the guide for the care and use of animals of the Association for Research in Vision and Ophthalmology (ARVO) and Committee for Animal Experiments of National Center. The protocol was approved by Ethics Committee of Nanjing Medical University. 8-week-old mice were housed in the Experimental Animal Facilities at Nanjing Medical University under specific-pathogen-free (SPF) conditions. Three groups each consisting of 12 male db/db mice along with 12 db/m mice (heterozygotes (Lepr$^{db/m}$) as littermate controls) were randomly assigned. The animals were fed with a normal diet and dosed daily by oral gavage, at 4.5 or 9 mg/kg of AS IV, or an equal amount of physiological saline.

Experimental design needed for the present in vivo study has been summarized as follows (Fig. 1):

Group 1 (Littermate controls, LC) consisted of normal db/m animals that received physiological saline only.

Group 2 (Negative control, NC) consisted of db/db mice that received saline orally.

Group 3 (AS IV Low-dose group, AL) consisted of db/db mice that were given As IV orally at a dose of 4.5 mg/kg body weight for 20 weeks.

Group 4 (AS IV High-dose group, AH) consisted of db/db mice that were given AS IV orally at a dose of 9 mg/kg body weight for 20 weeks.

4-weekly body weight measurement and blood glucose monitoring were conducted during the experiment period. The animals were allowed normal access to food and water and were maintained on a 12-h light/dark cycle at controlled temperature (20–25°C) and humidity (50%±5%). All reasonable efforts were made to minimize suffering.

Electroretinogram Recordings

The pattern ERG has specific potential to detect retinal ganglion cell (RGC) dysfunction or loss [29]. So functional outcomes are needed to follow the progression of db/db mice and assess the therapeutic effects of As IV neuroprotective treatments. We used the amplitude and latency of pattern ERG to monitor progressive RGC dysfunction. After 20 weeks gavage administration, pattern ERGs were recorded from 96 undilated eyes. 36 anesthetized (90 mg/kg ketamine and 6 mg/kg xylazine) db/db mice and 12 anesthetized db/m mice responded to contrast reversal of gratings that maximize pattern ERG amplitude (99% contrast, 1-Hz reversal, spatial frequency of 0.05 cyc/deg). The stimulus display contained four full cycles of the gratings. The center of visual stimulus was aligned with the projection of the pupil. Robust averaging (1800 sweeps) was used to isolate pattern ERG from background noise. The head of anesthetized mice was gently restrained in a modified stereotaxic console, a corneal electrode was placed on the test eye, positioning entailed minimal manipulation of the eye. Reference and ground electrodes were small stainless-steel needles inserted in the skin of the back of the head and the back of the body, respectively. A small drop of balanced saline was added to prevent corneal dryness, and the body of the mouse rested on a feedback controlled heating pad that maintained the body temperature at 37°C. A mouth bite and a small nose holder, which allows unobstructed vision, were used to restrain the anterior part of the head. Under these conditions, the eyes of the mice were naturally proptosed, with undilated pupils pointing laterally and upward. For pattern ERG, response amplitude was evaluated peak-to-trough, and the latency was the time-to-peak of the major positive deflection [29].

TUNEL Staining

Decreased population of cells is regarded as an important factor in the pathogenesis of various metabolic diseases [30,31]. To determine the effects of AS IV on RGCs, the apoptosis was determined using TUNEL assays. Only cells marked with green and blue fluorescence can be identified as apoptosis. TUNEL staining was performed according to the manufacturer's protocols to detect diabetic RGC death. After treatment for ERGs recording, animals were sacrificed. Eyes were enucleated and fixed in 4% paraformaldehyde (PFA, wuhan Boster Bio-engineering, Wuhan, China) for 8 h. The eye was cut at the ora serrata and the anterior portion of the eye and lens were removed. The eyecup (retina, choroid, and sclera) was placed in 30% sucrose solution at 4°C overnight for cryoprotection. Eyecups were then embedded in a supporting medium for frozen-tissue specimens (O.C.T. compound, Tissue-Tek, Naperville, IL) and stored in −20°C. The frozen sections will be cut at thicknesses of 8 μm for each sample before use. Slices were collected every 5 pieces and stored at −20°C until labeled. The sections were mounted on glass slides previously treated with poly-L-Lysine. These slides were examined under a laser scanning confocal microscope (LSM710; CarlZeiss, Oberkochen, Germany).

Retina Aldose reductase (AR) Activity Assay

To assess the reverse effects of AS IV on AR activity in blood and retina, blood sample and retinas were prepared. As for blood sample, AR was isolated from erythrocytes by a modification. The entire procedure was performed at 4°C. About 1 mL of heparinized whole blood obtained from each individual was centrifuged at 1000 rpm for 10 min. After removal of the buffy coat, the erythrocytes were suspended in 2 volumes of PBS and centrifuged again. This washing step was repeated once, and the packed erythrocytes were stored at −70°C until use. Retina complexes were micro-surgically isolated and placed immediately into 200 ul Radio-Immunoprecipitation Assay (RIPA) buffer supplemented with 1 mM protease inhibitor phenylmethane sulfonyl fluoride (PMSF) at 4°C. After mechanical disruption,

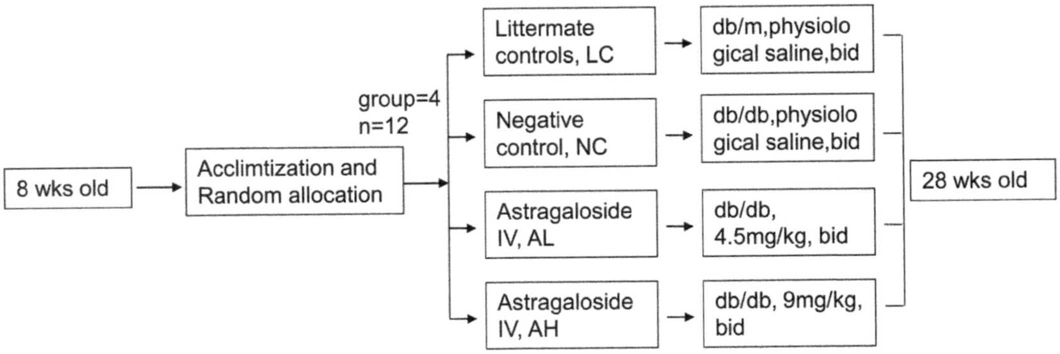

Figure 1. Schematic diagram of experimental design in vivo. 12 db/m mice were treated with physiological saline as a littermate control. Physiological saline was also given to 12 db/db mice as a negative control. 4.5 mg/kg and 9 mg/kg astragaloside IV were treated to see their effects on db/db mice eyes.

lysates were placed on ice for 20 minutes and centrifuged at 12,000 rpm for 10 minutes at 4°C. Protein concentrations were determined using a Bradford assay kit (Bio-Rad) with bovine serum albumin as a standard. AR activity was assayed by observing the decrease in the absorbance of NADPH at 367 nm using DL-glyceraldehyde as a substrate [32]. The assay mixture contained 30 mM potassium phosphate buffer (pH 6.5), 5 mM DL-glyceraldehyde (Lot No. 023k2512, Sigma Co.,St.Louis,Mo.), 0.2 M ammonium sulfate, and 1.0 mM β-NADPH (Lot#SLBC6718V, Sigma Co.,St.Louis,Mo.). Fluorescence was measured by fluorescence spectrometer (Thermo Scientific Varioskan Flash Spectral Scanning Multimode Reader, USA) at wavelengths of 367 nm for excitation and 455 nm for emission. One unit of enzyme activity was defined as the amount of enzyme able to oxidize 1 um of NADPH per min at 37°C versus total retina protein.

Western Blot

To identify possible cellular responses to AS IV in the diabetic model, extracellular signal regulated kinases ERK1/2 and nuclear transcription factor NF-κB were isolated. Following concentration and heating at 100°C for 5 min, 20 μg of protein was run on an SDS-PAGE gel and electro-blotted onto polyvinylidene fluoride membrane (PVDF). The membrane was blocked for 1 h in 5% skim milk in TBST (20 mM Tris-HCl, pH 7.6, 136 mM NaCl, and 0.1% Tween-20) and incubated in the primary antibody at 4°C overnight. After washed 3 times for 5 to 10 min in 50 mL of TBST at room temperature (RT), the membrane was incubated with goat anti-rabbit 1:2000 for 1 h at RT in 1× TBST, washed 3×10 min, and rinsed with dH_2O. Detection of the protein was determined by the use of the ECL kit (2 mL/membrane) according to standard procedures. p-ERK/ERK ratio and NF-κB in each group were therefore compared. GAPDH or Histone3 was used as a loading control.

Mouse Antibody Array-Detection of the Level of inflammatory cytokines and chemokines

Protein expression screening by the Label-based Mouse Antibody Array 1-the differential screening antibody microarray, which was designed and manufactured by RayBiotech, Inc. (Norcross, USA), contains 308 antibodies [33]. Retina protein obtained from db/db or db/m mice were pretreated and resultant supernatant was collected with measured protein contents. Each of the antibodies has two replicates that are printed on a coated glass microscope slide, along with multiple positive and negative controls. The antibody array experiment was performed by Wayen biotechnologies (Shanghai), according to the established protocol. Fluorescence Detection were scanned (GenePix 4000B,

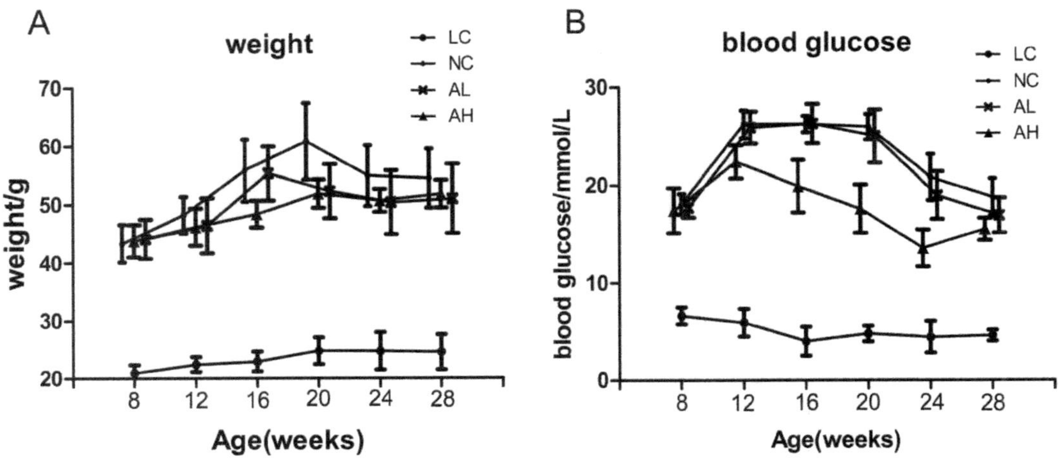

Figure 2. Animal general situations (collected every 4 weeks). A: body weight in all groups during treatment. B: Blood glucose in all groups during treatment.

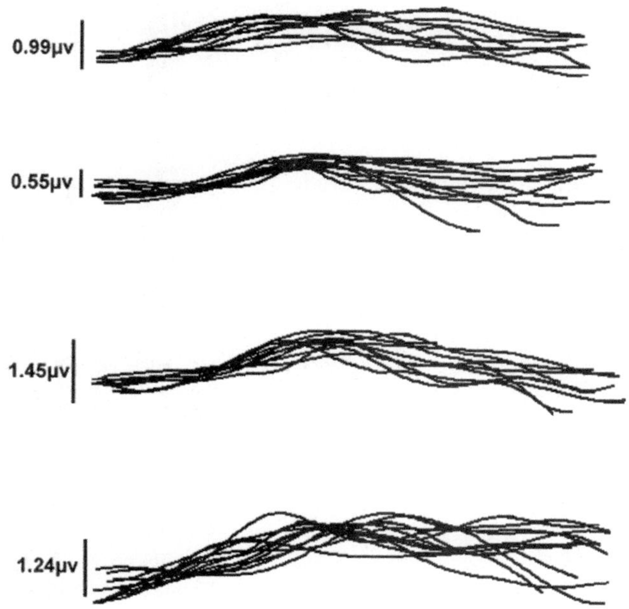

Figure 3. Pattern ERGs derived from each eye in response to pattern reversal of horizontal gratings in a population of 48 mice aged 28 weeks. Individual waveforms of each eye are shown superimposed in each group. Mean amplitude in each group is regarded as a consult. A: LC, B: NC, C: AL, D: AH.

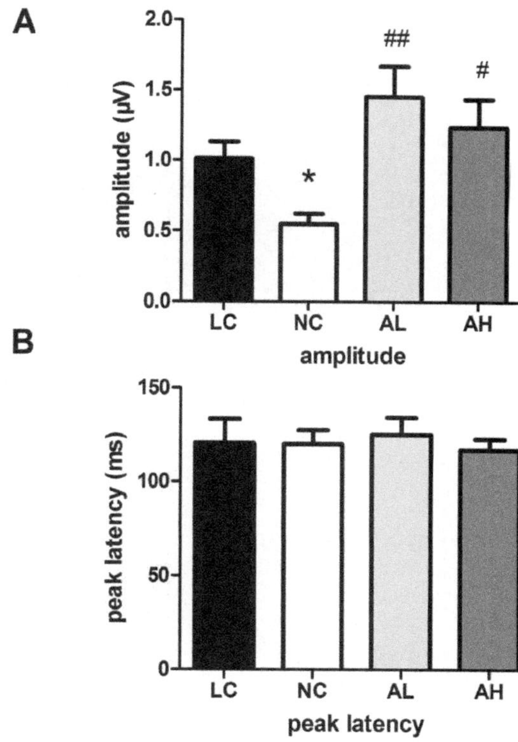

Figure 4. Effects of Astragaloside IV on pattern ERG outcomes. Data are expressed as the mean ± SD. A. Pattern ERG amplitudes in all groups. NC group received significantly decreased amplitudes compared with LC group (NC vs LC, p = 0.037, * p<0.05). Mice in Astragaloside IV treatment groups have increased amplitudes compared with NC group (AL, AH vs NC, p = 0.005, 0.037 respectively. ## p<0.01; # p<0.05). Amplitudes have no significance between AL and AH group. B. Pattern ERG latency in all groups. Astragaloside IV treatment changed the latency, but latency levels did not reveal a statistically significant difference.

Axon Instruments, USA) until glass chips were completely dry and the chips were scanned on a GenePix ×4000 scanner (GenePix 4000B, Axon Instruments, USA) and the images were analyzed with GenePix Pro 6.0 (Axon Inxtruments, USA). After subtracting background signals and normalization to positive controls, comparison of signal intensities between and among array images can be used to determine relative differences in expression levels of each protein between groups. Any ≥1.5-fold increase or ≤0.65-fold decrease in signal intensity for a single analyte between samples or groups may be considered a measurable and significant difference in expression, provided that both sets of signals are well above background.

Statistical Analysis

The results were expressed as mean ± SD. A comparison between two groups was performed using the two-sided t test and a comparison among multiple groups was subjected to one way analysis of variance (ANOVA) followed by a Kruskal–Wallis Test, with $P<0.05$ considered statistically significant. Data were analyzed using SPSS 19.0 version.

Results

Status of Body Weight and Blood Glucose

As can be seen from Fig 2A, mean weights of LC group were less than half of that in db/db mice groups from 8 weeks to 28 weeks. Compared with NC group, AL and AH groups showed less body weight gain from 12 weeks old. The blood glucose levels in NC group were significantly different from that of LC group since 8 weeks. At 8 weeks, there was no difference of glucose levels in all db/db mice groups (Fig. 2B). From 12-week-old to 24-week-old, mice in AH group had decreased blood glucose levels compared with NC group, while at 28-week-old, mice in each db/db mice group showed no difference (AL vs. NC, $P = 0.996$; AH vs. NC, $p = 0.082$, respectively). However, in AH group, blood glucose at 28 weeks showed a significant difference compared to baseline (AH: 28 weeks vs. 8 weeks, $p<0.01$).

Electroretinograms and TUNEL-Positive Cells

Individual waveforms of each eye are shown superimposed in each group (Fig. 3). Fig. 4 shows the measurement of the pattern ERG implicit time and amplitudes at 28 weeks after treatment in the mouse retina. In LC group, the mean amplitude of P_{50} was about 0.99±0.55 μV; the implicit time of P_{50} was about 120.86±33.62 ms. In NC group, the results were changed into 0.55±0.22 μV and 120.33±21.91 ms. In AL and AH groups, the results were changed into 1.45±0.72 μV, 125.45±30.32 ms; 1.24±0.53 μV, 117.50±17.98 ms, respectively. Amplitudes significantly reduced ($p = 0.037$) in NC group when compared with LC group, indicating the reduced activity of the survival RGCs or the lack of activity of lost RGCs. Amplitudes in AL and AH groups were significantly increased compared with NC group ($p = 0.005$, 0.037, respectively). AS IV treatment shortened pattern ERG latency, but the change latency levels did not reveal a statistically significance. In Fig. 5, the detection of DNA damage by TUNEL staining indicated that diabetes could induce the apoptosis of RGCs and AS IV decreased the apoptosis of RGCs in retina.

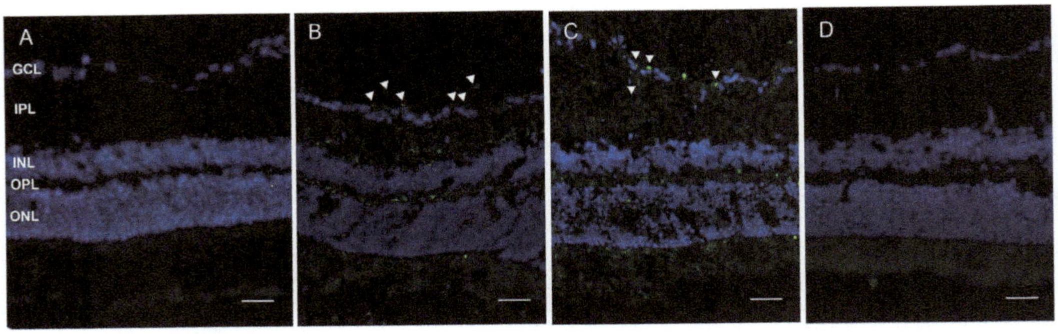

Figure 5. The effect of astragaloside IV on the apoptosis of retina cells. Apoptotic cells were marked with green fluorescence, the nuclei of cells are stained by blue fluorescence (DAPI). A: LC, B: NC, C: AL, D: AH. GCL, retinal ganglion cell layer; IPL, inner plexiform layer; INL, inner nuclear layer; OPL, outer plexiform layer; ONL, outer nuclear layer. Original magnification: ×20; scale bar, 100 mm. Triangles: Apoptotic cells.

AR Activity and Responses of Signal Regulators in DR

AR activity assay demonstrated a difference between NC group and LC group. AR activity in retina of LC, NC, AL, and AH groups were 17.53±1.12, 22.61±2.29, 20.51±1.58, and 18.07±1.63 U/g protein respectively. Statistic significance was found between LC and NC groups, NC and AH groups ($p = 0.026$, 0.025, respectively.). AR activity in blood was consistent with that in retina (Table 1). Further analysis of the NF-κB pathway implied the pathogenesis of diabetic retinopathy [34–36]. As demonstrated in Fig. 6, NF-κB was significantly upregulated in diabetic retinas compared to LC controls. NF-κB expression in the retinas of NC group was increased by about 75.6% compared to LC group. But in AL and AH groups, the expression were decreased. ERK1/2 phosphorylation was activated in NC group compared with LC group ($p = 0.038$), while in AH groups, it showed significantly decrease compared with NC group ($p = 0.025$). The analysis of downstream cytokines of NF-κB and ERK1/2 also showed increased expression of IL-1, IL-6,VEGF,VCAM-1,TNF-βand MMPs in LC compared with NC group (Table 2), but decreased expression in AH compared with NC group.

Discussion

AS IV has been shown to possess many pharmacological properties, including anti-diabetes [28], antivirus [37], anti-ischemic injury, [38] and anti-inflammation [39]. The anti-inflammatory effect of As IV in DN in STZ-induced diabetic rats has already been reported [27]. The present study demonstrated that AS IV, act as an inhibitor of AR, prevent the activation of ERK1/2 phosporylation and NF-kB, and further relieve the RGCs disfunction in db/db mice with DR.

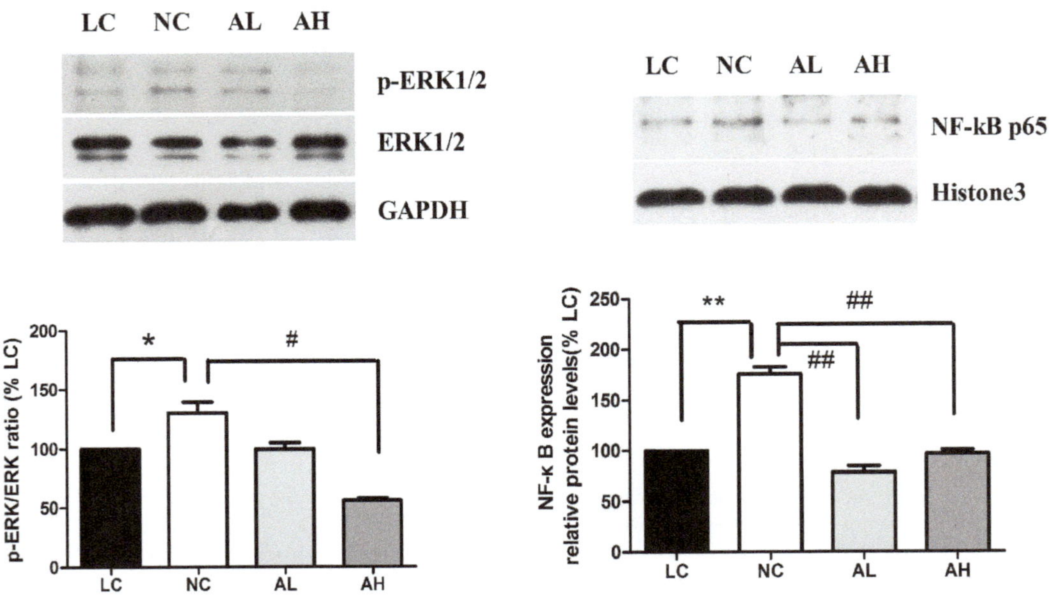

Figure 6. Effects of astragaloside IV on the changes in retina protein. p-ERK/ERK ratio (left) and NF-κB (right) expression in retina protein determined by Western blot. Upper panels are the representative immunoblots of proteins in this area. Bottom graphs show the mean p-ERK/ERK ratio or densitometric quantification of the corresponding bands. GAPDH or Histone3 was used as a loading control. The mean for proteins in db/m mice (LC group) retina was set at 100%. A. p-ERK/ERK ratio: NC vs. LC, $p = 0.038$. * $p < 0.05$; AL, AH vs NC, $p = 0.126$, 0.025 respectively. $n = 3$, # $p < 0.05$). B. NF-κB: NC vs. LC, $p = 0.001$. ** $p < 0.01$; AL, AH vs. NC, $p = 0.001$, 0.004 respectively. $n = 3$, ## $p < 0.01$).

Table 1. Effects of astragaloside IV on dissolve blood Aldose reductase (AR) and retina AR activity (mean with SD) in db/db mice.

Group	N	Blood AR activity (U/g HB)	Retina AR activity (U/g protein)
LC	12	1856.01±61.76	17.53±1.12
NC	12	2192.24±22.25**	22.61±2.29*
AL	12	2088.80±37.47##	20.51±1.58
AH	12	1845.47±39.46##	18.07±1.63#

There is a difference between NC and LC group in AR activity (NC vs. LC, p = 0.000, 0.026 in blood AR, retina AR respectively. ** $p<0.01$; * $p<0.05$). Astragaloside IV treatment showed a significance in AR activity compared with NC group. (blood AR: AL, AH vs. NC, p = 0.000, 0.000 respectively. Significance also showed in AL and AH groups. p = 0.000. ## $p<0.01$; retina AR: AL, AH vs. NC, p = 0.218, 0.025 respectively. No significance between AL and AH groups. p = 0.159. # $p<0.05$).

The db/db mouse is the most widely used mouse model of type 2 diabetes since 1966 [40], especially in DN [41]. As a successful DR model, db/db mouse has been used to investigate the pathogenesis progress in many studies [42–46]. Clements used db/db mice to state that Anti-glycated albumin therapy offered prophylaxis against the early changes of diabetic retinopathy [43]. Li used db/db mice to investigate the potential role of lovastatin in diabetic retinopathy in type 2 diabetes [44,45]. Xiao and Fletcher evaluated retinal neuronal dysfunction in db/db mice [46,47]. In our study, compared with LC group, higher weight gain and blood glucose levels in NC group indicated the success of this model.

Evidence suggests that retinal neurodegeneration is an early event in the pathogenesis of DR [11,47–49]. Several authors have also reported the presence of retinal neurodegeneration (apoptosis, glial activation and retinal thinning) in db/db mice[50,51]. Pattern ERG acts as an useful tool to detect the disfunction of RGCs. Recently, Bogdanov et al. [52] have obtained the features of the neurodegenerative process in db/db mice via ERG recording. Our pattern ERG demonstrated that AS IV treatment largely slowed down the dysfunction of RGCs, which is consistent with previous reports. Furthermore, the detection of DNA damage by Tunel staining has also concerned it.

So far, the mechanism of AS IV alleviates diabetes-induced neuronal injury was still unclear. Naeser et al. demonstrated that AR participated in the degeneration of the optic nerve [53], Yu et al. showed inhibitory effects of AS IV on diabetic peripheral neuropathy in rats, which related to the decrease of AR [28]. In the present study, AS IV treatment significantly inhibited activation of AR and the overexpression of NF-κB and ERK1/2 phosphorylation. MAPKs are stress-related kinases, and members of the MAPKs subfamily (JNK, p38, and ERK1/2) have been implicated in neuronal injury and diseases [54]. ERK1/2 is activated by oxidative stress, mitogens, and survival factors, and that regulates cell proliferation and differentiation [55]. Inhibitors of ERKs cooperatively regulated the transactivation potential of the NF-kB p65 subunit [56]. Researches have commented that ERK (MAPK) mediated alterations in early feature of DR [57]. ERK pathway plays a critical role in the induction of processes such as apoptosis. NF-κB is a major transcriptional factor regulating many proinflammatory cytokines, chemokines, and adhesion molecules. Down regulation of IL-1, IL-6, VEGF, VCAM-1, TNF-β and MMPs in our study might linked to the apoptosis of the RGCs.

In conclusion, our data demonstrated the anti-inflammatory and neuroprotective function of AS IV in db/db mice with DR. Therefore, we propose that AS IV, an inhibitor of AR, may act as an potential therapeutic approach for the treatment of DR. Further clinical trials are needed for investigating the clinical efficacy of AS IV.

Table 2. Partial list of related cytokine.

Cytokine	db/m	db/db	db/db + astragaloside IV (9 mg/kg)	ratio1 (NC/LC)	ratio2 (AH/NC)	tendency
IL-1α	2499	4096	2702	1.64	0.65	Down-regulation
IL-1β	1557	2710	1806	1.74	0.67	down-regulation
IL-6	8976	19529	12573	2.18	0.64	down-regulation
VEGF	1029	2241	1131	2.18	0.50	down-regulation
VEGF-D	1397	2236	1433	1.60	0.64	down-regulation
VCAM-1	1893	3083	2016	1.63	0.65	down-regulation
TNF-β	1804	3089	1976	1.71	0.64	down-regulation
MMP-2	1246	2494	1488	2.00	0.60	down-regulation
MMP-3	1273	2361	1471	1.85	0.62	down-regulation
MMP-12	1177	2313	1388	1.97	0.60	down-regulation
MMP-24	2357	4014	2506	1.70	0.62	down-regulation

Cytokine expression changed in db/db mice and reversed by Astragaloside IV.

Acknowledgments

We thank prof. Yindi Zhang at the Department of Pharmacology, Nanjing Medical University for technical assistance in confirming the daily dosage and making critical comments on this manuscript.

Author Contributions

Conceived and designed the experiments: YZD STY YL. Performed the experiments: YZD XYL PAM QH YF QLS DQY PX. Analyzed the data: YZD XYL RHZ QHL CZ. Contributed reagents/materials/analysis tools: STY PAM YF CZ. Wrote the paper: YZD STY YL QHL CZ.

References

1. Madsen-Bouterse SA, Kowluru RA (2008) Oxidative stress and diabetic retinopathy: pathophysiological mechanisms and treatment perspectives. Reviews in endocrine & metabolic disorders 9: 315–327.
2. Antonetti DA, Barber AJ, Bronson SK, Freeman WM, Gardner TW, et al. (2006) Diabetic retinopathy: seeing beyond glucose-induced microvascular disease. Diabetes 55: 2401–2411.
3. Cheung N, Mitchell P, Wong TY (2010) Diabetic retinopathy. Lancet 376: 124–136.
4. Romero-Aroca P, Sagarra-Alamo R, Basora-Gallisa J, Basora-Gallisa T, Baget-Bernaldiz M, et al. (2010) Prospective comparison of two methods of screening for diabetic retinopathy by nonmydriatic fundus camera. Clinical ophthalmology 4: 1481–1488.
5. Resnikoff S, Pascolini D, Etya'ale D, Kocur I, Pararajasegaram R, et al. (2004) Global data on visual impairment in the year 2002. Bulletin of the World Health Organization 82: 844–851.
6. The Diabetes Control and Complications Trial Research Group (1993) The effect of intensive treatment of diabetes on the development and progression of long-term complications in insulin-dependent diabetes mellitus. The New England journal of medicine 329: 977–986.
7. UK Prospective Diabetes Study (UKPDS) Group (1998) Intensive blood-glucose control with sulphonylureas or insulin compared with conventional treatment and risk of complications in patients with type 2 diabetes (UKPDS 33). Lancet 352: 837–853.
8. Newman EA (2003) New roles for astrocytes: regulation of synaptic transmission. Trends in neurosciences 26: 536–542.
9. Bearse MA Jr, Han Y, Schneck ME, Barez S, Jacobsen C, et al. (2004) Local multifocal oscillatory potential abnormalities in diabetes and early diabetic retinopathy. Investigative ophthalmology & visual science 45: 3259–3265.
10. Han Y, Adams AJ, Bearse MA Jr, Schneck ME (2004) Multifocal electroretinogram and short-wavelength automated perimetry measures in diabetic eyes with little or no retinopathy. Archives of ophthalmology 122: 1809–1815.
11. Barber AJ, Lieth E, Khin SA, Antonetti DA, Buchanan AG, et al. (1998) Neural apoptosis in the retina during experimental and human diabetes. Early onset and effect of insulin. The Journal of clinical investigation 102: 783–791.
12. Abu-El-Asrar AM, Dralands L, Missotten L, Al-Jadaan IA, Geboes K (2004) Expression of apoptosis markers in the retinas of human subjects with diabetes. Investigative ophthalmology & visual science 45: 2760–2766.
13. Park SH, Park JW, Park SJ, Kim KY, Chung JW, et al. (2003) Apoptotic death of photoreceptors in the streptozotocin-induced diabetic rat retina. Diabetologia 46: 1260–1268.
14. Zeng XX, Ng YK, Ling EA (2000) Neuronal and microglial response in the retina of streptozotocin-induced diabetic rats. Visual neuroscience 17: 463–471.
15. Krady JK, Basu A, Allen CM, Xu Y, LaNoue KF, et al. (2005) Minocycline reduces proinflammatory cytokine expression, microglial activation, and caspase-3 activation in a rodent model of diabetic retinopathy. Diabetes 54: 1559–1565.
16. Zhang J, Gerhardinger C, Lorenzi M (2002) Early complement activation and decreased levels of glycosylphosphatidylinositol-anchored complement inhibitors in human and experimental diabetic retinopathy. Diabetes 51: 3499–3504.
17. Gerhardinger C, Costa MB, Coulombe MC, Toth I, Hoehn T, et al. (2005) Expression of acute-phase response proteins in retinal Muller cells in diabetes. Investigative ophthalmology & visual science 46: 349–357.
18. Tang J, Kern TS (2011) Inflammation in diabetic retinopathy. Progress in retinal and eye research 30: 343–358.
19. Kuzumoto Y1, Kusunoki S, Kato N, Kihara M, Low PA. (2006) Effect of the aldose reductase inhibitor fidarestat on experimental diabetic neuropathy in the rat. Diabetologia. 49: 3085–3093.
20. Tiwari AK, Kumar DA, Sweeya PS, Chauhan HA, Lavanya V, et al. (2014) Vegetables' juice influences polyol pathway by multiple mechanisms in favour of reducing development of oxidative stress and resultant diabetic complications. Pharmacognosy Magazine. 10: 383–391.
21. Chang KC, Ponder J, Labarbera DV, Petrash JM (2014) Aldose reductase inhibition prevents endotoxin-induced inflammatory responses in retinal microglia. Investigative ophthalmology & visual science. 55: 2853–2861.
22. Noh HL, Hu Y, Park TS, DiCioccio T, Nichols AJ, Okajima K, et al. (2009) Regulation of plasma fructose and mortality in mice by the aldose reductase inhibitor lidorestat. journal of pharmacology and experimental therapeutics. 328: 496–503.
23. Sango K, Suzuki T, Yanagisawa H, Takaku S, Hirooka H, et al. (2006) High glucose-induced activation of the polyol pathway and changes of gene expression profiles in immortalized adult mouse Schwann cells IMS32. Journal of neurochemistry. 98: 446–458.
24. Lv L, Wu SY, Wang GF, Zhang JJ, Pang JX, et al. (2010) Effect of astragaloside IV on hepatic glucose-regulating enzymes in diabetic mice induced by a high-fat diet and streptozotocin. Phytotherapy research: PTR 24: 219–224.
25. Motomura K, Fujiwara Y, Kiyota N, Tsurushima K, Takeya M, et al. (2009) Astragalosides isolated from the root of astragalus radix inhibit the formation of advanced glycation end products. Journal of agricultural and food chemistry 7: 7666–7672.
26. Gui D, Guo Y, Wang F, Liu W, Chen J, et al. (2012) Astragaloside IV, a Novel Antioxidant, Prevents Glucose Induced Podocyte Apoptosis In Vitro and In Vivo. PLoS One. 2012; 7(6): e39824.
27. Gui D, Huang J, Guo Y, Chen J, Chen Y, et al. (2013) Astragaloside IV ameliorates renal injury in streptozotocin-induced diabetic rats through inhibiting NF-kappaB-mediated inflammatory genes expression. Cytokine 2013;61: 970–977.
28. Yu J, Zhang Y, Sun S, Shen J, Qiu J, et al. (2006) Inhibitory effects of astragaloside IV on diabetic peripheral neuropathy in rats. Canadian journal of physiology and pharmacology 84: 579–587.
29. Porciatti V, Saleh M, Nagaraju M (2007) The pattern electroretinogram as a tool to monitor progressive retinal ganglion cell dysfunction in the DBA/2J mouse model of glaucoma. Investigative ophthalmology & visual science 48: 745–751.
30. Li GY, Fan B, Su GF (2009) Acute energy reduction induces caspase-dependent apoptosis and activates p53 in retinal ganglion cells (RGC-5). Experimental eye research 89: 581–589.
31. Ji Y, Lu G, Chen G, Huang B, Zhang X, et al. (2011) Microcystin-LR Induces Apoptosis via NF-kappaB/iNOS Pathway in INS-1 Cells. International journal of molecular sciences 12: 4722–4734.
32. Yin X, Zhang Y, Wu H, Zhu X, Zheng X, et al. (2004) Protective effects of Astragalus saponin I on early stage of diabetic nephropathy in rats. Journal of pharmacological sciences 95: 256–266.
33. Huang R, Jiang W, Yang J, Mao YQ, Zhang Y, et al. (2010) A biotin label-based antibody array for high-content profiling of protein expression. Cancer genomics & proteomics 7: 129–141.
34. Dong N, Chang L, Wang B, Chu L. (2014) Retinal neuronal MCP-1 induced by AGEs stimulates TNF-α expression in rat microglia via p38, ERK, and NF-κB pathways. Mol Vis. 20: 616–628.
35. Basavarajappa HD, Lee B, Fei X, Lim D, Callaghan B, et al. (2014) Synthesis and mechanistic studies of a novel homoisoflavanone inhibitor of endothelial cell growth. PLoS One. 2014 Apr 21 9(4): e95694.
36. Kim J, Kim CS, Sohn E, Lee YM, Jo K, et al. (2014) Aminoguanidine protects against apoptosis of retinal ganglion cells in Zucker diabetic fatty rats. Eur Rev Med Pharmacol Sci. 18: 1573–1578.
37. Wang S, Li J, Huang H, Gao W, Zhuang C, et al. (2009) Anti-hepatitis B virus activities of astragaloside IV isolated from radix Astragali. Biological & pharmaceutical bulletin 32: 132–135.
38. Luo Y, Qin Z, Hong Z, Zhang X, Ding D, et al. (2004) Astragaloside IV protects against ischemic brain injury in a murine model of transient focal ischemia. Neuroscience letters 363: 218–223.
39. Zhang WJ, Hufnagl P, Binder BR, Wojta J (2003) Antiinflammatory activity of astragaloside IV is mediated by inhibition of NF-kappaB activation and adhesion molecule expression. Thrombosis and haemostasis. 90: 904–914.
40. Hummel KP, Dickie MM, Coleman DL (1966) Diabetes, a new mutation in the mouse. Science. 153: 1127–1128.
41. Tesch GH, Lim AK (2011) Recent insights into diabetic renal injury from the db/db mouse model of type 2 diabetic nephropathy. American journal of physiology Renal physiology. 300: 301–310.
42. Robinson R, Barathi VA, Chaurasia SS, Wong TY, Kern TS (2012) Update on animal models of diabetic retinopathy: from molecular approaches to mice and higher mammals. Dis Model Mech. 5: 444–456.
43. Clements RS Jr, Robison WG Jr, Cohen MP (1998) Anti-glycated albumin therapy ameliorates early retinal microvascular pathology in db/db mice. J Diabetes Complications. 12: 28–33.
44. Li J, Wang JJ, Chen D, Mott R, Yu Q, et al. (2009) Systemic administration of HMG-CoA reductase inhibitor protects the blood-retinal barrier and ameliorates retinal inflammation in type 2 diabetes. Exp Eye Res. 89: 71–78.
45. Li J, Wang JJ, Yu Q, Chen K, Mahadev K, et al. (2010) Inhibition of reactive oxygen species by Lovastatin downregulates vascular endothelial growth factor expression and ameliorates blood-retinal barrier breakdown in db/db mice: role of NADPH oxidase 4. Diabetes. 59: 1528–1538.
46. Xiao C, He M, Nan Y, Zhang D, Chen B, et al. (2012) Physiological effects of superoxide dismutase on altered visual function of retinal ganglion cells in db/db mice. PLoS One. 7:e30343.

47. Fletcher EL, Phipps JA, Ward MM, Puthussery T, Wilkinson-Berka JL, et al. (2007) Neuronal and glial cell abnormality as predictors of progression of diabetic retinopathy. Curr Pharm Des. 13: 2699–2712.
48. Barber AJ, Gardner TW, Abcouwer SF (2011) The significance of vascular and neural apoptosis to the pathology of diabetic retinopathy. Invest Ophthalmol Vis Sci. 52: 1156–1163.
49. Antonetti DA, Klein R, Gardner TW (2012) Diabetic retinopathy. N Engl J Med. 366: 1227–1239.
50. Cheung AK, Fung MK, Lo AC, Lam TT, So KF, et al. (2005) Aldose reductase deficiency prevents diabetes-induced blood-retinal barrier breakdown, apoptosis, and glial reactivation in the retina of db/db mice. Diabetes. 54: 3119–3125.
51. Tang L, Zhang Y, Jiang Y, Willard L, Ortiz E, et al. (2011) Dietary wolfberry ameliorates retinal structure abnormalities in db/db mice at the early stage of diabetes. Exp Biol Med (Maywood). 236: 1051–1063.
52. Bogdanov P, Corraliza L, Villena JA, Carvalho AR, Garcia-Arumí J, et al. (2014) The db/db mouse: a useful model for the study of diabetic retinal neurodegeneration. PLoS One. 9:e97302.
53. Naeser P, Brolin SE, Berggren PO (1987) The sorbitol shunt in the retina and the optic nerve of mice with inherited and STZ-induced diabetes. Acta Ophthalmol (Copenh). 65: 693–698.
54. Miloso M, Scuteri A, Foudah D, Tredici G (2008) MAPKs as mediators of cell fate determination: an approach to neurodegenerative diseases. Curr Med Chem 15: 538–548.
55. Luo Y, DeFranco DB (2006) Opposing roles for ERK1/2 in neuronal oxidative toxicity: distinct mechanisms of ERK1/2 action at early versus late phases of oxidative stress. J Biol Chem 281: 16436–16442.
56. Vanden-Berghe W, Plaisance S, Boone E, De Bosscher K, Schmitz ML, et al. (1995) P38 and extracellular signal-regulated kinase mitogen-activated protein kinase pathways are required for nuclear factor- kB p65 transactivation mediated by tumor necrosis factor. Science. 270: 2008–2011.
57. Kim JH, Kim JH, Jun HO, Yu YS, Kim KW (2010) Inhibition of protein kinase C delta attenuates blood-retinal barrier breakdown in diabetic retinopathy. Am J Pathol. 176: 1517–1524.

Glycemic Effects and Safety of L-Glutamine Supplementation with or without Sitagliptin in Type 2 Diabetes Patients

Dorit Samocha-Bonet[1,2]*, Donald J. Chisholm[1,2], Fiona M. Gribble[3], Adelle C. F. Coster[4], Kevin H. Carpenter[5], Graham R. D. Jones[2,6], Jens J. Holst[7], Jerry R. Greenfield[1,2,8]

1 Diabetes and Metabolism Division, Garvan Institute of Medical Research, Sydney, Australia, **2** Faculty of Medicine, UNSW (The University of New South Wales), Sydney, Australia, **3** Cambridge Institute of Medical Research and Department of Clinical Biochemistry, University of Cambridge, Cambridge, United Kingdom, **4** School of Mathematics and Statistics, UNSW (The University of New South Wales), Sydney, Australia, **5** Disciplines of Genetic Medicine & Paediatrics and Child Health, University of Sydney, Sydney, Australia, **6** Department of Chemical Pathology, St. Vincent's Hospital, Sydney, Australia, **7** NNF Center for Basic Metabolic Research, Department of Biomedical Sciences, University of Copenhagen, Panum Institute, Copenhagen, Denmark, **8** Department of Endocrinology and Diabetes Center, St. Vincent's Hospital, Sydney, Australia

Abstract

Background and Aims: L-glutamine is an efficacious glucagon-like peptide (GLP)-1 secretagogue *in vitro*. When administered with a meal, glutamine increases GLP-1 and insulin excursions and reduces postprandial glycaemia in type 2 diabetes patients. The aim of the study was to assess the efficacy and safety of daily glutamine supplementation with or without the dipeptidyl peptidase (DPP)-4 inhibitor sitagliptin in well-controlled type 2 diabetes patients.

Methods: Type 2 diabetes patients treated with metformin (n = 13, 9 men) with baseline glycated hemoglobin (HbA1c) 7.1±0.3% (54±4 mmol/mol) received glutamine (15 g bd)+ sitagliptin (100 mg/d) or glutamine (15 g bd) + placebo for 4 weeks in a randomized crossover study.

Results: HbA1c ($P = 0.007$) and fructosamine ($P = 0.02$) decreased modestly, without significant time-treatment interactions (both $P = 0.4$). Blood urea increased ($P < 0.001$) without a significant time-treatment interaction ($P = 0.8$), but creatinine and estimated glomerular filtration rate (eGFR) were unchanged ($P \geq 0.5$). Red blood cells, hemoglobin, hematocrit, and albumin modestly decreased ($P \leq 0.02$), without significant time-treatment interactions ($P \geq 0.4$). Body weight and plasma electrolytes remained unchanged ($P \geq 0.2$).

Conclusions: Daily oral supplementation of glutamine with or without sitagliptin for 4 weeks decreased glycaemia in well-controlled type 2 diabetes patients, but was also associated with mild plasma volume expansion.

Trial Registration: ClincalTrials.gov NCT00673894

Editor: Noel Christopher Barengo, University of Tolima, Colombia

Funding: The research was supported by a National Health and Medical Research Council (NHMRC) of Australia Project Grant no. 535949 (JRG), Diabetes Australia Research Trust (DART and JRG), and a research grant from the Investigator-Initiated Studies Program of Merck and Co. (Garvan Institute of Medical Research). JRG was supported by a Neil Hamilton Fairley Fellowship from NHMRC and the Don Chisholm Fellowship and DS-B by the Australian Diabetes Society (ADS), the Sachdev Foundation (the Garvan Research Foundation), and the Investigator-Initiated Studies Program of Merck and Co. grant awarded to the Garvan Institute of Medical Research. The funders had no role in study design, data collection and analysis, decision to publish, or preparation of the manuscript.

Competing Interests: Carpenter KH, Coster ACF, and Jones GRD have nothing to declare; Chisholm DJ has been a board member for Astra Zeneca/Bristol Myer Squibb (Member/Chairman of Australian and International Advisory Board) and has received speaker honoraria from Astra Zeneca/Bristol Myers Squibb and MSD; Gribble FM is a board member of BioKier, consultant for Roche, and has received speaker honoraria from Novo Nordisk and Merck, and travel/accommodation expenses from Merck. Holst JJ is a consultant to NovoNordisk and holds grants from Novartis and Merck. Greenfield JR was a Principal Investigator on an Investigator-Initiated Studies Program grant from Merck and Co., awarded to the Garvan Institute of Medical Research, and Samocha-Bonet D was partly supported by this grant.

* Email: d.samochabonet@garvan.org.au

Introduction

Impaired insulin secretion contributes to hyperglycemia in type 2 diabetes. Glucagon-like peptide (GLP)-1 is secreted from intestinal L-cells in response to nutrients and is rapidly degraded by dipeptidyl peptidase (DPP)-4. GLP-1 contributes to myriad of metabolic effects, including insulin secretion, beta cell proliferation, slowing of gastric emptying and increased satiety; all are desirable features of type 2 diabetes therapy [1–3]. GLP-1 receptor agonists and DPP-4 inhibitors are used to treat type 2 diabetes patients. However, enhancement of GLP-1 secretion with meals has the advantage of increasing GLP-1 concentrations in the intestinal milieu, where it is believed to act on vagal neurons and mediate its central effects. Moreover, the cleaved GLP-1 product (9–36), which suppresses hepatic glucose production and exerts antioxidant action [4], may also be enhanced by agents that increase GLP-1 secretion.

The amino acid L-glutamine is an efficacious GLP-1 secretagogue for the colonic L-cells model GLUTag [5] and primary murine colonic culture [6]. Well-controlled type 2 diabetes patients have intact GLP-1 response to glutamine ingestion [7] and glutamine (30 g) or glutamine (15 g) in combination with the DPP-4 inhibitor sitagliptin (100 mg) decreases postprandial glycaemia and increases circulating insulin and GLP-1 when administered with a meal [8].

The primary aim of this randomized crossover study was to determine the glycemic effect of 4 weeks of glutamine (15 bd) supplementation with sitagliptin (100 mg/d) or placebo in type 2 diabetes patients treated with metformin. We hypothesized that both treatments will decrease hemoglobin A1c (HbA1c) and fructosamine, with a greater effect exhibited in the combined glutamine-sitagliptin treatment, due to more pronounced postprandial increases in GLP-1 in the circulation. The secondary aim was to evaluate the safety of glutamine supplementation.

Methods

This study was conducted according to the principles expressed in the declaration of Helsinki. The study was approved by the Human Research and Ethics Committee at St Vincent's Hospital, Sydney. All participants gave written informed consent prior to commencement of the study. The protocol for this study and supporting CONSORT checklist are available as supporting information (Checklist S1 and Protocol S1). The study was registered at www.ClinicalTrials.gov (NCT00673894).

Participants

Type 2 diabetes patients were recruited through advertisements at the St Vincent's Hospital precinct, Sydney and in local newspapers. Participants were recruited and followed between January 2010 and November 2011. Inclusion criteria were age 40–70 years, short diabetes duration (5 years or less), treatment with metformin in a stable dose (≤2000 mg/d) for at least 3 months, HbA1c 6.5–9% (48–75 mmol/mol), BMI ≤40 kg/m^2 and stable body weight in the preceding 6 months (±2 kg). Exclusion criteria were treatment with oral hypoglycemic agents other than metformin, ethanol intake of 40 g/d or more, liver or kidney disease or abnormal full blood count, renal or liver function tests, use of weight loss medications, previous bowel surgery or documented malabsorption. Of the 108 individuals pre-screened for eligibility over the telephone, 22 were invited to a screening visit at the clinic. Fifteen participants (Caucasian, 10 men) were included and 13 (9 men) completed the study (Figure 1).

Trial design

The primary endpoints of this study were the glycemic control markers HbA1c and fructosamine, determined as below (Laboratory Analyses). Two treatments were considered in the study and randomized crossover design was applied (Figure 2). Participants received glutamine (15 g bd) with sitagliptin (100 mg) or placebo. Treatment allocation order was randomized according to a randomization sequence provided by Merck. A nurse not involved directly with the study was in charge of distribution of sequentially numbered containers of sitagliptin or placebo to participants and kept a list with participants' identification numbers and treatment

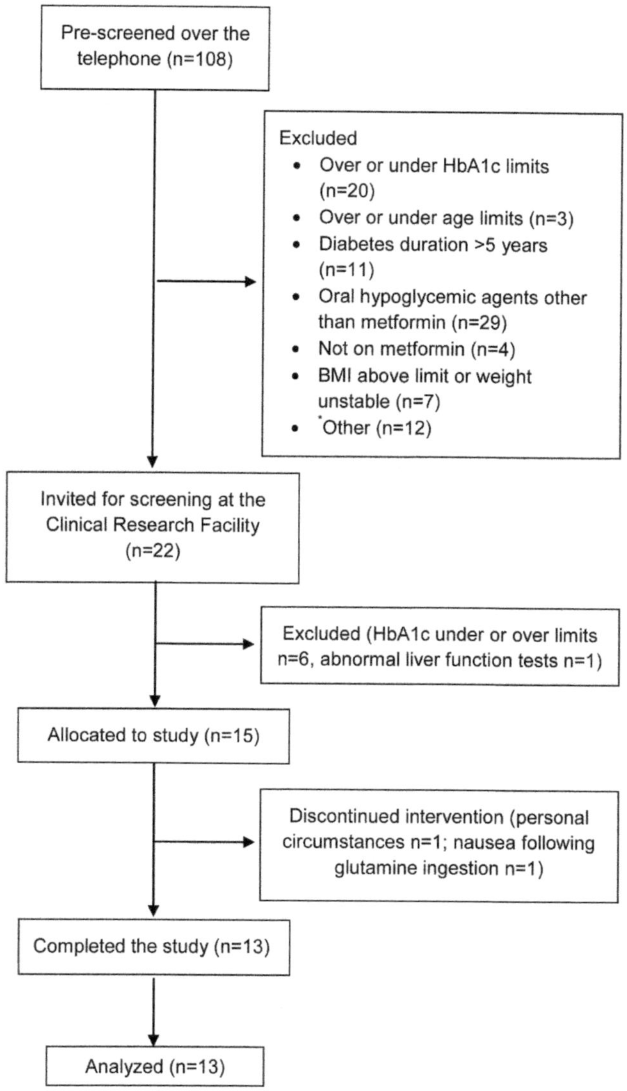

Figure 1. Flow of participants in the study. *Other reasons include participant not able to take time off work or other engagements (n = 3), family not approving (n = 2), underlying disease (n = 3), weight unstable or actively trying to lose weight (n = 2), change of mind (n = 1) and inability to provide informed consent (n = 1).

sequence allocation. Study participants, investigators and nurses were blinded to the treatment allocation order. HbA1c and fructosamine levels were determined at baseline (control). Participants were then administered their first treatment over a 4 week period. Endpoint levels were then determined. This period was followed by a 4–6 week washout period. The second treatment trial then followed using the same protocol.

Procedures

Screening study was performed at the Clinical Research Facility at the Garvan Institute of Medical Research and included weight, height and blood pressure measurements, and medical examination. Blood was drawn for renal and liver function tests, full blood count, and HbA1c. Participants were provided with lead-in placebo tablets and instructed to take 1 tablet 15 min before breakfast for two weeks preceding each baseline study (lead-in, Figure 2). On day 0 and 4-weeks of each study participants

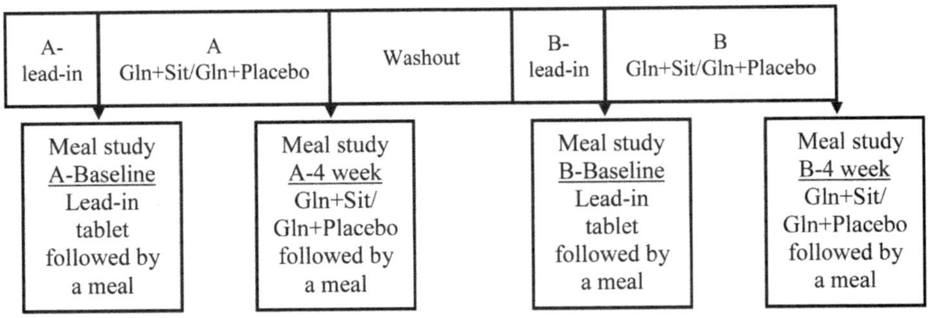

Figure 2. Study timeline. The effect of glutamine with sitagliptin or placebo was assessed in a randomized crossover study. Each study period (A and B) was initiated with 2-weeks lead-in followed by L-glutamine (Gln) 15 g with breakfast and dinner with either sitagliptin (Sit; 100 mg) or placebo for 4 weeks. Participants visited the Clinical Research Facility at day 0 (Baseline) and 4-weeks of studies A and B for a meal challenge. Treatments were randomly assigned with a 4–6 week washout period between A and B studies.

attended the Clinical Research Facility fasting from 22:00 h the previous night for a meal challenge (Figure 2). Weight, height and blood pressure were measured and indirect calorimetry performed following 30 min of supine rest (Parvomedics, UT, USA). Heart rate was measured by a SphygmoCor device (AtCor Medical, Australia). A large-bore intravenous indwelling cannula was inserted into a large antecubital vein for blood sampling. Blood was collected for glycemic markers, full blood count, liver and renal function tests and glutamine. After drawing blood twice 10 min apart at baseline for blood glucose, serum insulin and plasma GLP-1 measurements, the lead-in placebo tablet on day 0 or the tablet taken during the study on the 4-weeks visits was taken in 300 ml of cold water and followed by a low fat meal comprising 33 g Wheat-Bix (Sanitarium) and 250 mL low fat milk, providing 230 kcal (37 g carbohydrate, 1.3 g fat and 16 g protein), as described previously [8]. Meal was consumed within 8 min and blood samples were drawn at 15, 30, 45, 60, 90, 120, 150 and 180 min. At completion of A-Baseline and B-Baseline studies (Figure 2), participants were provided with 4 weeks' worth of study tablets and L-glutamine (Cambridge Commodities, Cambridge, United Kingdom) and instructed to fill compliance lists and diet diaries. At home, during A and B studies, participants took sitagliptin (100 mg) or placebo 15 min prior to L-glutamine (15 g), followed by their normal breakfast. L-glutamine (15 g) was taken again 15 min prior to dinner. Meal challenge at 4 weeks of A and B studies was repeated, but participants received not only the tablet they had been taking in the preceding 4 weeks, but also glutamine (15 g) followed by the meal (Figure 2).

Compliance, diet and physical activity monitoring

Participants were instructed not to change their eating habits and physical activity levels during the study to avoid confounding effects of diet and physical activity on glycemic control. They recorded food and drinks consumed during 6 days in the lead-in and study periods, filled daily compliance lists and were contacted by the research nurse weekly. On clinic study days, participants returned residual tablets and glutamine, and intake of protein-rich food items and physical activity level were assessed by 7-day questionnaires.

Laboratory analyses

HbA1c was analyzed by cation-exchange HPLC using the Variant II analyzer (Bio-Rad Laboratories, Gladesville, NSW, Australia), fructosamine by a nitro-blue tetrazolium method, fasting plasma glucose by a hexokinase method and other biochemistry tests using standard methods on a Roche Modular analyzer using Roche reagents (Roche Diagnostics Australia, Castle Hill, NSW Australia). Full blood count was measured using a Beckman Coulter analyzer (Beckman-Coulter, Gladesville NSW, Australia). Whole blood glucose was assayed immediately after collection by the glucose oxidase electrode (Yellow Springs Instrument Company; Life Sciences). Insulin was measured in sera stored at −80°C by radioimmunoassay (Millipore, St Charles, USA). Blood samples for plasma glutamine were collected into chilled heparin-coated tubes and immediately centrifuged (7 min at 4100 × g), snap frozen and stored at −80°C until analysis. Plasma glutamine was measured by reverse phase ultra-performance liquid chromatography with UV detection (Acquity UPLC, Waters, Rydalmere, NSW, Australia). Plasma was deproteinized with 10% s-sulphosalicylic acid containing norvaline as an internal standard. Amino acids were then derivatized with 6-aminoquinolyl-N-hydroxysuccinimidyl carbamate and separated by gradient elution. Blood samples for total and active GLP-1 were collected into chilled EDTA-coated tubes (with DPP-4 inhibitor and trasylol in the active GLP-1 testing tube) and immediately centrifuged (7 min at 4100 × g), snap-frozen and stored at −80°C until analysis. Total and active GLP-1 concentrations were measured as previously described [8]. Briefly, total GLP-1 was measured by radioimmunoassay after extraction of plasma with 70% ethanol (v:v, final concentration). Carboxy-terminal GLP-1 immunoreactivity was determined using antiserum 89390, which has an absolute requirement for the intact amidated carboxyl terminus of GLP-1 7–36 amide and cross-reacts <0.01% with carboxy-terminally truncated fragments and 89% with GLP-1 9–36 amide, the primary metabolite of DPP-4-mediated degradation. The sum of the two components, total GLP-1 concentration, reflects the rate of secretion of the L-cell [9]. Active GLP-1 was analyzed using an enzyme-linked immunosorbent assay on unextracted plasma, as reported previously [8].

Statistical analysis

Area under the curve (AUC) of postprandial glucose, insulin, insulin-to-glucose ratio, total and active GLP-1 concentrations were calculated using the trapezoidal rule. Insulin data were log10-transformed prior to statistical analysis. All values are presented as means ± standard deviation (SD), unless stated otherwise. An a priori power analysis for the ANOVA repeated measures within-between interaction design ($\alpha = 0.05$, power $= 0.8$) was performed (G*Power version 3.0.10) giving a minimum sample size of 6. The effects of the 4 week supplementation of glutamine with sitagliptin or glutamine with placebo were analyzed using repeated measure ANOVA. For this, the within subject factor was time – detecting differences in measured endpoints at 4 weeks supplementation compared to baseline. The between subjects factor was the treatment (supplementation) type – either glutamine with sitagliptin or glutamine with placebo. The significance (P-values) for both the within subject factor (time), and the interaction of time and treatment is reported. Normal probability plots of the P-values versus their rank were then examined to determine statistical significance (not shown). Relationships that were found to be non-linear were indicative of statistically significant results. The data below P of 0.05 were in the non-linear regions. Data were analyzed using SPSS version 21.

Results

Cohort characteristics

Participants were 65±6 years old with BMI 28±4 kg/m^2 on average. Type 2 diabetes duration was 3.3±1.7 years, HbA1c 7.1±0.3% (54±4 mmol/mol), fasting plasma glucose 7.1±1.0 mmol/L and glutamine 572±67 µmol/L (range 444–677 µmol/L).

The effects of the treatments on HbA1c, fructosamine, fasting plasma glucose and GLP-1

HbA1c and fructosamine decreased modestly, without significant time-treatment interactions. Fasting plasma glucose did not change significantly with the treatments, but there was a significant time-treatment effect (Table 1).

Fasting total GLP-1 increased (4.5±2.8 and 6.5±2.3 pmol/L with glutamine + placebo and 5.3±2.6 and 7.4±2.3 pmol/L with glutamine + sitagliptin at baseline and 4-weeks respectively, $P = 0.006$), without a significant time-treatment interaction ($P = 1$). Fasting active GLP-1 also increased with both treatments (0.4±0.6 and 1.0±1.2 pmol/L with glutamine + placebo and 0.8±1.0 and 2.3±1.6 pmol/L with glutamine + sitagliptin at baseline and 4 weeks, respectively, $P \leq 0.001$), without a significant time-treatment interaction ($P = 0.1$).

The effect of the treatments on postprandial blood glucose, serum insulin and plasma total and active GLP-1

Postprandial glucose AUC decreased ($P = 0.008$), with a significant time-treatment effect ($P = 0.003$, Figure 3A). Postprandial insulin AUC increased ($P < 0.001$), without a significant time-treatment effect ($P = 1$, Figure 3B). Insulin-to-glucose AUC increased ($P = 0.001$), with a significant time-treatment effect ($P = 0.003$, Figure 3C). Postprandial total GLP-1 AUC increased ($P = 0.008$, Figure 3D), without a significant time-treatment effect ($P = 0.2$) and active GLP-1 AUC increased ($P < 0.001$), with a significant time-treatment effect ($P = 0.001$, Figure 3E).

The effects of the treatments on weight, blood pressure, full blood count, electrolytes and renal and liver function

Weight, resting metabolic rate (RMR), respiratory quotient (RQ), systolic and diastolic blood pressure were unchanged. Resting heart rate decreased, without a significant time-treatment effect (Table 1). WBC, RBC, Hb and Hct all decreased, without significant time-treatment interactions (Table 2). There were no effects on the red blood cell characteristics mean corpuscular volume (MCV), mean corpuscular Hb (MCH), mean corpuscular Hb concentration (MCHC) and red cell distribution width (RDW; Table 2). Neutrophil count decreased, without significant time-treatment interaction and lymphocyte count decreased with a significant time-treatment interaction (Table 2). Total protein, albumin, alkaline phosphatase and gamma-glutamyl transpeptidase (GGT) all decreased, without significant time-treatment interactions, while alanine transaminase (ALT), aspartate transaminase (AST) and bilirubin were unchanged (Table 2). There were no significant changes in electrolytes, including sodium, potassium, chloride and bicarbonate (Table 2). Blood urea increased, without a significant time-treatment interaction, but creatinine, and therefore estimated glomerular filtration rate (eGFR), were unchanged (Table 2).

Diet and physical activity during the study

Dietary intake of protein-rich food was not different between baseline and 4-weeks ($P = 0.6$) or between treatment periods

Table 1. Effects of the treatments on glycemic markers, weight and blood pressure.

	Glutamine + Placebo		Glutamine + Sitagliptin		*P* value[1]	
	Baseline	**4-weeks**	**Baseline**	**4-weeks**	**Time**	**Time-Treatment interaction**
HbA1c (%)	7.0±0.4	6.9±0.4	6.9±0.3	6.7±0.3	**0.007**	0.4
HbA1c (mmol/mol)	53±4.3	52±4.3	52±3.6	50±3.6		
Fructosamine (µmol/L)	258±40	244±41	246±32	240±30	**0.02**	0.4
Fasting plasma glucose (mmol/L)	7.1±0.8	7.3±0.9	7.2±1.0	6.7±0.8	0.1	**0.003**
Weight (kg)	82.8±15.7	82.9±15.6	82.9±15.1	82.7±15.3	0.8	0.4
RMR (kcal/d)	1510±300	1480±320	1490±330	1540±400	0.8	0.3
Respiratory quotient	0.80±0.04	0.81±0.03	0.81±0.04	0.81±0.03	0.7	0.5
Systolic blood pressure (mmHg)	138±17	137±11	139±16	134±9	0.2	0.5
Diastolic blood pressure (mmHg)	84±9	84±7	84±12	79±6	0.2	0.2
Heart rate (bpm)	71±8	67±9	71±10	69±6	**0.02**	0.4

Data are means ± SD.
RMR, resting metabolic rate.
[1]Significance of the repeated measure ANOVA with time (within subjects factor) and the interaction of time with treatments (the between subjects factor) is given (n = 13). Bold values represent $P < 0.05$. Normal probability plots of the P-values versus their rank were examined to determine statistical significance. Relationships that were found to be non-linear were indicative of statistically significant results. The data below P of 0.05 were in the non-linear regions.

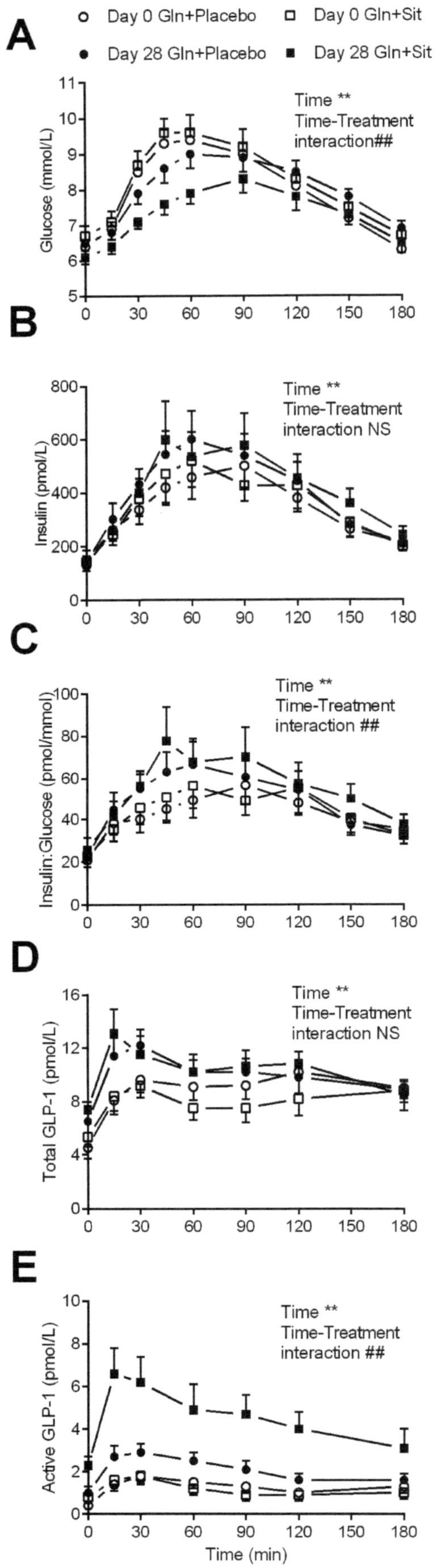

Figure 3. The effect of glutamine + sitagliptin and glutamine + placebo on postprandial circulating concentrations of glucose, insulin and glucagon-like peptide-1. Postprandial circulating concentrations of blood glucose (A), serum insulin (B), insulin to glucose ratio (C) and plasma total and active GLP-1 (D and E, respectively) at baseline (day 0; empty symbols) and 4-weeks (dark symbols) of glutamine + sitagliptin (Gln + Sit; squares) and glutamine + placebo (Gln + Placebo; circles) in type 2 diabetes patients (n = 13). Data are means ± SEM. Significance of the repeated measure ANOVA with time (within subjects factor, $^{**}P<0.01$) and the interaction of time with treatments (the between subjects factor, $^{\#\#}P\leq0.01$) in the AUC is given (n = 13).

($P = 0.7$). Participants were sedentary and physical activity levels were not different at baseline and 4-weeks ($P = 0.3$) or between treatment periods (243±14 and 245±15 metabolic equivalent of tasks (METs) hr/week for glutamine + placebo and 249±18 and 242±16 METs hr/week for glutamine + sitagliptin at baseline and 4-weeks respectively, $P = 0.1$).

Discussion

Daily ingestion of L-glutamine, with or without sitagliptin, for 4 weeks decreased HbA1c and fructosamine in well-controlled type 2 diabetes patients treated with metformin. However, glutamine treatment was also associated with modest decreases in concentrations of circulating blood cells, total protein and albumin, without changes in body weight or plasma electrolytes, suggesting mild plasma volume expansion.

Both glycemic control markers, the longer term HbA1c and the shorter term fructosamine decreased significantly with the treatments in the present study, without a significant difference between treatments. These findings suggest that the reduction in glycaemia was attributed to the glutamine. Notably, HbA1c reduction is expected to be larger if treatment was prolonged as the treatment period of 28 days is under the mean red blood cell age of about 50 days [10]. Fructosamine was added to the panel of glycemic markers because of its shorter half-life. The meal studies revealed that the combined glutamine and sitagliptin treatment was more effective in decreasing postprandial glycaemia and in increasing insulin-to-glucose ratio and active GLP-1. Accordingly, we predict that longer treatments would have likely resulted in more pronounced decreases in glycemic control markers with the combined glutamine-sitagliptin treatment. This is also in line with the decreases in fasting plasma glucose only with the sitagliptin combination, potentially attributed to glucagon inhibition [7,8,11]. Importantly, reductions in the proportion of HbA1c are unaffected by plasma volume expansion, however decreases in fructosamine may have been affected by the general decreases in circulating proteins in the present study.

Safety of glutamine supplementation of enteral or parenteral nutrition was widely studied in critically-ill patients where L-glutamine is used to maintain intestinal integrity, improve nitrogen balance, prevent infections, decrease oxidative stress and improve survival [12]. Glutamine supplementation in critically-ill patients resulted in conflicting findings, including decreased [12], increased [13] or no effect [14] on complications and mortality rates. Type 2 diabetes has been associated with decreases in circulating glutamine previously [15] but, in this well-controlled diabetic cohort plasma glutamine concentrations were within the reference range [15,16]. Glutamine supplementation at levels of 1–30 g/d are safe for several hours post ingestion in physically active healthy populations [16] and type 2 diabetes patients [8]. However, safety data of prolonged glutamine intake in non-critically-ill patients are scarce. Galera and colleagues [17] investigated the safety of 14

Table 2. Effects of the treatments on full blood count, renal and liver function and plasma electrolytes.

Marker (normal range)	Glutamine + Placebo		Glutamine + Sitagliptin		*P* value[1]	
	Baseline	**4-weeks**	**Baseline**	**4-weeks**	**Time**	**Time-Treatment interaction**
WBC (4.0–11.0 .10^9/L)	6.2±1.5	5.8±1.2	6.3±1.5	5.5±1.8	**0.004**	0.4
RBC (4.5–6.5 .10^{12}/L)	4.3±0.4	4.1±0.3	4.3±0.3	4.1±0.3	**0.003**	0.7
Hemoglobin (130–180 g/L)	135±13	129±10	134±12	129±11	**0.001**	0.8
Hematocrit (0.40–0.54%)	0.40±0.04	0.38±0.03	0.39±0.03	0.38±0.03	**0.001**	0.9
MCV (76–96 fL)	92±4	92±3	92±4	91±4	0.8	0.4
MCH (27.0–32.0 pg)	31.2±1.5	31.3±1.5	31.3±1.4	31.2±1.4	0.6	0.3
MCHC (320–360 g/L)	340±5	341±6	342±5	342±4	0.5	0.7
RDW (11.5–14.5%)	13.3±0.5	13.3±0.6	13.2±0.6	13.3±0.7	0.6	0.9
Platelets (150–400 10^9/L)	245±66	240±54	252±56	240±58	0.1	0.4
Neutrophils (2.0–7.5 10^9/L)	3.6±1.0	3.3±0.8	3.7±1.0	3.3±1.5	**0.05**	0.7
Lymphocytes (1.5–4.0 10^9/L)	1.8±0.6	1.8±0.6	1.9±0.5	1.6±0.5	**0.003**	**0.01**
Monocytes (0.2–1.0 10^9/L)	0.6±0.2	0.5±0.1	0.5±0.2	0.5±0.1	0.08	0.1
Total protein (60–82 g/L)	70±4	65±5	69±4	67±4	**<0.001**	0.1
Albumin (36–52 g/L)	45±2	43±3	45±2	44±1	**0.02**	0.4
Alkaline phosphatase (30–100 U/L)	62±21	58±17	64±19	57±18	**<0.001**	0.2
GGT (0–35 U/L)	25±13	22±11	25±17	22±13	**0.01**	0.7
ALT (0–30 U/L)	29±11	27±10	26±12	24±8	0.08	0.9
AST (0–30 U/L)	26±8	25±9	23±6	22±6	0.4	1
Total bilirubin (0–18 μmol/L)	11±7	9±4	10±6	10±6	0.2	**0.02**
Sodium (137–146 mmol/L)	142±2	142±2	141±2	141±2	0.5	0.4
Potassium (3.5–5.0 mmol/L)	4.4±0.3	4.4±0.3	4.7±0.3	4.5±0.2	0.2	0.4
Chloride (95–110 mmol/L)	104±3	105±4	104±2	104±2	0.7	0.2
Bicarbonate (24–31 mmol/L)	26±2	26±2	27±2	26±2	0.2	0.9
Urea (3.0–8.5 mmol/L)	6.1±1.1	7.4±2.0	6.4±0.9	7.8±1.5	**<0.001**	0.8
Creatinine (60–120 μmol/L)	76±17	73±13	75±14	76±14	0.6	0.2
eGFR (mL/min/1.73 m^2)	80±13	81±11	81±10	81±10	0.5	0.6

Data are means ± SD.
WBC, white blood cells; RBC, red blood cells; MCV, mean corpuscular volume; MCH, mean corpuscular hemoglobin; MCHC, mean corpuscular hemoglobin concentration; RDW, red cell distribution width; GGT, gamma-glutamyl transpeptidase; ALT, alanine transaminase; AST, aspartate transaminase.
[1]Significance of the repeated measure ANOVA with time (within subjects factor) and the interaction of time with treatments (the between subjects factor) is given (n = 13). Bold values represent $P<0.05$. Normal probability plots of the *P*-values versus their rank were examined to determine statistical significance. Relationships that were found to be non-linear were indicative of statistically significant results. The data below *P* of 0.05 were in the non-linear regions.

days of glutamine or casein supplementation in healthy, predominantly sedentary, middle age and elderly individuals in dosages slightly higher than those administered here (0.5 g/kg/d). Unlike the present study, serum creatinine concentrations increased and eGFR decreased with glutamine or casein [17], maybe due to the higher protein intake. Similarly to the present study however, blood urea concentrations increased [17], reflecting the increased dietary nitrogen intake. Interestingly, blood cells, Hb, Hct, total protein and albumin concentrations were all decreased with glutamine in the present study. The decreases in red blood cells without changes in MCV, MCH and MCHC and the general decreases in circulating macromolecules suggest intravascular fluid volume expansion, an effect previously documented in piglets with parenteral glutamine supplementation [18]. Notably, body weight and plasma electrolytes were unchanged in the present study, consistent with minor changes in plasma volume or changes in fluid distribution. The mechanisms involved in extracellular fluid volume expansion with glutamine are unclear, but have been suggested to involve increased glomerular sodium reabsorption [18], which with prolonged glutamine ingestion may alter electrolyte concentrations and acid-base regulation. Furthermore, modest decreases in Hb and Hct were also noted previously with high dose glutamine or casein supplementation for 14 days in healthy individuals [17], suggesting that these effects are not limited to glutamine or type 2 diabetes patients. In any case, further study is required to determine the mechanisms involved in the effect of glutamine on plasma volume expansion.

This is the first study to evaluate the effect of daily glutamine supplementation for a period of weeks on glycemic control and safety in type 2 diabetes patients. There are several strengths to the study, including the sitagliptin versus placebo crossover design that enabled investigation of possible interaction between glutamine and DPP-4 inhibition. Furthermore, the homogeneity of the cohort in terms of age, disease duration and background diabetes treatment increased the power to detect the effects of the treatment on the endpoints. The main limitation of the study is the lack of sitagliptin-alone arm. Furthermore, the relatively low baseline

HbA1c and short study duration may have limited the magnitude of change in outcome measures.

In conclusion, daily glutamine administration for 4 weeks decreased HbA1c, irrespective of sitagliptin treatment in well-controlled type 2 diabetes patients treated with metformin. Glutamine administration also resulted in an apparent plasma volume expansion in this population and requires further study.

Supporting Information

Checklist S1 Consort checklist.

Protocol S1 Trial protocol.

Acknowledgments

The authors wish to thank the Clinical Research Facility Head Nurse Ms Lynne Schofield and the study nurses Ms Olivia Wong, Ms Jennifer Evans and Ms Renee Richens, all from the Garvan Institute of Medical Research. We also thank Dr Amanda Brandon for helpful discussions.

Author Contributions

Conceived and designed the experiments: DS-B DJC JRG. Performed the experiments: DS-B JJH KHC GRDJ JRG. Analyzed the data: DS-B ACFC. Contributed reagents/materials/analysis tools: JJH KHC GRDJ. Wrote the paper: DS-B DJC JRG. Contributed to discussion: FMG JJH GRDJ.

References

1. Drucker DJ (2006) The biology of incretin hormones. Cell Metabolism 3: 153–165.
2. Holst JJ, Vilsboll T, Deacon CF (2009) The incretin system and its role in type 2 diabetes mellitus. Mol Cell Endocrinol 297: 127–136.
3. Nauck MA, Baller B, Meier JJ (2004) Gastric inhibitory polypeptide and glucagon-like peptide-1 in the pathogenesis of type 2 diabetes. Diabetes 53 Suppl 3: S190–196.
4. Thomas E, Habener JF (2010) Insulin-like actions of glucagon-like peptide-1: a dual receptor hypothesis. Trend Endocrinol Metab 21: 59–68.
5. Reimann F, Williams L, da Silva Xavier G, Rutter GA, Gribble FM (2004) Glutamine potently stimulates glucagon-like peptide-1 secretion from GLUTag cells. Diabetologia 47: 1592–1601.
6. Tolhurst G, Zheng Y, Parker HE, Habib AM, Reimann F, et al. (2011) Glutamine triggers and potentiates glucagon-like peptide-1 secretion by raising cytosolic Ca2+ and cAMP. Endocrinology 152: 405–413.
7. Greenfield JR, Farooqi IS, Keogh JM, Henning E, Habib AM, et al. (2009) Oral glutamine increases circulating glucagon-like peptide 1, glucagon, and insulin concentrations in lean, obese, and type 2 diabetic subjects. Am J Clin Nutr 89: 106–113.
8. Samocha-Bonet D, Wong O, Synnott EL, Piyaratna N, Douglas A, et al. (2011) Glutamine reduces postprandial glycemia and augments the glucagon-like peptide-1 response in type 2 diabetes patients. J Nutr 141: 1233–1238.
9. Orskov C, Rabenhoj L, Wettergren A, Kofod H, Holst JJ (1994) Tissue and plasma concentrations of amidated and glycine-extended glucagon-like peptide I in humans. Diabetes 43: 535–539.
10. Cohen RM, Franco RS, Khera PK, Smith EP, Lindsell CJ, et al. (2008) Red cell life span heterogeneity in hematologically normal people is sufficient to alter HbA1c. Blood 112: 4284–4291.
11. Solis-Herrera C, Triplitt C, Garduno-Garcia JdJ, Adams J, DeFronzo RA, et al. (2013) Mechanisms of Glucose Lowering of Dipeptidyl Peptidase-4 Inhibitor Sitagliptin When Used Alone or With Metformin in Type 2 Diabetes: A double-tracer study. Diabetes Care 36: 2756–2762.
12. Novak F, Heyland DK, Avenell A, Drover JW, Su X (2002) Glutamine supplementation in serious illness: a systematic review of the evidence. Crit Care Med 30: 2022–2029.
13. Heyland D, Drover J, Dhaliwal R (2006) Does the addition of glutamine to enteral feeds affect patient mortality? Crit Care Med 34: 2031–2032; author reply 2032.
14. Andrews PJD, Avenell A, Noble DW, Campbell MK, Croal BL, et al. (2011) Randomised trial of glutamine, selenium, or both, to supplement parenteral nutrition for critically ill patients. Br Med J 342
15. Menge BA, Schrader H, Ritter PR, Ellrichmann M, Uhl W, et al. (2010) Selective amino acid deficiency in patients with impaired glucose tolerance and type 2 diabetes. Regul Pept 160: 75–80.
16. Gleeson M (2008) Dosing and Efficacy of Glutamine Supplementation in Human Exercise and Sport Training. J Nutr 138: 2045S–2049S.
17. Galera SC, Fechine F, Teixeira MJ, Branco Coelho ZC, de Vasconcelos RC, et al. (2010) The safety of oral use of l-glutamine in middle-aged and elderly individuals. Nutrition 26: 375–381.
18. House JD, Pencharz PB, Ball RO (1994) Glutamine Supplementation to Total Parenteral Nutrition Promotes Extracellular Fluid Expansion in Piglets. J Nutr 124: 396–405.

19

The Sodium-Glucose Co-Transporter 2 Inhibitor Empagliflozin Improves Diabetes-Induced Vascular Dysfunction in the Streptozotocin Diabetes Rat Model by Interfering with Oxidative Stress and Glucotoxicity

Matthias Oelze[1,❡,¶], Swenja Kröller-Schön[1,❡,¶], Philipp Welschof[1], Thomas Jansen[1], Michael Hausding[1], Yuliya Mikhed[1], Paul Stamm[1], Michael Mader[1], Elena Zinßius[1], Saule Agdauletova[1], Anna Gottschlich[1], Sebastian Steven[1], Eberhard Schulz[1], Serge P. Bottari[2], Eric Mayoux[3], Thomas Münzel[1], Andreas Daiber[1]*

1 2nd Medical Clinic, Department of Cardiology, Medical Center of the Johannes Gutenberg University, Mainz, Germany, **2** Laboratory of Fundamental and Applied, Bioenergetics, INSERM U1055, Grenoble-Alpes Université et Pôle de Biologie, CHU, Grenoble, France, **3** Boehringer Ingelheim Pharma GmbH & Co. KG, Ingelheim, Germany

Abstract

Objective: In diabetes, vascular dysfunction is characterized by impaired endothelial function due to increased oxidative stress. Empagliflozin, as a selective sodium-glucose co-transporter 2 inhibitor (SGLT2i), offers a novel approach for the treatment of type 2 diabetes by enhancing urinary glucose excretion. The aim of the present study was to test whether treatment with empagliflozin improves endothelial dysfunction in type I diabetic rats via reduction of glucotoxicity and associated vascular oxidative stress.

Methods: Type I diabetes in Wistar rats was induced by an intravenous injection of streptozotocin (60 mg/kg). One week after injection empagliflozin (10 and 30 mg/kg/d) was administered via drinking water for 7 weeks. Vascular function was assessed by isometric tension recording, oxidative stress parameters by chemiluminescence and fluorescence techniques, protein expression by Western blot, mRNA expression by RT-PCR, and islet function by insulin ELISA in serum and immunohistochemical staining of pancreatic tissue. Advanced glycation end products (AGE) signaling was assessed by dot blot analysis and mRNA expression of the AGE-receptor (RAGE).

Results: Treatment with empagliflozin reduced blood glucose levels, normalized endothelial function (aortic rings) and reduced oxidative stress in aortic vessels (dihydroethidium staining) and in blood (phorbol ester/zymosan A-stimulated chemiluminescence) of diabetic rats. Additionally, the pro-inflammatory phenotype and glucotoxicity (AGE/RAGE signaling) in diabetic animals was reversed by SGLT2i therapy.

Conclusions: Empagliflozin improves hyperglycemia and prevents the development of endothelial dysfunction, reduces oxidative stress and improves the metabolic situation in type 1 diabetic rats. These preclinical observations illustrate the therapeutic potential of this new class of antidiabetic drugs.

Editor: Andrea Cignarella, University of Padova, Italy

Funding: The present work was supported by a vascular biology research grant from Boehringer Ingelheim Pharma GmbH & Co. KG (A.D. and T.M.) and by the Centre of Translational Vascular Biology (CTVB). Yuliya Miked holds a stipend from the International PhD Programme on the "Dynamics of Gene Regulation, Epigenetics and DNA Damage Response" from the Institute of Molecular Biology gGmbH, (Mainz, Germany) funded by the Boehringer Ingelheim Foundation. This paper contains results that are part of the doctoral thesis of Philipp Welschof. The funders had no role in data collection and analysis, decision to publish, or preparation of the manuscript. E.M. (Boehringer Ingelheim Pharma GmbH & Co. KG) was involved in the study design.

Competing Interests: T.M. and A.D. received research grants from Boehringer Ingelheim Pharma GmbH & Co. KG. E.M. is an employee of Boehringer Ingelheim Pharma GmbH & Co. KG. The remaining authors declare that they have no competing interests in connection with this manuscript.

* Email: andreas.daiber@bioredox.com

❡ These authors contributed equally to this work.

¶ MO and SKS should both be considered as first author.

Introduction

Diabetes mellitus is one of the major risk factors for the development of cardiovascular disease [1]. Several studies have demonstrated that endothelial dysfunction due to increased oxidative stress is frequently encountered in the diabetic state (for review see [2]). The vascular NADPH oxidase and an uncoupled endothelial nitric oxide synthase (eNOS, type 3) have been identified as enzymatic sources of increased vascular production of reactive oxygen species (ROS) [3]. Pharmacological treatment of diabetic animals with HMG-CoA-reductase inhibitors, AT_1-receptor blockers or heme oxygenase-1 induction by NO donor therapy with pentaerithrityl tetranitrate have been demonstrated to prevent the activation of the NADPH oxidase and to recouple the dysfunctional eNOS [4–6]. The mechanisms underlying eNOS uncoupling in vessels from diabetic animals include increased functional depletion of BH_4 due to the oxidation to the $^{\bullet}BH_3$ radical, oxidation of the zinc-sulfur-complex and S-glutathionylation of the enzyme [4,6]. Adverse phosphorylation of eNOS at Thr495 and Tyr657 may potentially play a significant role as well [7,8]. Another major concept of diabetic pathology is based on direct glucotoxicity, including increased formation of advanced glycation end products (AGE) and their signaling via specific receptors (RAGE) leading to vascular dysfunction and end organ damage [9,10]. Most importantly, oxidative stress and AGE/RAGE components interact with each other in a cross-talk fashion, wherein AGE/RAGE signaling can activate sources of reactive oxygen species (ROS) [11,12] and normalization of mitochondrial ROS formation in turn normalizes hyperglycemic damage by decreasing AGE/RAGE signaling [13]. In addition, increased vascular oxidative stress can lead to immune cell activation [14,15] or is even mediated by inflammatory cells, as was recently demonstrated in the angiotensin II infusion model [16].

A new class of anti-diabetic drugs targets the sodium-glucose co-transporter 2 (SGLT2), which is the main glucose transporter of the kidney, located in the S1 and S2 segments of the proximal tubule and is responsible for the reabsorption of >90% of the glucose from primary urine [17]. SGLT2 inhibition (SGLT2i) reduces the reabsorption of glucose and therefore enhances urinary glucose excretion, consequently decreasing both fasting and postprandial hyperglycemia. Since conventional anti-diabetic therapies rely on insulin secretion, their efficacy may get lost over time due to progressing β-cell dysfunction and desensitization to insulin signaling (especially with increasing age) [18]. Therapy with SGLT2i does not share these drawbacks, since its action is independent of insulin secretion and signaling. Likewise, in contrast to conventional anti-diabetics, SGLT2i removes excessive glucose from the body and thereby prevents glucotoxicity, which should represent a straight-forward strategy to prevent hyperglycemia-induced damage. Empagliflozin is a SGLT2i that was recently approved for clinical use in the United States of America and Europe. According to randomized, placebo-controlled, double-blind clinical studies, empagliflozin had a good safety and tolerability profile in healthy Japanese male subjects [19,20].

With the present study we sought to test whether treatment of diabetic animals with the SGLT2i empagliflozin improves endothelial dysfunction, oxidative stress, AGE/RAGE signaling and inflammation in a well-characterized rat model of type 1 diabetes mellitus [3].

Materials and Methods

Materials

The High-Capacity cDNA Reverse Transcription Kit was purchased from Applied Biosystems, Darmstadt, Germany. All oligonucleotides and dual labeled probes were purchased from MWG Biotech, Ebersberg, Germany. The Bradford reagent was obtained from BioRad, Munich, Germany. For isometric tension studies, nitroglycerin (GTN) was used from a Nitrolingual infusion solution (1 mg/ml) from G.Pohl-Boskamp (Hohenlockstedt, Germany). SGLT2-inhibitor (SGLT2i, empagliflozin) was a kind gift from Boehringer Ingelheim Pharma GmbH & Co KG (Biberach, Germany). For induction of diabetes we used streptozotocin (STZ) from Fluka (Steinheim, Germany). L-012 (8-amino-5-chloro-7-phenylpyrido[3,4-d]pyridazine-1,4-(2H,3H)dione sodium salt) was purchased from Wako Pure Chemical Industries (Osaka, Japan). All other chemicals were of analytical grade and were obtained from Sigma-Aldrich, Fluka or Merck.

Animals and in vivo treatment

All animals were treated in accordance with the Guide for the Care and Use of Laboratory Animals as adopted by the U.S. National Institutes of Health and approval was granted by the Ethics Committee of the University Hospital Mainz and the Landesuntersuchungsamt Rheinland-Pfalz (Koblenz, Germany; permit number: 23 177-07/G 12-1-025). All surgery was performed under isoflurane or ketamine/xylazine anesthesia, and all efforts were made to minimize suffering. A total number of 48 male Wistar Rats (6 weeks old, 300 g, Charles River Laboratories, Sulzfeld, Germany) were divided into 4 treatment groups: untreated controls (Ctr), streptozotocin-induced diabetes mellitus type 1 with placebo (STZ), SGLT2i low dose (10 mg/kg/d p.o.) or SGLT2i high dose (30 mg/kg/d p.o.) therapy. Given the maximal acute glucosuric effect of empagliflozin, the dose of 10 mg/kg/d was chosen according to previous animal studies [21–23]. Moreover, considering the higher metabolism of rats, the dose of 30 mg/kg/d allowed a higher 24 h drug exposure as already observed in previous study with chronic treatment [24]. The study was performed as 3 sub-studies with 4, 5 and 3 animals per group. Not all animals were used for all assays. For induction of diabetes mellitus type 1, rats were injected with a single dose of STZ into the vena dorsalis penis (60 mg/kg s.c., in 5 mM pH 4.5 citrate buffer). Control animals were injected with the solvent. SGLT2i treatment by drinking water, containing the requested concentrations of the drug to reach the desired doses of 10 and 30 mg/kg/d, was started 1 week after STZ-injection and continued for 7 weeks. After 8 weeks of total treatment duration, animals were killed under isoflurane anesthesia by transection of the diaphragm and removal of the heart and thoracic aorta. For protein and mRNA expression also the abdominal part and the arch of the aorta were used as well. Diabetes was diagnosed by measuring glucose levels and glycosylated hemoglobin (HbA1c) in whole blood (for STZ-treated rats it was diluted 1:5 with NaCl solution) using the ACCU-CHEK Sensor system from Roche Diagnostics GmbH (Mannheim, Germany) and A1C Now^{+} system from Bayer HealthCare Diabetes Care (Basel, Switzerland), respectively. STZ treatment was previously shown to be a valid type 1 diabetes model and hyperglycemic complications such as vascular dysfunction and oxidative stress were completely reversed by insulin administration [25].

Detection of serum cholesterol, triglyceride and interferon-γ levels

Serum cholesterol, triglyceride and interferon-γ levels were analysed in the Department of Clinical Chemistry, University Hospital Mainz, Germany, using the daily routine facilities for in-patient care. Total cholesterol in serum was also assessed by HF5 (Superon GmbH, Dernbach, Germany). More detailed information on determination of cholesterol by Field-Flow Fractionation (FFF) can be found in the online supplemental data in File S1.

Immunohistochemistry of pancreatic tissue

Pancreatic segments were fixed in paraformaldehyde (4%), paraffin-embedded and stained with primary antibodies against glucagon (1:4000, Abcam, UK) and insulin (1:200, LifeSpan BioSciences, Seattle, USA); depending upon the species of primary antibodies, appropriate biotinylated secondary antibodies were used at dilutions according to the manufacturer's instructions. For immunochemical detection ABC reagent (Vector) and then DAB reagent (peroxidase substrate Kit, Vector) were used as substrates.

Detection of insulin serum levels by ELISA and by RIA

Venous blood was transferred into serum-vials, left on ice for 30 min and centrifuged for 10 min at 2000 g. The supernatant (serum) was stored at −80°C. Quantitative measurement of serum insulin levels was performed using a rat insulin ELISA (DRG Instruments GmbH, Marburg, Germany) and a rat insulin RIA (Cat. # SRI-13K, Millipore, St. Charles, Missouri, USA) according to the manufacturer's instructions.

Histological staining of aortic rings and pancreatic tissue

Sirius red staining for vascular fibrosis and trichrom staining was performed with paraffin-embedded samples of aortic tissue upon deparaffination [26]. The nuclei were prestained with hemalum prior to staining for 1 hour in 0.1% with Sirius red solution in saturated picric acid (1.2%) [26]. Finally, tissue samples were dehydrated with 70%, 96% and 100% isopropanol and coverslipped with Entellan. Trichrom staining (according to Goldner et al.) was performed with paraffin-embedded samples of pancreatic tissue upon deparaffination [26]. After prestaining of the nuclei with haematoxylin (according to Harris et al.), the samples were stained for 5 minutes with mallory red in 100% acetic acid, fuchsin acid and Orange G (Merck, Darmstadt, Germany), followed by 15 minutes in 1% molybdatophosphoric acid hydrate (VWR, Darmstadt, Germany) and 5 minutes in acid light green. Finally tissue samples were dehydrated in glacial acetic acid and 100% ethanol and coverslipped in Entellan.

Isometric tension studies

Vasodilator responses to acetylcholine (ACh) and nitroglycerin (GTN) and vasoconstrictor responses to KCl were assessed with endothelium-intact isolated rat aortic rings mounted for isometric tension recordings in organ chambers, preconstricted with phenylephrine (PheE), as described previously [5,27].

Detection of oxidative stress in whole blood, cardiac membrane fractions and aorta

Whole blood leukocyte-dependent ROS formation was measured in fresh blood (in citrate tubes) which was diluted 1:50 in PBS with Ca^{2+}/Mg^{2+} (each 1 mM) and L-012. The oxidative burst (activation of the phagocytic NADPH oxidase) was triggered by the phorbol ester PDBu (10 μM) or the fungal endotoxin zymosan A (50 μg/ml) and assessed with L-012 (100 μM) enhanced chemiluminescence (ECL) [28]. NADPH oxidase activity in cardiac membrane fractions was determined by lucigenin (5 μM) ECL in the presence of NADPH (200 μM) using a Lumat LB9507 single photon counter as described [5,29]. Vascular ROS formation was determined using dihydroethidium (DHE, 1 μM)-dependent fluorescence microtopography in aortic cryo-sections as described [5,29]. To investigate involvement of eNOS uncoupling in ROS production and endothelial dysfunction within the endothelial monolayer, aortic rings were preincubated with the NOS inhibitor L-NAME [5,25,29]. ROS-derived red fluorescence was detected using a Zeiss Axiovert 40 CFL microscope, Zeiss lenses and Axiocam MRm camera. Intensity of the DHE oxidation products' fluorescence was evaluated by densitometry.

Western blot and dot blot analysis

Protein expression and modification was assessed by standard Western and dot blot analysis using established protocols [5,25,29]. Isolated aortic tissue was frozen and homogenized in liquid nitrogen. Proteins were separated by SDS-Page and blotted onto nitrocellulose membranes. After blocking, immunoblotting was performed with the following antibodies: monoclonal mouse α-actinin (100 kDa) as a control for loading and transfer, polyclonal rabbit NADPH oxidase isoform 1 (Nox1) (1:500, Abcam, UK) and monoclonal mouse NADPH oxidase isoform 2 (Nox2) ($gp91^{phox}$, 1:1000, BD Biosciences, USA), monoclonal mouse eNOS (1:1000, BD Biosciences, USA), polyclonal rabbit phospho-Ser1177-eNOS (1:1000, Upstate Biotechnology, MA, USA), monoclonal mouse dihydrofolate reductase (1 μg/ml, Abnova Corp., Germany), monoclonal mouse heme oxygenase-1 (HO-1) (4 μg/ml, Stressgen, San Diego, CA), polyclonal goat cGMP-dependent protein kinase (cGK-I, 1:200, Santa Cruz Biotechnologies, USA), vasodilator stimulated phosphoprotein (VASP) phosphorylated on serine239 (P-VASP, clone 16C2, 1.5 μg/ml, Calbiochem, UK), polyclonal rabbit monocyte-chemoattractant-protein-1 (MCP-1 or CCL-2, Serotec, UK), polyclonal rabbit receptor for advanced glycation end products (RAGE, 1:1000, Cell Signaling Technology, Danvers, MA). Detection and quantification were performed by ECL with peroxidase conjugated anti–rabbit/mouse (1:10000, Vector Lab., Burlingame, CA) and anti-goat (1:5000, Santa Cruz Biotechnologies, USA) secondary antibodies. Densitometric quantification of antibody-specific bands was performed with a ChemiLux Imager (CsX-1400 M, Intas, Göttingen, Germany) and Gel-Pro Analyzer software (Media Cybernetics, Bethesda, MD).

Advanced glycation end products (AGE) positive proteins were assessed by dot blot analysis of aortic protein homogenate, which was transferred to a Protran BA85 (0.45 μm) nitrocellulose membrane (Schleicher & Schuell, Dassel, Germany) by a Minifold I vacuum dot-blot system (Schleicher&Schuell, Dassel, Germany). Each slot was washed with 250 μl PBS and the membrane was dried for 15 min at 60°C. For detection of AGE's, a mouse monoclonal AGE antibody (Antibodies-online GmbH, Aachen, Germany) was used at a dilution of 1:1000. Positive dots were detected by enhanced chemiluminescence after incubation with a peroxidase-coupled secondary antibody (1:10000, Vector Lab., Burlingame, CA). All incubation and washing steps were performed according to the manufacturer's instructions. Densitometric quantification of the dots was performed as described in the Western blot section.

Detection of serum methylglyoxal levels and liver ALDH-2 activity by HPLC-based quantification

Methylglyoxal serum levels were quantified by an HPLC-based method upon derivatization of the reactive aldehyde as adapted from a previously described protocol [30]. Briefly, 500 µl serum was filtrated by size exclusion centrifugation in a 30 kDa filter device (Millipore, Billierica, MA, USA) for 60 min at 17000 g. The eluate (350 µl) was mixed with 70 µl 7M $HClO_4$, 10 µl 100 µM 2,3-dimethylquinoxaline (internal standard) and 70 µl 9.2 mM 1,2-diaminobenzene (derivatization reagent) for 30 min at 25°C. 50 µl of each sample were subjected to HPLC analysis. The system consisted of a Jasco HPLC system and a C_{18}-Nucleosil 125×4 100-3 reversed phase column from Macherey & Nagel (Düren, Germany). The mobile phase consisted of solvent A (50 mM citric acid pH 2.2) and solvent B (acetonitrile (90 v/v%) and water (10 v/v%)). The substrate and its products were eluted at a flow rate of 1 ml/min using a gradient (0 min: 37% B; 12 min: 60% B; 12.5 min: 90% B; 13 min: 37% B; 15 min: 37% B), detected by their absorption at 315 nm, and quantified using internal and external standards (methylglyoxal derivatization product served as external standard and 2,3-dimethylquinoxaline was the internal standard). The typical retention times were 3.9 and 4.4 min, respectively.

The activity of ALDH-2 in isolated mitochondria was determined by measuring the conversion of 2-hydroxy-3-nitro-benzaldehyde to 2-hydroxy-3-nitro-benzoic acid as described previously [31]. Briefly, liver samples were homogenized in HEPES buffer (composition in mM: 50 HEPES, 70 sucrose, 220 mannitol, 1 EGTA and 0.033 BSA) and centrifuged at 1500 g (10 min at 4°C) and 2000 g for 5 min (the pellets were discarded). The supernatant was then centrifuged at 20000 g for 20 min, and the pellet resuspended in 1 ml of HEPES buffer. The latter step was repeated and the pellet resuspended in 1 ml of Tris buffer (composition in mM: 10 Tris, 340 sucrose, 100 KCl and 1 EDTA). The mitochondrial fraction (total protein approximately 5–10 mg/ml) was kept on ice and diluted to approximately 1 mg/ml protein in 0.25 ml of PBS and preincubated for 10 min at room temperature. For measurement of ALDH-2 dehydrogenase activity, 2-hydroxy-3-nitro-benzaldehyde (100 µM) was added and the samples were incubated for another 30 min at 37°C. Samples were sonicated, centrifuged at 20000 g (4°C) for 20 min, and the supernatant was purified by size exclusion centrifugation in a 10 kDa filter device (Millipore). 50 µl of each sample were subjected to HPLC analysis. The system consisted of a Jasco HPLC system and a C_{18}-Nucleosil 125×4 100-3 reversed phase column from Macherey & Nagel (Düren, Germany). The mobile phase consisted of solvent A (50 mM citric acid pH 2.2) and solvent B (acetonitrile (90 v/v%) and water (10 v/v%)). The substrate and its products were eluted at a flow rate of 1 ml/min using a gradient (0 min: 25% B; 7 min: 50% B; 8 min: 100% B; 9 min: 25% B; 11 min: 25% B), detected by their absorption at 360 nm, and quantified using internal and external standards (2-hydroxy-3-nitro-benzoic acid and 2-hydroxy-3-nitro-benzaldehyde). The typical retention times were 2.4 and 3.7 min, respectively.

Quantitative reverse transcription real-time PCR (qRT-PCR)

mRNA expression was analyzed with quantitative reverse transcription real-time PCR (qRT-PCR) as previously described [32]. Briefly, total RNA from rat aorta was isolated (RNeasy Fibrous Tissue Mini Kit; Qiagen, Hilden, Germany), and 50 ng of total RNA was used for real-time RT-PCR analysis with the QuantiTect Probe RT-PCR kit (Qiagen). TaqMan Gene Expression assays for monocyte chemoattractant protein-1 (MCP-1 or CCL-2), monocyte/macrophage-specific protein CD68, cytokine interleukin-6 (IL-6), immune-signaling proteins interferon-γ (IFN-γ) and tumor necrosis factor-α (TNF-α), intercellular adhesion molecule-1 (ICAM-1), cyclooxygenase-2 (COX-2) and the receptor for advanced glycation end products (RAGE) as well as TBP were purchased as probe-and-primer sets (Applied Biosystems, Foster City, CA). The comparative Ct method was used for relative mRNA quantification. Gene expression was normalized to the endogenous control, TATA box binding protein (TBP) mRNA, and the amount of target gene mRNA expression in each sample was expressed relative to the control.

Statistical analysis

Results are expressed as the means ±SEM. Two-way ANOVA (with Bonferroni's correction for comparison of multiple means) was used for comparisons of concentration-relaxation curves. In addition, one-way ANOVA (with Bonferroni's or Dunn's correction for comparison of multiple means) was used for comparisons of vasodilator potency (EC_{50}, pD_2 see Table 1) and efficacy (max. relaxation see Table 1). One-way ANOVA (with Bonferroni's or Dunn's correction for comparison of multiple means) was used for comparisons of weight gain, blood glucose, HbA1c levels, other serum parameters, such as insulin, triglycerides and methylglyoxal levels, histological data, aortic and cardiac ROS formation, protein and mRNA expression, vasoconstriction and hepatic ALDH-2 activity. p values <0.05 were considered as statistically significant. The number of replicates in the different assays may vary due to the death of some rats in the different sub-studies and since some values were excluded when they exceeded a deviation of 2xSD from the means.

Results

Diabetes-related parameters (Table 2)

During the treatment period 3 (STZ), 1 (SGLT2i low dose) and 1 (SGLT2i high dose) rats died. The weight gain was significantly decreased in the STZ-treated diabetic rats and not significantly affected by a low dose but increased by a high dose SGLT2i therapy. Diabetic animals had higher triglyceride and total cholesterol levels compared to controls and to diabetic animals treated with SGLTi. Blood glucose was higher in all STZ-treated groups (approximately 4-fold as compared to the control group) when measured 3 days after STZ injection, clearly excluding any interference of the drug therapy (which was started 7 days after STZ injection) with the induction of diabetes. Blood glucose levels were determined 8 weeks after STZ injection and the untreated STZ rats showed an almost 5-fold increase in this parameter, which was dose-dependently decreased by SGLT2i therapy in non-fasting rats. In fasting rats, blood glucose levels were increased almost 4-fold in the untreated STZ rats and were reduced by low and high dose SGLT2i therapy to near control levels. The parameter for long-term glycemic conditions, HbA1c, was increased more than 4-fold by STZ injection and was dose-dependently decreased by SGLT2i therapy. Trichrome staining of pancreatic tissue revealed morphological changes in the islet cells in untreated diabetic rats (Figure S1 in File S1). Glucagon production as detected by immunohistochemical staining of pancreatic tissue, showed no obvious change in control, diabetic and SGLT2i treated groups (if at all a moderate increase in staining in the STZ group) (Figure 1A). In contrast, immunohistochemical staining for insulin showed a clear decrease in the STZ group as compared to the controls with only minor part of the islets producing any insulin at all (not shown) and even in these "active" islets only few β-cells were producing insulin. Low dose SGLT2i therapy showed some improvement of islet insulin production which was clearly increased by high dose SGLT2i therapy (Figure 1B). In accordance with these observations, the

Table 1. Potencies and efficacies of the endothelium-dependent vasodilator acetylcholine and the endothelium-independent vasodilator nitroglycerin in rat aorta.

	In vivo treatment group			
Parameter[a]	Ctr	STZ	STZ+low SGLT2i	STZ+high SGLT2i
Potency (pD2), ACh	7.52±0.07 (n = 12)	7.12±0.06 (n = 9)*	7.33±0.06 (n = 10)#	7.28±0.05 (n = 9)*#
Efficacy (%), ACh	90.3±1.4 (n = 12)	80.3±2.3 (n = 9)*	91.5±0.7 (n = 10)#	85.5±2.4 (n = 9)§
Potency (pD2), GTN	7.81±0.07 (n = 12)	7.62±0.11 (n = 9)*	7.73±0.08 (n = 10)	7.70±0.12 (n = 9)
Efficacy (%), GTN	99.4±0.2 (n = 12)	96.7±1.6 (n = 9)*	99.2±0.1 (n = 10)	98.8±0.3 (n = 9)

[a]Potency is –log EC_{50} and EC_{50} is the concentration that induces half-maximal relaxation with respect to the maximal relaxation achieved with the highest concentration of the vasodilator used. Efficacy is defined as maximal relaxation obtained with the highest concentration of the vasodilator used. The data are the means ± SEM of the indicated number of animals/group.

*, p<0.05 vs. control and #, p<0.05 vs. STZ-injected and §, p<0.05 vs. low dose SGLT2i treated.

serum insulin levels were significantly decreased to background concentrations (measured both by ELISA and RIA) in the STZ group and dose-dependently normalized by SGLT2i therapy (Figure 1C and D). Interferon-γ levels showed no significant changes (Table 2).

Vascular parameters

Histological staining for collagen (sirius red) and aortic wall (media) thickness revealed no significant increase in thickening (remodeling) in the STZ group but substantial reduction of these parameters by both doses of SGLT2i (Figure 2A). STZ injection caused endothelial dysfunction (acetylcholine [ACh]-dependent relaxation), which was improved by both SGLT2i doses (Figure 2B). The effects on endothelium-independent (nitroglycerin [GTN]) relaxation were less pronounced (Figure 2C). Vasodilator potency (EC_{50}, pD_2) and efficacy (max. relaxation) are presented in Table 1. KCl-induced vasoconstriction did not change in any group but the phenylephrine-induced constriction was increased in almost all STZ groups and interestingly not corrected by SGLT2i therapy (Figure S2 in File S1).

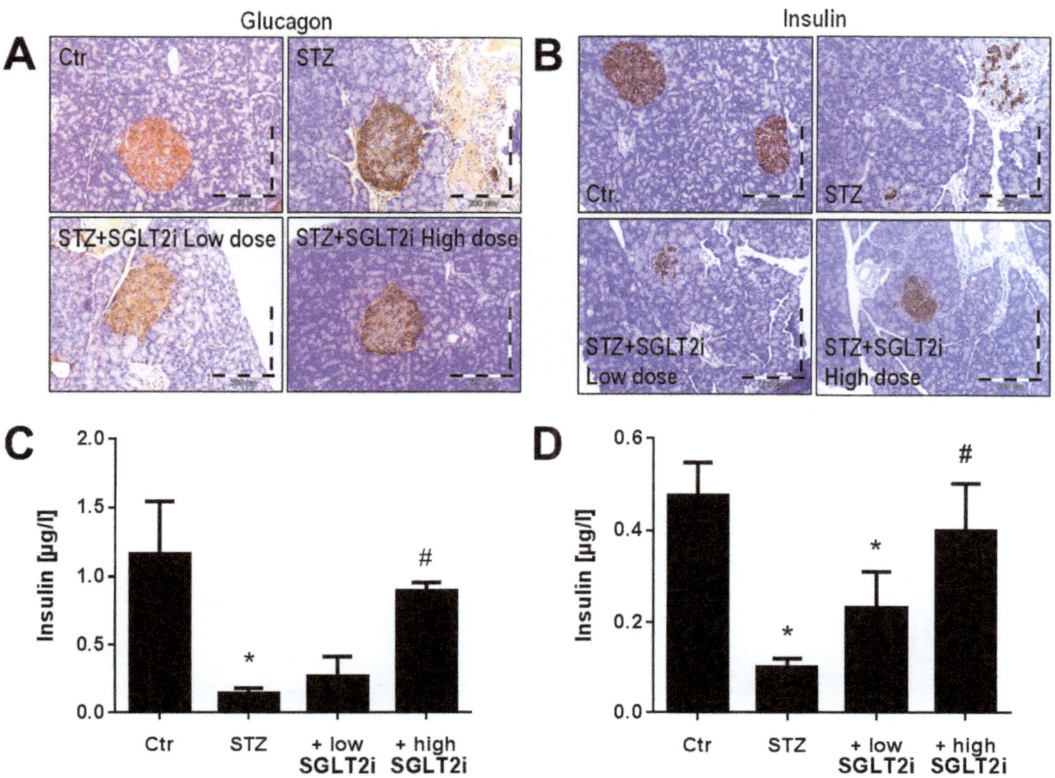

Figure 1. Glucagon and insulin measurements in controls and diabetic rats 8 weeks after STZ injection and 7 weeks of SGLT2i (low and high dose) treatment. Representative immunohistochemical stainings of pancreatic tissue for glucagon (**A**), insulin (**B**) and ELISA (**C**) or RIA (**D**) based determination of insulin serum levels. The data are the means ±SEM of 3–4 (**A,B**), 3–5 (**C**) or 9–11 (**D**) animals/group. *, p<0.05 vs. control and #, p<0.05 vs. STZ-injected group.

Table 2. Weight gain, and blood and serum parameters in controls and diabetic rats.

	In vivo treatment group			
Parameter[a]	**Ctr**	**STZ**	**STZ+low SGLT2i**	**STZ+high SGLT2i**
Weight gain [g]	137±10 (n=12)	27±19 (n=8)*	43±19 (n=9)*	97±14 (n=10)$^{\#§}$
Blood glucose [mg/dl], 3d post STZ, non-fasting, before SGLT2i treatment	120±6 (n=7)	441±22 (n=9)*	457±22 (n=11)*	447±26 (n=11)*
Blood glucose [mg/dl], 8w post STZ, non-fasting	132±8 (n=11)	509±20 (n=9)$^{*\#}$	336±49 (n=10)$^{*\#}$	230±30(n=10)$^{*\#§}$
Blood glucose [mg/dl], 8w post STZ, fasting	117±4 (n=11)	395±42 (n=9)*	185±15 (n=10)$^{\#}$	168±19 (n=10)$^{\#}$
HbA1c [mmol/mol]	24±2 (n=10)	99±12 (n=8)*	68±8 (n=8)$^{*\#}$	40±6 (n=8)$^{*\#§}$
HbA1c [%]	4.3±2.3	11.2±3.2	8.4±2.9	5.8±2.7
Cholesterol [mg/dl], ELISA	83±6 (n=9)	105±8 (n=7)*	93±4(n=7)	83±5 (n=7)$^{\#}$
Cholesterol [mg/dl], HF5[b]	102±5(n=11)	125±4 (n=9)*	108±4 (n=9)$^{\#}$	105±3 (n=9)$^{\#}$
Triglycerides [mg/dl]	87±7(n=7)	273±79 (n=5)*	178±31 (n=6)	95±15 (n=7)$^{\#}$
Interferon-γ [pg/dl]	n.d.(n=5)	6±3 (n=4)	2±2 (n=4)	n.d. (n=3)

[a]Weight gain was calculated from the difference of values prior and 8 weeks post STZ injection. Blood glucose was determined three days after STZ injection without SGLT2i treatment; fasting and non-fasting blood glucose as well as HbA1c levels were measured 8 weeks post STZ injection. The data are the means ± SEM of the indicated number of animals/group; n.d. means not detectable.

*, $p<0.05$ vs. control and #, $p<0.05$ vs. STZ-injected and §, $p<0.05$ vs. low dose SGLT2i treated.

[b]Separation of HDL and LDL using HF5 (Hollow Fiber Flow Field Flow Fractionation).

Oxidative stress parameters

Oxidative burst in whole blood in response to zymosan A was increased in the diabetic rats and normalized by both SGLT2i doses and a similar pattern was observed in response to the synthetic phorbol ester analogue PDBu (mainly reflecting leukocyte NADPH oxidase activity) without displaying significant changes (Figure 3A and C). The signal in the STZ group was largely suppressed by the NADPH oxidase inhibitor VAS2870 (highest affinity for Nox2 isoform) and the intracellular calcium chelator BAPTA-AM, indicating the involvement of the phagocytic NADPH oxidase and $[Ca^{2+}]_i$ in this process (Figure 3B). NADPH oxidase activity from heart membranes was increased in the STZ group and dose-dependently inhibited by SGLT2i therapy (Figure 3D). In line with this, activity of the redox-sensitive enzyme mitochondrial aldehyde dehydrogenase (ALDH-2) was decreased in diabetic rats but not significantly impaired under SGLT2i therapy (Figure S3 in File S1).

Aortic reactive oxygen species formation was increased in the STZ group and reduced by high dose of SGLT2i, although still increased as compared to the control (Figure 3E). An almost similar pattern was observed for endothelial dihydroethidium staining of aortic cryo-sections, however, without significant reduction in the endothelial dihydroethidium fluorescence signal by either SGLT2i dose (Figure 3F). Experiments with the eNOS inhibitor L-NAME reduced the superoxide signal in the endothelial cell layer of vessels from the STZ group, compatible with eNOS uncoupling. SGLT2i treatment showed a mixed effect suggesting that eNOS uncoupling is not completely prevented. The dihydroethidium staining signal was sensitive to low concentration SOD treatment and high concentration catalase pre-incubation (Figure S4 in File S1).

Protein expression

We have shown previously that eNOS and dihydrofolate reductase (DHFR) expression was increased in aorta from diabetic animals suggesting compensatory up-regulation of these enzymes due to the dysfunction/uncoupling of eNOS and oxidative depletion of its co-factor tetrahydrobiopterin (BH_4) with subsequent induction of dihydrofolate reductase, the BH_2 recycling enzyme. STZ treatment significantly increased eNOS and dihydrofolate reductase expression and SGLT2i therapy decreased it dose-dependently suggesting that SGLT2i therapy normalized these adverse effects of hyperglycemia, thereby preventing the compensatory up-regulation of these enzymes (Figure 4 A and C). It should be noted that eNOS up-regulation per se is a beneficial event but if overexpressed in an oxidized environment (with depleted BH_4 levels or in S-glutathionylated state) the enzyme might be uncoupled and might further aggravate the phenotype. Phosphorylation of eNOS at Ser1177, which increases eNOS activity, was impaired in STZ-treated rats and dose-dependently improved with SGLT2i therapy (Figure 4B). The expression of cGMP-dependent kinase was slightly increased in the STZ group and reduced to control levels by high dose SGLT2i therapy (Figure 4D, Figure S6D in File S1). Likewise, the phosphorylation of VASP at Ser239 (as a read-out of activation of the cGMP-dependent kinase) was decreased in the STZ-treated rats and normalized by high dose SGLT2i therapy (Figure 4D, Figure S6D in File S1). As a consequence, the ratio of P-VASP/cGK-I was significantly decreased in diabetic rats and improved dose-dependently by SGLT2i therapy with no significant impairment as compared to controls under low dose SGLT2i therapy and significant improvement as compared to STZ group under high dose SGLT2i therapy (Figure 4D). The expression of NADPH oxidase isoforms Nox1 and Nox2 was increased in diabetes and significantly reduced by high dose SGLT2i therapy (Figure 4E and F). As a general stress response, the antioxidant enzyme heme oxygenase-1 (HO-1) was up-regulated in diabetic rats without therapy and significantly reduced by high dose SGLT2i therapy (Figure 4G). The inflammatory protein monocyte chemoattractant protein-1 (MCP-1 or CCL-2) was up-regulated in untreated STZ rats, and normalized by high dose SGLT2i therapy (Figure 4H).

AGE/RAGE signaling

Quantification of advanced glycation end products (AGE)-positive proteins by dot blot analysis (Figure 5A) and AGE signaling was assessed by expression levels of their receptor

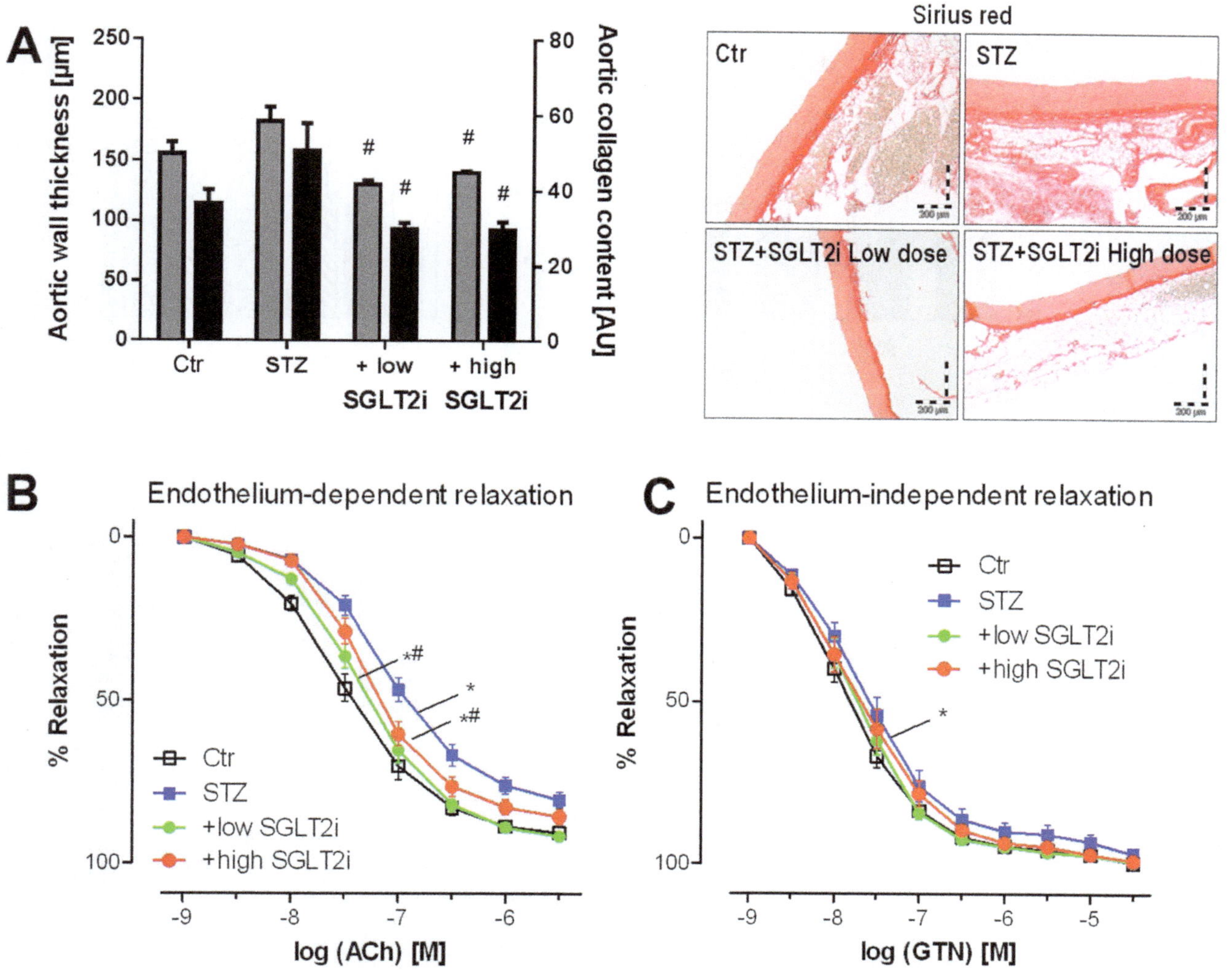

Figure 2. Effects of SGLT2i treatment on vascular parameters in diabetic rats. Microscopic determination of wall thickness (grey) and collagen content (black) by sirius red staining of paraffinated aortic sections (**A**). Representative microscope images are shown along with the densitometric quantification. Effects of SGLT2i therapy on endothelium-dependent and independent vascular relaxation by the vasodilators acetylcholine (ACh, **B**) and nitroglycerin (GTN, **C**), respectively. Data are the means±SEM from 6–7 (**A**) and 9–12 (**B,C**) animals/group. Each single value for an animal corresponds to the means of 4 individual aortic rings from this animal. *, $p<0.05$ vs. control and #, $p<0.05$ vs. STZ-injected group. For the vascular function data the significance levels were determined by two-way-ANOVA and significances for the entire curves are indicated when at least one compared concentration condition showed significant differences. Vasodilator potency (EC_{50}, pD_2) and efficacy (max. relaxation) were also calculated and subjected to statistical analysis using one-way-ANOVA. The data and results are presented in Table 1.

(RAGE) at mRNA and protein level (Figure 5B and C). Aortic RAGE protein expression and levels of AGE-positive proteins was increased in the STZ group and normalized by a high dose SGLT2i therapy. Aortic RAGE mRNA expression showed similar results. In agreement with this, serum levels of the AGE precursor methylglyoxal were significantly increased in the STZ group and improved by high dose SGLT2i therapy (Figure 5D).

mRNA expression

We also determined a number of inflammation markers by RT-PCR-based measurement of mRNA levels. The already mentioned monocyte chemoattractant protein-1 (MCP-1 or CCL-2, Figure 6A), the monocyte/macrophage-specific protein CD68 (Figure 6B) and the cytokine interleukin-6 (IL-6, Figure 6C) were up-regulated at the mRNA level in the aorta and significantly reduced by at least one SGLT2i dose. Likewise, the immune-signaling protein tumor necrosis factor-α (TNF-α, Figure 6E) was up-regulated in STZ-treated rats and reduced by both doses of SGLT2i, a pattern that was mirrored for interferon-γ (IFN-γ) and intercellular adhesion molecule-1 (ICAM-1) expression without reaching significant differences (Figure 6D and 6F). The general marker of inflammation, cyclooxygenase-2 (COX-2, Figure S5 in File S1) was increased in diabetic rats without treatment and normalized by both doses of SGLT2i.

Discussion

With the present study we demonstrate that chronic treatment of STZ-treated rats with the SGLT2i empagliflozin prevents the development of endothelial dysfunction, oxidative stress, AGE/RAGE signaling and inflammation in a well characterized animal model of type I diabetes mellitus. These beneficial effects are mainly due to antioxidant and anti-inflammatory effects of this compound, such as an inhibition of the activity of NADPH oxidase

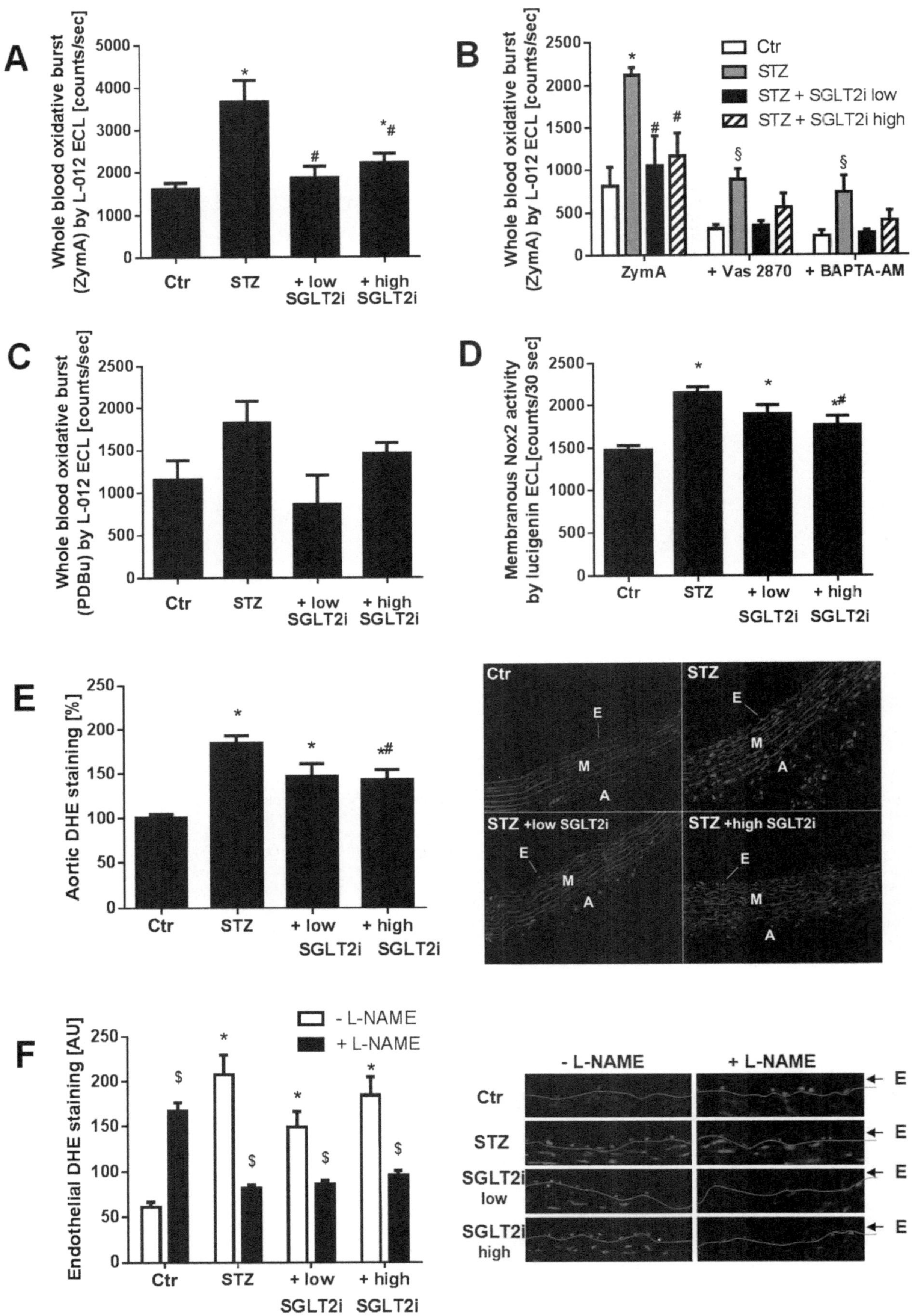
A
Whole blood oxidative burst (ZymA) by L-012 ECL [counts/sec]
5000
4000
3000
2000
1000
0
*
#
*#
Ctr
STZ
+ low SGLT2i
+ high SGLT2i
B
Whole blood oxidative burst (ZymA) by L-012 ECL [counts/sec]
2500
2000
1500
1000
500
0
Ctr
STZ
STZ + SGLT2i low
STZ + SGLT2i high
*
#
#
§
§
ZymA
+ Vas 2870
+ BAPTA-AM
C
Whole blood oxidative burst (PDBu) by L-012 ECL [counts/sec]
2500
2000
1500
1000
500
0
Ctr
STZ
+ low SGLT2i
+ high SGLT2i
D
Membranous Nox2 activity by lucigenin ECL[counts/30 sec]
2500
2000
1500
1000
500
0
*
*
*#
Ctr
STZ
+ low SGLT2i
+ high SGLT2i
E
Aortic DHE staining [%]
250
200
150
100
50
0
*
*
*#
Ctr
STZ
+ low SGLT2i
+ high SGLT2i
Ctr
STZ
STZ +low SGLT2i
STZ +high SGLT2i
E
M
A
F
Endothelial DHE staining [AU]
250
200
150
100
50
0
- L-NAME
+ L-NAME
*
$
*
$
*
$
*
$
Ctr
STZ
+ low SGLT2i
+ high SGLT2i
- L-NAME
+ L-NAME
Ctr
STZ
SGLT2i low
SGLT2i high
E

Figure 3. Effects of SGLT2i treatment on oxidative stress parameters in diabetic rats. Leukocyte-derived ROS (oxidative burst) in whole blood at 30 min upon zymosan A (**A**) stimulation along with the effects of the NADPH oxidase isoform 2 (Nox2) inhibitor VAS2870 and the intracellular calcium chelator BAPTA-AM (**B**) and upon PDBu stimulation (**C**). **(D)** Quantification of cardiac NADPH oxidase activity in membrane preparations by lucigenin (5 μM)-derived chemiluminescence. Dihydroethidium (DHE, 1 μM)-fluorescence microtopography was used to assess the effects of SGLT2i treatment on vascular (**E**) and endothelial (**F**) ROS production with and without incubation with the eNOS inhibitor L-NAME. Representative microscope images are shown along with the densitometric quantification. Red fluorescence indicates ROS formation whereas green fluorescence represents basal laminae autofluorescence. Data are the means±SEM from 6–7 (**A,B**), 5 (**C**), 7–8 (**D**), 9 (**E**) or 5–6 (**F**) animals/group. *, $p<0.05$ vs. control and #, $p<0.05$ vs. STZ-injected and §, $p<0.05$ vs. low dose SGLT2i treated and $, $p<0.05$ vs. w/o L-NAME.

and decreased serum levels of the AGE precursor methylglyoxal. These antioxidant and anti-inflammatory effects are likely due to glucose lowering effects. Glucose lowering is likely due to removal of glucose by the kidney via SGLT2 inhibition but may also be secondary to improved glucose utilization by restored insulin production and signaling, all of which prevent AGE formation, AGE/RAGE signaling, metabolic dysfunction, oxidative stress and impairment of vascular function. As expected, SGLT2i-dependent glucose lowering decreases cellular glucotoxicity and thereby contributes to the survival of pancreatic islet cells and preserves insulin production (Figure 7).

Diabetes is the most common cause of blindness, non-traumatic amputations and end-stage renal disease and the sixth most common cause of death. Yet only limited knowledge exists about the pathogenesis, the cardiovascular consequences and the prevention of this disease. Previous data suggests that the cardiovascular consequences of diabetes mellitus are secondary to oxidative stress [3,6,25], as previously shown for hypercholesterolemia, hypertension or established atherosclerosis. NADPH oxidases, mitochondria, xanthine oxidase, as well as uncoupled eNOS have been identified as major sources of these reactive oxygen and nitrogen species [4,5,33,34]. Importantly, the efficacy of the current anti-diabetic treatments vanishes over time, leading to a progression of the disease [18]. This phenomenon is mostly explained by the reduction of the ß-cells' capacity to secrete insulin and by a desensitization of the insulin signalling pathways, while most of the treatments aim to induce insulin release or to improve insulin sensitivity. Mode of action of SGLT2 inhibitors is insulin independent, thus efficacy of empagliflozin should be preserved independently of the advancement of the ß-cell failure. Along these lines SGLT2 inhibitors have been demonstrated to be effective in diabetes mellitus type II [35] and are anticipated to be also effective in type 1 diabetic patients. The proof of concept that empagliflozin is effective in lowering glucose and sparing insulin has been recently demonstrated in a preclinical model of STZ-induced type 1 diabetes [22] but also in human studies [36,37].

In contrast to the classical anti-diabetic therapies, SGLT2i treatment removes the glucose from the body and is thereby highly efficient in preventing so-called glucotoxicity, increased methylglyoxal levels, formation of AGE and induction of RAGE. Importantly, methylglyoxal has recently been demonstrated to play an essential role in the development and progression of diabetic neuropathy in diabetic mice and patients and therefore represents a target of special interest for pharmacological modulation [38]. Increased AGE/RAGE signaling in STZ rats has been established [39] and its contribution to increased oxidative stress and vascular complications under hyperglycemic conditions was identified [40]. In 2001, it was demonstrated that macrophages from gp91phox deficient mice responded less to AGE stimulation providing a direct link between AGE/RAGE signaling and NADPH oxidase expression/activity [12]. The same authors also demonstrated a connection between AGE/RAGE signaling and inflammation by increased VCAM-1 and tissue factor expression in human endothelial cells in response to AGE treatment. Increased tissue levels of macrophages were identified by MCP-1 and CD68 staining in STZ rats [41]. Increased TNF-α, IFN-γ expression as well as ROS producing enzymes in STZ rats were normalized by multiple antioxidant therapy [42]. Therefore, hyperglycemia via increased AGE/RAGE signaling leads to oxidative stress from NADPH oxidases, impaired NO/cGMP

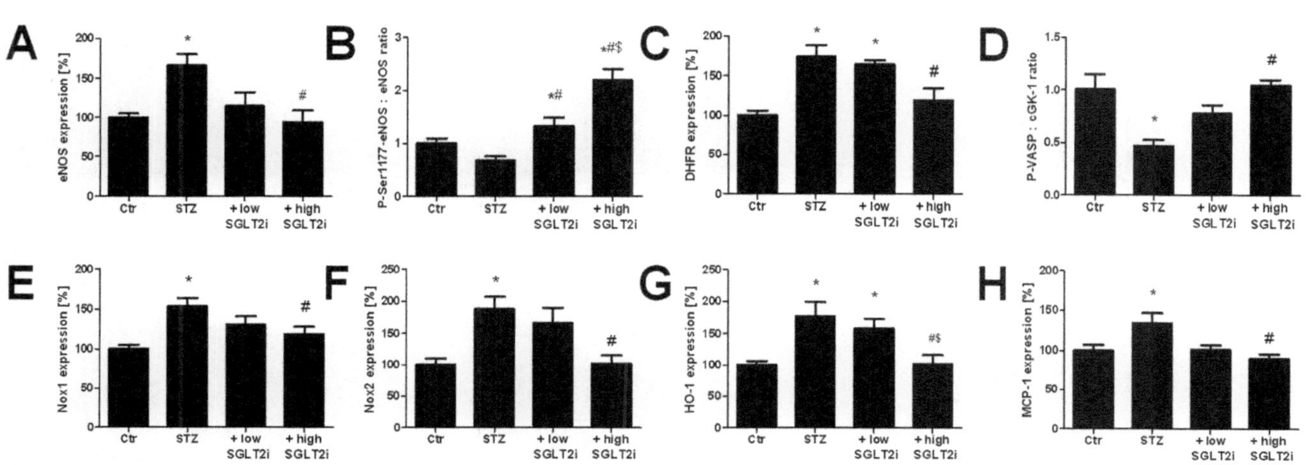

Figure 4. Effects of SGLT2i treatment on aortic protein expression of the NO/cGMP signaling cascade as well as oxidative stress and inflammatory pathways in diabetic rats. Expression of endothelial nitric oxide synthase (eNOS, **A**), serine1177 phosphorylated eNOS (**B**), dihydrofolate reductase (DHFR, **C**), ratio of cGK-I and serine239 phosphorylated VASP (**D**) were assessed by Western blotting analysis and specific antibodies. Expression of NADPH oxidases Nox1 (**E**) and Nox2 (**F**), heme oxygenase-1 (HO-1) (**G**) and monocyte-chemoattractant-protein-1 (MCP-1 or CCL-2, **H**) were assessed by Western blotting analysis and specific antibodies. Representative blots for all proteins are shown in supplemental Figure S6 in File S1. The data are expressed as % of control and are the means ± SEM from 8–9 (**A**), 5–6 (**B**), 7 (**C**), 4 (**D**), 6–7 (**E**), 7–9 (**F**), 7–9 (**G**) and 4–6 (**H**) animals/group. *, $p<0.05$ vs. control and #, $p<0.05$ vs. STZ-injected and $, $p<0.05$ vs. low dose SGLT2i treated.

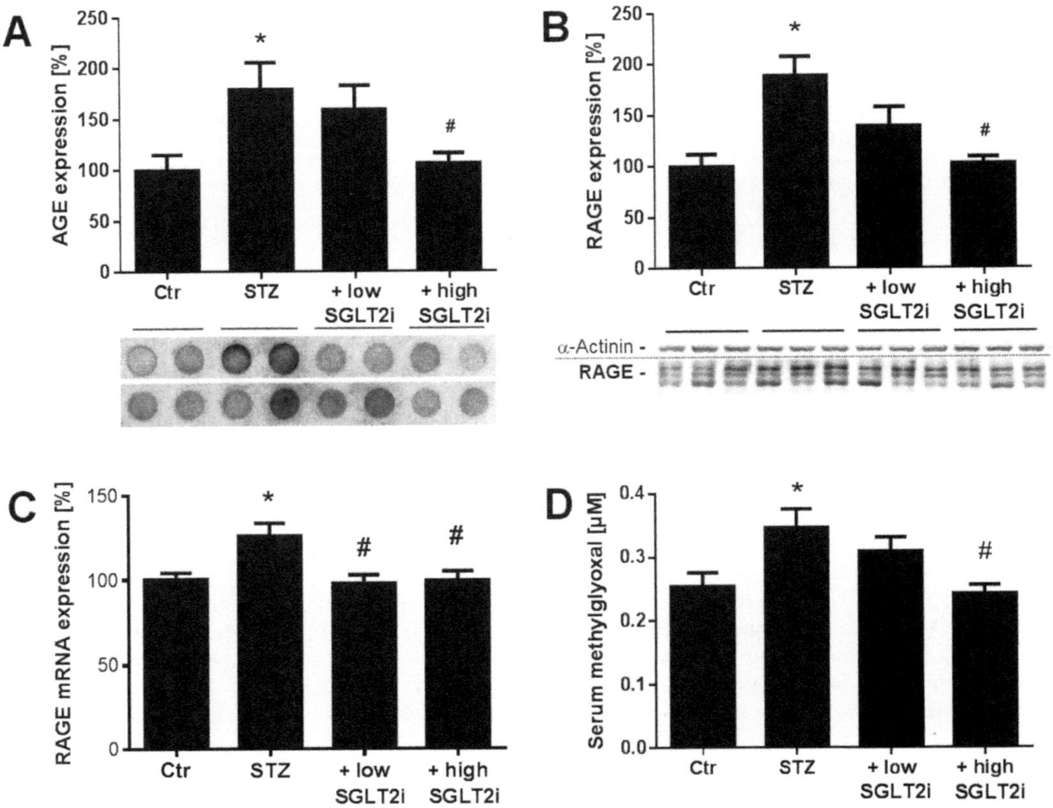

Figure 5. Effects of SGLT2i treatment on AGE/RAGE signaling in diabetic rats. Quantification of AGE-positive proteins by dot blot analysis (**A**) and RAGE expression was assessed by Western blotting analysis with specific antibodies (**B**) and quantitative RT-PCR analysis (**C**). Representative blots are shown at the bottom of the densitometric quantifications. Serum methylglyoxal levels were assessed by HPLC-based quantification (**D**). Representative chromatograms are shown in supplemental Figure S7 in File S1. The data are expressed as % of control and are the means ±SEM from 7 (**A**), 6–7 (**B**) and 8–11 (**C,D**) animals/group. *, $p<0.05$ vs. control and #, $p<0.05$ vs. STZ–injected.

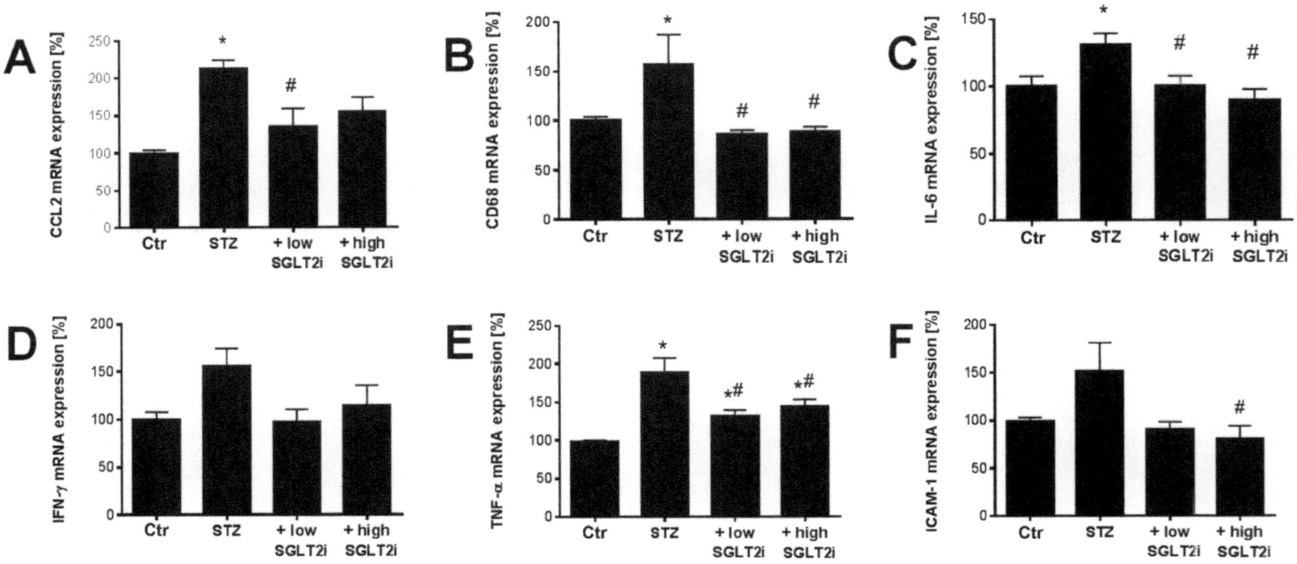

Figure 6. Effects of SGLT2i treatment on aortic mRNA expression of pro-inflammatory genes in diabetic rats. Expression of the monocyte chemoattractant protein-1 (CCL-2, **A**), the monocyte/macrophage-specific protein CD68 (**B**), the cytokine interleukin-6 (IL-6, **C**), the immune-signaling proteins interferon-γ (IFN-γ, **D**) and tumor necrosis factor-α (TNF-α, **E**) and the intercellular adhesion molecule-1 (ICAM-1, **F**) was assessed by quantitative RT-PCR. The data are expressed as % of control and are the means ±SEM from 7–9 (**A–C**), 9–10 (**D–E**) and 6–7 animals/group. *, $p<0.05$ vs. control and #, $p<0.05$ vs. STZ-injected.

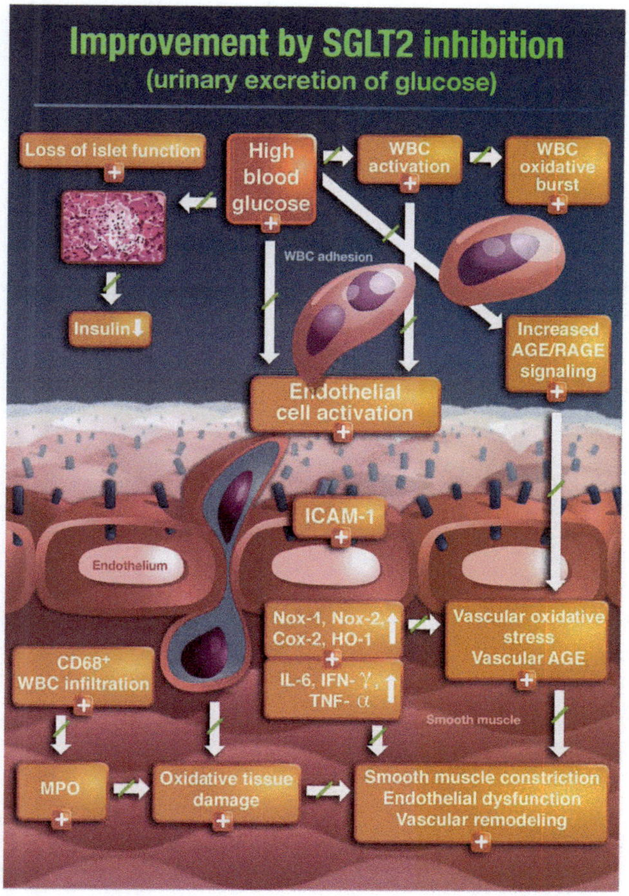

Figure 7. Summary of beneficial effects of SGLT2i treatment on diabetes induced vascular dysfunction and other adverse effects of hyperglycemia in rats.

signaling and low-grade inflammation as supported by the present protein and mRNA expression data and oxidative stress measurements. All of these adverse effects were normalized by SGLT2i treatment.

In line with this, the burden of oxidative stress was decreased by SGLT2i at all levels (whole blood, aorta, heart) supporting the concept of a cross-talk between AGE/RAGE signaling and ROS formation in diabetes mellitus. The contribution of calcium signaling in this process was demonstrated by the inhibitory effect of intracellular calcium chelation in the present work and the overall importance of calcium for the interaction of mitochondrial ROS with the activation of NADPH oxidases (Nox1 and Nox2) was demonstrated recently [15]. Related to the oxidative stress concept, the redox regulated mitochondrial aldehyde dehydrogenase (ALDH-2) is not only important as a nitroglycerin bioactivating enzyme [43,44] but also is an important antioxidant enzyme by degrading toxic aldehydes such as acetaldehyde, malondialdehyde and 4-hydroxynonenal [45,46]. More recently it has been shown that ALDH-2 plays an important role for the reduction of myocardial damage during ischemia/reperfusion by reducing the infarct size [47] and conferring cardio-protection in an experimental diabetes/MI model [48]. Therefore, the inactivation of ALDH-2 in the STZ group substantially supports the cardio-toxic phenotype of hyperglycemia and improved activity of this redox-sensitive enzyme by a high dose SGLT2i therapy clearly points to cardio-protective and anti-oxidant properties of this drug.

Limitations of the study

There are some limitations in the present study. We used not all animals for all assays. Therefore, to ensure that the treatment with STZ and other drugs was comparable among all rats, some parameters were measured in all of them (e.g. blood glucose, HbA1c, cholesterol, insulin by RIA, vascular function and oxidative stress (dihydroethidium staining)). The here observed increase in leukocyte activity (oxidative burst) in diabetic rats, which also nicely correlates with all other measured markers of inflammation, is at variance with previous reports indicating impaired oxidative burst in neutrophils [49] and monocytes [50] in diabetic individuals, which correlates with the impaired phagocytic clearance of bacterial pathogens in these individuals. The major limitation of the study is that STZ treatment kills only some part of the islet cells directly. The remaining β-cells probably die due to glucotoxicity within the first 2 weeks after the injection of STZ. This represents a clear difference as compared to human T1DM where all islet cells are lost due to autoimmune-driven killing of these cells. This limitation will complicate the translation of our findings to the clinical situation. It is also unclear, whether the present results from T1DM can be translated to T2DM, which is the much more frequent form of diabetes in humans. Therefore, our future studies will address whether 1) much later onset of SGLT2i therapy (6 weeks after STZ for weeks 7 and 8 after STZ) will improve the diabetic complications even when all islet cells have died and 2) early onset of SGLT2i therapy (only the first 2 weeks after STZ, w/o treatment for weeks 3-8 after STZ) will still have a beneficial effect by preserving islet cell function. Finally, similar studies on SGLT2i therapy in a T2DM model (e.g. ZDF rats) and assessment of parameters of diabetic complications at all levels are highly recommended.

Conclusions and clinical implications

The results of the present study confirm previous findings that vascular dysfunction in the setting of diabetes is associated with increased vascular oxidative stress, AGE/RAGE signaling and low-grade inflammation (Figure 7). The clinical implications of the present findings originate from the complex interaction of redox and inflammatory pathways in cardiovascular pathogenesis [15,16] requiring multi-targeted therapy to improve the disease progression at all levels. The presented data clearly shows that SGLT2i therapy leading to enhanced glucose excretion improves glucose-induced vascular dysfunction by reducing glucotoxicity, oxidative stress, low-grade inflammation and restoring insulin signaling, ultimately improving endothelial dysfunction as an important determinant of future cardiovascular events.

Supporting Information

File S1 Online supplemental data.

Acknowledgments

We thank Philip Wenzel (University Medical Center Mainz, 55101 Mainz, Germany) for helpful discussions. We are also indebted to Angelica Karpi (University Medical Center Mainz, 55101 Mainz, Germany), Jörg Schreiner (University Medical Center Mainz, 55101 Mainz, Germany), Jessica Rudolph (University Medical Center Mainz, 55101 Mainz, Germany) and Bettina Mros (University Medical Center Mainz, 55101 Mainz, Germany) for expert technical assistance. The graphical assistance of Thilo Weckmüller is gratefully acknowledged. We thank Dr. Ulrich Rösch (Superon GmbH, Dernbach, Germany) for the Field-Flow Fractionation (FFF) measurements. This work contains data that are part of the thesis of Philipp Welschof.

Author Contributions

Conceived and designed the experiments: MO EM AD. Performed the experiments: MO SKS PW MH YM PS MM EZ SA AG SS SPB AD. Analyzed the data: MO SKS PW MH YM SPB AD. Contributed reagents/materials/analysis tools: EM. Wrote the paper: MO TJ YM ES SPB TM AD.

References

1. Nathan DM, Cleary PA, Backlund JY, Genuth SM, Lachin JM, et al. (2005) Intensive diabetes treatment and cardiovascular disease in patients with type 1 diabetes. N Engl J Med 353: 2643–2653.
2. Jay D, Hitomi H, Griendling KK (2006) Oxidative stress and diabetic cardiovascular complications. Free Radic Biol Med 40: 183–192.
3. Hink U, Li H, Mollnau H, Oelze M, Matheis E, et al. (2001) Mechanisms Underlying Endothelial Dysfunction in Diabetes Mellitus. Circ Res 88: E14–E22.
4. Wenzel P, Daiber A, Oelze M, Brandt M, Closs E, et al. (2008) Mechanisms underlying recoupling of eNOS by HMG-CoA reductase inhibition in a rat model of streptozotocin-induced diabetes mellitus. Atherosclerosis 198: 65–76.
5. Wenzel P, Schulz E, Oelze M, Muller J, Schuhmacher S, et al. (2008) AT1-receptor blockade by telmisartan upregulates GTP-cyclohydrolase I and protects eNOS in diabetic rats. Free Radic Biol Med 45: 619–626.
6. Schuhmacher S, Oelze M, Bollmann F, Kleinert H, Otto C, et al. (2011) Vascular Dysfunction in Experimental Diabetes Is Improved by Pentaerithrityl Tetranitrate but not Isosorbide-5-Mononitrate Therapy. Diabetes 60: 2608–2616.
7. Lin MI, Fulton D, Babbitt R, Fleming I, Busse R, et al. (2003) Phosphorylation of threonine 497 in endothelial nitric-oxide synthase coordinates the coupling of L-arginine metabolism to efficient nitric oxide production. J Biol Chem 278: 44719–44726.
8. Loot AE, Schreiber JG, Fisslthaler B, Fleming I (2009) Angiotensin II impairs endothelial function via tyrosine phosphorylation of the endothelial nitric oxide synthase. J Exp Med 206: 2889–2896.
9. Forbes JM, Cooper ME, Thallas V, Burns WC, Thomas MC, et al. (2002) Reduction of the accumulation of advanced glycation end products by ACE inhibition in experimental diabetic nephropathy. Diabetes 51: 3274–3282.
10. Yamamoto Y, Yamagishi S, Yonekura H, Doi T, Tsuji H, et al. (2000) Roles of the AGE-RAGE system in vascular injury in diabetes. Ann N Y Acad Sci 902: 163-170; discussion 170–162.
11. Coughlan MT, Thorburn DR, Penfold SA, Laskowski A, Harcourt BE, et al. (2009) RAGE-induced cytosolic ROS promote mitochondrial superoxide generation in diabetes. J Am Soc Nephrol 20: 742–752.
12. Wautier MP, Chappey O, Corda S, Stern DM, Schmidt AM, et al. (2001) Activation of NADPH oxidase by AGE links oxidant stress to altered gene expression via RAGE. Am J Physiol Endocrinol Metab 280: E685–694.
13. Nishikawa T, Edelstein D, Du XL, Yamagishi S, Matsumura T, et al. (2000) Normalizing mitochondrial superoxide production blocks three pathways of hyperglycaemic damage. Nature 404: 787–790.
14. Schulz E, Wenzel P, Munzel T, Daiber A (2014) Mitochondrial redox signaling: Interaction of mitochondrial reactive oxygen species with other sources of oxidative stress. Antioxid Redox Signal 20: 308–324.
15. Kroller-Schon S, Steven S, Kossmann S, Scholz A, Daub S, et al. (2014) Molecular mechanisms of the crosstalk between mitochondria and NADPH oxidase through reactive oxygen species-studies in white blood cells and in animal models. Antioxid Redox Signal 20: 247–266.
16. Wenzel P, Knorr M, Kossmann S, Stratmann J, Hausding M, et al. (2011) Lysozyme M-positive monocytes mediate angiotensin II-induced arterial hypertension and vascular dysfunction. Circulation 124: 1370–1381.
17. Rieg T, Masuda T, Gerasimova M, Mayoux E, Platt K, et al. (2014) Increase in SGLT1-mediated transport explains renal glucose reabsorption during genetic and pharmacological SGLT2 inhibition in euglycemia. Am J Physiol Renal Physiol 306: F188–193.
18. Evans JL, Goldfine ID (2013) Aging and insulin resistance: just say iNOS. Diabetes 62: 346–348.
19. Sarashina A, Koiwai K, Seman LJ, Yamamura N, Taniguchi A, et al. (2013) Safety, tolerability, pharmacokinetics and pharmacodynamics of single doses of empagliflozin, a sodium glucose cotransporter 2 (SGLT2) inhibitor, in healthy Japanese subjects. Drug Metab Pharmacokinet 28: 213–219.
20. Ferrannini E, Seman L, Seewaldt-Becker E, Hantel S, Pinnetti S, et al. (2013) A Phase IIb, randomized, placebo-controlled study of the SGLT2 inhibitor empagliflozin in patients with type 2 diabetes. Diabetes Obes Metab 15: 721–728.
21. Hansen HH, Jelsing J, Hansen CF, Hansen G, Vrang N, et al. (2014) The sodium glucose cotransporter type 2 inhibitor empagliflozin preserves beta-cell mass and restores glucose homeostasis in the male zucker diabetic fatty rat. J Pharmacol Exp Ther 350: 657–664.
22. Luippold G, Klein T, Mark M, Grempler R (2012) Empagliflozin, a novel potent and selective SGLT-2 inhibitor, improves glycaemic control alone and in combination with insulin in streptozotocin-induced diabetic rats, a model of type 1 diabetes mellitus. Diabetes Obes Metab 14: 601–607.
23. Grempler R, Thomas L, Eckhardt M, Himmelsbach F, Sauer A, et al. (2012) Empagliflozin, a novel selective sodium glucose cotransporter-2 (SGLT-2) inhibitor: characterisation and comparison with other SGLT-2 inhibitors. Diabetes Obes Metab 14: 83–90.
24. Vickers SP, Cheetham SC, Headland KR, Dickinson K, Grempler R, et al. (2014) Combination of the sodium-glucose cotransporter-2 inhibitor empagliflozin with orlistat or sibutramine further improves the body-weight reduction and glucose homeostasis of obese rats fed a cafeteria diet. Diabetes Metab Syndr Obes 7: 265–275.
25. Oelze M, Knorr M, Schuhmacher S, Heeren T, Otto C, et al. (2011) Vascular dysfunction in streptozotocin-induced experimental diabetes strictly depends on insulin deficiency. J Vasc Res 48: 275–284.
26. Oelze M, Kroller-Schon S, Steven S, Lubos E, Doppler C, et al. (2013) Glutathione Peroxidase-1 Deficiency Potentiates Dysregulatory Modifications of Endothelial Nitric Oxide Synthase and Vascular Dysfunction in Aging. Hypertension.
27. Daiber A, Oelze M, Coldewey M, Bachschmid M, Wenzel P, et al. (2004) Oxidative stress and mitochondrial aldehyde dehydrogenase activity: a comparison of pentaerythritol tetranitrate with other organic nitrates. Mol Pharmacol 66: 1372–1382.
28. Kroller-Schon S, Knorr M, Hausding M, Oelze M, Schuff A, et al. (2012) Glucose-independent improvement of vascular dysfunction in experimental sepsis by dipeptidyl-peptidase 4 inhibition. Cardiovasc Res 96: 140–149.
29. Oelze M, Daiber A, Brandes RP, Hortmann M, Wenzel P, et al. (2006) Nebivolol inhibits superoxide formation by NADPH oxidase and endothelial dysfunction in angiotensin II-treated rats. Hypertension 48: 677–684.
30. Shiryaeva YK, Krylin VV, Titov VN (2012) Chromatographic determination of methyl glyoxal in blood plasma as the test for glycotoxicity and accumulation of glycation end-products. Bull Exp Biol Med 153: 114–117.
31. Wenzel P, Hink U, Oelze M, Seeling A, Isse T, et al. (2007) Number of nitrate groups determines reactivity and potency of organic nitrates: a proof of concept study in ALDH-2-/- mice. Brit J Pharmacol 150: 526–533.
32. Hausding M, Jurk K, Daub S, Kroller-Schon S, Stein J, et al. (2013) CD40L contributes to angiotensin II-induced pro-thrombotic state, vascular inflammation, oxidative stress and endothelial dysfunction. Basic Res Cardiol 108: 386.
33. Pricci F, Leto G, Amadio L, Iacobini C, Cordone S, et al. (2003) Oxidative stress in diabetes-induced endothelial dysfunction involvement of nitric oxide and protein kinase C. Free Radic Biol Med 35: 683–694.
34. Yu Y, Lyons TJ (2005) A lethal tetrad in diabetes: hyperglycemia, dyslipidemia, oxidative stress, and endothelial dysfunction. Am J Med Sci 330: 227–232.
35. Ferrannini E, Muscelli E, Frascerra S, Baldi S, Mari A, et al. (2014) Metabolic response to sodium-glucose cotransporter 2 inhibition in type 2 diabetic patients. J Clin Invest 124: 499–508.
36. Perkins BA, Cherney DZ, Partridge H, Soleymanlou N, Tschirhart H, et al. (2014) Sodium-Glucose Cotransporter 2 Inhibition and Glycemic Control in Type 1 Diabetes: Results of an 8-Week Open-Label Proof-of-Concept Trial. Diabetes Care 37: 1480–1483.
37. Cherney DZ, Perkins BA, Soleymanlou N, Har R, Fagan N, et al. (2014) The effect of empagliflozin on arterial stiffness and heart rate variability in subjects with uncomplicated type 1 diabetes mellitus. Cardiovasc Diabetol 13: 28.
38. Bierhaus A, Fleming T, Stoyanov S, Leffler A, Babes A, et al. (2012) Methylglyoxal modification of Nav1.8 facilitates nociceptive neuron firing and causes hyperalgesia in diabetic neuropathy. Nat Med 18: 926–933.
39. Sun M, Yokoyama M, Ishiwata T, Asano G (1998) Deposition of advanced glycation end products (AGE) and expression of the receptor for AGE in cardiovascular tissue of the diabetic rat. Int J Exp Pathol 79: 207–222.
40. Wautier JL, Wautier MP, Schmidt AM, Anderson GM, Hori O, et al. (1994) Advanced glycation end products (AGEs) on the surface of diabetic erythrocytes bind to the vessel wall via a specific receptor inducing oxidant stress in the vasculature: a link between surface-associated AGEs and diabetic complications. Proc Natl Acad Sci U S A 91: 7742–7746.
41. Jeong KH, Lee TW, Ihm CG, Lee SH, Moon JY, et al. (2009) Effects of sildenafil on oxidative and inflammatory injuries of the kidney in streptozotocin-induced diabetic rats. Am J Nephrol 29: 274–282.
42. Kumar S, Prasad S, Sitasawad SL (2013) Multiple antioxidants improve cardiac complications and inhibit cardiac cell death in streptozotocin-induced diabetic rats. PLoS One 8: e67009.
43. Chen Z, Zhang J, Stamler JS (2002) Identification of the enzymatic mechanism of nitroglycerin bioactivation. Proc Natl Acad Sci U S A 99: 8306–8311.
44. Sydow K, Daiber A, Oelze M, Chen Z, August M, et al. (2004) Central role of mitochondrial aldehyde dehydrogenase and reactive oxygen species in nitroglycerin tolerance and cross-tolerance. J Clin Invest 113: 482–489.
45. Oelze M, Knorr M, Schell R, Kamuf J, Pautz A, et al. (2011) Regulation of human mitochondrial aldehyde dehydrogenase (ALDH-2) activity by electrophiles in vitro. J Biol Chem 286: 8893–8900.
46. Wenzel P, Hink U, Oelze M, Schuppan S, Schaeuble K, et al. (2007) Role of reduced lipoic acid in the redox regulation of mitochondrial aldehyde dehydrogenase (ALDH-2) activity. Implications for mitochondrial oxidative stress and nitrate tolerance. J Biol Chem 282: 792–799.

47. Chen CH, Budas GR, Churchill EN, Disatnik MH, Hurley TD, et al. (2008) Activation of aldehyde dehydrogenase-2 reduces ischemic damage to the heart. Science 321: 1493–1495.
48. Wang J, Wang H, Hao P, Xue L, Wei S, et al. (2011) Inhibition of aldehyde dehydrogenase 2 by oxidative stress is associated with cardiac dysfunction in diabetic rats. Mol Med 17: 172–179.
49. Osar Z, Samanci T, Demirel GY, Damci T, Ilkova H (2004) Nicotinamide effects oxidative burst activity of neutrophils in patients with poorly controlled type 2 diabetes mellitus. Exp Diabesity Res 5: 155–162.
50. Chang FY, Shaio MF (1995) Respiratory burst activity of monocytes from patients with non-insulin-dependent diabetes mellitus. Diabetes Res Clin Pract 29: 121–127.

Influence of the Time of Day and Fasting Duration on Glucose Level following a 1-Hour, 50-Gram Glucose Challenge Test in Pregnant Women

Panchalli Wang[1], Mei-Chun Lu[1,2], Cheng-Wei Yu[3], Yuan-Horng Yan[2,4,5]*

1 Department of Obstetrics and Gynecology, Ditmanson Medical Foundation Chia-Yi Christian Hospital, Chia-Yi City, Taiwan, **2** Department of Medical Research, Ditmanson Medical Foundation Chia-Yi Christian Hospital, Chia-Yi City, Taiwan, **3** Department of Nutrition, Ditmanson Medical Foundation Chia-Yi Christian Hospital, Chia-Yi City, Taiwan, **4** Department of Internal Medicine, Ditmanson Medical Foundation Chia-Yi Christian Hospital, Chia-Yi City, Taiwan, **5** Institute of Occupational Medicine and Industrial Hygiene, College of Public Health, National Taiwan University, Taipei, Taiwan

Abstract

Background: Previous studies have shown that the time of day (TD) of glucose measurement and the fasting duration (FD) influence the glucose levels in adults. Few studies have examined the effects of the TD and FD on the glucose level following a 1-hour, 50-gram glucose challenge test (GCT) in pregnant women in screening for or diagnosing gestational diabetes mellitus (GDM). The objective of this study was to investigate the influence of the TD (morning, afternoon, night) and the FD (the time of the last food ingestion as follows: ≤1 hour, 1–2 hours, and >2 hours) by examining their combined effects on the glucose levels following a 50-gram GCT in pregnant women.

Methods and Results: We analyzed the data of 1,454 non-diabetic pregnant Taiwanese women in a prospective study. Multiple linear regression and multiple logistic regression were used to estimate the relationships between the 9 TD-FD groups and the continuous and binary glucose levels (cut-off at 140 mg/dL) following a 50-gram GCT, after adjusting for maternal age, nulliparity, pre-pregnancy body mass index, and weight gain. Different TD and FD groups were associated with variable glucose responses to the 50-gram GCT, some of which were significant. The estimate coefficients (β) of the TD-FD groups "night, ≤1 hr" and "night, 1–2 hr" revealed significantly lower glucose concentrations [β (95% confidence interval [CI]): −6.46 (−12.53, −0.38) and −6.85 (−12.50, −1.20)] compared with the "morning, >2 hr" group. The TD-FD groups "afternoon, ≤1 hr" and "afternoon, 1–2 hr" showed significantly lower odds ratios (OR) of a positive GCT; the adjusted ORs (95% CI) were 0.54 (0.31–0.95) and 0.58 (0.35–0.96), respectively.

Conclusions: Our findings demonstrate the importance of standardizing the TD and FD for the 1-hour, 50-gram GCT. In screening for and diagnosing GDM, the TD and FD are modifiable factors that should be considered in clinical practice and epidemiological studies.

Editor: Sisira Siribaddana, Rajarata Univeresity of Sri Lanka, Sri Lanka

Funding: The authors received no specific funding for this work.

Competing Interests: The authors have declared that no competing interests exist.

* Email: d97841006@ntu.edu.tw

Introduction

Previous studies have shown that the time of day (TD) of glucose measurement and the fasting duration (FD) influence the glucose level in adults [1–4]. Studies in pregnant women have shown the effects of the TD (or circadian or diurnal variations) on the results of a gestational 1-hour, 50-gram glucose challenge test (GCT) [5–8]. Previous studies have demonstrated that the fasting duration (FD) (or the time since the last caloric intake) might influence the gestational GCT [6,9]. Few studies have investigated the effects of the TD and the FD on the glucose levels following gestational GCT in pregnant women [6].

The two-step approach for the diagnosis of gestational diabetes mellitus (GDM), which consists of a 1-hour, 50-gram GCT combined with a 100-gram oral glucose tolerance test (OGTT), is supported by the American College of Obstetricians and Gynecologists (ACOG); it has been widely used in nearly all the hospitals in Taiwan for more than 10 years. In Taiwan, the general recommendation is that all pregnant women complete the 1-hour, 50-gram GCT, which is covered by the National Health Insurance (NHI) policy. The 1-hour, 50-gram GCT portion of the current two-step approach for the diagnosis of GDM does not specify the parameters for the TD or the FD, and the instructions regarding whether pregnant women should fast for this test are inconsistent. Appointment schedules for outpatient services in Taiwan are very busy and include morning, afternoon, and night appointments in clinics where pregnant women can undergo the 1-hour, 50-gram GCT.

Recently, based on the Hyperglycemia and Adverse Pregnancy Outcome (HAPO) study, the International Association of Diabetes and Pregnancy Study Groups [10] presented new consensus guidelines for the diagnosis of GDM using a 1-step, 2-hour, 75-gram OGTT [10,11]. The HAPO study and the IADPSG guidelines do not consider the TD or FD. To our knowledge, no study has investigated the associations between the TD, FD, and glucose measurements with the 2-hour, 75-gram OGTT. The 1-hour, 50-gram GCT and the 2-hour, 75-gram OGTT are glucose tolerance tests, and they should be used carefully in pregnant women [12]. Understanding the modifiable factors that might cause variations in glucose tolerance test results is important. Thus, the objective of this study was to investigate the influence of the TD and FD on glucose levels following a 1-hour, 50-gram GCT in pregnant Taiwanese women.

Materials and Methods

Study participants

This hospital-based prospective study was conducted in a 1000-bed teaching hospital in southern Taiwan. During the study period, March - October 2011, all patients who underwent a 50-gram GCT at 24–28 weeks of gestation at the obstetric clinic at the Ditmanson Medical Foundation Chia-Yi Christian Hospital (DMF-CYCH) were enrolled. The patients with pre-pregnancy diabetes, multi-fetal pregnancies, and a history of GDM were excluded. The DMF-CYCH institutional review board (IRB) approved this study (CYCH-IRB No. 100030), and all the study participants provided written informed consent to participate in the study.

Measurements of the TD, FD and glucose level

The venous plasma glucose levels were measured by the glucose oxidase method using a Hitachi 7170 automatic analyzer (Hitachi Co., Tokyo, Japan) in the DMF-CYCH central laboratory, according to a standard clinical protocol. The TD was defined as the time of the blood draw minus one hour; the times of all blood draws were obtained from the same computer in the DMF-CYCH central laboratory. Nurses from the Department of Community Health at DMF-CYCH administered a face-to-face interview questionnaire to the patients to collect basic data (including maternal age, parity, pre-pregnancy body mass index [BMI], and weight gain) and FD data.

Statistics

The patients were stratified into 9 groups, designated as the TD-FD groups, by the TD (morning: 9 AM–12 PM, afternoon: 12–5 PM, and night: 5–10 PM) and FD (the time elapsed from the patient's last food ingestion prior to the GCT: ≤1 hr, 1–2 hr, and >2 hr). The chi-square test was used to analyze the distribution of the known risk factors for the glucose levels in each TD-FD group. The known risk factors included maternal age, nulliparity, pre-pregnancy BMI, and weight gain. BMI was calculated as weight [3]/[height (m)]^2 and was categorized according to the criteria of the Bureau of Health Promotion of the Department of Health in Taiwan. Weight gain was defined as the percentage of gestational weight gain = [(weight at the time of the 50-gram GCT − pre-pregnancy weight)/pre-pregnancy weight] * 100 and was classified into four groups based on increments of 10%.

In the univariate analysis, the association between each TD-FD group and the risk factors for the mean glucose level was analyzed using analysis of variance or Student's t test, as appropriate; and the association between each TD-FD group and the risk factors for the glucose cut-off level of 140 mg/dL was analyzed using a chi-square test. In the multivariate analysis, first, a multiple linear regression model was used to estimate the relationship between each TD-FD group and the glucose levels response to the GCT (continuous variables), adjusted for other risk factors. Second, we used the multiple logistic regression model to further describe the impact of TD-FD on a positive GCT (glucose level ≥140 mg/dL as the event). The significance level was set at 0.05, and all tests were two-tailed. SAS 9.2 software was used for the data analysis (SAS Institute, Cary, NC, USA).

Results

Of the 1681 patients at 24–28 weeks of gestation without pre-pregnancy diabetes, 91% (n = 1530) underwent a 50-gram GCT and were enrolled in this study. Thirty-three women without information regarding their FD, 29 women with multi-fetal pregnancies, and 14 women with a history of GDM were excluded from the analysis. In total, 1454 women were included in the analysis (**Figure 1**).

Table 1 shows the distribution of risk factors across the TD-FD groups. These risk factors, with the exception of pre-pregnancy BMI, differed significantly across the TD-FD groups.

Table 2 shows the results of the univariate analysis. The mean glucose level did not differ among the TD-FD groups. With the exception of nulliparity, the mean glucose level differed significantly among the risk factors. The results were similar using the continuous and categorical 50-gram GCT glucose levels. There was a trend of increasing glucose level with increasing maternal age and pre-pregnancy BMI. The relationship between glucose level and weight gain showed a J-shape, and the women with a weight gain of 20%–30% had the lowest glucose concentration; the mean±SD was 121.0±27.8 mg/dL, and 63 subjects (21.7%) had a level ≥140 mg/dL.

Table 3 shows the results of the multivariate analysis. First, in the multiple linear regression model, after adjusting for the risk factors, the estimate coefficients (β) of the "night, ≤1 hr" and

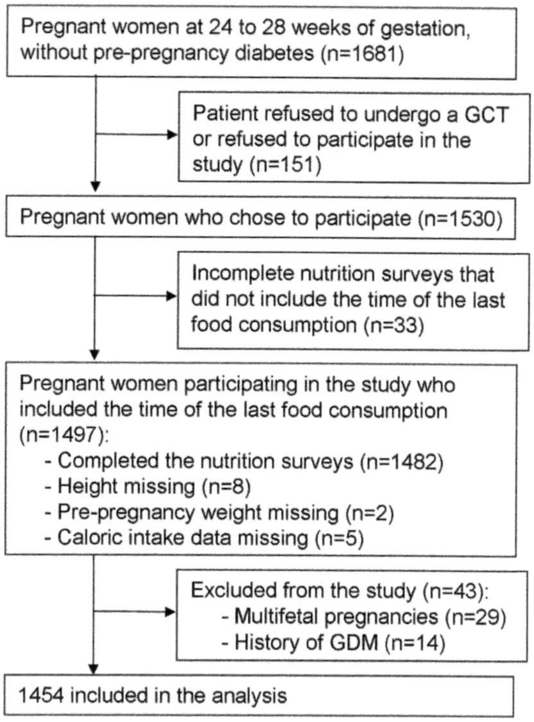

Figure 1. Flowchart of methods.

Table 1. Distribution of risk factors across the TD-FD groups.

Variable	Number	Morning (9 AM–12 AM)			Afternoon (12–5 PM)			Night (5–10 PM)			P*
		≤1 hr	1–2 hr	>2 hr	≤1 hr	1–2 hr	>2 hr	≤1 hr	1–2 hr	>2 hr	
Cases No.	1454	151	158	179	124	162	180	140	179	181	
Nulliparous status											0.01
Yes	737	85 (56.3)	70 (44.3)	83 (46.4)	63 (50.8)	76 (46.9)	83 (46.1)	92 (65.7)	94 (52.5)	91 (50.3)	
No	717	66 (43.7)	88 (55.7)	96 (53.6)	61 (49.2)	86 (53.1)	97 (53.9)	48 (34.3)	85 (47.5)	90 (49.7)	
Maternal age (y)											
<25	153	14 (9.3)	13 (8.2)	15 (8.4)	21 (16.9)	16 (9.9)	28 (15.6)	12 (8.6)	14 (7.8)	20 (11.1)	0.049
25–30	510	59 (39.1)	48 (30.4)	57 (31.8)	45 (36.3)	53 (32.7)	59 (32.8)	55 (39.3)	70 (39.1)	64 (35.4)	
30–35	564	53 (35.1)	59 (37.3)	75 (41.9)	41 (33.1)	61 (37.7)	68 (37.8)	57 (40.7)	77 (43.0)	73 (40.3)	
≥35	227	25 (16.6)	38 (24.1)	32 (17.9)	17 (13.7)	32 (19.8)	25 (13.9)	16 (11.4)	18 (10.1)	24 (13.3)	
Pre-pregnancy BMI (kg/m^2)											
<18.5	221	27 (17.9)	19 (12.0)	25 (14.2)	29 (23.6)	29 (18.0)	29 (16.3)	14 (10.1)	20 (11.2)	29 (16.1)	0.65
18.5–24	925	98 (64.9)	103 (65.2)	111 (63.1)	71 (57.7)	100 (62.1)	117 (65.7)	93 (67.4)	117 (65.4)	115 (63.9)	
24–27	178	18 (11.9)	20 (12.7)	21 (11.9)	15 (12.2)	20 (12.4)	21 (11.8)	17 (12.3)	24 (13.4)	22 (12.2)	
≥27	120	8 (5.3)	16 (10.1)	19 (10.8)	8 (6.5)	12 (7.5)	11 (6.2)	14 (10.1)	18 (10.1)	14 (7.8)	
Missing	10										
Weight gain (%)†											
<10	289	18 (11.9)	38 (24.1)	46 (25.7)	23 (18.6)	39 (24.1)	44 (24.6)	17 (12.1)	29 (16.2)	35 (19.4)	0.001
10–20	825	98 (64.9)	78 (49.4)	103 (57.5)	68 (54.8)	77 (47.5)	101 (56.4)	92 (65.7)	109 (60.9)	99 (55.0)	
20–30	291	32 (21.2)	37 (23.4)	28 (15.6)	23 (18.6)	36 (22.2)	29 (16.2)	28 (20.0)	36 (20.1)	42 (23.3)	
≥30	47	3 (2.0)	5 (3.2)	2 (1.1)	10 (8.1)	10 (6.2)	5 (2.8	3 (2.1)	5 (2.8)	4 (2.2)	
Missing	2										

TD-FD, time of day glucose was measured and fasting duration; GCT, glucose challenge test; BMI, body mass index.
*Data are presented as n (%) and were analyzed using the chi-square test.
†Percentage of gestational weight gain = [(weight at time of GCT − pre-pregnancy weight)/pre-pregnancy weight] * 100.

Table 2. The association between TD-FD group and risk factors for the mean glucose level and a cut-off level of 140 mg/dL.

Variable		Number	Glucose level (mg/dL)				
			Mean ± SD	P*	≥140 mg/dL, n (%)		P†
TD-FD group				0.37			0.39
Morning	≤1 hr	151	124.7±28.3		39	(25.8)	
	1–2 hr	158	124.7±26.8		40	(25.3)	
	>2 hr	179	129.4±29.4		56	(31.3)	
Afternoon	≤1 hr	124	123.5±23.9		25	(20.2)	
	1–2 hr	162	124.6±26.0		35	(21.6)	
	>2 hr	180	126.9±30.1		54	(30.0)	
Night	≤1 hr	140	122.6±31.2		35	(25.0)	
	1–2 hr	179	122.4±26.2		44	(24.6)	
	>2 hr	181	123.8±27.8		50	(27.6)	
Nulliparous status				0.11			0.58
Yes		737	123.7±27.3		187	(25.4)	
No		717	126.0±28.5		191	(26.6)	
Maternal age (y)				<0.001			<0.001
<25		153	115.4±24.5		23	(15.0)	
25–30		510	120.9±25.8		111	(21.8)	
30–35		564	127.0±27.5		165	(29.3)	
≥35		227	134.8±31.9		79	(34.8)	
Pre-pregnancy BMI (kg/m^2)				<0.001			0.02
<18.5		221	120.6±25.8		49	(22.2)	
18.5–24		925	123.5±27.5		230	(24.9)	
24–27		178	129.6±28.2		55	(30.9)	
≥27		120	136.6±31.0		42	(35.0)	
Missing		10	-				
Weight gain (%)‡				0.004			0.02
<10		289	128.9±31.4		90	(31.1)	
10–20		825	124.5±26.5		208	(25.2)	
20–30		291	121.0±27.8		63	(21.7)	
≥30		47	130.1±25.7		17	(36.2)	
Missing		2	-				

TD-FD, time of day glucose was measured and fasting duration; GCT, glucose challenge test; BMI, body mass index.
*Data were analyzed using analysis of variance or Student's t test as appropriate.
†Data were analyzed using the chi-square test.
‡Percentage of gestational weight gain = [(weight at time of GCT − pre-pregnancy weight)/pre-pregnancy weight] * 100.

Table 3. Multivariate analysis of the TD-FD groups and the GCT adjusted for risk factors (n = 1444).

Variable		Multiple linear regression			Multiple logistic regression		
		β	95% Confidence interval	*P*	Odds ratio	95% Confidence interval	*P*
Intercept		67.06	(53.04–81.09)	<0.001			
TD-FD group							
Morning	≤1 hr	−4.11	(−10.02, 1.81)	0.17	0.78	(0.48, 1.28)	0.33
	1–2 hr	−5.95	(−11.79, −0.11)	0.046	0.68	(0.42, 1.11)	0.12
	>2 hr	0			1		
Afternoon	≤1 hr	−4.74	(−11.02, 1.54)	0.14	0.54	(0.31, 0.95)	0.03
	1–2 hr	−4.58	(−10.39, 1.24)	0.12	0.58	(0.35, 0.96)	0.03
	>2 hr	−1.61	(−7.26, 4.04)	0.58	0.99	(0.62, 1.56)	0.95
Night	≤1 hr	−6.46	(−12.53, −0.38)	0.04	0.73	(0.44, 1.22)	0.23
	1–2 hr	−6.85	(−12.50, −1.20)	0.02	0.72	(0.45, 1.15)	0.17
	>2 hr	−4.65	(−10.29, 0.99)	0.11	0.88	(0.55, 1.39)	0.57
Nulliparous status							
Yes		1.29	(−1.63, 4.21)	0.38	1.15	(0.90, 1.48)	0.27
No		0			1		
Maternal age (y)		1.28	(0.96, 1.61)	<0.001	1.08	(1.05, 1.11)	<0.001
Pre-pregnancy BMI		1.00	(0.55, 1.45)	<0.001	1.04	(1.00, 1.08)	0.04
Weight gain (%)*							
<10		1.42	(−3.50, 6.34)	0.57	1.25	(0.82, 1.91)	0.30
10–20		0.96	(−2.74, 4.66)	0.61	1.06	(0.76, 1.48)	0.73
20–30		0			1		
≥30		10.39	(1.99, 18.79)	0.02	2.38	(1.22, 4.67)	0.01

TD-FD, time of day glucose was measured and fasting duration; GCT, glucose challenge test; β, regression coefficient; BMI, body mass index.
*Percentage of gestational weight gain = [(weight at time of GCT − pre-pregnancy weight)/pre-pregnancy weight] * 100.

"night, 1–2 hr" TD-FD groups revealed significantly lower glucose concentrations [β (95% confidence interval [CI]): −6.46 (−12.53, −0.38) and −6.85 (−12.50, −1.20)] compared with the "morning, >2 hr" group. Second, for further describing the impact of TD-FD on a positive GCT for potential clinical practice, a multiple logistic regression model was used. The TD-FD groups "afternoon, ≤1 hr" and "afternoon, 1–2 hr" showed significantly lower odds ratios (OR) of a positive GCT compared with the "morning, >2 hr" group; the adjusted ORs (95% CI) were 0.54 (0.31–0.95) and 0.58 (0.35–0.96), respectively.

Discussion

Our findings suggest that the TD and FD influence the glucose level following a 1-hour, 50-gram GCT in pregnant women. The patients who were examined in the afternoon and at night without a sufficient fasting interval have had significantly lower glucose measurements in the multivariate analysis. Because the TD and FD are modifiable factors in screening for and diagnosing GDM, they should be considered in clinical practice and epidemiological studies [5,7,8,13–15].

We used linear and logistic regression models to determine whether TD and FD were predictors of the glucose concentrations of 50-g GCT and the magnitude of this relation in the current study. The two models both showed the glucose concentrations of 50-g GCT, which performing in the afternoon and night, were lower than that performing in the morning. Although afternoon groups in linear model and the night groups in logistic regression model did not reach the statistical significance, the trends were consistent. We speculated the differences between the two models were caused by the type of outcomes (continuous and binary variables) and the type of results they produced [16].

Additionally, the findings might have implications for the IADPSG guidelines for GDM for both the 2-step approach and the 1-step, 2-hour, 75-gram OGTT. The universal standard for the glucose cut-off value of the 1-hour, 50-gram GCT should be further validated [17,18]. Although the effects of the TD and FD on the glucose level were mild, these slight changes could affect the diagnosis of GDM at the threshold glucose levels [19]. Our findings indicate that the TD and FD should be considered when screening for and diagnosing GDM in clinical practice. Thus, standardizing the TD and FD for the 1-hour, 50-gram GCT, as well as other glucose tolerance tests, is an important goal.

Maternal glucose metabolism during pregnancy differs from that in non-pregnancy. Previous studies have examined the diurnal glycemic profile and the influence of food intake during pregnancy, using continuous glucose monitoring systems (CGMS) that measure the interstitial glucose levels in subcutaneous tissues every 5 minutes for 72 consecutive hours [20]. The roles of systemic inflammation and insulin resistance in glucose regulation during pregnancy have been investigated [21]. The novel metabolomics approach has recently been used to further explore maternal metabolism during pregnancy [22]. Metabolomics data from 67 mothers of Northern European ancestry from the HAPO study revealed perturbations in the metabolism of major macronutrients and amino acid degradation pathways in mothers with high- versus low-fasting glucose [23]. Further mechanistic studies on the effects of the TD and FD on maternal metabolism during pregnancy are needed.

In addition, we showed that age, pre-pregnancy BMI, and weight gain affect the relationships among the TD, FD and glucose measures. The findings regarding age, maternal obesity, and parity are consistent with previous findings [2,5]. Our findings support prior evidence that weight gain during pregnancy is an important factor [24–27]. Our findings support the recommendation that the TD and FD be standardized in epidemiological studies.

The strength of our study is its detailed assessment, using a relatively large population, of the TD and FD, which are modifiable factors that are important in screening for and diagnosing GDM. The limitations of our study are that other factors might influence the glucose level and that detailed diet records and physical activity data were lacking [28]. Further research is needed to examine the generalizability of our findings to other ethnic groups.

Conclusions

Our results demonstrate the importance of standardizing the TD and FD for the 1-hour, 50-gram GCT; these factors have previously been ignored in clinical practice and epidemiological investigations. To avoid bias and misclassification when using a glucose tolerance test to screen for and diagnose GDM, the TD and FD should be considered [22].

Acknowledgments

The authors thank the staff members of the Department of Community Health for their assistance with interviews of the pregnant women and collection of the questionnaire.

Author Contributions

Conceived and designed the experiments: PW MCL CWY YHY. Performed the experiments: CWY MCL. Analyzed the data: MCL. Contributed reagents/materials/analysis tools: YHY. Wrote the paper: MCL YHY. Discussed the results and commented on the manuscript: PW MCL CWY YHY.

References

1. Moebus S, Göres L, Lösch C, Jöckel K-H (2011) Impact of time since last caloric intake on blood glucose levels. Eur J Epidemiol 26: 719–728.
2. Hulmán A, Færch K, Vistisen D, Karsai J, Nyári T, et al. (2013) Effect of time of day and fasting duration on measures of glycaemia: analysis from the Whitehall II Study. Diabetologia 56: 294–297.
3. Emberson J, Whincup P, Walker M, Thomas M, Alberti K (2002) Biochemical measures in a population-based study: effect of fasting duration and time of day. Ann Clin Biochem 39: 493–501.
4. Troisi RJ, Cowie CC, Harris MI (2000) Diurnal variation in fasting plasma glucose: Implications for diagnosis of diabetes in patients examined in the afternoon. JAMA 284: 3157–3159.
5. Goldberg RJ, Ye C, Sermer M, Connelly PW, Hanley AJ, et al. (2012) Circadian Variation in the Response to the Glucose Challenge Test in Pregnancy Implications for screening for gestational diabetes mellitus. Diabetes care 35: 1578–1584.
6. Mayer KH, Stamler J, Dyer A, Freinkel N, Stamler R, et al. (1976) Epidemiologic findings on the relationship of time of day and time since last meal to glucose tolerance. Diabetes 25: 936–943.
7. Jarrett RJ, Keen H (1969) Diurnal Variation of Oral Glucose Tolerance: a Possible Pointer to the Evolution of Diabetes Mellitus. Br Med J 2: 341–344.
8. McElduff A, Hitchman R (2002) Screening for gestational diabetes: the time of day is important. Med J Aust 176: 136.
9. Sermer M, Naylor CD, Gare DJ, Kenshole AB, Ritchie JWK, et al. (1994) Impact of time since last meal on the gestational glucose challenge test: The Toronto Tri-Hospital Gestational Diabetes Project. Am J Obstet Gynecol 171: 607–616.
10. Metzger BE, Gabbe SG, Persson B, Buchanan TA, Catalano PA, et al. (2010) International association of diabetes and pregnancy study groups recommendations on the diagnosis and classification of hyperglycemia in pregnancy. Diabetes Care 33: 676–682.

11. Metzger BE, Lowe LP, Dyer AR, Trimble ER, Chaovarindr U, et al. (2008) Hyperglycemia and adverse pregnancy outcomes. N Engl J Med 358: 1991–2002.
12. O'Sullivan JB, Mahan CM (1966) Glucose tolerance test. Variability in pregnant and nonpregnant women. Am J Clin Nutr 19: 345–351.
13. Aparicio NJ, Joao MA, Cortelezzi M, Guz M, Sturgeon C, et al. (1998) Pregnant women with impaired tolerance to an oral glucose load in the afternoon: evidence suggesting that they behave metabolically as patients with gestational diabetes. Am J Obstet Gynecol 178: 1059–1066.
14. Dokus K, Dokusova S (2013) Comment on: Goldberg, et al. Circadian Variation in the Response to the Glucose Challenge Test in Pregnancy: Implications for Screening for Gestational Diabetes Mellitus. Diabetes Care 2012; 35: 1578–1584. Diabetes care 36: e38.
15. Goldberg RJ, Ye C, Sermer M, Connelly PW, Hanley AJ, et al. (2013) Response to Comment on: Goldberg et al. Circadian Variation in the Response to the Glucose Challenge Test in Pregnancy: Implications for Screening for Gestational Diabetes Mellitus. Diabetes Care 2012; 35: 1578–1584. Diabetes care 36: e39.
16. Worster A, Fan J, Ismaila A (2007) Understanding linear and logistic regression analyses. CJEM 9: 111–113.
17. Miyakoshi K, Tanaka M, Ueno K, Uehara K, Ishimoto H, et al. (2003) Cutoff value of 1 h, 50 g glucose challenge test for screening of gestational diabetes mellitus in a Japanese population. Diabetes Res Clin Pract 60: 63–67.
18. Yee LM, Cheng YW, Liddell J, Block-Kurbisch I, Caughey AB (2011) 50-Gram glucose challenge test: is it indicative of outcomes in women without gestational diabetes mellitus? J Matern Fetal Neonatal Med 24: 1102–1106.
19. d'Emden M (2014) Do the new threshold levels for the diagnosis of gestational diabetes mellitus correctly identify women at risk? Diabetes Care 37: e30.
20. Yogev Y, Ben-Haroush A, Chen R, Rosenn B, Hod M, et al. (2004) Diurnal glycemic profile in obese and normal weight nondiabetic pregnant women. Am J Obstet Gynecol 191: 949–953.
21. Guillemette L, Lacroix M, Battista MC, Doyon M, Moreau J, et al. (2014) TNFalpha dynamics during the oral glucose tolerance test varies according to the level of insulin resistance trimester in pregnant women. J Clin Endocrinol Metab: doi: 10.1210/jc.2013-4016.
22. Lowe WL, Jr., Karban J (2014) Genetics, genomics and metabolomics: new insights into maternal metabolism during pregnancy. Diabet Med 31: 254–262.
23. Scholtens DM, Muehlbauer MJ, Daya NR, Stevens RD, Dyer AR, et al. (2014) Metabolomics reveals broad-scale metabolic perturbations in hyperglycemic mothers during pregnancy. Diabetes Care 37: 158–166.
24. Colditz GA, Willett WC, Rotnitzky A, Manson JE (1995) Weight gain as a risk factor for clinical diabetes mellitus in women. Ann Intern Med 122: 481–486.
25. Sommer C, Morkrid K, Jenum AK, Sletner L, Mosdol A, et al. (2014) Weight gain, total fat gain and regional fat gain during pregnancy and the association with gestational diabetes: a population-based cohort study. Int J Obes (Lond) 38: 76–81.
26. Tomedi LE, Simhan HN, Chang CC, McTigue KM, Bodnar LM (2013) Gestational Weight Gain, Early Pregnancy Maternal Adiposity Distribution, and Maternal Hyperglycemia. Matern Child Health J.
27. Li N, Liu E, Guo J, Pan L, Li B, et al. (2013) Maternal prepregnancy body mass index and gestational weight gain on pregnancy outcomes. PLoS One 8: e82310.
28. Baptiste-Roberts K, Ghosh P, Nicholson WK (2011) Pregravid physical activity, dietary intake, and glucose intolerance during pregnancy. J Womens Health (Larchmt) 20: 1847–1851.

The 5-Year Onset and Regression of Diabetic Retinopathy in Chinese Type 2 Diabetes Patients

Peiyao Jin[1], Jinjuan Peng[1], Haidong Zou[1,2]*, Weiwei Wang[3], Jiong Fu[3], Binjie Shen[3], Xuelin Bai[3], Xun Xu[1], Xi Zhang[1]

1 Department of Ophthalmology, Shanghai First People's Hospital, Shanghai Jiao Tong University, Shanghai, 20080, China, **2** Department of Preventative Ophthalmology, Shanghai Eye Disease Prevention and Treatment Center, Shanghai, 200040, China, **3** Beixinjing Community Health Service Center, Shanghai, China

Abstract

Purpose: To determine the rate and risk factors of diabetic retinopathy (DR) onset and regression in Chinese type 2 diabetes mellitus patients.

Methods: This is a 5-year community-based prospective study. The demographic information, systemic examination results and ophthalmological test results of each participant were collected. The study outcomes were DR incidence, defined as the onset of DR in at least one eye, and DR regression, defined as full regression from existing DR to no retinopathy without invasive treatments. The associations between each potential risk factor and the outcomes were studied.

Results: In total, 778 participants were enrolled. There were 322 patients without DR at baseline, of which 151 participants developed DR during follow-up (DR incidence rate = 46.89%). Baseline hyperglycemia and high blood pressure were two independent risk factors associated with DR incidence. Among the 456 participants with existing DR at entry, 110 fully recovered after 5 years (DR regression rate = 24.12%). Low baseline glucose and low serum triglyceride were two independent factors associated with DR regression.

Conclusions: DR incidence occurred more frequently in patients with hyperglycemia and high blood pressure. DR regression occurred mostly in patients with lower glucose and lower serum triglyceride levels among Chinese type 2 diabetes patients.

Editor: Demetrios Vavvas, Massachusetts Eye & Ear Infirmary, Harvard Medical School, United States of America

Funding: This work was funded by the Chinese National Natural Science Foundation (Project number 81371069), the Shanghai Pujiang Program (Project number PJ (2012) 0001652), and the Shanghai New Hundred Talents Program from the Shanghai Medical and Family Planning Committee (Project number 13B141). The funders had no role in study design, data collection and analysis, decision to publish, or preparation of the manuscript.

Competing Interests: The authors have declared that no competing interests exist.

* Email: zouhaidong@hotmail.com

Introduction

Diabetic retinopathy (DR) is a common complication of diabetes mellitus. Although many treatments are available, DR remains the most common cause of blindness among people 30 to 69 years of age in several Western countries. [1,2] It is universally believed that the key to controlling diabetic retinal complications is to prevent them from happening. To achieve this target, it is necessary to identify the factors associated with DR onset.

According to a recent Chinese population-based study [3], the age-standardized prevalence of diabetes in Chinese adults in 2010 was 9.7%, representing at least 92 million Chinese diabetes patients, which might be greater than that found in any other country. Most of these patients are suffering from type 2 diabetes. However, many classic DR incidence studies have been conducted among type 1 diabetes patients [4,5], while studies targeting type 2 diabetes patients are relatively fewer. Moreover, a previous study suggested that large differences may exist in DR onset among various populations [6]. Most former studies were undertaken in Caucasian populations [4,7–9], whereas data regarding the incidence of DR in Asian races, especially in the Chinese population, are scarce. To the best of our knowledge, only one with a Chinese population has been conducted to date in a hospital setting in Hong Kong and found a 20.3% 4-year cumulative DR incidence in a total of 212 type 2 diabetes patients [10]. Thus, a community-based prospective study with a larger population will provide more evidence to reveal the risk factors of DR incidence in Chinese type 2 diabetes patients.

Since 2003, our study group has been helping diabetes residents in the Beixinjing community to prevent and control DR progression through glucose control [11]. During our work, we have witnessed fully regressed retinopathy in several DR patients. The interesting part was that the regression happened without invasive treatments such as photocoagulation, intraocular medicine injection or surgery. These patients only accepted systematic treatments to improve microcirculation and to control high glucose levels, hypertension and hyperlipidemia. Although many studies have discussed the effect of photocoagulation or intravitreal bevacizumab (Avastin) treatments in DR regression [12–14], studies concerning DR regression without invasive treatments are limited. A few observational studies [15,16] and case reports [17,18] have reported the phenomenon of DR regression without discussing the factors associated with it. A famous randomized controlled trial (RCT) reported the influence of Candesartan in DR regression in type 2 diabetes patients [19]. Although the reliability of observational studies is not as good as RCTs in determining the effect of a treatment, observational studies can obtain the DR regression rate in a community population. As far as we know, no observational population study has reported the systemic factors associated with DR regression in a community population before. Although late stage DR can be contained by photocoagulation, intraocular medicine or vitreoretinal surgery, it is often at the expense of functional retina and visual performance and often results in poor prognoses [20,21]. By studying the factors associated with DR regression, we can provide early stage DR patients with more options to not only slow the progression of retinopathy but also to reverse the existing disease, thus avoiding late-stage retinopathy and achieving better prognoses.

The results we report here were based on a 5-year prospective study of 778 participants in a community-setting cohort in Shanghai, China. The aim of this study was to determine the onset and regression rate of DR and the associated factors in Chinese type 2 diabetes patients.

Methods

Setting and participants

The Beixinjing community is located in the southwestern corner of the Shanghai urban district. The population of this community has generally remained stable over the past 20 years. In 1995, a health information database including almost all of the residents was created and has been updated annually by the Beixinjing Community Health Service Center [11].

During follow-up, participants took necessary medicines to control systemic diseases. For example, individualized anti-hyperglycemia therapy, including metformin, sulfonylureas, meglitinides, glitazones and insulin injections, or behavioral therapy, such as exercise, diet control, and smoking cessation, were used to help control hyperglycemia. Patients' blood glucose levels were monitored by capillary blood glucose determination once a week, and their hemoglobin A1c (HbA1c) levels were measured once per year. Participants who also had high blood pressure continued their antihypertensive therapy during follow-up using common drugs including diuretics, β-adrenoceptor blocking drugs, angiotensin-converting enzyme inhibitor (ACEI), angiotensin II receptor antagonist (ARB), and calcium channel blocking drugs. Participants with hyperlipemia or hypercholesterolemia took drugs such as statins to lower their lipid levels. Many patients also used calcium dobesilate drugs to improve microcirculation.

As the clinical profile of DR suggests [22], most DR patients in this community with severe non-proliferative DR or proliferative retinopathy accepted photocoagulation, intraocular medicine injection or surgery to control DR progression. Because those treatments would influence the outcome of our study, patients who accepted invasive treatment before or during the study period were excluded. Only those patients without obvious DR, mild non-proliferative DR or moderate non-proliferative DR and those with severe DR but who refused to undertake invasive treatments were included.

The inclusion criteria for the present study were as follows: patients with diagnosed type 2 diabetes according to the WHO definition [23], more than 18 years of age, no previous eye surgery, no history of photocoagulation or intraocular medicine, willingness to accept a general physical examination, and willingness to sign the informed consent form. The exclusion criteria were as follows: suffering from severe systemic disease other than diabetes (such as severe heart/brain vessel disease and cancer), suffering from severe eye diseases other than DR (such as severe cornea opacity, severe cataracts, glaucoma, or retinal detachment), and accepting eye surgery, intraocular injection or photocoagulation as DR treatment during follow-up.

This study was conducted according to the tenets of the Declaration of Helsinki and was approved by the Institutional Review Board of the Shanghai First People's Hospital, Shanghai Jiao Tong University. All of the participants understood the study protocol and provided written informed consent to take part in this study.

Anthropometric and Laboratory Measurements

The baseline survey was conducted in 2007. We acquired some of the participants' information from the community health information database, including age, gender, diabetes duration, diabetes onset age, occupation, education level, and general and ophthalmological medical history. The diabetes duration was the interval between the diagnosis of diabetes and the baseline examination. The patients' heights, weights, and systolic and diastolic blood pressures were measured by trained doctors. The blood pressure was measured in a supine position on the right arm using a standard mercury sphygmomanometer. Hypertension was defined as a systolic blood pressure value ≥140 mmHg and/or a diastolic blood pressure value ≥90 mmHg. BMI was calculated as weight (kg)/height $(m)^2$. According to the guidelines released by the Chinese Ministry of Health, the definition of obesity was BMI≥28 [24]. Laboratory tests included measurements of serum triglycerides, total cholesterol, serum creatinine, urinary microalbumin and HbA1c. Serum creatinine, total cholesterol and triglycerides were measured using an enzymatic assay. Urinary microalbumin was analyzed by nephelometry. HbA1c was measured by ion exchange chromatography. Serum triglyceride levels ≥1.7 $mmol*L^{-1}$ were considered hyperlipidemia, and serum total cholesterol levels ≥5.2 $mmol*L^{-1}$ were considered hypercholesterolemia. Microalbuminuria levels ≥30 mg/L and serum creatinine levels ≥104 $umol*L^{-1}$ suggested renal dysfunction. During follow-up, the HbA1c value of each participant was measured once per year, and the average HbA1c of the five years was recorded. All control values were consistent with the standards recommended by the Shanghai Clinical Testing Center.

General Eye Examinations and Retinopathy Assessments

Eye examinations were conducted during the baseline survey (2007) and the final survey (2012). Visual acuity was tested by EDTRS tables with a 300-lux light. The eyelid, conjunctiva, cornea, iris, and lens were examined with a slit-lamp microscope (YZ-5, Liuliu Medical Instrument Company, Suzhou, China). All of the participants were screened for DR using the standardized protocol described in our previous paper [25]. The procedure was generally as follows. First, the patient's vitreous and fundus were examined by a direct ophthalmoscope, and the posterior pole was then photographed with a non-mydriatic funduscopic camera (CR-DGI, Canon, Tokyo, Japan). Two 45-degree digital retinographs were obtained per eye. The retinographs were taken using the technique described in the EURODIAB study [26], with one centering on the macula and the other nasal to the optic disk. Once DR was suspected by our screening exams, the patient received a series of further exams in our hospital, including optical coherence tomography and fundus fluorescein angiography, to confirm the diagnosis and severity. Two trained ophthalmological doctors independently classified the DR grades according to the well-accepted "International Clinical Diabetic Retinopathy and Diabetic Macular Edema Disease Severity Scale" [27]. This system has five DR grades: no obvious DR (grade 0), mild non-proliferative DR (grade 1), moderate non-proliferative DR (grade 2), severe non-proliferative DR (grade 3), and proliferative retinopathy (grade 4). The two assessors were masked during the reading procedure. A sample of retinal photographs was graded again to assess the validity. Overall, there was a high degree of agreement on the assessment of retinopathy with respect to internal and inter-observer reliability (k1 = 0.874 and k2 = 0.869). Any unresolved disagreements between the two assessors were referred to the group leader (H.Z.) for arbitration.

There were two main outcomes assessed in the present study: DR incidence, defined as the onset of DR from grade 0 to grade 1–4 in at least one eye, and DR regression, defined as the decrease of DR severity from grade 1–4 to grade 0 in at least one eye and no DR worsening in the other eye.

Statistical Analysis

The data were independently input by two staff members into an Access database. SAS (version 9.3 SAS Institute, Cary, NC, USA) was used for all statistical analyses. The baseline characteristics are presented as the means ± standard deviation for continuous variables and as rates (proportions) for categorical data. The data distribution was examined using the Kolmogorov-Smirnov Test. For normally distributed continuous variables, t tests were used to compare the means between groups. For variables that did not follow Gaussian distribution, a Kruskal-Wallis H test was used. The categorical variables were compared with the Chi-square test. From the univariate logistic analyses, variables with p values under 0.5 were considered for entry into multiple logistic regression analysis. Stepwise multiple logistic regression analysis was used to determine whether potential risk factors (including age, gender, diabetes duration, diabetes onset age, occupation, education level, BMI, baseline HbA1c, average HbA1c, high blood pressure, serum triglycerides, total cholesterol, serum creatinine and urinary microalbumin) were associated with DR onset and regression (inclusion value = 0.05 and exclusion value = 0.05). Statistical significance was defined as $p<0.05$ (two tailed).

Results

In 2007, a total of 811 diabetes patients were enrolled in our study, of which 778 completed the whole study. Among the 33 excluded patients, 6 had refractive media opacity that affected the quality of their retinal photographs, and 27 patients, including 15 patients with grade 4 DR and 12 patients with grade 3 DR, accepted surgery or photocoagulation during follow-up. A total of 623 of the included diabetes patients were also suffering from high blood pressure; and most of these patients took medicine such as angiotensin converting enzyme inhibitors (ACEI), angiotensin receptor blockers (ARB) and traditional Chinese medicine to control their hypertension. However, most of them could not provide us with the exact dosage of their drugs. A total of 322 participants did not have DR in either eye at entry and were studied for DR incidence. The remaining 456 participants had existing DR in at least one eye at entry, and they were studied for DR regression. No missing cases were found during the five-year follow-up period.

Risk factors for the onset of DR

At the time of the baseline survey in 2007, there were 322 DR-free participants, of which 142 (44.10%) were male. The youngest participant was 19 years of age, and the oldest was 88 years of age. A total of 85.09% of the participants were more than 60 years old. In 6 participants, diabetes had been diagnosed within the last year, and the longest duration of diabetes was 30 years. A total of 50.93% of the patients had diabetes for more than ten years. All participants' microalbuminuria values were less than 30 mg/L. Detailed information of all of the baseline DR-free participants are summarized in Table 1.

After five years, 151 patients developed DR in at least one eye (DR incidence rate = 46.89%), including 87 patients (57.62%) with grade 1 DR, 36 (23.84%) with grade 2 DR, 21 (13.91%) with grade 3 DR, and 7 (4.63%) with grade 4 DR. Among patients who developed DR, 94.04% (n = 142) developed DR in both eyes. The data indicated that patients with greater age, later diabetes onset, higher blood pressure, higher baseline glucose and higher average glucose were more likely to develop DR (Table 1). From the univariate logistic regression, participant age, age of diabetes onset, BMI, blood pressure, serum creatinine baseline HbA1c and average HbA1c were entered into the multivariate logistic analysis ($p<0.5$). Multivariate regression analysis suggested that both high blood pressure (OR = 1.80, 95% CI 1.14–2.86, $p = 0.01$) and high baseline HbA1c (OR = 1.12, 95% CI 1.01–1.24, $p = 0.03$) were independent factors associated with DR incidence.

Factors related to DR regression

There were 456 participants with existing DR at entry, and 40.36% (n = 184) of them were male. Their ages ranged from 20 years of age to 90 years of age, and 84.65% were more than 60 years of age. Their diabetes duration ranged from 1 year to 33 years, and 43.42% of them had diabetes for more than ten years. All participants had microalbuminuria values less than 30 mg/L. Detailed information of the baseline characteristics of the participants with pre-existing DR is summarized in Table 2.

One hundred and five patients exhibited DR regression in both eyes, and another 5 patients had DR regression in one eye and no DR worsening of the other eye. A total of 110 participants had their DR severity grade regressed to grade 0 in the five-year follow-up period (DR regression rate = 24.12%), including 80 patients from grade 1 DR (72.73%) and 30 patients from grade 2 DR (27.27%). No patients from grade 3 or grade 4 exhibited full regression to grade 0.

DR regression often occurred in patients with shorter diabetes duration, normal serum triglyceride levels, lower baseline HbA1c levels and lower average HbA1c levels (Table 2). From the univariate logistic regression, participant age, diabetes duration, serum creatinine, serum triglyceride, serum total cholesterol, baseline HbA1c and average HbA1c were entered into the multivariate logistic analysis ($p<0.5$). The multivariate regression analysis suggested that low baseline HbA1c (OR = 0.53, 95% CI 0.44–0.63, $p<0.01$) and low serum triglyceride levels (OR = 0.77, 95% CI 0.60–0.99, $p = 0.04$) were two independent factors related to DR regression.

Discussion

To the best of our knowledge, the present study was not only the first prospective study of DR incidence in a community setting cohort of Chinese type 2 diabetes patients but also the first observational study aimed at exploring the systemic factors related to DR regression in a community population.

Table 1. Characteristics of baseline DR-free patients and comparison of the clinical characteristics between patients with DR development during follow-up and patients without DR development.

	Total	DR development	No DR development	Statistical value	P value
Number of participants	322	151 (46.89)	171 (53.11)		
Age (years)	66.07±13.18	67.47±13.38	64.84±12.90	2.52*	0.01
age<60	48 (14.91)	20 (13.25)	28 (16.37)	4.19†	0.04
60≤age<70	116 (36.02)	49 (32.45)	67 (39.18)		
70≤age<80	136 (42.23)	67 (44.37)	69 (40.35)		
age>80	22 (6.83)	15 (9.93)	7 (4.09)		
Male gender	142 (44.10)	64 (42.38)	78 (45.61)	0.34†	0.56
High school degree or above	205 (63.66)	96 (63.58)	109 (63.74)	<0.01†	0.98
Diabetes onset age (years)	55.13±14.90	56.72±15.25	53.72±14.48	2.08*	0.04
Diabetes duration (years)	10.95±7.89	10.75±7.89	11.12±7.90	−0.48*	0.63
duration<10	158 (49.07)	78 (51.66)	80 (46.78)	0.02†	0.90
10≤duration<20	102 (31.68)	41 (27.15)	61 (35.67)		
20≤duration<30	60 (18.63)	31 (20.53)	29 (16.96)		
duration≥30	2 (0.62)	1 (0.66)	1 (0.58)		
Obesity	37 (11.49)	20 (13.25)	17 (9.94)	0.86†	0.35
High blood pressure	129 (40.06)	70 (46.36)	59 (34.50)	4.69†	0.03
High serum creatinine	12 (3.73)	7 (4.64)	5 (2.92)	0.65†	0.42
Hyperlipidemia	114 (35.40)	55 (36.42)	59 (34.50)	0.13†	0.72
Hypercholesterolemia	202 (62.73)	93 (61.59)	109 (63.74)	0.16†	0.69
Baseline HbA1c (%)	7.42±2.19	7.65±2.09	7.22±2.27	2.52*	0.01
Average HbA1c (%)	6.84±1.43	6.96±1.48	6.74±1.38	2.02*	0.04

Note: *Wilcoxon two-sample test †Chi-Square test.

Previous studies have found several risk factors of DR incidence in type 2 diabetes patients, including hypertension, hyperglycemia, long diabetes duration, smoking, insulin therapy, and obesity. Our research suggested that high blood pressure and high glucose are two independent risk factors for DR in Chinese diabetes patients, which is consistent with the findings of previous research conducted in other populations [7,9,28–32]. The complex pathogenesis of hyperglycemia and hypertension in retinal damage remains unclear, but significant evidence has indicated that chronic hyperglycemia and hypertension lead to oxidative injury, microthrombi formation, cell adhesion molecule activation, leukostasis and cytokine activation including vascular endothelial growth factor, insulin-like growth factor-1, angiopoetin-1 and -2, stromal-derived factor-1, fibroblast growth factor-2 and tumor necrosis factor. The combination of these cytokines leads to further retinal damage [33]. Although diabetes duration is recognized as a risk factor associated with diabetes retinopathy in Caucasian populations, there is no evidence in the present study that could independently associate diabetes duration with DR onset. This discrepancy might result from the inaccuracy of diabetes duration determinations. Because the onset of type 2 diabetes is often unknown, the disease could exist long before the patient is diagnosed.

Although DR incidence of type 2 diabetes patients has been reported in several countries [5,7,9,28–30,34], there is a large difference between the incidence values, which vary from 3.9% (for 5 years) [34] to 47.5% (for 4 years) [30]. The 5-year cumulative incidence of DR presented in our study was 46.89%, which is similar to that found in a study conducted in Iran [30]. Former studies have suggested that the Asian population is more sensitive to high glucose than Caucasian patients and is thus more likely to develop DR [35,36]. The racial difference might explain the higher incidence rate reported in Iran and in our study compared with several studies conducted in Western countries. Moreover, although diabetes duration is not an independent factor associated with DR onset in our study, the mean diabetes duration of our participants is similar to that of the participants in the Iranian research study and is much longer than that found in other studies conducted in Asian populations [10,31]. This might contribute to the high incidence rate.

Despite the high incidence rate, DR regression cases were quite common in our study, especially in patients with well-controlled glucose and mild baseline DR. Spontaneous diabetic retinopathy reversal has been noted by many ophthalmologists and reported by some researchers [15–18]; however, few have discussed its association with systemic factors. Compared with the 4.9% regression rate found in the Netherlands [15] and the 6.6% regression rate found in Hong Kong [10], the 24.12% DR regression rate in the present research is very high. This difference could be explained by the better systemic condition of our participants, which suggests that they had less severe diabetes complications. The inclusion criteria of our study ensured that the participants had no severe heart/brain vessel diseases, whereas the other two studies did not exclude patients with severe circulation problems. Furthermore, no patients in our study had abnormal microalbuminuria, whereas 24.4% of the participants in the Hong Kong study had albuminuria or proteinuria. The mean baseline HbA1c of our participants was 7.20%±2.25% (55±24.6 mmol/mol), which is significantly lower than the mean levels of 8.1%±1.5% (65±16.4 mmol/mol) and 7.8%±1.7%

Table 2. Characteristics of patients with DR at baseline and comparison of the clinical characteristics between patients with DR regression during follow-up and patients without DR regression.

	Total	DR regression	No DR regression	Statistical value	P value
Number of participants	456	110	346		
Age (years)	68.76±12.27	67.15±13.72	69.27±11.75	−1.39*	0.16
age<60	52 (11.40)	18 (16.36)	34 (9.83)	1.44†	0.23
60≤age<70	135 (29.61)	28 (25.45)	107 (30.92)		
70≤age<80	211 (46.27)	53 (48.18)	158 (45.66)		
age>80	58 (12.72)	11 (10.00)	47 (13.58)		
Male gender	184 (40.35)	43 (39.09)	141 (40.75)	0.10†	0.76
High school degree or above	261 (57.24)	64 (58.18)	197 (56.94)	0.05†	0.81
Diabetes onset age (years)	56.98±13.51	56.88±15.02	57.01±13.01	0.66*	0.51
Diabetes duration (years)	11.78±8.01	10.26±7.53	12.27±8.11	−2.55*	0.01
duration<10	208 (45.61)	61(55.45)	147 (42.49)	4.71†	0.03
10≤duration<20	149 (32.68)	30 (27.27)	119 (34.39)		
20≤duration<30	93 (20.39)	18 (16.36)	75 (21.68)		
duration≥30	6 (1.32)	1 (0.91)	5 (1.45)		
Obesity	80 (17.54)	20 (18.18)	60 (17.34)	0.04†	0.84
High blood pressure	194 (42.54)	46 (41.82)	148 (42.77)	0.03†	0.86
High serum creatinine	9 (1.97)	0	9 (2.60)	2.92†	0.09
Hyperlipidemia	182 (39.91)	35 (31.82)	147 (42.49)	3.96†	0.04
Hypercholesterolemia	292 (64.04)	67 (60.91)	225 (65.03)	0.62†	0.43
Baseline HbA1c (%)	7.20±2.25	5.66±1.76	7.68±2.18	−10.69*	<0.01
Average HbA1c (%)	6.73±1.41	5.99±0.87	7.05±1.48	−9.35*	<0.01

Note: *Wilcoxon two-sample test †Chi-Square test.

(62±18.6 mmol/mol) in the other two studies. Because our results indicated that the maintenance of euglycemia is associated with DR regression, the strict glucose target could lead to less worsening and further regression of retinopathy. Another possible explanation of the high regression rate found in the present study is that the drugs our patients used to control hypertension and to improve microcirculation may also promote DR regression. Previous studies have suggested that ACEI therapy has an additional protective effect in promoting the regression of DR [19,37,38], and it has been reported that pycnoyenol prevents progression of retinopathy and partly recovers visual acuity [39,40]. Although there were previous case reports about PDR reversal [17], full reversal to grade 0 was not observed in late-stage DR patients in our study, which is consistent with a former RCT study about the effect of candesartan in patients with DR [19]. The study also reported that DR regression only occurred in participants with early retinopathy. Another possible reason is the lack of subjects because 15 PDR patients were excluded from the study for receiving invasive treatments during the follow-up, and only 2 PDR patients completed the study.

Our results suggested that if a DR patient's HbA1c was decreased by 1% (10.9 mmol/mol), the chance of a full regression would be almost doubled. It has been reported that background retinopathy is not merely a process of cumulative increase in the number of microaneurysms but also reflects a dynamic balance between microaneurysm formation and disappearance. In patients with good glucose control, microaneurysm formation showed a decreasing trend, but the disappearance rate was not directly connected with glucose control [41,42]. We speculated that this phenomenon could explain the reversal in our patients. Long-term maintenance of euglycemia leads to a lower rate of new microaneurysm formation, and the existing background microaneurysms eventually disappeared completely.

According to our results, low serum triglyceride is another systemic factor that is independently related to DR regression, which is in accordance with previous studies. Several studies have reported that serum lipid levels are associated with the severity of hard exudates [43]. Moreover, strict lipid-lowering therapy was found to be associated with hard exudate regression in clinically significant macular edema [44], and fibrate drugs have been reported to be able to reduce the need for photocoagulation in DR patients [43]. A review of previous research studies showed that animal experiments suggest that the reversibility of retinal flow abnormalities, which is the earliest change of DR damage, can only be observed in short disease-duration subjects [45,46]. However, although the mean diabetes duration of the regression patients in our study was significantly shorter than those who did not regress, there was no evidence to independently relate diabetes disease duration to DR regression.

Our participants paid more attention to controlling glucose after the enrollment of the study, a large part of them had a decrease in HbA1c level during the follow-up period. Results showed that baseline HbA1c, instead of 5-year average HbA1c, are related to DR development and DR regression. We speculated that this might result from the "metabolic memory" phenomenon. In 1990, Roy and his colleagues coined the term "metabolic memory" to describe the hypothesis that systemic metabolic imbalance may continue to develop in patients who no longer have hyperglycemia [47]. Two well-known studies have proved this negative metabolic memory in Western populations, "The Diabetes Control and

Complications Trial/Epidemiology of Diabetes Interventions and Complications Research Group" (DCCT) study in type 1 diabetes [48] and the "United Kingdom Prospective Diabetes Study" (UKPDS) in type 2 diabetes [49]. They found that among patients with similar glucose level, DR often occurred in those with higher initial HbA1c. We suspect that this might also apply to the positive metabolic memory of low glucose, which could explain the reason why DR reversal often occurred in patients with lower baseline HbA1c levels in our study.

Our research has some limitations. First, the study population was limited to one community and was not sufficiently large to represent all diabetes patients in Shanghai. Second, the retinographs were taken centering on only the macula and the optic disk; thus, retinopathy outside of these areas might have been missed. Third, this research only covered a 5-year period. The DR regression observed might be hard to maintain for a longer duration. Future longer-term, multicenter studies should be conducted to verify these results. In conclusion, DR incidence often occurred in patients with baseline hyperglycemia and high blood pressure. DR regression occurred mostly in patients with lower baseline glucose and lower serum triglyceride levels among Chinese type 2 diabetes patients.

Author Contributions

Conceived and designed the experiments: HZ XX XZ. Performed the experiments: JP WW JF BS. Analyzed the data: PJ JP XB. Contributed reagents/materials/analysis tools: BS XB HZ. Contributed to the writing of the manuscript: PJ HZ.

References

1. Klein K, Eden B (2007) Overview of epidemiologic studies of diabetic retinopathy. Ophthalmic epidemiology 14: 179–183.
2. Younis N, Broadbent DM, Vora JP, Harding SP, Liverpool Diabetic Eye S (2003) Incidence of sight-threatening retinopathy in patients with type 2 diabetes in the Liverpool Diabetic Eye Study: a cohort study. Lancet 361: 195–200.
3. Yang W, Lu J, Weng J, Jia W, Ji L, et al. (2010) Prevalence of diabetes among men and women in China. New England Journal of Medicine 362: 1090–1101.
4. Klein R, Klein BE, Moss SE, Davis MD, DeMets DL (1989) The Wisconsin Epidemiologic Study of Diabetic Retinopathy: X. Four-Year Incidence and Progression of Diabetic Retinopathy When Age at Diagnosis Is 30 Years or More. Archives of ophthalmology 107: 244.
5. Zhang L, Krzentowski G, Albert A, Lefebvre PJ (2001) Risk of developing retinopathy in Diabetes Control and Complications Trial type 1 diabetic patients with good or poor metabolic control. Diabetes Care 24: 1275–1279.
6. Scanlon PH, Aldington SJ, Stratton IM (2013) Epidemiological issues in diabetic retinopathy. Middle East African journal of ophthalmology 20: 293.
7. Stratton IM, Kohner EM, Aldington SJ, Turner RC, Holman RR, et al. (2001) UKPDS 50: risk factors for incidence and progression of retinopathy in Type II diabetes over 6 years from diagnosis. Diabetologia 44: 156–163.
8. Perol J, Balkau B, Guillausseau P-J, Massin P (2012) A study of the 3-year incidence of diabetic retinopathy in a French diabetic population seen at Lariboisière Hospital, Paris. Diabetes & metabolism 38: 225–229.
9. Cikamatana L, Mitchell P, Rochtchina E, Foran S, Wang J (2007) Five-year incidence and progression of diabetic retinopathy in a defined older population: the Blue Mountains Eye Study. Eye 21: 465–471.
10. Tam VH, Lam EP, Chu BC, Tse KK, Fung LM (2009) Incidence and progression of diabetic retinopathy in Hong Kong Chinese with type 2 diabetes mellitus. J Diabetes Complications 23: 185–193.
11. Wang N, Xu X, Zou H, Zhu J, Wang W, et al. (2007) The status of diabetic retinopathy and diabetic macular edema in patients with type 2 diabetes: a survey from Beixinjing District of Shanghai city in China. Ophthalmologica 222: 32–36.
12. Arevalo JF, Wu L, Sanchez JG, Maia M, Saravia MJ, et al. (2009) Intravitreal bevacizumab (Avastin) for proliferative diabetic retinopathy: 6-months follow-up. Eye (Lond) 23: 117–123.
13. Yang CS, Hung KC, Huang YM, Hsu WM (2013) Intravitreal bevacizumab (Avastin) and panretinal photocoagulation in the treatment of high-risk proliferative diabetic retinopathy. J Ocul Pharmacol Ther 29: 550–555.
14. Mirshahi A, Roohipoor R, Lashay A, Mohammadi SF, Abdoallahi A, et al. (2008) Bevacizumab-augmented retinal laser photocoagulation in proliferative diabetic retinopathy: a randomized double-masked clinical trial. Eur J Ophthalmol 18: 263–269.
15. Zavrelova H, Hoekstra T, Alssema M, Welschen LM, Nijpels G, et al. (2011) Progression and regression: distinct developmental patterns of diabetic retinopathy in patients with type 2 diabetes treated in the diabetes care system west-friesland, the Netherlands. Diabetes Care 34: 867–872.
16. Gerritzen F (1973) The course of diabetic retinopathy: a longitudinal study. Diabetes 22: 122–128.
17. Han JR, Ju WK, Park IW (2004) Spontaneous regression of neovascularization at the disc in diabetic retinopathy. Korean Journal of Ophthalmology 18: 41–46.
18. White M, Kohner E, Pickup J, Keen H (1981) Reversal of diabetic retinopathy by continuous subcutaneous insulin infusion: a case report. British Journal of Ophthalmology 65: 307–311.
19. Sjolie AK, Klein R, Porta M, Orchard T, Fuller J, et al. (2008) Effect of candesartan on progression and regression of retinopathy in type 2 diabetes (DIRECT-Protect 2): a randomised placebo-controlled trial. Lancet 372: 1385–1393.
20. Aiello LP, Edwards AR, Beck RW, Bressler NM, Davis MD, et al. (2010) Factors associated with improvement and worsening of visual acuity 2 years after focal/grid photocoagulation for diabetic macular edema. Ophthalmology 117: 946–953.
21. Theodossiadis GP, Boudouri A, Georgopoulos G, Koutsandrea C (1990) Central visual field changes after panretinal photocoagulation in proliferative diabetic retinopathy. Ophthalmologica 201: 71–78.
22. López F, Rodríguez M, Marticorena J, Gómez-Ulla F (2007) Diabetic Retinopathy Treatment. European Ophthalmic Review: 68–70.
23. Consultation W (1999) Definition, diagnosis and classification of diabetes mellitus and its complications: Part.
24. Wu Y (2006) Overweight and obesity in China: the once lean giant has a weight problem that is increasing rapidly. BMJ: British Medical Journal 333: 362.
25. Peng J, Zou H, Wang W, Fu J, Shen B, et al. (2011) Implementation and first-year screening results of an ocular telehealth system for diabetic retinopathy in China. BMC health services research 11: 250.
26. Gibbins R, Owens D, Allen J, Eastman L (1998) Practical application of the European Field Guide in screening for diabetic retinopathy by using ophthalmoscopy and 35 mm retinal slides. Diabetologia 41: 59–64.
27. Wilkinson CP, Ferris FL 3rd, Klein RE, Lee PP, Agardh CD, et al. (2003) Proposed international clinical diabetic retinopathy and diabetic macular edema disease severity scales. Ophthalmology 110: 1677–1682.
28. Varma R, Choudhury F, Klein R, Chung J, Torres M, et al. (2010) Four-year incidence and progression of diabetic retinopathy and macular edema: the Los Angeles Latino Eye Study. Am J Ophthalmol 149: 752–761 e751–753.
29. Leske MC, Wu S-Y, Hennis A, Nemesure B, Hyman L, et al. (2003) Incidence of diabetic retinopathy in the Barbados Eye Studies. Ophthalmology 110: 941–947.
30. Manaviat M, Rashidi M, Afkhami-Ardekani M (2008) Four years incidence of diabetic retinopathy and effective factors on its progression in type II diabetes. European journal of ophthalmology 18: 572–577.
31. Kawasaki R, Tanaka S, Yamamoto T, Sone H, Ohashi Y, et al. (2011) Incidence and progression of diabetic retinopathy in Japanese adults with type 2 diabetes: 8 year follow-up study of the Japan Diabetes Complications Study (JDCS). Diabetologia 54: 2288–2294.
32. Tapp RJ, Zimmet PZ, Harper CA, McCarty DJ, Chitson P, et al. (2006) Six year incidence and progression of diabetic retinopathy: results from the Mauritius diabetes complication study. Diabetes research and clinical practice 73: 298–303.
33. Grant MB, Afzal A, Spoerri P, Pan H, Shaw LC, et al. (2004) The role of growth factors in the pathogenesis of diabetic retinopathy. Expert opinion on investigational drugs 13: 1275–1293.
34. Younis N, Broadbent DM, Vora JP, Harding SP (2003) Incidence of sight-threatening retinopathy in patients with type 2 diabetes in the Liverpool Diabetic Eye Study: a cohort study. The Lancet 361: 195–200.
35. Bao Y, Ma X, Li H, Zhou M, Hu C, et al. (2010) Glycated haemoglobin A1c for diagnosing diabetes in Chinese population: cross sectional epidemiological survey. BMJ 340.
36. Raymond NT, Varadhan L, Reynold DR, Bush K, Sankaranarayanan S, et al. (2009) Higher prevalence of retinopathy in diabetic patients of South Asian ethnicity compared with White Europeans in the Community A cross-sectional study. Diabetes care 32: 410–415.
37. Ruggenenti P, Iliev I, Filipponi M, Tadini S, Perna A, et al. (2010) Effect of trandolapril on regression of retinopathy in hypertensive patients with type 2 diabetes: a prespecified analysis of the benedict trial. Journal of ophthalmology 2010.
38. Zheng Z, Chen H, Ke G, Fan Y, Zou H, et al. (2009) Protective Effect of Perindopril on Diabetic Retinopathy Is Associated With Decreased Vascular Endothelial Growth Factor–to–Pigment Epithelium–Derived Factor Ratio Involvement of a Mitochondria–Reactive Oxygen Species Pathway. Diabetes 58: 954–964.
39. Steigerwalt R, Belcaro G, Cesarone MR, Di Renzo A, Grossi MG, et al. (2009) Pycnogenol improves microcirculation, retinal edema, and visual acuity in early diabetic retinopathy. J Ocul Pharmacol Ther 25: 537–540.

40. Schonlau F, Rohdewald P (2001) Pycnogenol for diabetic retinopathy. A review. Int Ophthalmol 24: 161–171.
41. Sjolie AK, Klein R, Porta M, Orchard T, Fuller J, et al. (2011) Retinal microaneurysm count predicts progression and regression of diabetic retinopathy. Post-hoc results from the DIRECT Programme. Diabet Med 28: 345–351.
42. Hellstedt T, Immonen I (1996) Disappearance and formation rates of microaneurysms in early diabetic retinopathy. British journal of ophthalmology 80: 135–139.
43. Gordon B, Chang S, Kavanagh M, Berrocal M, Yannuzzi L, et al. (1991) The effects of lipid lowering on diabetic retinopathy. Am J Ophthalmol 112: 385–391.
44. Kameda Y, Kumakawa M, Endo N, Iwamoto Y, Kitano S (2010) Association of systemic health and functional outcomes with changes in hard exudates associated with clinically significant macular oedema over the natural course of the disease. British Journal of Ophthalmology 94: 725–729.
45. Higashi S, Clermont AC, Dhir V, Bursell S-E (1998) Reversibility of retinal flow abnormalities is disease-duration dependent in diabetic rats. Diabetes 47: 653–659.
46. Engerman RL (1989) Pathogenesis of diabetic retinopathy. Diabetes 38: 1203–1206.
47. Roy S, Sala R, Cagliero E, Lorenzi M (1990) Overexpression of fibronectin induced by diabetes or high glucose: phenomenon with a memory. Proc Natl Acad Sci U S A 87: 404–408.
48. White NH, Sun W, Cleary PA, Danis RP, Davis MD, et al. (2008) Prolonged effect of intensive therapy on the risk of retinopathy complications in patients with type 1 diabetes mellitus: 10 years after the Diabetes Control and Complications Trial. Arch Ophthalmol 126: 1707–1715.
49. Holman RR, Paul SK, Bethel MA, Matthews DR, Neil HA (2008) 10-year follow-up of intensive glucose control in type 2 diabetes. N Engl J Med 359: 1577–1589.

Measurement of Visceral Fat: Should We Include Retroperitoneal Fat?

Chi-Sheng Hung[1]⁹, Jen-Kuang Lee[2]⁹, Chung-Yi Yang[3], Hung-Ren Hsieh[4], Wen-Ya Ma[5], Mao-Shin Lin[1], Pi-Hua Liu[6], Shyang-Rong Shih[1], Jyh-Ming Liou[1], Lee-Ming Chuang[1], Ming-Fong Chen[1], Jou-Wei Lin[7], Jung-Nan Wei[8]¶, Hung-Yuan Li[1]*¶

1 Department of Internal Medicine, National Taiwan University Hospital, Taipei, Taiwan, **2** Department of Clinical Pathology, Far Eastern Memorial Hospital, New Taipei City, Taiwan, **3** Department of Medical Imaging, National Taiwan University Hospital and National Taiwan University College of Medicine, Taipei, Taiwan, **4** Department of Radiology, National Taiwan University Hospital Yun-Lin Branch, Yun-Lin, Taiwan, **5** Division of Endocrinology, Department of Internal Medicine, Cardinal Tien Hospital, Xindian, Taiwan, **6** Clinical Informatics and Medical Statistics Research Center, Chang Gung University, Gueishan, Taiwan, **7** Department of Internal Medicine, National Taiwan University Hospital Yun-Lin Branch, Yun-Lin, Taiwan, **8** Chia Nan University of Pharmacy and Science, Tainan, Taiwan

Abstract

Objective: Whether retroperitoneal fat should be included in the measurement of visceral fat remains controversial. We compared the relationships of fat areas in peritoneal, retroperitoneal, and subcutaneous compartments to metabolic syndrome, adipokines, and incident hypertension and diabetes.

Methods: We enrolled 432 adult participants (153 men and 279 women) in a community-based cohort study. Computed tomography at the umbilicus level was used to measure the fat areas.

Results: Retroperitoneal fat correlated significantly with metabolic syndrome (adjusted odds ratio (OR), 5.651, $p<0.05$) and the number of metabolic abnormalities ($p<0.05$). Retroperitoneal fat area was significantly associated with blood pressure, plasma glycemic indices, lipid profile, C-reactive protein, adiponectin ($r=-0.244$, $P<0.05$), and leptin ($r=0.323$, $p<0.05$), but not plasma renin or aldosterone concentrations. During the 2.94±0.84 years of follow-up, 32 participants developed incident hypertension. Retroperitoneal fat area (hazard ration (HR) 1.62, $p=0.003$) and peritoneal fat area (HR 1.62, $p=0.009$), but not subcutaneous fat area ($p=0.14$) were associated with incident hypertension. Neither retroperitoneal fat area, peritoneal fat area, nor subcutaneous fat areas was associated with incident diabetes after adjustment.

Conclusions: Retroperitoneal fat is similar to peritoneal fat, but differs from subcutaneous fat, in terms of its relationship with metabolic syndrome and incident hypertension. Retroperitoneal fat area should be included in the measurement of visceral fat for cardio-metabolic studies in human.

Editor: Cordula M. Stover, University of Leicester, United Kingdom

Funding: This work was supported in part by a grant (NSC 98-2314-B-002-024-MY3) from the National Science Council, Taiwan, and a grant (DAROC2012YPI-0001) from the Diabetes Association of the Republic of China, Taiwan. The funders had no role in study design, data collection and analysis, decision to publish, or preparation of the manuscript.

Competing Interests: The authors have declared that no competing interests exist.

* Email: larsli@ntuh.gov.tw

⁹ These authors contributed equally to this work.

¶ These authors also contributed equally to this work

Introduction

Metabolic syndrome (MS) is a combination of risk factors mainly related to abdominal obesity and insulin resistance, according to the National Cholesterol Education Program's Adult Treatment Panel III report (ATP III) [1]. Participants with MS have a higher risk of fatal and nonfatal cardiovascular diseases [2]. Abdominal or central obesity plays an important role in the development of MS. Indeed, central obesity is a requirement to meet the criteria of MS as defined by the International Diabetes Federation [3]. Abdominal adipose tissue is not only a fat storage site, but also acts as an endocrine organ that secretes various adipokines such as adiponectin and leptin as well as several inflammatory cytokines. In addition, the free fatty acid flux from abdominal adipose tissue to the liver results in disturbances in glucose and lipid metabolism [4], which contribute to the development of insulin resistance and dyslipidemia in participants with MS [5]. [6].

In the abdominal cavity, there are 3 different compartments of fat: omental, mesenteric, and retroperitoneal fat. Blood from fat tissue in the peritoneal region, including omental and mesenteric fat, is drained through the portal vein into the liver, while the blood from fat in the retroperitoneal region is drained into the kidney, pancreas, or directly to the vena cava [7]. Furthermore, the composition and amount of adipokines released from different compartments can differ, and along with their endocrine effects, these adipokines can have paracrine effects on adjacent organs. Therefore, peritoneal and retroperitoneal fats may play different roles in our metabolism. Two recent reports in animals have shown that peritoneal and retroperitoneal fat have different immuno-modulatory roles and respond differently to exercise training [8,9]. However, most human studies using CT or MRI to assess the degree of visceral obesity have included the retroperitoneal fat area [10–12]. In the literature, retroperitoneal and peritoneal fat depots were quantified together as visceral fat, to study their relationships to cardiometabolic diseases. To the best of our knowledge, there is no report investigating the role of retroperitoneal fat, independent to other part of visceral fat, in metabolic abnormalities in humans. Therefore, we conducted this study to compare the relationships of retroperitoneal fat area, peritoneal fat area, and subcutaneous fat area to metabolic syndrome, adipocytokines, and incident hypertension and diabetes. Patterns of the relationships can help us to answer if we should include retroperitoneal fat when measuring visceral fat area in humans.

Methods and Materials

Ethic statement

The study was approved by the Institutional Review Board of the National Taiwan University Hospital, and complied with the Helsinki Declaration. Written informed consent was obtained from each patient before enrollment.

Participants

From 2006 to 2012, residents from the Yunlin county, Taiwan, aged ≥18 years, who did not report the presence of diabetes during an interview, were invited to join this prospective study, named the Taiwan Lifestyle Study [13,14]. There were 3 visits for this prospective study, separated by 1–3 years. Individuals underwent abdominal CT exam at the 2nd visit, which was defined as the baseline visit in the present study. The 3rd visit was defined as the follow-up visit. The new diabetes or hypertension was defined by comparing the status between baseline and follow-up visit. Written informed consent was obtained from every participant. The study was review and approved by the Institutional Review Board.

A questionnaire was administered by trained nurses in order to obtain data on the demographic characteristics, medical history, and health habits of the participants. Body height and weight were recorded to the nearest 0.5 cm and 0.1 kg, respectively. BMI was calculated from body weight in kilogram divided by the square of body height in meters. Waist circumferences were measured according to the method by the World Health Organization and the International Diabetes Federation to the nearest 0.1 cm [15]. Blood pressure was recorded using a mercury sphygmomanometer to the nearest 2 mmHg with the arm supported at the heart level after the subject sat calmly for 10 min; trained nurses took 3 separate readings at 1-min intervals, and the average of the second and the third readings was used for analysis. A standard 75-g oral glucose tolerance test (OGTT) was performed after fasting overnight for 8 h. All study participants were contacted by telephone, e-mail, or postal mail every 1 to 3 years after the initial visit, and follow-up visits were scheduled according to the respondent's availability. Abdominal computer tomography was done at baseline visit to measure abdominal fat. Clinical questionnaires, physical examination, and blood tests including OGTT were repeated to know the development of incident hypertension or incident diabetes at the time of follow-up.

Plasma glucose and fasting serum total cholesterol, triglycerides, high-density lipoprotein cholesterol, and low-density lipoprotein cholesterol concentrations were measured using an automatic analyzer (Toshiba TBA 200 FR; Toshiba Medical Systems Co., Ltd., Tokyo, Japan). Plasma hemoglobin A1c (HbA1c) concentrations were measured using another automatic analyzer (HLC-723 G7 HPLC systems; Tosoh Corporation, Tokyo, Japan). Hepatitis B surface antigen and hepatitis C virus antibody were measured by the AxSYM System (Abbott Laboratories, North Chicago, IL). The laboratory attends and is qualified by an external quality assurance program by the Taiwan Society of Laboratory Medicine twice a year. The HbA1c assay was certified by the National Glycohemoglobin Standardization Program [16] and standardized to the Diabetes Control and Complications Trial reference assay.

Definitions

Diabetes was diagnosed according to the American Diabetes Association (ADA) recommendations in 2010 (HbA1c concentration ≥6.5% (48 mmol/mol), fasting plasma glucose (FPG) concentration ≥126 mg/dL, or OGTT 2h plasma glucose (OGTT-2h-PG) concentration ≥200 mg/dL). MS was diagnosed using the criteria defined in the ATP III, with a modification of waist circumference for Asians [17]. Participants were classified as having MS if they met 3 or more of the following 5 criteria: (1) high blood pressure: systolic and/or diastolic blood pressure ≥130/85 mmHg or receiving blood pressure-lowering medications; (2) hyperglycemia: fasting plasma glucose concentration ≥100 mg/dL (5.6 mmol/L) or receiving glucose-lowering medications; (3) hypertriglyceridemia: fasting plasma triglyceride concentration ≥150 mg/dL (1.69 mmol/L); (4) HDL cholesterol concentration <40 mg/dL in men and <50 mg/dL in woman; and (5) waist circumference ≥90 cm in men and ≥80 cm in women.

Measurements of abdominal adipose tissue

Abdominal adiposity was assessed using a 16-slice multidetector CT scanner (LightSpeed 16; GE Healthcare, Milwaukee, WI) in the supine position (120 kVp, 400 mAs, slice thickness of 5 mm). Image analysis software (ImageJ, version 1.44; National Institutes of Health, Bethesda, MD) was used to quantify the subcutaneous and visceral adipose fat areas, on one cross-sectional scan obtained at the level of umbilicus and expressed in millimeters squared. [11] After applying threshold with an attenuation range of −50 to −250 Hounsfield units, a fat-density mask was generated. A total fat mask was created after manual exclusion of non-adipose area (such as the CT table, air-object interface or fecal material) from the fat-density mask (Figure 1). The visceral fat area was determined by cutting areas other than visceral fat, and the subcutaneous fat area was calculated with the total fat area subtracted by the visceral fat area. The visceral fat area was further divided into peritoneal and retroperitoneal areas along the boundary comprised of posterior surface of small bowel, ascending colon, descending colon, mesenteric vessels and gonadal veins (Figure 1). The interfascial plane could be visualized as a thin line in some participants and this could help outline of the boundary.

Statistical analysis

The sample size estimation was based on the following assumptions that was modified from a previous study(18): a 2-sided α level of 0.05 and power of 95% and retroperitoneal fat

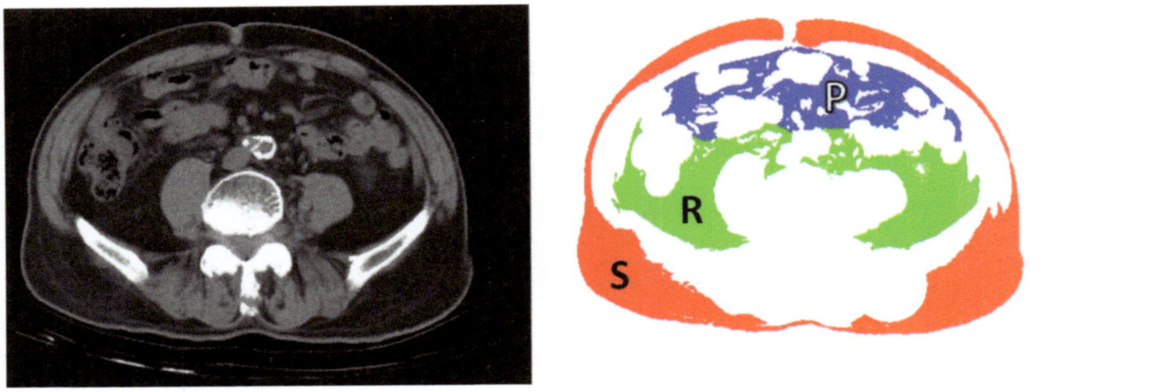

Figure 1. Image demonstration of determining abdominal fat distribution on a CT scan. Left, sample CT image obtained at the umbilicus level. Right, fat masks created for determining areas of subcutaneous fat (red, "S"), peritoneal fat (blue, "P") and retroperitoneal fat (green, "R") using methods described in the Materials and Methods section.

area of 5000 mm^2 in MS group and 4000 mm^2 in non-MS group with a SD of 2500 mm^2. The MS to non-MS group ratio was set at 1:3 according to a prevalence of MS at around 25–30%. Accordingly, a sample size of 400 patients (100 patients in MS group and 300 patients in non-MS group) was calculated.

All variables are expressed as the mean and standard deviation (SD). Two-sample *t*-tests and Pearson's chi-square tests were used to compare the demographic and metabolic parameters between participants with and without MS. The different fat areas were logarithmically transformed to approximate normal distributions. Logistic regression models were used to evaluate the relationship between MS and different fat areas using age, gender, and BMI as potential confounders. We also performed this analysis with standardized fat areas as follows: standardized fat area = (log fat area – mean of log fat area)/(SD of log fat area). Pearson's correlation coefficients were used to assess the relationship between metabolic parameters and different fat areas. Partial correlation coefficients were calculated after adjusting for age and gender. Bootstrap resampling was used to compare the correlation coefficient of each metabolic variable and the retroperitoneal fat area with the correlation coefficient of each metabolic variable and the subcutaneous or peritoneal fat area. The differences in numbers of metabolic abnormalities were assessed by analysis of variance. The relationship between adipokines and the retroperitoneal fat area was expressed by Pearson's correlation coefficients. Cox proportional hazard models were used to assess the relationship of abdominal fat areas and the development of incident hypertension or incident diabetes during follow-up, adjusted for age, sex, and family history of hypertension or diabetes. The fat areas in the Cox regression models were normalized by the standard deviation, to show the hazard ratios for every 1 standard deviation increase in fat areas. Kaplan-Meier failure curves were used to estimate the cumulative incidence of hypertension and diabetes in participants with fat areas above and below the median value. A two-tailed p value <0.05 was regarded as significant. Statistical analyses were performed with Stata/SE 11.0 for Windows (StataCorp LP, College Station, TX).

Results

A total of 432 participants (153 men and 279 women), with a mean age of 52.6±12.0 years, were enrolled in this study. Of the 432, 125 participants fulfilled the criteria for MS. The mean fat areas in men and women were as follows: 14,757 mm^2 and 19,659 mm^2, respectively, of subcutaneous fat area ($p<0.001$); 7,187 mm^2 and 4,855 mm^2, respectively, of peritoneal fat area ($p<0.001$); and 5,233 mm^2 and 3,784 mm^2, respectively, of retroperitoneal fat area ($p<0.001$). As shown in Table 1, participants with MS were older; more obese; more likely to have hypertension and diabetes; had higher plasma triglyceride, glutamyl pyruvic transaminase (GPT), leptin, and C-reactive protein (CRP) concentrations, had lower plasma adiponectin concentrations, and had higher subcutaneous, peritoneal, and retroperitoneal fat areas.

Retroperitoneal fat area is associated with metabolic syndrome

As shown in Figure 2, participants with higher fat areas had more metabolic abnormalities in all compartments of abdominal fat (all $p<0.05$). In multivariate logistic regression analysis (Table 2), retroperitoneal and peritoneal fat areas, but not the subcutaneous fat area, were significant predictors for the presence of MS, independent of age, gender, and BMI (retroperitoneal fat: OR, 5.651; 95% CI, 2.707–11.79; $p<0.05$; peritoneal fat: OR, 3.991; 95% CI, 2.181–7.304; $p<0.05$; subcutaneous fat: OR, 2.569; 95% CI, 0.935–7.053; $p>0.05$). The odds ratios for every 1 SD increase in fat area, adjusted for age, gender, and BMI, were 1.562 ($p>0.05$) for the subcutaneous fat area, 3.489 ($p<0.05$) for the peritoneal fat area, and 2.849 ($p<0.05$) for the retroperitoneal fat area.

Retroperitoneal fat area is associated with adipocytokines

Of the study population, 353 participants did not take any medication for hypertension, diabetes, or dyslipidemia. In these participants, there were significant correlations between metabolic variables and the retroperitoneal as well as peritoneal fat area (Table 3). The retroperitoneal fat area was significantly associated with blood pressure, BMI, waist circumference, plasma glycemic indices, lipid profile, CRP concentration s, GPT concentrations, leptin concentrations, and adiponectin concentrations, but not with plasma renin and aldosterone concentrations. The associations between retroperitoneal fat area and blood pressure, BMI, waist circumference, fasting glucose, total cholesterol, and LDL cholesterol were independent to peritoneal fat area. The

Table 1. Clinical characteristics of participants with and without metabolic syndrome (MS).

	No MS	MS	*p* value
N	307	125	
Age (years)	50.8 (12.2)	57.1 (10.2)	<0.001
Gender (male (%))	97 (31)	56 (44.8)	<0.001
Systolic blood pressure (mmHg)	121 (16)	133 (15)	<0.001
Diastolic blood pressure (mmHg)	77 (9)	83 (10)	<0.001
Medications for hypertension (n, %)	24 (7.8)	37 (29.6)	<0.001
Hypertension (n, %)	68 (22.1)	68 (54.4)	<0.001
Body mass index (kg/m^2)	23.1 (3.0)	26.4 (2.9)	<0.001
Waist circumference (cm)	80.4 (7.3)	89.8 (7.1)	<0.001
Fasting plasma glucose (mg/dL)	91.2 (10.2)	102.2 (21.2)	<0.001
OGTT-2h-PG (mg/dL)	116.5 (36.2)	158.9 (71)	<0.001
Hemoglobin A1c (%)	5.7 (0.4)	6.0 (1.0)	<0.001
Hemoglobin A1c (mmol/mol)	39(2.7)	42(6.8)	<0.001
HOMA2%B	81.6 (34.9)	87.9 (41.2)	0.1
HOMA2%S	156.8 (72.2)	108.6 (60)	<0.001
Medications for diabetes (n, %)	4 (1.3)	9 (7.2)	0.003
Diabetes (n, %)	26 (8.5)	34 (27.2)	<0.001
Total cholesterol (mg/dL)	193.7 (35.7)	196.4 (36.1)	0.243
Triglyceride (mg/dL) [a]	93.2 (62–111)	189.3 (113–209)	<0.001
HDL cholesterol (mg/dL)	53.4 (10.5)	42.3 (8.2)	<0.001
LDL cholesterol (mg/dL)	118.7 (31.8)	122.3 (35.8)	0.149
Medications for dyslipidemia (n, %)	4 (1.3)	16 (12.8)	<0.001
Glutamate oxalate transaminase (IU/L)	23.1 (12.4)	23.6 (7.5)	0.35
Glutamate pyruvate transaminase (IU/L)	22.6 (20.7)	27.3 (16.8)	0.012
Leptin (pg/mL) [a]	9645 (3873–12844)	12093 (5576–15835)	0.002
Adiponectin (ng/mL) [a]	8040 (3678–10850)	5441 (2489–7647)	<0.001
Renin (pg/mL) [a]	27.6 (9.3–37.3)	32.3 (10.5–40.7)	0.24
Aldosterone (pg/mL) [a]	48.5(22.1–61.5)	43.4 (20.3–54.1)	0.47
C-reactive protein (mg/dL) [a]	0.13 (0.04–0.15)	0.24 (0.06–0.24)	<0.001
Subcutaneous fat (mm^2) [a]	16588 (6935)	21203 (6769)	<0.001
Peritoneal fat (mm^2) [a]	4610 (3075)	8303 (3448)	<0.001
Retroperitoneal fat (mm^2) [a]	3629 (1925)	5927 (2154)	<0.001

Means (standard deviations) are shown.

[a]Medians (interquartile ranges) of variables not normally distributed are shown. Statistical analyses were performed after log transformation.

OGTT-2h-PG, plasma glucose at 2 h during oral glucose tolerance test; HOMA, homeostasis model assessment; HDL, high-density lipoprotein; LDL, low-density lipoprotein.

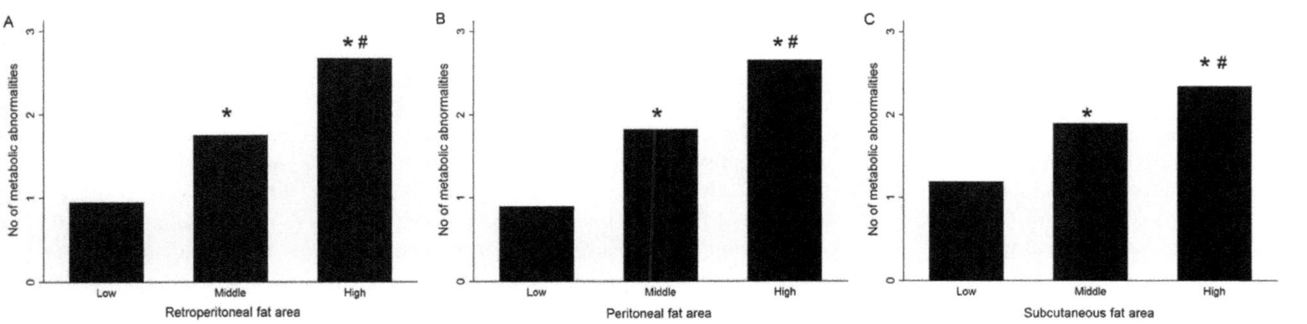

Figure 2. Clustering of metabolic abnormalities defined by MS in participants with body fat areas in the lowest, middle, or highest tertiles. (A) Retroperitoneal fat, (B) peritoneal fat, and (C) subcutaneous fat. *p<0.05 vs. lowest tertile, #p<0.05 vs. middle tertile.

Table 2. The relationship between metabolic syndrome and body fat in logistic regression models, using metabolic syndrome as the dependent variable.

	Model 1	Model 2	Model 3
Age	1.045[a] (1.022–1.068)	1.032[a] (1.008–1.057)	1.034[a] (1.009–1.058)
Male gender	1.615 (0.840–3.106)	0.797 (0.471–1.345)	0.79 (0.465–1.343)
Body mass index	1.292[a] (1.147–1.463)	1.241[a] (1.121–1.373)	1.245[a] (1.126–1.377)
Subcutaneous fat	2.569 (0.935–7.053)		
Peritoneal fat		3.991[a] (2.181–7.304)	
Retroperitoneal fat			5.651[a] (2.707–11.79)

Body fat was logarithmically transformed for statistical analyses. Odds ratios (95% CI) were shown.
[a]$p<0.05$.

retroperitoneal fat area correlated better with diastolic blood pressure and waist circumference as compare to the peritoneal fat area, whereas the peritoneal fat area correlated better with low HDL cholesterol, triglyceride, glutamyl oxaloacetic transaminase (GOT), and GPT concentrations. In contrast, the subcutaneous fat area was not significantly associated with blood pressure, fasting plasma glucose, HbA1c concentration, or lipid profile. The subcutaneous fat area correlated significantly with BMI, waist circumference, OGTT-2h-PG, plasma leptin concentration, adiponectin concentration, and CRP concentration. The retroperitoneal fat area correlated better with the systolic and diastolic blood pressure, waist circumference, plasma glycemic indices, lipid profile, CRP concentration, GOT concentration, GPT concentration, and leptin and adiponectin concentrations, as compared to the relationship with subcutaneous fat area. In participants with positive hepatitis B surface antigen or positive hepatitis C antibody (i.e., not hepatitis B carriers and did not have hepatitis C infection), the remaining 267 participants still showed a better correlation between the peritoneal fat area and GOT concentration (peritoneal fat vs. GOT, $r = 0.1940$, $p<0.05$; retroperitoneal fat vs. GOT, $r = 0.0958$, $p>0.05$ between 2 correlation coefficients) or GPT concentration (peritoneal fat vs. GPT, $r = 0.2648$, $p<0.05$; retroperitoneal fat vs. GPT, $r = 0.2140$, $p<0.05$ between 2 correlation coefficients).

Retroperitoneal and peritoneal fat areas were associated with incident hypertension

After a mean duration of 2.94±0.84 years, 297 (69%) of the 432 participants were followed successfully. Among the 199 participants who did not have hypertension at baseline and have been followed successfully, 32 participants developed incident hypertension. Among the 236 participants who did not have diabetes at baseline, 18 patients developed incident diabetes. Participants with retroperitoneal fat area above the median showed higher risk for incident hypertension, compared with participants with retroperitoneal fat area lower than the median ($p = 0.004$, Figure 3A). Similar trend can be found for peritoneal fat areas (Figure 3B and 3C), but not for subcutaneous fat areas. In Table 4, retroperitoneal and peritoneal fat areas were associated with the development of incident hypertension in adjusted models, which is different from subcutaneous fat areas (HR for retroperitoneal fat, 1.62 (1.18 2.22), $p = 0.003$, HR for peritoneal fat, 1.62 (1.12 2.34), $p = 0.009$, HR for subcutaneous fat, 1.38 (0.90 2.01), $p = 0.14$). Neither retroperitoneal fat area, peritoneal fat area, nor subcutaneous fat areas was associated with incident diabetes after the adjustment for age, gender and family history of diabetes, which may result from the limited event of incident diabetes in the present study.

Discussion

In the present study, we found that retroperitoneal fat area is associated with MS, plasma adipokines, systemic inflammation, and incident hypertension. Retroperitoneal fat is similar to peritoneal fat, but differs from subcutaneous fat, in its relationship with metabolic syndrome, adipokines, and incident hypertension. Our results indicate that the retroperitoneal fat area should be included as part of visceral fat assessment. Compared with peritoneal fat, retroperitoneal fat is more closely associated with blood pressure and waist circumference, whereas peritoneal fat correlates better with low HDL cholesterol concentration, high triglyceride concentration, and abnormal liver function.

In the literature, there is only one previous study investigating the independent role of retroperitoneal fat to other part of visceral fats in MS [18]. Supporting our findings, the authors of that study also reported a significant association between retroperitoneal fat and MS. However, since all study participants in that study had adrenal diseases (19 had adrenal-dependent Cushing's syndrome, 12 had subclincal Cushing's syndrome, and 30 had nonfunctional adrenal incidentaloma), it remained unknown whether the relationship only holds true for participants with adrenal diseases or if the relationship is a consequence of adrenal diseases. In the present study, we included generally healthy participants from the community and confirmed that there is a significant relationship between retroperitoneal fat and MS in the general population.

The mechanisms underlying how visceral adiposity induces metabolic abnormalities are not fully understood. Several hypotheses have been proposed, including increased portal free fatty acid, endocrine function of visceral adipose tissue (adipokines), and visceral obesity as a marker of dysfunctional adipose tissue leading to ectopic fat deposition [4]. For peritoneal and retroperitoneal fat, the blood supply and venous drainage systems are different. Peritoneal fat drains into the portal vein, which may result in increased free fatty acid flux to the liver. High concentration of free fatty acid to the liver leads to the development of fatty liver, insulin resistance, high triglyceride concentrations, and low HDL cholesterol concentrations [19,20]. Indeed, when epididymal fat pads were transplanted into the mesenterium (portal drainage) or parietal peritoneum (systemic drainage) in mice, only mice with fat transplanted into the mesenterium developed impaired glucose tolerance and hepatic insulin resistance [21]. However, retroperitoneal fat can drain into the renal vein or directly into the inferior

Table 3. Correlation coefficients (r) between body fat and metabolic variables in participants without medications for hypertension, diabetes, or dyslipidemia (N = 353).

	Retroperitoneal fat	p1[a]	p2[b]	Peritoneal fat	p1[a]	p3[c]	Subcutaneous fat	p1[a]	p3[c]
Systolic BP	0.397[a]	<0.001	<0.001	0.350[a]	<0.001	0.07	0.055[b]	0.31	<0.001
Diastolic BP	0.387[a]	<0.001	<0.001	0.325[ab]	<0.001	0.01	0.106[b]	0.05	<0.001
BMI	0.670[a]	<0.001	<0.001	0.645[a]	<0.001	0.14	0.609[a]	<0.001	0.11
WC	0.730[a]	<0.001	<0.001	0.694[ab]	<0.001	0.04	0.542[ab]	<0.001	<0.001
FPG	0.243[a]	<0.001	0.01	0.203[a]	<0.001	0.08	0.067[b]	0.21	0.001
OGTT-2h-PG	0.290[a]	<0.001	0.06	0.279[a]	<0.001	0.67	0.141[ab]	0.008	0.001
HbA1c	0.215[a]	<0.001	0.128	0.202[a]	<0.001	0.65	0.044[b]	0.41	<0.001
Total cholesterol	0.230[a]	<0.001	0.008	0.185[a]	<0.001	0.1	0.074[b]	0.17	0.002
HDL cholesterol	−0.354[a]	<0.001	0.768	−0.399[ab]	<0.001	0.07	−0.082[b]	0.13	<0.001
LDL cholesterol	0.290[a]	<0.001	0.01	0.259[a]	<0.001	0.2	0.084[b]	0.11	<0.001
Triglyceride	0.269[a]	<0.001	0.728	0.299[ab]	<0.001	0.07	0.080[b]	0.13	<0.001
GOT	0.089	0.1	0.03	0.168[ab]	0.002	<0.001	−0.024[b]	0.65	0.03
GPT	0.213[a]	0.001	0.672	0.258[ab]	<0.001	0.03	0.090[b]	0.09	0.04
HOMA2%B	0.206[a]	0.001	0.353	0.215[a]	<0.001	0.74	0.239[a]	<0.001	0.47
HOMA2%S	−0.400[a]	<0.001	0.467	−0.400[a]	<0.001	0.98	−0.360[a]	<0.001	0.44
CRP[d]	0.335[a]	<0.001	0.72	0.376[a]	<0.001	0.14	0.194[ab]	0.07	0.18
Plasma adiponectin[d]	−0.244[a]	<0.001	0.14	−0.237[a]	<0.001	0.755	−0.016[b]	0.05	<0.001
Plasma leptin[d]	0.323[a]	<0.001	0.124	0.327[a]	<0.001	0.97	0.741[ab]	<0.001	<0.001
Plasma renin[d]	0.049	0.21	0.768	0.065	0.06	0.21	0.035	0.45	0.56
Plasma aldosterone[d]	−0.005	0.22	0.01	−0.070[b]	0.03	0.08	−0.012	0.87	0.3

Body fat area was logarithmically transformed for statistical analysis.
BP, blood pressure; BMI, body mass index; WC, waist circumference; FPG, fasting plasma glucose; OGTT-2h-PG, plasma glucose at 2 h during oral glucose tolerance test; HbA1c, hemoglobin A1c; GOT, glutamic oxaloacetic transaminase; GPT, glutamic pyruvic transaminase; HDL, high-density lipoprotein; LDL, low-density lipoprotein; CRP, C-reactive protein.
[a]p1: retroperitoneal fat, peritoneal fat or subcutaneous fat area vs the indicated metabolic variable.
[b]p2: retroperitoneal fat vs the indicated metabolic variable, adjusted for peritoneal fat.
[c]p3: compare with the correlation coefficient between retroperitoneal fat and the indicated metabolic variable.
[d]log-transformed.

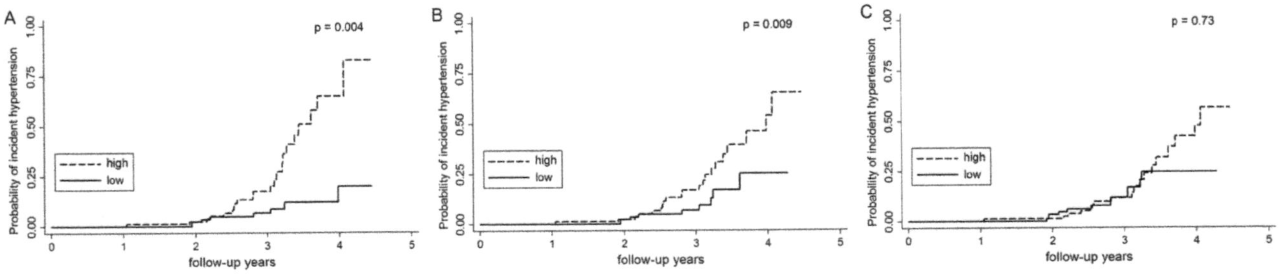

Figure 3. Different fat compartments to predict the probability of incident hypertension. Kaplan-Meier failure curves for the probability of developing hypertension in subgroups divided by the median of (A) retroperitoneal fat area, (B) peritoneal fat area, and (C) subcutaneous fat area. P values by log-rank tests are shown.

vena cava, which may lead to "fatty kidney." Fatty kidney, as defined by higher renal sinus fat area on CT, has been shown to be associated with hypertension [22]. In addition, there are further differences between different compartments of abdominal fat. Mesenteric pre-adipocytes are found to be distinct from omental pre-adipocytes in their replication potential, mechanism of lipid accumulation, and response to tumor necrosis factor-alpha–induced apoptosis [23]. Retroperitoneal fat has been shown to contain increased amount of brown adipose tissue in humans, as reported by Betz MJ *et al* [24]. In mice, Cohen CA *et al.* found that intra-abdominal fat depots from different compartments showed distinct patterns in terms of leukocyte to monocyte ratio and gene expression profiles [8]. Indeed, we found different relationships of diastolic blood pressure and plasma HDL cholesterol, triglyceride, GOT, and GPT concentrations with peritoneal and retroperitoneal fat in humans. However, an even greater difference was noted between retroperitoneal fat and subcutaneous fat. The association trends between retroperitoneal fat, metabolic profiles, adipokine concentrations, CRP concentrations, and incident hypertension and diabetes were similar to those of peritoneal fat, but differed from those of subcutaneous fat in the present study.

Taken together, these data suggest that differences exist in the biologic functions of retroperitoneal fat and peritoneal fat. However, compared to subcutaneous fat, retroperitoneal fat and peritoneal fat behave more similarly. Therefore, when the visceral fat area is measured by CT or MRI in human studies for cardiovascular and metabolic diseases, the retroperitoneal fat area should be included.

To the best of our knowledge, the present study is the first comprehensive research to investigate if retroperitoneal fat should be included in the measurement of visceral fat in humans. We analyzed the relationship between retroperitoneal fat, MS, each metabolic abnormality, adipokines, a marker of systemic inflammation, and incident hypertension and diabetes. We also compared the pattern of these relationships among retroperitoneal fat, peritoneal fat, and subcutaneous fat. In addition, the use of CT to measure abdominal adiposity enabled us to compare different compartments of abdominal fat in detail. By contrast, the present study was limited in its follow-up rate of 69%. Although it is not likely that the relationships of retroperitoneal fat to incident hypertension and diabetes will be different in subjects who lost of follow-up, we cannot exclude the possibility completely.

Conclusion

Retroperitoneal fat is associated with MS, plasma adipokine concentrations, systemic inflammation, and incident hypertension. Retroperitoneal fat is similar to peritoneal fat, but differs from subcutaneous fat, in its relationship with metabolic syndrome, adipokines, and incident hypertension. Our results indicate that the retroperitoneal fat area should be included in the measurement of visceral fat area. In addition, since the relationships between these factors and different compartments of abdominal fat are different, further research is needed to explore the pathophysiologic implications of these findings.

Table 4. Hazard ratios (HRs) and 95% confidence interval (95% CI) of different fat components to predict the development of incident hypertension and incident diabetes during follow-up.

	Retroperitoneal fat	Peritoneal fat	Subcutaneous fat
Incident hypertension			
Crude (unadjusted)	1.64[a] (1.25–2.15)	1.77[a] (1.29–2.41)	1.21 (0.83–1.78)
Model 1	1.62[a] (1.18–2.22)	1.62[a] (1.12–2.34)	1.38 (0.90–2.01)
Incident diabetes			
Crude (unadjusted)	1.43[a] (1.01–2.02)	1.38 (0.91–2.0)	0.72 (0.41–1.2)
Model 2	1.42 (0.89–2.24)	1.46 (0.91–2.35)	0.90 (0.51–1.60)

Hazard ratios were normalized to show the effect of every 1 standard deviation increase in fat areas.
[a]$p<0.05$.
Model 1: adjusted for age, sex, and family history of hypertension.
Model 2: adjusted for age, sex, and family history of diabetes.

Supporting Information

Dataset S1 Cross sectional dataset.

Dataset S2 Longitudinal dataset.

Acknowledgments

H.-Y.L. had full access to all of the data in the study and takes responsibility for the integrity of the data and the accuracy of the data analysis. The authors would like to thank Ms. Chien-Yin Su, Ms. Kuan-Yi Wu, Ms. Ying-Jhu Liao, and the staff of the Eighth Core Lab, Department of Medical Research, and National Taiwan University Hospital, for their technical and computing assistance.

Author Contributions

Conceived and designed the experiments: CSH JKL MSL JML JNW HYL. Performed the experiments: CSH CYY WYM HYL SRS. Analyzed the data: CSH PHL HYL CYY JWL. Contributed reagents/materials/analysis tools: HRH HYL. Contributed to the writing of the manuscript: JML LMC MFC JNW.

References

1. National Cholesterol Education Program Expert Panel on Detection E, Treatment of High Blood Cholesterol in A (2002) Third Report of the National Cholesterol Education Program (NCEP) Expert Panel on Detection, Evaluation, and Treatment of High Blood Cholesterol in Adults (Adult Treatment Panel III) final report. Circulation 106: 3143–3421.
2. Dekker JM, Girman C, Rhodes T, Nijpels G, Stehouwer CD, et al. (2005) Metabolic syndrome and 10-year cardiovascular disease risk in the Hoorn Study. Circulation 112: 666–673.
3. Alberti KG, Zimmet P, Shaw J (2006) Metabolic syndrome-a new world-wide definition. A Consensus Statement from the International Diabetes Federation. Diabet Med 23: 469–480.
4. Cornier MA, Despres JP, Davis N, Grossniklaus DA, Klein S, et al. (2011) Assessing adiposity: a scientific statement from the American Heart Association. Circulation 124: 1996–2019.
5. Despres JP, Lemieux I (2006) Abdominal obesity and metabolic syndrome. Nature 444: 881–887.
6. Ross R, Aru J, Freeman J, Hudson R, Janssen I (2002) Abdominal adiposity and insulin resistance in obese men. Am J Physiol Endocrinol Metab 282: E657–663.
7. Tchernof A, Despres JP (2013) Pathophysiology of human visceral obesity: an update. Physiol Rev 93: 359–404.
8. Cohen CA, Shea AA, Heffron CL, Schmelz EM, Roberts PC (2013) Intra-abdominal fat depots represent distinct immunomodulatory microenvironments: a murine model. PLoS One 8: e66477.
9. Chapados N, Collin P, Imbeault P, Corriveau P, Lavoie JM (2008) Exercise training decreases in vitro stimulated lipolysis in a visceral (mesenteric) but not in the retroperitoneal fat depot of high-fat-fed rats. Br J Nutr 100: 518–525.
10. Fox CS, Massaro JM, Hoffmann U, Pou KM, Maurovich-Horvat P, et al. (2007) Abdominal visceral and subcutaneous adipose tissue compartments: association with metabolic risk factors in the Framingham Heart Study. Circulation 116: 39–48.
11. Yoshizumi T, Nakamura T, Yamane M, Islam AH, Menju M, et al. (1999) Abdominal fat: standardized technique for measurement at CT. Radiology 211: 283–286.
12. Borel AL, Boulet G, Nazare JA, Smith J, Almeras N, et al. (2013) Improved plasma FFA/insulin homeostasis is independently associated with improved glucose tolerance after a 1-year lifestyle intervention in viscerally obese men. Diabetes Care 36: 3254–3261.
13. Hung CS, Lee PC, Li HY, Ma WY, Lin MS, et al. (2011) Haemoglobin A1c is associated with carotid intima-media thickness in a Chinese population. Clin Endocrinol (Oxf) 75: 780–785.
14. Li HY, Lin MS, Shih SR, Hua CH, Liu YL, et al. (2011) The performance of risk scores and hemoglobin A1c to find undiagnosed diabetes with isolated postload hyperglycemia. Endocr J 58: 441–448.
15. Ma WY, Yang CY, Shih SR, Hsieh HJ, Hung CS, et al. (2013) Measurement of Waist Circumference: midabdominal or iliac crest? Diabetes Care 36: 1660–1666.
16. Little RR, Rohlfing CL, Wiedmeyer HM, Myers GL, Sacks DB, et al. (2001) The national glycohemoglobin standardization program: a five-year progress report. Clin Chem 47: 1985–1992.
17. Tan CE, Ma S, Wai D, Chew SK, Tai ES (2004) Can we apply the National Cholesterol Education Program Adult Treatment Panel definition of the metabolic syndrome to Asians? Diabetes Care 27: 1182–1186.
18. Ersoz F, Erbil Y, Sari S, Salmaslioglu A, Issever H, et al. (2011) Predictive value of retroperitoneal fat area measurement for detecting metabolic syndrome in patients undergoing adrenalectomy. World J Surg 35: 986–994.
19. Yoshii H, Lam TK, Gupta N, Goh T, Haber CA, et al. (2006) Effects of portal free fatty acid elevation on insulin clearance and hepatic glucose flux. Am J Physiol Endocrinol Metab 290: E1089–1097.
20. Kabir M, Catalano KJ, Ananthnarayan S, Kim SP, Van Citters GW, et al. (2005) Molecular evidence supporting the portal theory: a causative link between visceral adiposity and hepatic insulin resistance. Am J Physiol Endocrinol Metab 288: E454–461.
21. Rytka JM, Wueest S, Schoenle EJ, Konrad D (2011) The portal theory supported by venous drainage-selective fat transplantation. Diabetes 60: 56–63.
22. Foster MC, Hwang SJ, Porter SA, Massaro JM, Hoffmann U, et al. (2011) Fatty kidney, hypertension, and chronic kidney disease: the Framingham Heart Study. Hypertension 58: 784–790.
23. Tchkonia T, Tchoukalova YD, Giorgadze N, Pirtskhalava T, Karagiannides I, et al. (2005) Abundance of two human preadipocyte subtypes with distinct capacities for replication, adipogenesis, and apoptosis varies among fat depots. Am J Physiol Endocrinol Metab 288: E267–277.
24. Betz MJ, Slawik M, Lidell ME, Osswald A, Heglind M, et al. (2013) Presence of brown adipocytes in retroperitoneal fat from patients with benign adrenal tumors: relationship with outdoor temperature. J Clin Endocrinol Metab 98: 4097–4104.

Differential Regulation of Human Aortic Smooth Muscle Cell Proliferation by Monocyte-Derived Macrophages from Diabetic Patients

Te-Chuan Chen[1], Mao-Ling Sung[2], Hsing-Chun Kuo[3,4], Shao-Ju Chien[5], Chia-Kuang Yen[2], Cheng-Nan Chen[6]*

1 Division of Nephrology, Kaohsiung Chang Gung Memorial Hospital and Chang Gung University College of Medicine, Kaohsiung, Taiwan, **2** Department of Cardiology, St. Martin De Porres Hospital, Chiayi, Taiwan, **3** Institute of Nursing and Department of Nursing, Chang Gung University of Science and Technology, Chronic Diseases and Health Promotion Research Center, CGUST, Taoyuan, Taiwan, **4** Research Center for Industry of Human Ecology, Chang Gung University of Science and Technology, Taoyuan, Taiwan, **5** Division of Pediatric Cardiology, Department of Pediatrics, Kaohsiung Chang Gung Memorial Hospital, Chang Gung University College of Medicine, Kaohsiung, Taiwan, **6** Department of Biochemical Science and Technology, National Chiayi University, Chiayi, Taiwan

Abstract

Macrophage accumulation in the arterial wall and smooth muscle cell (SMC) proliferation are features of type 2 diabetes mellitus (DM) and its vascular complications. However, the effects of diabetic monocyte-derived macrophages on vascular SMC proliferation are not clearly understood. In the present study, we investigated the pro-proliferative effect of macrophages isolated from DM patients on vascular SMCs. Macrophage-conditioned media (MCM) were prepared from macrophages isolated from DM patients. DM-MCM treatment induced HASMC proliferation, decreased $p21^{Cip1}$ and $p27^{Kip1}$ expressions, and increased microRNA (miR)-17-5p and miR-221 expressions. Inhibition of either miR-17-5p or miR-221 inhibited DM-MCM-induced cell proliferation. Inhibition of miR-17-5p abolished DM-MCM-induced $p21^{Cip1}$ down-regulation; and inhibition of miR-221 attenuated the DM-MCM-induced $p27^{Kip1}$ down-regulation. Furthermore, blocking assays demonstrated that PDGF-CC in DM-MCM is the major mediators of cell proliferation in SMCs. In conclusion, our present data support the hypothesis that SMC proliferation stimulated by macrophages may play critical roles in vascular complications in DM patients and suggest a new mechanism by which arterial disease is accelerated in diabetes.

Editor: Jozef Dulak, Faculty of Biochemistry, Poland

Funding: Grants CZRPG880253, CMRPF6A0073, CMRPG891581, CMRPG6C0071, CMRPG6C0011 and EZRPF6C0011 from Chang Gung Memorial Hospital-Kaohsiung Medical Center, Chang Gung Memorial Hospital, and Chang Gung University of Science and Technology, Chia-Yi Campus, Taiwan, and by the National Science Council, Taiwan (NSC101-2320-B-415-003-MY3, NSC102-2314-B-750-001, NSC101-2622-B-255-001-CC3, NSC102-2313-B-255-002). The funders had no role in study design, data collection and analysis, decision to publish, or preparation of the manuscript.

Competing Interests: The authors have declared that no competing interests exist.

* Email: cnchen@mail.ncyu.edu.tw

Introduction

Diabetes mellitus (DM) is associated with an increased risk for atherothrombotic complications such as peripheral artery disease, coronary artery disease, and myocardial infarction [1,2]. It is well documented that macrophage accumulation is a common feature of type 2 diabetes and its complications [3,4]. Recruitment of monocytes from the peripheral blood to the intima of the vessel wall and the monocytes' subsequent differentiation into macrophages are critical events in atherogenesis. In addition, pathological environments, such as hyperglycemia, may promote macrophage activation and secretion within DM tissues. It has been demonstrated that high-glucose (HG) treatments of human monocytes lead to the increased expression of inflammatory cytokine and chemokine genes [5]. Our previous study also reported that the macrophage inflammatory protein (MIP)-1α and 1β released by HG-treated monocyte-derived macrophages are major mediators for the induction of E-selectin expression in vascular endothelial cells (ECs) [6]. However, the effect of monocyte-derived macrophages isolated from diabetic patients on vascular smooth-muscle-cell (SMC) activation has not been completely understood.

The proliferation and phenotypic changes of vascular SMCs are key events in the development of atherosclerosis and its complications [7]. During the development of atherosclerotic plaque, SMCs migrate from the media into the intimal layer of the arterial wall, where they proliferate and produce an extracellular matrix (ECM), resulting in the formation of intimal hyperplasia [8]. Growth factors, inflammatory cytokines, and chemokines have been implicated as factors that mediate such SMC proliferation [9]. Among these factors, the platelet-derived growth factor (PDGF) family possesses the most potent mitogenic effects for SMC [10]. The G1-to-S phase transit of the cell cycle requires activation of the cyclin-cyclin-dependent kinase (CDK) complex. The cyclin-dependent kinase inhibitors (CKI) such as $p21^{Cip1}$ and $p27^{Kip1}$ have been shown to regulate the activity of these complexes in the G1 phase [11]. $p21^{Cip1}$ and $p27^{Kip1}$ are expressed in quiescent SMCs and are down-regulated following mitogen stimulation [12]. It has been shown that a hyperglycemic environment can activate vascular SMCs and cause vascular dysfunction [13]. In addition, it has also been found that hyperglycemic conditions have mitogenic effects on vascular SMCs [14]. Therefore, examining the proliferative response of vascular SMCs to hyperglycemia may potentially extend our understanding of the pathogenic mechanisms of vascular complications in diabetes.

The functions of SMCs may be modulated by their interaction with other vascular cells such as monocyte-derived macrophages. It has been reported that interactions between monocytes and vascular SMCs may contribute to monocyte retention within the vasculature [15]. Moreover, macrophages can release a wide range of regulatory factors that are growth mediators to affect cell proliferation. Previous studies have indicated that human monocyte-derived macrophages have an inhibitory effect on SMC growth [16,17]. Evidence also shows that palmitate-stimulated macrophages promote SMC proliferation via the secretion of bone morphogenetic protein (BMP) 2 and BMP4 [18]. Although there is considerable research on the role of macrophages in the development of atherosclerotic lesions, the contribution of macrophages under hyperglycemic conditions to SMC proliferation remains unclear.

SMCs in the media of the artery are encompassed by a network of ECM such as fibrillar collagen. Culturing SMCs on fibrillar collagen promotes the maintenance of the SMC contractile phenotype and exerts an anti-proliferative effect [19]. Since proliferation and accumulation of SMCs are believed to play important roles in the progression of macrophage-rich lesions to fibroatheromas [4], it was hypothesized that monocyte-derived macrophages differentiated from diabetic patients may alter gene expression and affect SMC proliferation. We found that the SMC proliferation induced by macrophages in hyperglycemia is mediated through the up-regulation of microRNA (miR)-17-5p and miR-221. This study presents evidence for a novel mechanism in which miRNAs act synergistically to induce SMC proliferation.

Methods

Materials

All culture materials were purchased from Gibco (Grand Island, NY, USA). Rat tail type I collagen was purchased from BD Biosciences (San Diego, CA). Mouse monoclonal antibodies (mAbs) against $p21^{Cip1}$ and rabbit polyclonal antibodies (pAbs) against $p27^{Kip1}$ were purchased from Cell Signaling Technology (Beverly, MA). mAbs against osteopontin (OPN) matrix gla protein (MGP) were purchased from Santa Cruz Biotech (*Santa Cruz*, CA, USA). Other chemicals of reagent grade were obtained from Sigma (St Louis, MO).

Subjects

The Ethics Committees of St. Martin De Porres Hospital (Chiayi City, Taiwan) approved the study protocol, and written informed consents were obtained from all patients before enrollment. The study group consisted of 13 patients with type 2 diabetes and 9 healthy control subjects. The patients had a mean (±SEM) age of 53.4±8.5 years, body mass index of 31.4±2.5 kg/m^2, fasting glucose of 185±12.4 mg/dL, triglyceride level of 182.9±16.1 mg/dL, LDL cholesterol level of 94.3±7.8 mg/dL, and hemoglobin $A1_C$ of 7.6±1.1%. All patients were treated with glyburide and metformin. None of the patients was primarily insulin dependent. In addition, we recruited 9 volunteers, who were admitted to the St. Martin De Porres Hospital for the purpose of routine physical examinations, as the control subject group. They had a mean (±SEM) age of 49.2±7.9 years, body mass index of 22.7±1.3 kg/m^2, fasting glucose of 84.6±1.7 mg/dL, triglyceride level of 147.1±8.7 mg/dL, LDL cholesterol level of 95.2±3.8 mg/dL, and hemoglobin $A1_C$ of 4.7±0.4%. None of the normal subjects had infectious or inflammatory conditions, or cardiac, renal, or pulmonary decompensated diseases. Volunteers who smoked cigarettes, used alcohol or were under medications (hormonal replacement therapy, nonsteroidal anti-inflammatory drugs, corticosteroids, and anticoagulant drugs) were excluded from this normal subject group.

Human monocyte isolation

Human monocytes were isolated as previously described [6]. Peripheral blood mononuclear cells (PBMCs) were isolated by Histopaque 1077 density-gradient centrifugation. Monocytes were purified from PBMCs by negative selection using the magnetic-activated cell sorting (MACS) monocyte isolation kit (Miltenyi Biotech, Auburn, CA); PBMCs were first treated with FcγR blocking reagent (human IgG), followed by a hapten/antibody mixture (mixture of hapten-conjugated monoclonal anti-CD3, anti-CD7, anti-CD19, anti-CD45RA, anti-CD56, and anti-IgE antibodies). After treatment with MACS antihapten magnetic microbeads conjugated to monoclonal antihapten antibody, the labeled cells were passed over a MACS column, and the effluent was collected as the negative fraction representing enriched monocytes (>95% purity).

Preparation of macrophage-conditioned medium (MCM)

Differentiation of monocyte-derived macrophages from diabetes patients or normal control subjects was achieved by culturing the freshly isolated monocytes (5×10^5 cells/mL) in RPMI-1640 medium supplemented with 10% autologous serum. After 4 days in culture, monocyte-derived macrophages were incubated for another 48 h in fresh serum-free RPMI medium. The conditioned medium was collected, centrifuged, filtered, and defined as diabetic (DM)-MCM and normal control (NC)-MCM.

Cell culture

Human aortic SMCs (HASMCs) were obtained commercially (Clonetics, Palo Alto, CA) and maintained in F12K medium supplemented with 10% FBS. Cells at passages 3 to 6 were used. Growth of the cells was arrested by incubating in F12K medium with 0.5% FBS for 48 hours before use.

Collagen matrices

Fibrillar collagen (0.1%) was prepared by mixing 4 mg/ml rat tail type I collagen (25%), 0.1 M NaOH (5%), 2× F12K medium (40%), FBS (10%), and complete medium (F12K with 10% FBS; 20%). The mixture (0.15 ml/cm^2) was allowed to form fibrillar collagen matrices for at least 1 h at 37°C. SMCs were cultured on the surface of fibrillar collagen as described [19].

MTT assay and flow cytometric analysis for cell proliferation

Cells were cultured on type I fibrillar collagen in 96-well plates. Cell proliferation was determined by 3-(4,5-dimethylthiazol-2-yl)-2,5-diphenyltetrazolium bromide (MTT) assay. After the incubation period, MTT solution was added to each well to a final concentration of 0.5 mg/mL, and the mixture was incubated at 37°C for 3 hours to allow MTT reduction. The formazan crystals were dissolved by adding dimethylsulfoxide (DMSO) and absorbance was measured at 570 nm with a spectrophotometer.

Cell-cycle distribution was determined by flow cytometry. Cells stained with propidium iodide were analyzed with a FACScalibur

(Becton Dickinson), and the data were analyzed by using a mod-fit cell cycle analysis program [19].

Real-time quantitative PCR

Total RNA preparation and the RT reaction were carried out as described previously [6]. Regular real-time quantitative PCR was performed to confirm PCR array results. PCRs were performed using an ABI Prism 7900HT according to the manufacturer's instructions. Amplification of specific PCR products was detected using the SYBR Green PCR Master Mix (Applied Biosystems). In addition, the designed primers in this study were: p21^{Cip1} forward primer, 5′-CTGAA AGATG GACGC TCAAT-3′; p21^{Cip1} reverse primer, 5′-CGTTT CA-GAA GCCAG AAGAG-3′; p27^{Kip1} forward primer, 5′-CTGAA AGATG GACGC TCAAT-3′; p27^{Kip1} reverse primer, 5′-CGTTT CAGAA GCCAG AAGAG-3′; OPN forward primer, 5′- TTGCA GCCTT CTCAG CCAA-3′; OPN reverse primer, 5′- GGAGG CAAAA GCAAA TCACT G-3′; MGP forward primer, 5′- GCTCA ATAGG GAAGC CTGTG AT-3′; MGP reverse primer, 5′- TTTCT TCCCT CAGTC TCATT TGG-3′; 18S rRNA forward primer, 5′-CGGCG ACGAC CCATT CGAAC-3′, 18S rRNA reverse primer, 5′-GAATC GAACC CTGAT TCCCC GTC-3′. Quantification was performed using the $2^{-\Delta\Delta Ct}$ method [6].

Western blot analysis

SMCs were lysed with a buffer containing 1% NP-40, 0.5% sodium deoxycholate, 0.1% SDS, and a protease inhibitor mixture (PMSF, aprotinin, and sodium orthovanadate). The total cell lysate (50 μg of protein) was separated by SDS-polyacrylamide gel electrophoresis (PAGE) (12% running, 4% stacking) and analyzed by using the designated antibodies and the Western-Light chemiluminescent detection system (Bio-Rad, Hercules, CA), as previously described [19].

Inhibition of miR-17-5p and miR-221

Anti-miR inhibitors for miR-17-5p, miR-221, and corresponding negative controls were purchased from Ambion, Life Technologies (Austin, TX, USA). The SMCs were then transfected with the miRNA inhibitors or miRNA inhibitor negative control by Oligofectamine Transfection Reagent from Invitrogen, Life Technologies, in accordance with the manufacturer's procedure. The final concentration for miRNA inhibitor was 200 nmol/L. The transfection efficiency of miRNA inhibitors was further verified by Real-time quantitative PCR assay. After transfection with the miR-17-5p and miR-221 inhibitors, the expression levels of miR-17-5p and miR-221 were decreased by 75.3% and 78.7%, respectively.

ELISA for PDGF-BB and PDGF-CC

The levels of PDGF-BB and PDGF-CC in the MCM were determined by using sandwich ELISA (sensitivity 18 pg/mL; R&D) according to manufacturer's protocols, as previously described [19].

Statistical analysis

The results are expressed as mean ± standard error of the mean (SEM). Statistical analysis was performed by using an independent Student t-test for two groups of data and analysis of variance (ANOVA) followed by Scheffe's test for multiple comparisons. *P* values less than 0.05 were considered significant.

Results

The effect of DM-MCM on SMC proliferation

The effects of monocyte-derived macrophages from DM patients on cell proliferation were studied by treating SMCs cultured on fibrillar collagen with DM-MCM (vs. NC-MCM). SMCs were stimulated with the two types of MCM at different concentrations for 24 h, or 1× DM-MCM for the times indicated. Cell proliferation was analyzed by MTT assays. As shown in Figure 1A, proliferation of SMC was significantly increased (38%, 56% and 89% after cultivation for 24, 48 and 72 h, respectively) when cultivated with DM-MCM. SMCs cultured with NC-MCM had limited proliferation capacities (Figure 1A). SMCs treated with DM-MCM at different concentrations for 24 h showed a significantly higher growth rate when compared to the control cells (Figure 1B). Table 1 summarizes the flow cytometry analysis of cell distribution in the cell cycle phases. SMCs stimulated with DM-MCM for 24 and 48 h had marked decreases of cells in the G_0/G_1 phases and increases in the S-phase (Table 1).

DM-MCM decreased p21^{Cip1} and p27^{Kip1} and increased synthetic differentiation marker expression in SMCs

We examined the effects of DM-MCM on the expression of cell-cycle regulatory proteins p21^{Cip1} and p27^{Kip1}. As shown in Figure 2B, SMCs with DM-MCM stimulation decreased the expressions of p21^{Cip1} and p27^{Kip1}. However, there was no effect on p21^{Cip1} and p27^{Kip1} expression in SMCs cultured with NC-MCM (Figure 2A). Figure 2C shows that DM-MCM induced decreases in the mRNA expression of p21^{Cip1} and p27^{Kip1} after 12 h of DM-MCM stimulation.

We also examined the effect of DM-MCM on the expression of synthetic differentiation markers in SMCs. SMCs were cultured on fibrillar collagen, and the mRNA and protein expression of OPN and MGP was analyzed at various time points after cultivation. Real-time PCR analysis indicated the time-dependent increase in the levels of mRNA expression for OPN (Figure 3A) and MGP (Figure 3B) in SMCs on fibrillar collagen. The cultivation of SMCs by DM-MCM also caused significant increases in the OPN and MGP expression at 72 h on fibrillar collagen (Figure 3C).

miR-17-5p and miR-221 are involved in the regulation of HASMC proliferation

Recent studies have demonstrated that miRNAs are involved in regulating SMC gene expression and proliferation [20]. We therefore examined the effects of DM-MCM on the expression of miRNAs. Stimulation of SMCs with DM-MCM increased the expression of the miR-17-5p (Figure 4A) and miR-221 (Figure 4B), in a time-dependent manner.

To determine whether DM-MCM-induced cell proliferation was mediated by the up-regulation of miR-17-5p and miR-221, SMCs were pretreated with miR-17-5p and miR-221 inhibitors and subsequently stimulated with DM-MCM. The DM-MCM-induced SMC proliferation was significantly inhibited by pretreatments with miR-17-5p and miR-221 inhibitors (Figure 4C). The DM-MCM-induced decrease in the percentage of cells in the G_0/G_1 phases and the increase in the percentage of cells in the S-phase were also significantly inhibited by miR-17-5p and miR-221 inhibitors (Figure 4D).

In addition, SMCs were incubated with specific inhibitors of miR-17-5p and miR-221 for 1 h before and during stimulation with DM-MCM, and the expressions of p21^{Cip1} and p27^{Kip1} were analyzed. As shown in Figure 4E, miR-17-5p inhibitor significantly inhibited the DM-MCM-induced expression of p21^{Cip1},

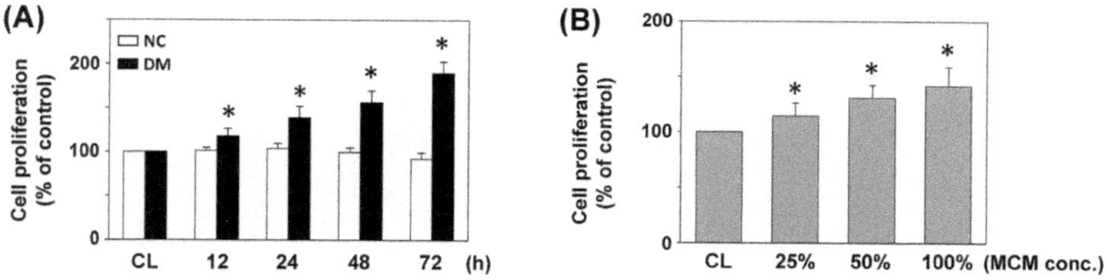

Figure 1. Effect of DM-MCM on cell viability of HASMCs. Bar graphs represent folds of controls (CL) SMCs, mean ± standard error of the mean (SEM) of 5 independent experiments. *$P<0.05$ versus CL SMCs. (A) SMCs were kept as CL or stimulated with NC-MCM or DM-MCM at the indicated time periods, or (B) stimulated with different concentrations of DM-MCM for 24 h. Cell proliferation was assayed by the MTT test.

whereas miR-221 inhibitor inhibited the DM-MCM-induced expression of $p27^{Kip1}$.

DM-MCM induced SMC proliferation was mediated by PDGF-CC

The effect of DM-MCM on SMC proliferation suggests that macrophages under a DM environment may release soluble mediators and exert paracrine effects on SMCs to induce cell proliferation. PDGF was identified in a search for serum factors that stimulate SMC proliferation [10]. As shown in Figure 5A, the incubation of SMCs with PDGF-CC neutralizing antibody, but not PDGF-BB, significantly inhibited DM-MCM-induced SMC proliferation. To confirm these results, the protein levels of PDGF-BB and PDGF-CC in NC- and DM-MCM were analyzed by ELISA. As shown in Figure 5B, culturing of monocyte-derive macrophages caused significant increases of PDGF-BB and PDGF-CC protein secretion in macrophages isolated from diabetic patients.

To further characterize the effect of the PDGF-BB or PDGF-CC in MCM on SMC proliferation and to determine the optimal PDGF concentrations, we examined the responses of SMC to 50% DM-MCM with different concentrations of the PDGF-BB and PDGF-CC (0–100 ng/mL) and their neutralizing antibodies. The results shown in Figure 5D indicated that PDGF-CC promoted SMC proliferation, and the effect was significantly inhibited by neutralizing antibody against PDGF-CC, while PDGF-BB had no significant effect on SMC proliferation (Figure 5C). Figure 5D also indicated that the optimal concentration of PDGF-CC was 50 ng/mL.

Discussion

Diabetic patients have an increased susceptibility to the development of atherosclerosis [21]. Atherosclerotic lesions in patients with diabetes are characterized by excessive macrophage infiltration, suggesting that the accumulation of monocyte-derived macrophages into the vasculature may be augmented under hyperglycemic conditions [3]. In addition, the migration and proliferation of SMCs are believed to play important roles in the progression of macrophage-rich lesions to fibroatheromas, and diabetic conditions have been shown to enhance this process [22]. It has been suggested that the macrophage-SMC coexistence as neighbors within the vessel walls induces regulatory signals involved in atherogenesis [23]. There is also evidence that hyperglycemia may enhance the interaction of macrophages and SMCs [24]. However, the pathophysiological mechanism of macrophage-SMC interaction remains poorly understood. The present study characterized the roles of two major monocyte-derived macrophage-induced mediators from diabetic patients in the regulation of $p21^{Cip1}$ and $p27^{Kip1}$ expressions by HASMCs. Several lines of evidence from the current study indicate that the effect of macrophages from DM patients on SMC proliferation was mediated by the down-regulation of expressions of $p21^{Cip1}$ and $p27^{Kip1}$ and that this down-regulation was mediated through the differential regulation of the miR-17-5p and miR-221. First, stimulation by DM-MCM induced decreased expression of $p21^{Cip1}$ and $p27^{Kip1}$, as well as increased cell proliferation. Second, stimulation of SMCs by DM-MCM induced expression of miR-17-5p. Pretreatment of the cells with miR-17-5p inhibitor suppressed the DM-MCM-induced down-regulation of $p21^{Cip1}$

Table 1. Cell cycle analysis of SMCs stimulated with NC- and DM-MCM.

	Duration (h)	% cells (mean ± SEM) G_0/G_1	S-phase	G_2/M
Control	**0**	87.4±2.1	6.5±0.8	6.1±1.2
NC-MCM	**24**	92.3±2.7	5.1±0.6	2.6±1.0
	48	92.9±1.9	3.9±0.4	3.2±0.8
	72	90.3±2.6	5.6±0.6	4.1±1.1
DM-MCM	**24**	72.1±4.8*	19.2±2.4*	8.7±1.4
	48	70.6±4.3*	22.3±2.7*	7.1±1.3
	72	65.7±6.6*	27.9±4.2*	6.4±0.9

SMCs were kept as controls or on fibrillar collagen with NG- or HG-MCM treatment. Cells were analyzed for DNA content by flow cytometry to show percentages in G_0/G_1, synthetic, or G_2/M phases of cell cycle. Data are mean ± SEM from three independent experiments.
*$P<0.05$ vs. control cells.

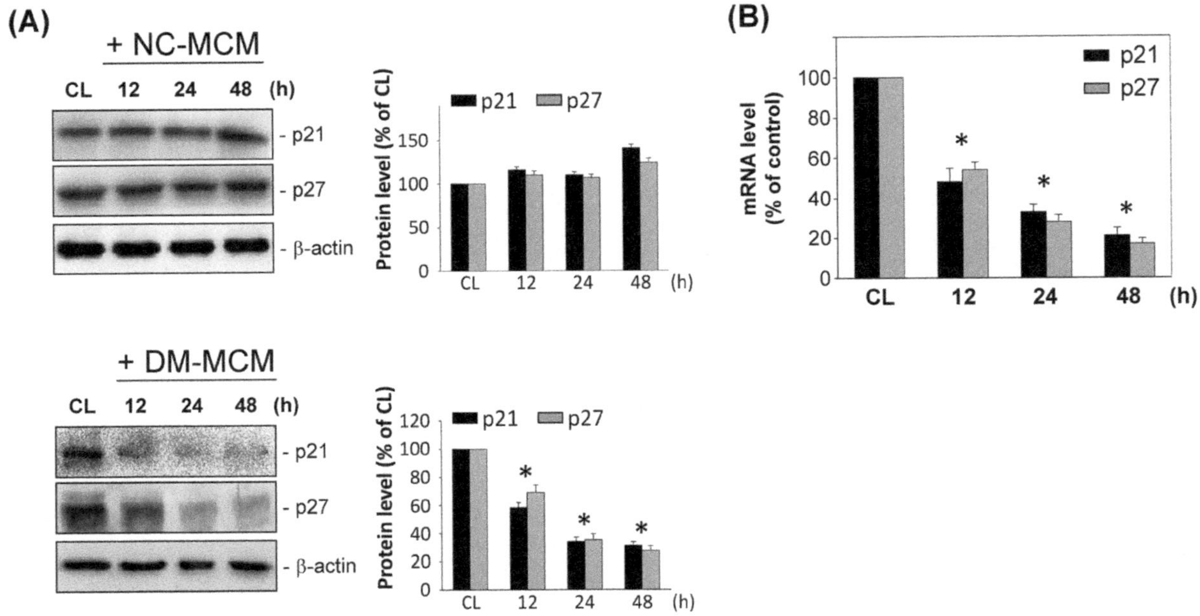

Figure 2. Effects of DM-MCM on p21^{Cip1} and p27^{Kip1} expression. Bar graphs represent folds of CL SMCs, mean ± SEM from 3 independent experiments. *$P<0.05$ versus CL SMCs. (A) SMCs were kept as CL or stimulated with NC-MCM or DM-MCM for the times indicated. Protein expressions were determined by Western blot analysis. Expression levels of p21^{Cip1} and p27^{Kip1} are presented as band densities (normalized to β-actin) relative to CL. (B) mRNA expressions were determined by real-time PCR analysis and normalized to 18S rRNA.

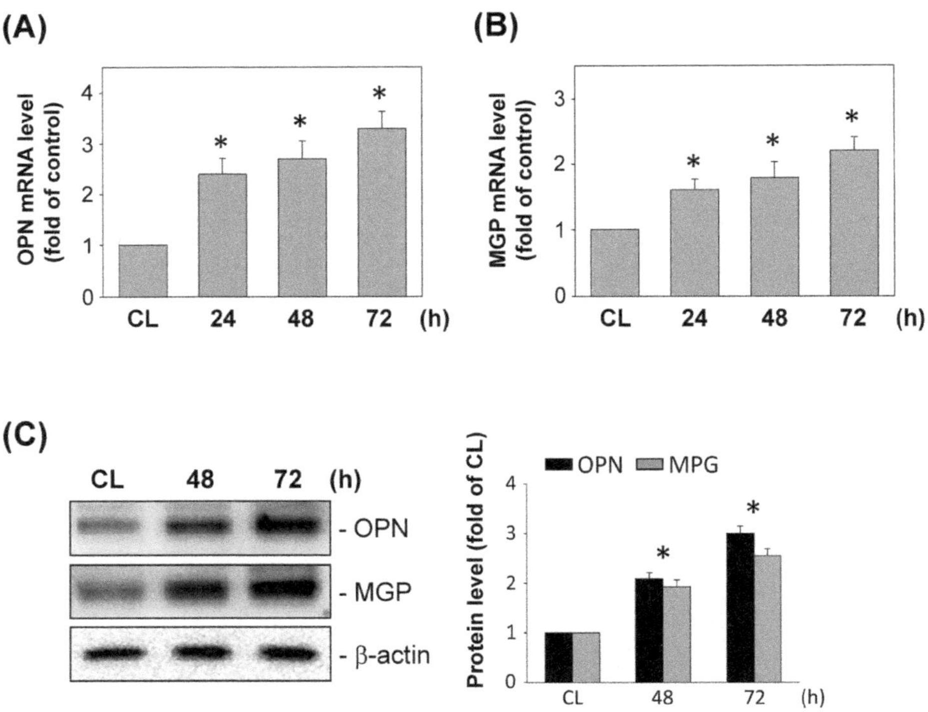

Figure 3. Effects of DM-MCM on synthetic differentiation marker expression in SMCs. Bar graphs represent folds of CL SMCs, mean ± SEM from 3 independent experiments. *$P<0.05$ versus CL SMCs. (A, B) DM-MCM induced mRNA expressions of osteopontin (OPN) and matrix gla protein (MGP) in SMCs. SMCs were kept as controls (CL) or stimulated with DM-MCM for the times indicated, and the mRNA expressions of OPN (A) and MGP (B) were determined using real-time PCR analysis and normalized to 18S rRNA. (C) SMCs were kept as CL or stimulated with DM-MCM for the times indicated. Protein expressions of OPN and MGP were determined by Western blot analysis. Expression levels of OPN and MGP are presented as band densities (normalized to β-actin) relative to CL.

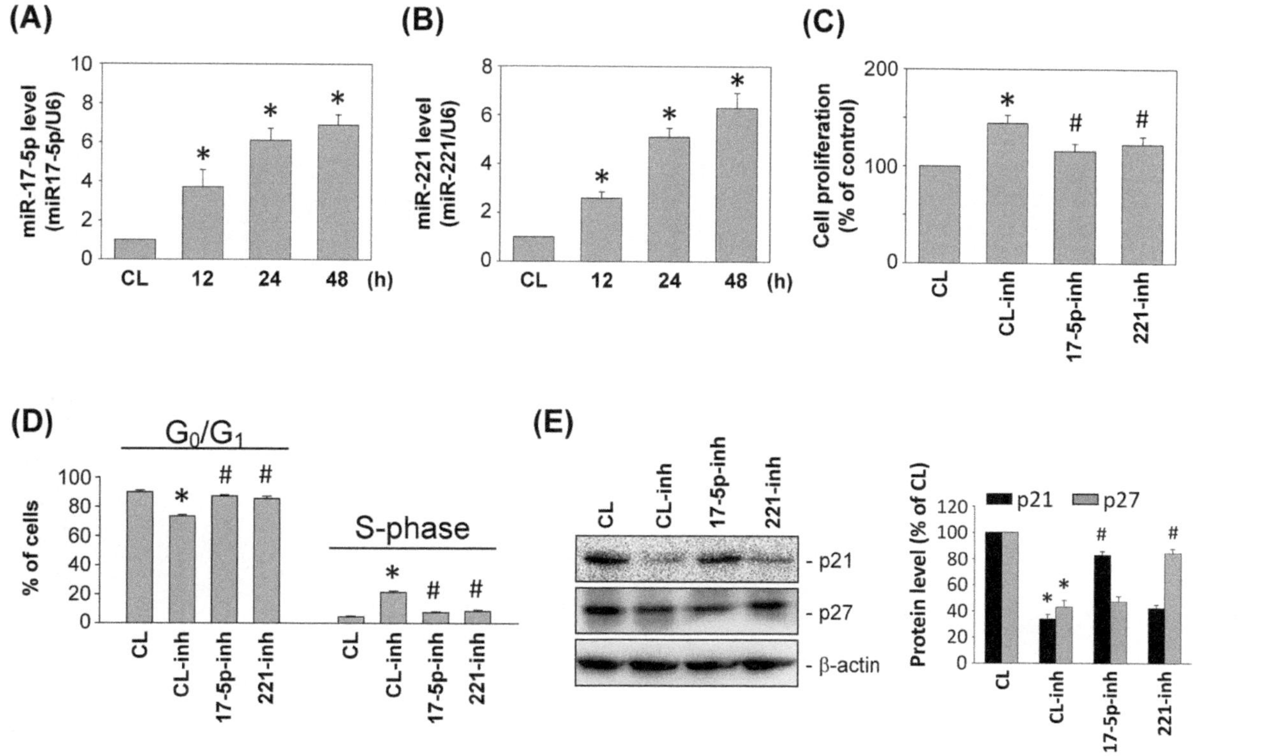

Figure 4. miR-17-5p and miR-221 are involved in the regulation of HASMC proliferation. (A, B) HASMCs were kept as controls (CL) or stimulated with DM-MCM for the times indicated. Relative miR-17-5p (A) and miR-221 (B) levels were determined through real-time PCR in HASMCs and normalized to U6 snRNA from 3 independent experiments. *$P<0.05$ versus CL SMCs. (C–E) SMCs were kept as CL or pretreated with miR-17-5p inhibitor (17-5p inh), miR-221 inhibitor (221 inh), or miRNA control inhibitor (CL inh) for 24 h, and then stimulated with DM-MCM for 24 h. The results are mean ± SEM from 3 independent experiments. *$P<0.05$ versus CL. $^{\#}P<0.05$ versus CL inhibitor (CL inh)-treated SMCs with DM-MCM stimulation. Cell proliferation was assayed by the MTT test (C). The distribution of the cell cycle was analyzed by flow cytometry (D). Protein expressions were determined by Western blot analysis. Expression levels of $p21^{Cip1}$ and $p27^{Kip1}$ are presented as band densities (normalized to β-actin) relative to CL (E).

and proliferation of the SMCs. Third, stimulation of SMCs with DM-MCM also induced expression of miR-221. Pretreatment of the cells with miR-221 inhibitor decreased the DM-MCM-induced down-regulation of $p27^{Kip1}$ and SMC proliferation.

It is believed that extravasation of macrophages in the arterial wall promotes formation of atherosclerotic lesions. It has also been suggested that diabetes-elicited SMC proliferation occurs secondary to the increased macrophage infiltration into the arterial wall [22]. The effects of HG levels on the proliferative capacity of arterial SMCs are controversial. While several studies have demonstrated that HG levels can stimulate SMC proliferation [14,25], others have found no stimulatory effect [26,27]; yet another study has shown an inhibitory effect of HG levels on SMC proliferation [28]. By culturing HASMCs on fibrillar collagen that promotes the maintenance of SMC in a non-proliferative phenotype [19], we have been able to elucidate the factors that signal and control the modulation of HASMC proliferation. The present findings in HASMC cultures showed that treatment with DM-MCM had a stimulatory effect on the proliferation of HASMCs. During cell cycle progression, $p21^{Cip1}$ and $p27^{Kip1}$ have been shown to mediate cell cycle arrest by inhibiting Cdk activities [29]. In this study, mRNA and protein expressions of $p21^{Cip1}$ and $p27^{Kip1}$ were down-regulated in DM-MCM-stimulated HASMCs. Our data also demonstrated that treatment of SMCs with DM-MCM increased the percentage of cells in the S-phase, while the percentage of cells in the G_0/G_1 phases decreased.

Several studies have revealed the effects of miRNAs on the modulation of functions of SMCs [20,30,31], but the mechanism underlying the DM-MCM-induced proliferation of SMC remains largely unclear. Different miRNAs have been implicated in the regulation of the mitogenic response in SMCs [31,32]. miR-17-5p is one of the critical miRNAs for cell proliferation [33], and its up-regulation has been shown to modulate $p21^{Cip1}$ expression in cancer cells [34]. miR-221 has also been implicated in the regulation of SMC proliferation and neointimal hyperplasia [35], and it has been reported to play an important role in the regulation of $p27^{Kip1}$ down-regulation in SMCs [36]. The present study demonstrated that DM-MCM stimulates SMC proliferation through at least two miRNAs, as indicated by the DM-MCM-induction of increases in miR-17-5p and miR-221, which may be involved in the mitogenic action. We further showed that the inhibition of miR-17-5p inhibited the DM-MCM-induced down-regulation of $p21^{Cip1}$ but had no effect on $p27^{Kip1}$, while the inhibition of miR-221 affected the down-regulation of $p27^{Kip1}$ but had no effect on $p21^{Cip1}$. It has previously been shown that the differential regulation of cell-cycle regulatory proteins occurs by different mechanisms [37]. On the basis of these studies and our findings, it is reasonable to propose that DM-MCM may stimulate SMC proliferation through the differential regulation of $p21^{Cip1}$ and $p27^{Kip1}$ expressions regulated by different miRNAs.

It has been reported that a variety of regulatory molecules with the ability to regulate SMC or stem cell function in a paracrine fashion are released from macrophages [18,38]. It is thus

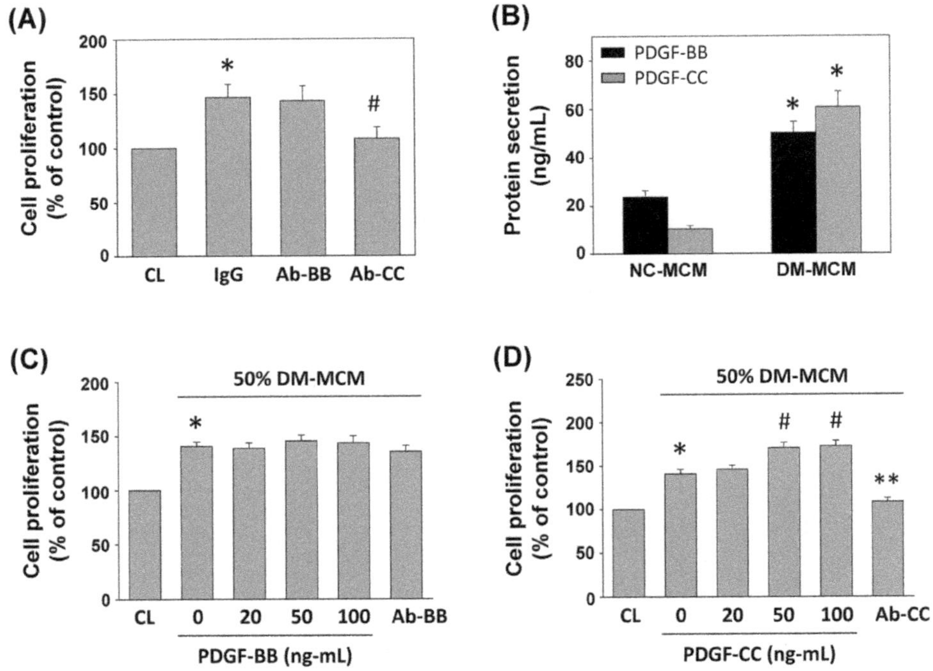

Figure 5. PDGF-CC is the major factor underlying DM-MCM-induced SMC proliferation. (A) Prior to culturing under control conditions (CL) or stimulation with DM-MCM, the DM-MCM and SMCs were pre-incubated with isotype-matched IgG or neutralizing antibodies against PDGF-BB (Ab-BB) or PDGF-CC (Ab-CC) individually for 2 h, and then stimulated with DM-MCM for 24 h. Cell proliferation was assayed by the MTT test from 3 independent experiments. $^*P<0.05$ versus CL. $^{\#}P<0.05$ versus IgG-treated SMCs under DM-MCM stimulation. (B) The expression levels of PDGF-BB and PDGF-CC in MCM were determined by sandwich ELISA from 3 independent experiments. $^*P<0.05$ versus NC-MCM. (C, D) SMCs were kept as CL or stimulated with 50% DM-MCM for 48 h. The proliferation of SMCs was obviously promoted by PDGF-CC at 50 and 100 ng/mL, and the promoting effect was inhibited by the neutralizing antibody against PDGF-CC (Ab-CC) (D). PDGF-BB has no significant effect on promoting SMC proliferation (C). Cell proliferation was assayed by the MTT assay from 3 independent experiments. $^*P<0.05$ versus CL. $^{\#}P<0.05$ versus 50% DM-MCM-treated SMCs. $^{**}P<0.05$ versus 50% DM-MCM-treated SMCs.

postulated that the elicited SMC growth in atherosclerotic lesions in diabetic conditions is due to the secretion of mediators from macrophages, and that macrophages may be directly affected by the diabetic environments. In our previous study, we observed that MIP-1α and 1β are significantly increased only in macrophages after differentiation under an HG environment [6]. In addition, it has been shown that levels of IGF-I in macrophage-rich regions in lesions of atherosclerosis from diabetic pigs were increased compared to non-diabetic controls [39]. Our present data demonstrated that MCM from DM patients significantly enhanced SMC proliferation, and this induction of cell proliferation by DM-MCM was inhibited following the neutralization of the PDGF-CC in DM-MCM. Hence, we suggest that the accumulation of macrophages in the arterial wall thereby increases the PDGF-CC level and contributes to SMC proliferation.

Taken together, our findings contribute new information about the mechanisms by which DM macrophages induce SMC proliferation. Treatment of SMCs with DM-MCM resulted in differential regulation of SMC–proliferation-mediated miRNAs. Activation of the miR-17-5p led to down-regulation of $p21^{Cip1}$, whereas activation of the miR-221 led to decreased expression of $p27^{Kip1}$. These findings provide insights into the mechanisms underlying the interplay between hyperglycemic macrophages with SMCs in modulating SMC function and gene expression, which may well be involved in the development of vascular complications in patients with diabetes.

Study limitations

There are some inherent limitations to this study. Although this study demonstrated that monocyte-derived macrophages differentiated from diabetic patients may affect SMC proliferation, the overall number of controls and patients was small. This association may therefore be correspondingly under- or over-estimated.

Author Contributions

Conceived and designed the experiments: TCC CNC. Performed the experiments: TCC MLS HCK SJC CKY. Analyzed the data: TCC MLS CNC. Contributed reagents/materials/analysis tools: MLS HCK. Wrote the paper: CNC.

References

1. Giacco F, Brownlee M (2010) Oxidative stress and diabetic complications. Circ Res 107: 1058–1070.
2. Rask-Madsen C, King GL (2013) Vascular complications of diabetes: mechanisms of injury and protective factors. Cell Metab 17: 20–33
3. Liang CP, Han S, Senokuchi T, Tall AR (2007) The macrophage at the crossroads of insulin resistance and atherosclerosis. Circ Res 100: 1546–1555.
4. Kanter JE, Johansson F, LeBoeuf RC, Bornfeldt KE (2007) Do glucose and lipids exert independent effects on atherosclerotic lesion initiation or progression to advanced plaques? Circ Res 100: 769–781.
5. Shanmugam N, Reddy MA, Guha M, Natarajan R (2003) High glucose-induced expression of proinflammatory cytokine and chemokine genes in monocytic cells. Diabetes 52: 1256–1264.

6. Chen TC, Chien SJ, Kuo HC, Huang WS, Sheen JM, et al. (2011) High glucose-treated macrophages augment E-selectin expression in endothelial cells. J Biol Chem 286: 25564–25573.
7. Lacolley P, Regnault V, Nicoletti A, Li Z, Michel JB (2012) The vascular smooth muscle cell in arterial pathology: a cell that can take on multiple roles. Cardiovasc Res 95: 194–204.
8. Owens GK, Kumar MS, Wamhoff BR (2004) Molecular regulation of vascular smooth muscle cell differentiation in development and disease. Physiol Rev 84: 767–801.
9. Tedgui A, Mallat Z (2006) Cytokines in atherosclerosis: pathogenic and regulatory pathways. Physiol Rev 86: 515–581.
10. Raines EW (2004) PDGF and cardiovascular disease. Cytokine Growth Factor Rev 15: 237–254.
11. Ahuja P, Sdek P, MacLellan WR (2007) Cardiac myocyte cell cycle control in development, disease, and regeneration. Physiol Rev 87: 521–544.
12. Findeisen HM, Gizard F, Zhao Y, Qing H, Heywood EB, et al. (2011) Epigenetic regulation of vascular smooth muscle cell proliferation and neointima formation by histone deacetylase inhibition. Arterioscler Thromb Vasc Biol 31: 851–860.
13. Bornfeldt KE, Tabas I (2011) Insulin resistance, hyperglycemia, and atherosclerosis. Cell Metab 14: 575–585.
14. Jeong IK, Oh da H, Park SJ, Kang JH, Kim S, et al. (2011) Inhibition of NF-κB prevents high glucose-induced proliferation and plasminogen activator inhibitor-1 expression in vascular smooth muscle cells. Exp Mol Med 43: 684–692.
15. Cai Q, Lanting L, Natarajan R (2004) Growth factors induce monocyte binding to vascular smooth muscle cells: implications for monocyte retention in atherosclerosis. Am J Physiol Cell Physiol 287: C707–714.
16. Proudfoot D, Fitzsimmons C, Torzewski J, Bowyer DE (1999) Inhibition of human arterial smooth muscle cell growth by human monocyte/macrophages: a co-culture study. Atherosclerosis 145: 157–165.
17. Schubert SY, Benarroch A, Ostvang J, Edelman ER (2008) Regulation of endothelial cell proliferation by primary monocytes. Arterioscler Thromb Vasc Biol 28: 97–104.
18. Chung JH, Jeon HJ, Hong SY, Lee da L, Lee KH, et al. (2012) Palmitate promotes the paracrine effects of macrophages on vascular smooth muscle cells: the role of bone morphogenetic proteins. PLoS One 7: e29100.
19. Chen CN, Li YS, Yeh YT, Lee PL, Usami S, et al. (2006) Synergistic roles of platelet-derived growth factor-BB and interleukin-1β in phenotypic modulation of human aortic smooth muscle cells. Proc Natl Acad Sci U S A 103: 2665–2670.
20. Robinson HC, Baker AH (2012) How do microRNAs affect vascular smooth muscle cell biology? Curr Opin Lipidol 23: 405–411.
21. Osório J (2010) Diabetes: Severe hypoglycemia associated with risk of vascular events and death. Nat Rev Cardiol 7: 666.
22. Askari B, Renard CB, Bornfeldt KE (2002) Regulation of smooth muscle cell accumulation in diabetes-accelerated atherosclerosis. Histol Histopathol 17: 1317–1328.
23. Matsumoto T, Kobayashi T, Kamata K (2010) Diabetic conditions act as matchmaker for monocytes and vascular smooth muscle cells. Am J Physiol Heart Circ Physiol 298: H731–733.
24. Febbraio M, Hajjar DP, Silverstein RL (2001) CD36: a class B scavenger receptor involved in angiogenesis, atherosclerosis, inflammation, and lipid metabolism. J Clin Invest 108: 785–791.
25. Yu S, Xi Z, Hai-Yan C, Ya-Li C, Shao-Hu X, et al. (2012) Interferon regulatory factor-1 as a positive regulator for high glucose-induced proliferation of vascular smooth muscle cells. J Cell Biochem 113: 2671–2678.
26. Suzuki LA, Poot M, Gerrity RG, Bornfeldt KE (2001) Diabetes accelerates smooth muscle accumulation in lesions of atherosclerosis: lack of direct growth-promoting effects of high glucose levels. Diabetes 50: 851–860.;
27. Indolfi C, Torella D, Cavuto L, Davalli AM, Coppola C, et al. (2001) Effects of balloon injury on neointimal hyperplasia in streptozotocin-induced diabetes and in hyperinsulinemic nondiabetic pancreatic islet-transplanted rats. Circulation 103: 2980–2986.
28. Peiró C, Lafuente N, Matesanz N, Cercas E, Llergo JL, et al. (2001) High glucose induces cell death of cultured human aortic smooth muscle cells through the formation of hydrogen peroxide. Br J Pharmacol 133: 967–974.
29. Tanner FC, Boehm M, Akyürek LM, San H, Yang ZY, et al. (2000) Differential effects of the cyclin-dependent kinase inhibitors $p27^{Kip1}$, $p21^{Cip1}$, and $p16^{Ink4}$ on vascular smooth muscle cell proliferation. Circulation 101: 2022–2025
30. Li P, Zhu N, Yi B, Wang N, Chen M, et al. (2013) MicroRNA-663 Regulates Human Vascular Smooth Muscle Cell Phenotypic Switch and Vascular Neointimal Formation. Circ Res 113: 1117–1127.
31. Sun Y, Chen D, Cao L, Zhang R, Zhou J, et al. (2013) MiR-490-3p modulates the proliferation of vascular smooth muscle cells induced by ox-LDL through targeting PAPP-α. Cardiovasc Res 100: 272–279.
32. Liu X, Cheng Y, Chen X, Yang J, Xu L, et al. (2011) MicroRNA-31 regulated by the extracellular regulated kinase is involved in vascular smooth muscle cell growth via large tumor suppressor homolog 2. J Biol Chem 286: 42371–42380.
33. Cloonan N, Brown MK, Steptoe AL, Wani S, Chan WL, et al. (2008) The miR-17-5p microRNA is a key regulator of the G1/S phase cell cycle transition. Genome Biol 9: R127.
34. Ballarino M, Jobert L, Dembélé D, de la Grange P, Auboeuf D, et al. (2013) TAF15 is important for cellular proliferation and regulates the expression of a subset of cell cycle genes through miRNAs. Oncogene 32: 4646–4655.
35. Liu X, Cheng Y, Zhang S, Lin Y, Yang J, et al. (2009) A necessary role of miR-221 and miR-222 in vascular smooth muscle cell proliferation and neointimal hyperplasia. Circ Res 104: 476–487.
36. Davis BN, Hilyard AC, Nguyen PH, Lagna G, Hata A (2009) Induction of microRNA-221 by platelet-derived growth factor signaling is critical for modulation of vascular smooth muscle phenotype. J Biol Chem 284: 3728–3738.
37. Chiang JK, Sung ML, Yu HR, Chang HI, Kuo HC, et al. (2011) Homocysteine induces smooth muscle cell proliferation through differential regulation of cyclins A and D1 expression. J Cell Physiol 226: 1017–1026.
38. Lee MJ, Kim MY, Heo SC, Kwon YW, Kim YM, et al. (2012) Macrophages regulate smooth muscle differentiation of mesenchymal stem cells via a prostaglandin $F_{2\alpha}$-mediated paracrine mechanism. Arterioscler Thromb Vasc Biol 32: 2733–2740.
39. Askari B, Carroll MA, Capparelli M, Kramer F, Gerrity RG, et al. (2002) Oleate and linoleate enhance the growth-promoting effects of insulin-like growth factor-I through a phospholipase D-dependent pathway in arterial smooth muscle cells. J Biol Chem 277: 36338–36344.

24

Possible Contribution of Taurine to Distorted Glucagon Secretion in Intra-Islet Insulin Deficiency: A Metabolome Analysis Using a Novel α-Cell Model of Insulin-Deficient Diabetes

Megumi Bessho[1], Yuko Murase-Mishiba[1]*, Akihisa Imagawa[1,2], Jungo Terasaki[1], Toshiaki Hanafusa[1]

1 Department of Internal Medicine (I), Osaka Medical College, Osaka, Japan, **2** Department of Metabolic Medicine, Graduate School of Medicine, Osaka University, Osaka, Japan

Abstract

Glycemic instability is a serious problem in patients with insulin-deficient diabetes, and it may be due in part to abnormal endogenous glucagon secretion. However, the intracellular metabolic mechanism(s) involved in the aberrant glucagon response under the condition of insulin deficiency has not yet been elucidated. To investigate the metabolic traits that underlie the distortion of glucagon secretion under insulin deficient conditions, we generated an αTC1-6 cell line with stable knockdown of the insulin receptor (IRKD), i.e., an *in vitro* α-cell model for insulin-deficient diabetes, which exhibits an abnormal glucagon response to glucose. A comprehensive metabolomic analysis of the IRKD αTC1-6 cells (IRKD cells) revealed some candidate metabolites whose levels differed markedly compared to those in control αTC1-6 cells, but also which could affect the glucagon release in IRKD cells. Of these candidates, taurine was remarkably increased in the IRKD cells and was identified as a stimulator of glucagon in αTC1-6 cells. Taurine also paradoxically exaggerated the glucagon secretion at a high glucose concentration in IRKD cells and islets with IRKD. These results indicate that the metabolic alterations induced by IRKD in α-cells, especially the increase of taurine, may lead to the distorted glucagon response in IRKD cells, suggesting the importance of taurine in the paradoxical glucagon response and the resultant glucose instability in insulin-deficient diabetes.

Editor: Amar Abderrahmani, University of Lille Nord de France, France

Funding: This work was supported in part by KAKENHI from Japan Society for the Promotion of Science (JSPS) to YMM (25461367). No additional funding was received for this study. The funders had no role in study design, data collection and analysis, decision to publish, or preparation of the manuscript.

Competing Interests: The authors have declared that no competing interests exist.

* Email: in1254@poh.osaka-med.ac.jp

Introduction

Glycemic instability is a crucial clinical problem in patients with insulin-deficient (type 1 and advanced type 2) diabetes. The wide fluctuations of glucose are due not only to the insulin deficiency, which has been considered to be one of the leading causes of glycemic volatility [1,2], but also may be at least partly due to abnormal glucagon secretion [3]; namely, a deficient glucagon response to hypoglycemia [4] and an inappropriately high glucagon response to hyperglycemia [5]. However, the effects of distorted glucagon secretion on the glycemic excursion have been largely overlooked. We recently reported that arginine-stimulated glucagon secretion is positively associated with the degree of glucose fluctuation in type 1 diabetic patients whose endogenous insulin was completely depleted [6]. Therefore, the aberrant increase in glucagon might contribute to glycemic instability, independent of deficient endogenous insulin.

However, little is known about the pathogenesis of the aberrant glucagon response in the pancreatic α-cells in insulin-deficient type 1 diabetic patients, which has so far been attributed to altered neuronal control [7], impairment of intrinsic glucose sensing by the α-cells themselves [8], and/or the local paracrine defects. Substances released from the neighboring endocrine cells, such as insulin, islet amyloid polypeptide, Zn^{2+}, ATP and GABA from β-cells, and somatostatin from δ-cells, have been reported to regulate glucagon secretion [9–12]. Of all these molecules, the actions of insulin or its signaling pathway may be key modulators for α-cell function, because extensive physiological and molecular biological approaches have demonstrated its importance among the mechanisms that regulate glucagon secretion in an intra-islet manner [13]. Indeed, hyperglucagonemia is suggested to develop in parallel with hypoinsulinemia [14]. The suppression of insulin signaling by insulin receptor (IR) silencing through a siRNA approach in α-cells has been reported to disturb the glucagon secretion in response to glucose [15]. In addition, an α-cell-specific insulin receptor knockout mouse has been demonstrated to exhibit an exaggerated glucagon response under both normo- and hypoglycemic conditions [16]. These studies strongly suggested that a lack of paracrine control by insulin on α-cells could account for the dysregulated glucagon secretion in insulin-deficient type 1 diabetes, although the intracellular metabolic mechanism(s) involved have not been elucidated.

To explore the cellular metabolic changes in α-cells under pathophysiological conditions of insulin-deficient diabetes, we generated a clonal mouse αTC1-6 cell line with a stably knocked-down IR, as a model of α cells in insulin deficiency, and performed a comprehensive *in vitro* intracellular metabolomic analysis. We herein provide evidence that metabolic alterations in the α-cell model of insulinopenic diabetes may lead to a paradoxical glucagon response, which would thereby lead to glycemic instability in insulin-deficient type 1 diabetes.

Materials and Methods

Cell culture

αTC1-6 cells (kindly provided as a gift by Dr. Y. Moriyama, Okayama University, Japan) [17–19], a mouse α-cell line, were used in the present study. The αTC1-6 cells were originally isolated from αTCl cells, an α-cell-derived multiclonal cell line established using a transgene strategy [17]. Although the original αTCl cells were composed of heterologous cell populations that seemed to contain α-cells and their progenitors, the αTCl-6 clone totally lacked insulin mRNA, and thus was similar to the differentiated α-cells *in vivo* [17]. The cells were maintained in DMEM (Invitrogen Inc., Carlsbad, CA) containing 25 mM glucose supplemented with 10% FCS (Sigma-Aldrich, St. Louis, MO), 100 units/ml penicillin, 100 μg/ml streptomycin, 0.25 mg/l fungizone (Invitrogen) and 55 μg/ml sodium pyruvate at 37°C in a humidified atmosphere (5% CO_2, 95% air).

Islet preparation and culture

Islets from male ICR mice (aged 7–8 weeks) were obtained from Cosmo Bio Co., Tokyo, Japan. Briefly, islets were isolated by the collagenase digestion of the pancreas as described previously [20], with some modifications. The animals were anesthetized by the intraperitoneal injection of pentobarbital sodium at 80 mg/kg. The abdomen was opened, and collagenase (3 mg/ml) dissolved in 6 ml of 5 mM Ca^{2+}-containing Krebs-Ringer bicarbonate buffer solution was injected into the common bile duct at the distal end after ligation of the duct proximal to the pancreas. The pancreas was dissected out and incubated at 37°C for 17 min. Isolated islets were handpicked and cultured in RPMI-1640 media (11 mM glucose) at 37°C and 5% CO_2. This study was conducted under the approval of the institutional animal care and use committee of Osaka Medical College.

Lentiviral transduction to generate shRNA-mediated stable knockdown cell lines and primary islets

MISSION lentiviral transduction particles expressing short hairpin RNA (shRNA) targeting the IR (TRCN0000023574, TRCN0000023575, TRCN0000023576, TRCN0000023577, TRCN0000023578) or a scrambled non-target negative control (SHC002V) were purchased from Sigma-Aldrich. Stably transduced cell lines were generated according to the manufacturer's instructions. Briefly, cells were seeded on 96-well plates. On the following day, the cells were infected with 50 MOI (multiplicity of infection) of the lentivirus. After 24 h, the medium was changed. The selection of stable clones started 24 h later with the addition of 1 μg/ml of puromycin. Surviving clones were screened for mRNA knockdown. Of the five IR-targeted lentiviral clones tested, the maximal knockdown was achieved with clone TRCN0000023575 (CCGGCCCTGAAGGATGGAGTCTTT-ACTCGAGTAAAGACTCCATCCTTCAGGGTTTTT). This clone was therefore selected and used for further studies. We performed functional assays 72–96 h post-transduction to determine the optimal transduction efficiency using the MISSION TurboGFP Control Transduction Particles (SIGMA) at various MOI (1, 5, 10 and 50) before assaying them with shRNA constructs. As a result, a MOI of 50 was found to be the best for transduction, with transfection efficiencies that reached >80%. We did not observe any non-specific cell death at a MOI of 50.

For islets, lentivirus infection was carried out the day after isolation. Briefly, isolated islets were plated in 96-well plates, 10–20 islets/well, with 120 μl of RPMI islet culture medium containing 11 mM glucose for 1–2 h at 37°C. The islets were infected with 20 MOI of the lentivirus expressing shRNA targeting IR (TRCN0000023575) or the scrambled sequence control shRNA (SHC002V), then were incubated overnight at 37°C. On the following day, the islets were transferred to new plates, washed twice and further cultured at 37°C, with the medium changed on a daily basis. Functional assays were performed 72 h post-transduction. The transduction and transfection efficiencies, as determined by GFP fluorescence, reached >80% under these conditions.

Western blot analysis

For extraction of the total protein, cell samples were homogenized in ice-cold lysis buffer (Cell Signaling Technology, Beverly, MA). Lysates were subjected to SDS-PAGE and blotted using antibodies against insulin receptor-β (Santa Cruz Biotechnology, Santa Cruz, CA), β-actin, Akt, phospho-Akt (Ser473), mammalian target of rapamycin (mTOR), phospho-mTOR (Ser2448), AMP-activated protein kinase (AMPK) α, phospho-AMPKα (Thr172), glycogen synthase kinase-3β (GSK-3β), phosho-GSK-3β (Ser9), extracellular signal-related kinase 1/2 (Erk1/2) or phospho-Erk1/2 (Thr202/Tyr204) (Cell signaling Technology). The densitometric analysis was performed using the Image J software program.

Insulin stimulation

Insulin receptor knock down (IRKD) and scrambled non-target negative control (control) αTC1-6 cells were plated in 10 cm culture plates at 80% confluency, and were serum starved for 24 h in DMEM. Subsequently, the cells were stimulated with 100 nM insulin for 15 min at 37°C in a humidified atmosphere (5% CO_2, 95% air). After the reaction was stopped by washing the cells twice with ice-cold PBS, we added 500 μl ice-cold lysis buffer (Cell Signaling Technology) and collected samples from each dish in microtubes. Cell lysates were prepared as described above for the Western blot analysis.

Cell viability, cytotoxicity and apoptosis assays

The cell viability (GF-AFC cleavage), cytotoxicity (bis-AAF-R110 cleavage) and apoptosis (caspase 3/7 activity) were measured simultaneously via the Apotox-Glo Triplex assay (Promega, Madison, WI). IRKD cells and control cells were plated (10^4 cells/100 μl/well) in 96 well plates in complete growth media. Samples were assayed 0, 1, 2, 4 and 6 days after plating, as indicated, and were processed according to the manufacturer's instructions. The GF-AFC and bis-AAF-R110 substrates were added, and fluorescence was measured by the GloMax-Multi Detection System (Promega) (excitation 400 nm/emission 485 nm and 505 nm/520 nm, respectively) after a 30 min incubation at 37°C. Luminescence was detected after a 30 min incubation with the Caspase-Glo 3/7 Substrate (Promega). After the background for each assay was subtracted, the data were represented as the fold-change from baseline (day 0).

Cell proliferation assay

Cell proliferation was measured by the BrdU (5-bromo-2′-deoxyuridine) incorporation assay using a CycLex Cellular BrdU ELISA Kit (CycLex, Nagano, Japan) according to the manufacturer's instructions. Briefly, IRKD and control cells (10^4 cells/100 μl/well) were cultured in 96-well plates in complete growth media. Samples were assayed 1, 2, 3 and 4 days after plating, as indicated. BrdU, at a concentration of 10 μM, was added to the medium and incubated for another two hours. Denatured cells were exposed to an anti-BrdU monoclonal antibody, followed by horseradish peroxidase-conjugated goat anti-mouse IgG. The reaction product was quantified by measuring the absorbance using a scanning multi-well spectrophotometer (ELISA reader) at 450 nm with a reference wavelength of 540 nm.

Glucagon secretion assay

Both IRKD αTC1-6 cells (IRKD cells) and control αTC1-6 cells were plated in 24-well culture plates at 80% confluency. Forty-eight hours later, the cells were preincubated in Krebs-Ringer bicarbonate buffer (KRB) containing 115 mM NaCl, 5 mM KCl, 24 mM $NaHCO_3$, 2.5 mM $CaCl_2$, 1 mM $MgCl_2$, 10 mM HEPES and 2% bovine serum albumin with 5.6 mM glucose for 1 h at 37°C. Subsequently, the cells were treated with 1000 μl of KRB buffer containing either 1.5 mM, 5.6 mM or 30 mM glucose for 2 h at 37°C. Aliquots (500 μl) from each treatment were taken at the end of the 2-h incubation to assess the glucagon secretion by an ELISA (YK090 Glucagon EIA; Yanaihara Institute Inc., Shizuoka, Japan). Following the secretion assay, the cellular glucagon content was assessed by acid ethanol extraction (0.15 M HCl in 75% ethanol in H_2O). The secretion data and content data from the assays were normalized to the total protein content measured by the bicinchoninic acid (BCA) protein assay (Pierce BCA Protein Assay Kit; Thermo scientific, Rockford, IL). For the taurine and/or insulin supplementation experiments, the cells were prepared as described above, and then were subsequently supplemented with taurine and/or insulin for 2 h. The taurine treatment for the control αTC1-6 cells was up to100 mM based on the fact that the plasma taurine concentrations in most vertebrate species are usually lower than 1 mM, while the intracellular taurine concentration ranges from 10 to 50 mM [21], and the concentration of added taurine was in the tens of millimolar range in some previous *in vitro* experiments [22].

Batches of 10–20 isolated islets with IRKD or transfected with the control were preincubated for 60 min at 37°C in a humidified atmosphere containing 5% CO_2 in 500 μl KRB buffer supplemented with 5.6 mM glucose. The islets were then incubated for 2 h at 37°C with 500 μl of KRB buffer containing 1.5 mM, 5.6 mM or 30 mM glucose. Finally, the glucagon secretion and intracellular contents were assessed by the above-mentioned ELISA, and these values were normalized to the islet numbers.

Metabolome analysis

IRKD and control αTC1-6 cells were plated in 10 cm culture plates at 80% confluency. Forty-eight hours later, the cells were preincubated in KRB buffer with 5.6 mM glucose for 1 h at 37°C. Subsequently, the cells were treated with KRB buffer containing 1.5 mM, 5.6 mM or 30 mM glucose for 2 h at 37°C. The culture medium was aspirated from the dish, and the cells were washed twice with a 5% mannitol solution (10 ml first and then 2 ml). The cells were then treated with 800 μl of methanol and left to rest for 30 sec in order to inactivate enzymes. Next, the cell extract was treated with 550 μl of Milli-Q water containing 10 μM internal standards (H3304-1002, Human Metabolome Technologies, Inc., Tsuruoka, Japan) and left to rest for another 30 sec. The extract was obtained and centrifuged at 2,300×g and 4°C for 5 min, and then 800 μl of the upper aqueous layer was centrifugally filtered through a Millipore 5-kDa cutoff filter at 9,100×g and 4°C for 120 min to remove proteins. The filtrate was centrifugally concentrated and re-suspended in 50 μl of Milli-Q water for a CE-MS analysis. Metabolome measurements were carried out by Human Metabolome Technology Inc., Tsuruoka, Japan.

The CE-TOF-MS was carried out using an Agilent CE Capillary Electrophoresis System equipped with an Agilent 6210 time-of-flight mass spectrometer, an Agilent 1100 isocratic HPLC pump, an Agilent G1603A CE-MS adapter kit and an Agilent G1607A CE-ESI-MS sprayer kit (Agilent Technologies, Waldbronn, Germany). The systems were controlled by the Agilent G2201AA ChemStation software program, version B.03.01 for CE (Agilent Technologies, Waldbronn, Germany). The metabolites were analyzed by using a fused silica capillary (50 μm i.d.×80 cm total length), with commercial electrophoresis buffer (Solution ID: H3301-1001 for the cation analysis and H3302-1021 for the anion analysis, Human Metabolome Technologies) as the electrolyte. The sample was injected at a pressure of 50 mbar for 10 sec (approximately 10 nl) in the cation analysis and 25 sec (approximately 25 nl) in the anion analysis. The applied voltage was set at 27 kV. ESI-MS proceeded in the positive ion mode, and the capillary was set at 4,000 V. The spectrometer was scanned from a mass/electric charge ratio (*m/z*) of 50 to 1,000. The other conditions used were the same as were described previously [23–25].

The raw data obtained by CE-TOF-MS were processed using the MasterHands ver. 2.13.0.8.h software program (developed at Keio University, Japans). Signal peaks corresponding to isotopomers, adduct ions and other product ions of known metabolites were excluded, all signal peaks potentially corresponding to authentic compounds were extracted and then their migration times (MT) were normalized against those of the internal standards. Thereafter, peaks were aligned according to the *m/z* and normalized MT values. Finally, the peak areas were normalized to those of the internal standards, methionine sulfone and D-Camphor-10-sulfonic acid, for cations and anions, respectively. The resultant relative area values were further normalized by the cell count. All experiments were conducted independently three times.

Quantitative real-time PCR

Total RNA isolation and cDNA synthesis were performed using the TaqMan Gene Expression Cell-to-CT Kit (Applied Biosystems, Foster City, CA) according to the manufacturer's protocol. The resulting pre-amplified cDNA preparations were analyzed by real-time PCR in a Step One Plus Real-time PCR System (Applied Biosystems) using the TaqMan Gene Expression Assay in combination with TaqMan Gene Expression Master Mix containing ROX (Applied Biosystems), according to the manufacturer's instructions. All of the probes were purchased from Applied Biosystems. The data were normalized to the β-actin level.

Taurine and amino acid uptake assay

The taurine and amino acid uptake were measured by a previously described method, with the following modifications [26]: In brief, confluent cells in 24-well plates were preincubated in KRB buffer with 5.6 mM glucose for 2 h at 37°C. The cells were supplemented and incubated with tritiated taurine or amino acids (taurine, L-arginine, L-glutamine or L-leucine; 0.44 μCi/well) (American Radiolabeled Chemicals, Inc., St. Louis, MO), together

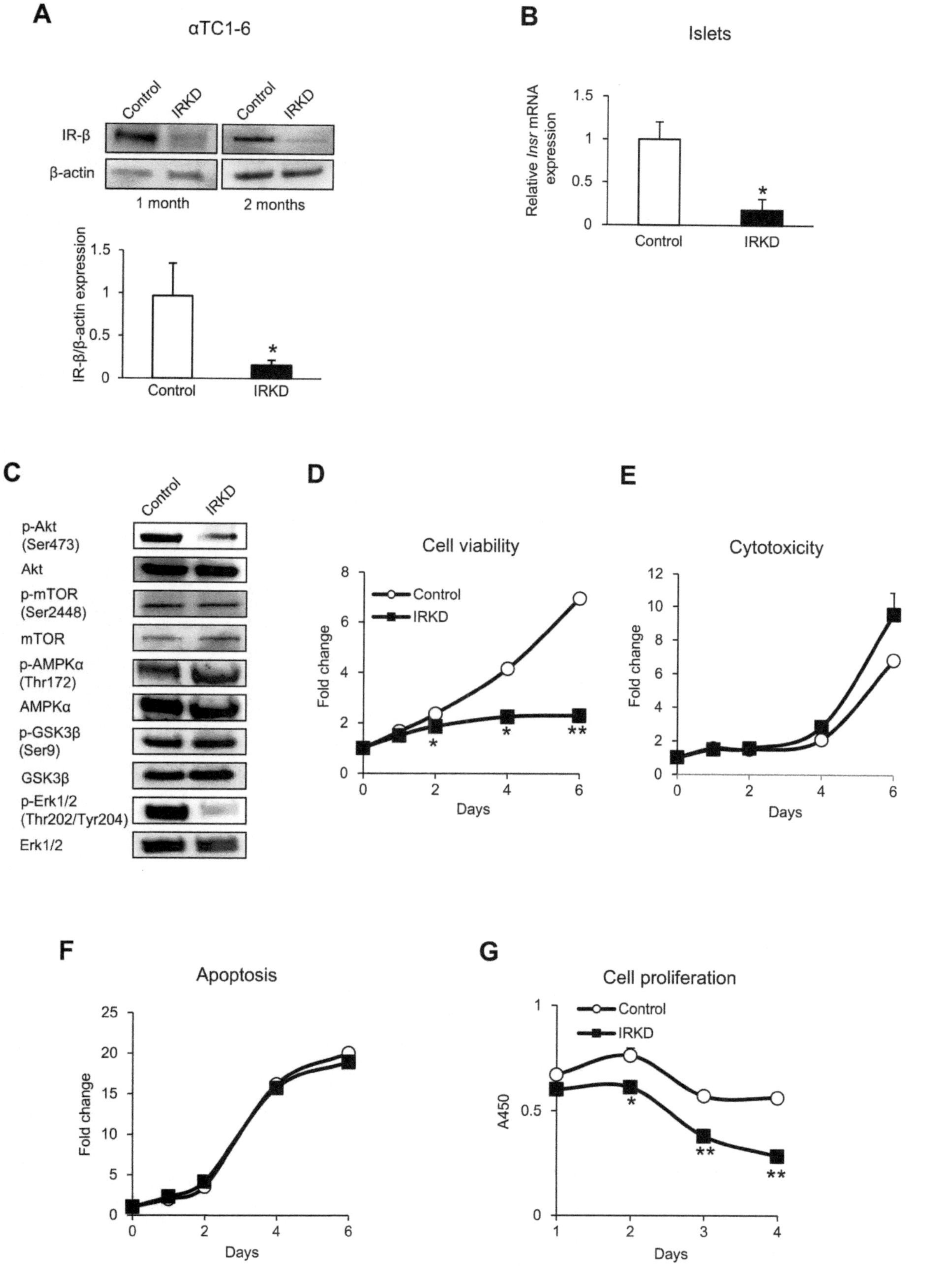

Figure 1. Results of an analysis of the effect of stable IR knockdown in αTC1-6 cells and IR knockdown in mouse islets. (**A**) An immunoblot analysis of the insulin receptor (IR) expression in αTC1-6 cells after the transduction with lentiviruses expressing control shRNA (control) and shRNA-IR (IRKD). αTC1-6 cells were infected with lentiviruses (see details in the "Materials and Methods"), and were cultured in medium containing 1 μg/ml puromycin for one month to generate homogenous stable cell lines. Cells were then analyzed by a Western blot analysis using

specific polyclonal antibodies against the β-subunit of the IR (IR-β). Stable αTC1-6 cells maintained in culture for two months were also examined. Blots are shown on the *top*, and the relative amount of IRβ protein normalized to the β-actin level is shown on the *bottom* ($n = 3$. The bars represent the means± SEM; *$P<0.05$, control vs. IRKD). (**B**) The relative expression of the *Insr* gene in isolated mouse islets infected with lentiviruses expressing control and IRKD ($n = 6$. The bars represent the means± SEM; *$P<0.05$, control vs. IRKD). (**C**) The results of the immunoblot analysis of the activation of insulin signal transduction pathways in control and IRKD αTC1-6 cells. Cells were serum-starved for 24 h in DMEM and were subsequently stimulated with 100 nM of insulin for 15 min. Samples were analyzed by a Western blot analysis using specific antibodies against phospho- and non-phospho-proteins, as indicated. (**D–F**) The time course of the changes in cell viability, cytotoxicity and apoptosis assessed using the ApoTox-Glo Triplex Assay (Promega) in the control and IRKD cells. $n = 3$ in each group. The data are expressed as the means ± SEM; *$P<0.05$, **$P<0.01$, control vs. IRKD. (**G**) The time course of BrdU incorporation in the control and IRKD cells. $n = 3$ in each group. The data are expressed as the means ± SEM; *$P<0.05$, **$P<0.01$, control vs. IRKD.

with 1 mM unlabelled taurine or amino acids, for 1, 10, 30, 60, 90 or 120 min. The incubation was stopped by removing the incubation medium and washing the cells three times with ice-cold PBS. The cells were then lysed with 300 μl of 0.1% Triton X-100. The radioactivity in the whole-cell lysates was counted with a Packard Tri-Carb 2200 CA liquid scintillation analyzer.

Statistical analysis

All data are the means ± SEM. Student's *t*-test or Welch's *t*- test was performed for comparisons of two groups, as appropriate. Comparisons of more than two groups were made using a one-way ANOVA. Differences were considered to be statistically significant at $P<0.05$.

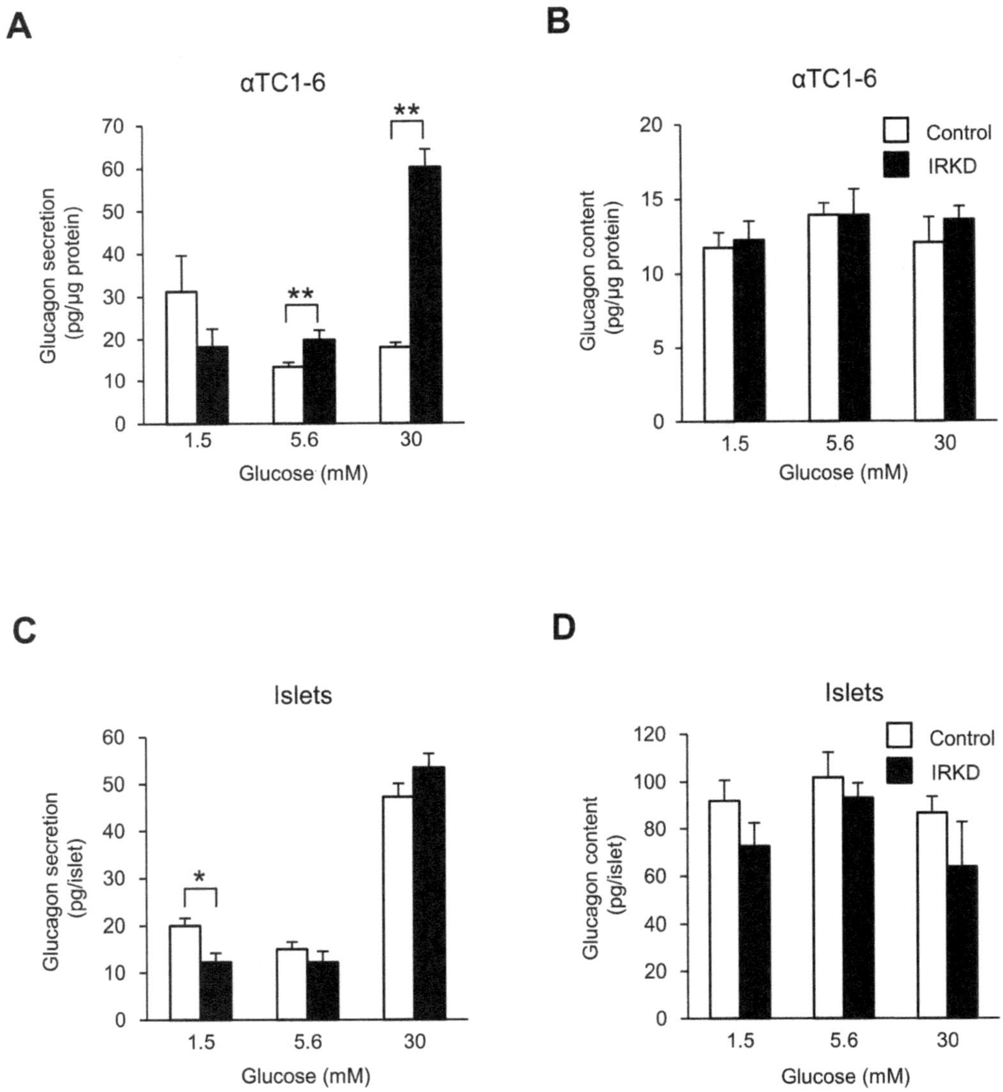

Figure 2. Glucose-stimulated glucagon secretion and cellular content of glucagon in αTC1-6 cells and islets after the expression of control shRNA and shRNA-IRKD. (**A, C**) Glucagon secretion in αTC1-6 cells (**A**) or islets (**C**) was assessed following a 2 h incubation in KRB with 1.5, 5.6 or 30 mM glucose after preincubation for 1 h with 5.6 mM glucose. $n = 6$ (**A**) or 3 (**C**) in each group. (**B, D**) The total protein content and total glucagon content in αTC1-6 cells (**B**) or islets (**D**). $n = 6$ (**B**) or 3 (**D**) in each group. The bars represent the means ± SEM; *$P<0.05$, **$P<0.01$, control vs. IRKD.

A

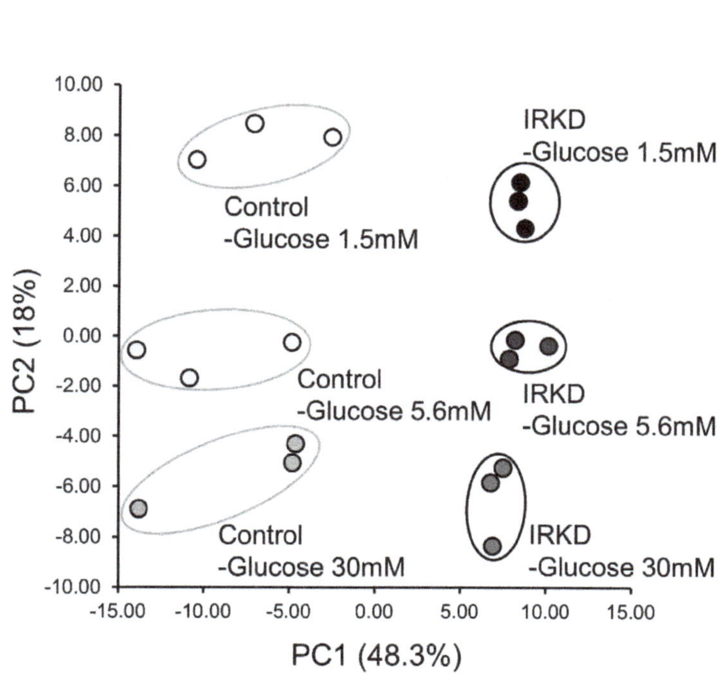

B

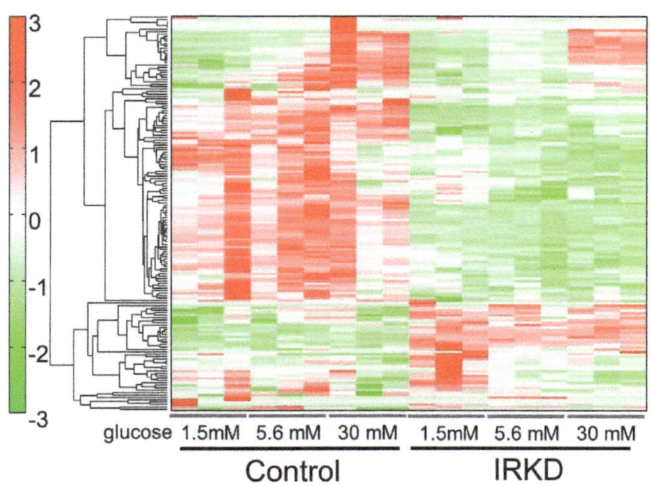

Figure 3. Comparison of the metabolic profile of control and IRKD αTC1-6 cells, as determined by CE-TOFMS. A principal component analysis (PCA) score plot (**A**) and heat map (**B**) from the metabolic data of the control and IRKD αTC1-6 cells treated with three different concentrations of glucose (1.5, 5.6 or 30 mM) ($n = 3$ in each group).

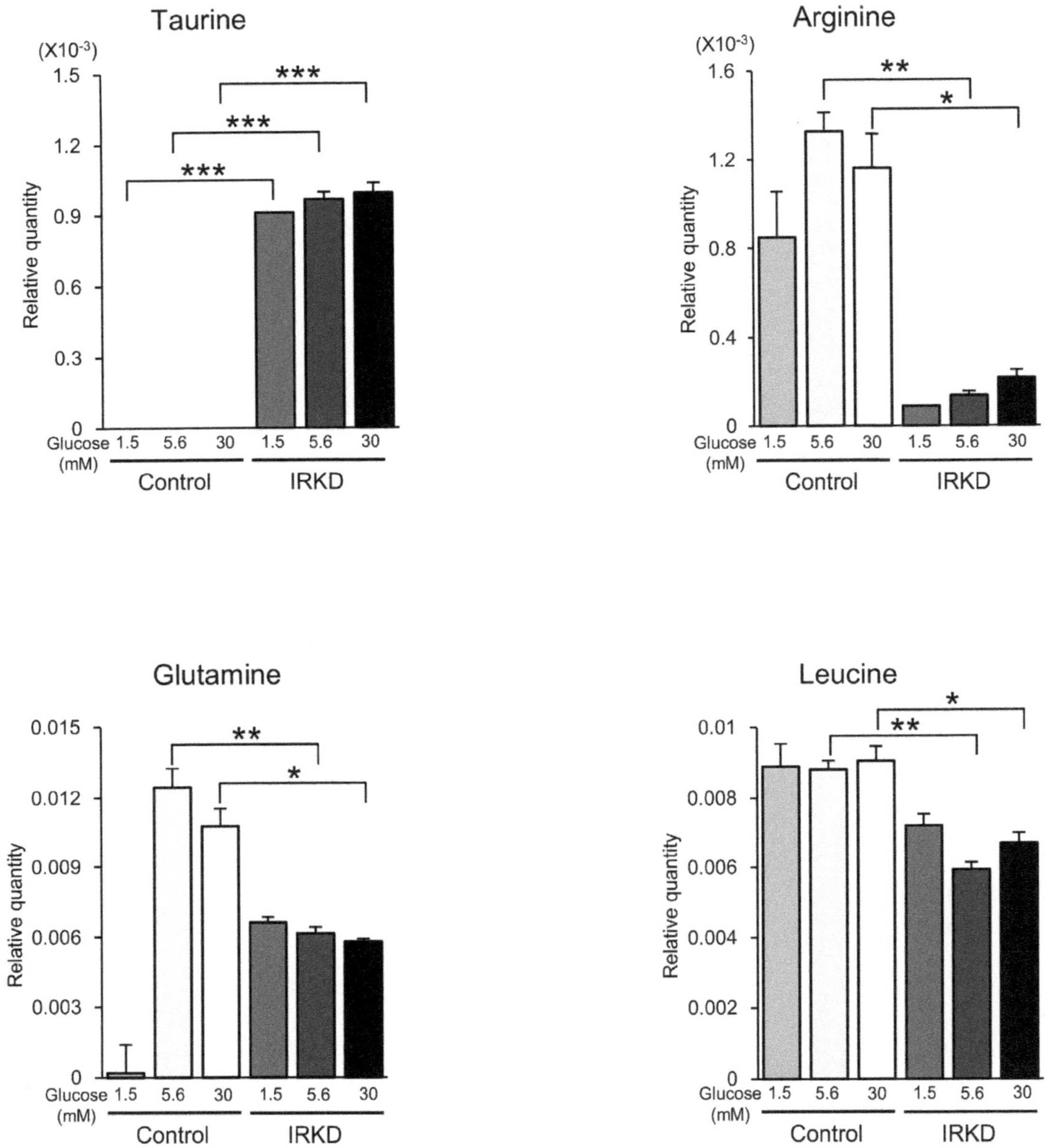

Figure 4. Metabolic quantities of taurine, arginine, glutamine and leucine between control and IRKD αTC1-6 cells. A comparison was made between control and IRKD αTC1-6 cells at three different concentrations of glucose (1.5, 5.6, 30 mM). $n = 3$ in each group. The bars represent the means ± SEM; *$P<0.05$, **$P<0.01$, control vs. IRKD.

Results

Generation of stable IR knockdown αTC1-6 cells and IR knockdown in mouse islets

To achieve stable expression of shRNA in cultured cell lines, a lentiviral vector was used to transduce the αTC1-6 cells. The effectiveness of knockdown in the stable cell lines was confirmed by a Western blot analysis using cells at six and 12 passages post-infection (one month and two months), and a maximum of 80% IR-knockdown at the protein level was observed in the cells at both of these passages (Fig. 1A). Similarly, isolated islets infected with a shRNA lentivirus targeting the IR showed an 82.1% decrease in *Insr* expression (Fig. 1B).

To evaluate the effect of the IR knockdown on insulin signal transduction, we examined the activation of pathways downstream of insulin signaling. The degree of insulin-induced phosphorylation of Akt was decreased in IRKD cells compared to control αTC1-6 cells, whereas the levels of mTOR, GSK3β and AMPKα were similar in αTC1-6 cells with and without IR (Fig. 1C). Erk1/2, a key mediator of the mitogenic potential of growth factors, was less activated in IRKD cells than in control cells, which was supported by the observation of reduced cellular proliferation in IRKD cells.

Effects of IR knockdown on the viability, apoptosis, cytotoxicity and proliferation of αTC1-6 cells

The cell viability was significantly more decreased with time from day 2 in the IRKD cells compared to the control cells (Fig. 1D), although the levels of cytotoxicity and apoptosis were

Table 1. A comparison of the biosynthetic metabolites between the control and IRKD αTC1-6 cells, as determined by CE-TOFMS.

Biosynthetic pathway(s)	Metabolite	Control-1.5	Control-5.6	Control-30	IRKD-1.5	IRKD-5.6	IRKD-30	Control-1.5 vs. IRKD-1.5	Control-5.6 vs. IRKD-5.6	Control-30 vs. IRKD-30
		Mean ± SEM	Mean ± SEM	Mean ± SEM	Mean ± SEM	Mean ± SEM	Mean ± SEM	Ratio¶	Ratio¶	Ratio¶
Glycolysis/ gluconeogenesis, pentose phosphate pathway, TCA cycle	Sedoheptulose 7-phosphate	2.3E-04±1.4E-05	2.6E-04±3.5E-05	3.1E-04±8.7E-06	1.4E-04±4.8E-06	1.6E-04±5.1E-06	1.9E-04±8.6E-06	0.6*	0.6	0.62***
	Ribulose 5-phosphate	1.6E-04±1.6E-05	1.7E-04±1.3E-05	2.2E-04±3.0E-05	5.7E-05±3.2E-06	5.9E-05±5.0E-06	1.4E-04±4.0E-06	0.36*	0.36**	0.61
	PRPP	3.4E-04±4.4E-05	4.7E-04±4.7E-05	3.9E-04±1.8E-05	3.2E-05±0.0E+00	5.5E-05±4.5E-06	5.3E-05±8.4E-06	0.09	0.12*	0.13***
	cis-Aconitic acid	1.2E-03±1.5E-04	1.8E-03±1.1E-04	1.9E-03±1.1E-04	8.6E-04±1.2E-04	1.1E-03±5.1E-05	1.2E-03±3.6E-05	0.71	0.6*	0.63*
	2-Oxoglutaric acid	1.3E-03±4.1E-05	1.7E-03±1.2E-04	1.7E-03±9.2E-05	8.0E-04±3.3E-05	9.1E-04±4.9E-05	8.6E-04±6.6E-05	0.6***	0.55*	0.52**
Purine metabolism, pyrimidine metabolism	UDP	2.7E-03±4.9E-05	2.1E-03±9.5E-05	1.3E-03±2.0E-04	1.3E-03±8.3E-05	1.0E-03±7.0E-05	7.4E-04±2.0E-05	0.47***	0.5**	0.57
	GMP	3.4E-04±3.9E-06	3.1E-04±2.1E-05	2.6E-04±2.9E-05	2.5E-04±6.0E-06	1.9E-04±1.0E-05	1.9E-04±6.8E-06	0.73***	0.61*	0.73
	GDP	1.5E-03±4.6E-05	1.3E-03±9.4E-05	9.3E-04±1.1E-04	8.5E-04±5.8E-05	8.4E-04±3.6E-05	6.7E-04±3.6E-05	0.58**	0.65*	0.72
	CDP	7.1E-04±1.8E-05	6.1E-04±6.3E-05	4.0E-04±3.9E-05	3.9E-04±3.8E-05	2.8E-04±2.0E-05	2.1E-04±5.9E-06	0.55**	0.46*	0.54*
	UMP	7.0E-04±4.0E-05	6.8E-04±1.0E-04	4.1E-04±9.6E-06	3.2E-04±8.5E-06	2.5E-04±1.5E-05	2.1E-04±1.4E-05	0.45**	0.38	0.52***
	ADP	1.3E-02±3.9E-04	1.2E-02±1.5E-03	8.0E-03±5.7E-04	7.7E-03±7.6E-04	7.1E-03±4.3E-04	5.0E-03±9.7E-05	0.61*	0.58	0.63*
	CTP	8.8E-03±6.1E-04	1.1E-02±1.4E-03	1.0E-02±5.6E-04	5.5E-03±9.4E-05	5.0E-03±1.6E-04	5.1E-03±1.3E-04	0.63*	0.48	0.51**
	CMP	3.0E-04±2.1E-05	2.8E-04±2.3E-05	2.4E-04±1.5E-05	1.9E-04±1.8E-06	1.5E-04±8.1E-06	1.4E-04±8.3E-06	0.61*	0.55*	0.6**
	UTP	2.8E-02±2.1E-03	3.0E-02±3.3E-03	2.6E-02±9.0E-04	1.8E-02±5.2E-04	1.7E-02±6.4E-04	1.7E-02±5.1E-05	0.65*	0.56	0.64**
	dCTP	4.6E-04±2.2E-05	4.5E-04±2.8E-05	4.3E-04±7.0E-06	3.7E-04±1.9E-05	3.4E-04±5.5E-06	3.6E-04±3.6E-06	0.82*	0.75	0.83**
Amino acid metabolism (Asp, Ala, Lys)	Asp	2.2E-01±1.7E-02	1.8E-01±7.5E-03	1.2E-01±1.3E-02	1.4E-01±6.2E-03	1.1E-01±4.1E-04	8.5E-02±1.6E-03	0.65*	0.62*	0.74
	Lys	1.4E-02±1.2E-03	1.3E-02±3.0E-04	1.2E-02±9.1E-04	9.3E-03±2.6E-04	7.9E-03±3.8E-04	7.5E-03±2.9E-04	0.69	0.6***	0.64*
	O-Acetylcarnitine	5.2E-04±7.8E-05	9.9E-04±5.1E-05	1.3E-03±7.1E-05	6.0E-04±3.8E-05	7.5E-04±4.1E-05	9.0E-04±4.3E-05	1.17	0.76*	0.67*
Amino acid metabolism (Gly, Ser, Cys)	CDP-choline	1.3E-04±7.4E-06	1.7E-04±2.3E-05	1.6E-04±2.0E-05	3.6E-04±5.5E-06	3.4E-04±1.8E-05	4.0E-04±2.9E-05	2.73***	2.05**	2.46**
	Choline	1.2E-02±5.7E-04	1.3E-02±2.2E-04	1.5E-02±5.6E-04	2.7E-02±2.4E-03	2.3E-02±1.2E-03	2.9E-02±1.7E-03	2.29*	1.82*	1.98**
	Hypotaurine	3.8E-03±4.6E-04	4.0E-03±2.4E-04	3.6E-03±2.7E-04	6.8E-03±3.5E-04	6.6E-03±4.3E-04	6.1E-03±1.2E-04	1.77**	1.66*	1.69**
	Taurine	0.0E+00±0.0E+00	0.0E+00±0.0E+00	0.0E+00±0.0E+00	9.1E-04±0.0E+00	9.7E-04±3.0E-05	9.9E-04±4.1E-05	1<***	1<***	1<***
Amino acid metabolism (Branched chain)	Val	9.9E-03±7.2E-04	1.0E-02±5.0E-04	9.9E-03±3.5E-04	7.8E-03±2.1E-04	7.0E-03±2.2E-04	7.7E-03±1.5E-04	0.79	0.69*	0.78*
	Leu	8.9E-03±6.5E-04	8.8E-03±2.6E-04	9.1E-03±4.1E-04	7.2E-03±3.4E-04	5.9E-03±2.1E-04	6.7E-03±3.0E-04	0.81	0.67**	0.74*
	Ile	4.0E-03±3.1E-04	4.0E-03±2.1E-04	4.1E-03±9.3E-05	3.4E-03±2.1E-04	2.6E-03±9.5E-05	3.3E-03±8.3E-05	0.86	0.66*	0.81**

Table 1. Cont.

Biosynthetic pathway(s)	Metabolite	Control-1.5	Control-5.6	Control-30	IRKD-1.5	IRKD-5.6	IRKD-30	Control-1.5 vs. IRKD-1.5	Control-5.6 vs. IRKD-5.6	Control-30 vs. IRKD-30
		Mean ± SEM	Mean ± SEM	Mean ± SEM	Mean ± SEM	Mean ± SEM	Mean ± SEM	Ratio¶	Ratio¶	Ratio¶
Urea cycle, amino acid metabolism (Glu, Gln, His, Pro)	Argininosuccinic acid	4.8E-04±5.5E-05	5.2E-04±3.3E-05	4.5E-04±6.0E-05	2.1E-04±1.3E-05	2.0E-04±1.3E-05	2.1E-04±1.5E-05	0.42*	0.38**	0.46*
	Arg	8.5E-04±2.1E-04	1.3E-03±8.6E-05	1.2E-03±1.5E-04	8.8E-05±0.0E+00	1.4E-04±1.9E-05	2.2E-04±3.6E-05	0.1	0.1**	0.19*
	Guanidoacetic acid	8.2E-04±7.5E-05	8.6E-04±4.3E-05	8.1E-04±4.5E-05	4.6E-04±1.7E-05	4.1E-04±3.0E-05	3.7E-04±3.2E-05	0.56*	0.48**	0.46**
	Pro	1.0E-01±7.9E-03	1.0E-01±6.8E-03	9.1E-02±6.4E-03	6.6E-02±1.8E-03	5.8E-02±2.6E-03	5.8E-02±2.6E-03	0.66*	0.57*	0.64*
	Gln	1.2E-02±1.2E-03	1.2E-02±8.1E-04	1.1E-02±7.6E-04	6.6E-03±2.4E-04	6.1E-03±2.7E-04	5.8E-03±1.1E-04	0.57	0.49**	0.54*
	5-Oxoproline	3.4E-04±3.6E-05	3.4E-04±1.9E-05	3.8E-04±3.1E-05	2.5E-04±1.7E-05	2.1E-04±4.2E-06	1.8E-04±5.5E-06	0.73	0.6*	0.46*
	Ornithine	4.2E-03±3.8E-04	4.3E-03±1.7E-04	4.1E-03±2.4E-04	3.4E-03±7.9E-05	2.8E-03±1.6E-04	2.7E-03±1.8E-04	0.81	0.64**	0.66*
	His	2.7E-03±3.3E-04	2.8E-03±4.8E-05	2.7E-03±2.5E-04	2.1E-03±1.3E-04	1.8E-03±9.5E-05	1.8E-03±1.3E-04	0.77	0.66**	0.65*

Control, shRNA control αTC1-6 cells; IRKD, shRNA insulin receptor knockdown αTC1-6 cells; −1.5, treated with 1.5 mM glucose; −5.6, treated with 5.6 mM glucose; −30, treated with 30 mM glucose.
*$P<0.05$,
**$P<0.01$,
***$P<0.001$ (Control vs. IRKD).
¶Control/IRKD ratio.

not significantly different between these two cell types (Figs. 1E and F). Cell proliferation was studied using the BrdU incorporation assay, and a significant reduction in the proliferation in IRKD cells was found (Fig. 1G). The observation that IRKD cells were significantly delayed in their transition from the G0/G1 to S phase, which was not accompanied by an increase in apoptosis, suggests that insulin signaling is responsible for cell cycle regulation in this cell line.

Effects of IR knockdown on the glucose-regulated glucagon secretion in αTC1-6 cells and islets

To assess the effects of IR disruption on the α-cell function, we studied the glucose-regulated glucagon release of IRKD cells. Figure 2A shows a comparison of the glucagon secretion in response to varying glucose concentrations (from 1.5 to 30 mM) between control and IRKD cells. The IRKD cells tended to secrete less glucagon compared to the controls at the 1.5 mM glucose concentration ($P=0.13$). On the other hand, the IRKD cells exhibited significantly higher glucagon secretion in response to the 5.6 and 30 mM glucose concentrations than controls. The glucagon content in the cells was not significantly different between the control and IRKD cells at any of the three different glucose concentrations (Fig. 2B).

In islets with IRKD, the glucagon secretion in response to 1.5 mM glucose concentration was significantly decreased, while at the 30 mM glucose concentration, the glucagon secretion tended to be increased ($P=0.06$) compared to the islets expressing control shRNA (Fig. 2C). The glucose-stimulated glucagon content in the islets was not affected by the knockdown of IR expression (Fig. 2D).

Differences between the metabolic profiles of the control and IRKD αTC1-6 cells detected using CE-TOFMS

To further investigate the metabolic traits that underlie the abnormal glucagon secretion in IR knockdown α cells, we analyzed the metabolomic profiles of control and IRKD cells using CE-TOFMS. Based on their *m/z* values and migration times, 163 metabolites (75 cations and 88 anions) were detected and visualized on a metabolome-wide pathway map using the VANTED (Visualization and Analysis of Networks containing Experimental Data) software program (http://vanted.ipk-gatersleben.de/). The metabolic pathways associated with all the detected metabolites are illustrated in Figure S1. These metabolites were associated with glycolysis/gluconeogenesis, the pentose phosphate pathway, the TCA cycle, the urea cycle, pyrimidine metabolism, nicotinate and nicotinamide metabolism and amino acid metabolism. The results of the comparison of the metabolic profiles between the control and IRKD cells are provided in Figure 3.

A principal component analysis (PCA) showed a clear distinction between the intracellular metabolites of control and IRKD cells according to glucose concentrations (Fig. 3A). The first component (PC1) indicated that 48.3% of the total variation was due to the differences between control and IRKD cells. Furthermore, a heatmap analysis indicated that the metabolic pattern of IRKD cells was remarkably different from that of the control cells (Fig. 3B). The cellular contents of 33 metabolites in the control and IRKD cells were significantly different, with P values less than 0.05 for at least two points at each concentration of glucose (Table 1). We observed a decrease of some metabolites associated with the pentose phosphate, TCA cycle, purine-pyrimidine and amino acid metabolism in αTC1-6 cells due to knocking down the IR. In contrast, taurine and choline were

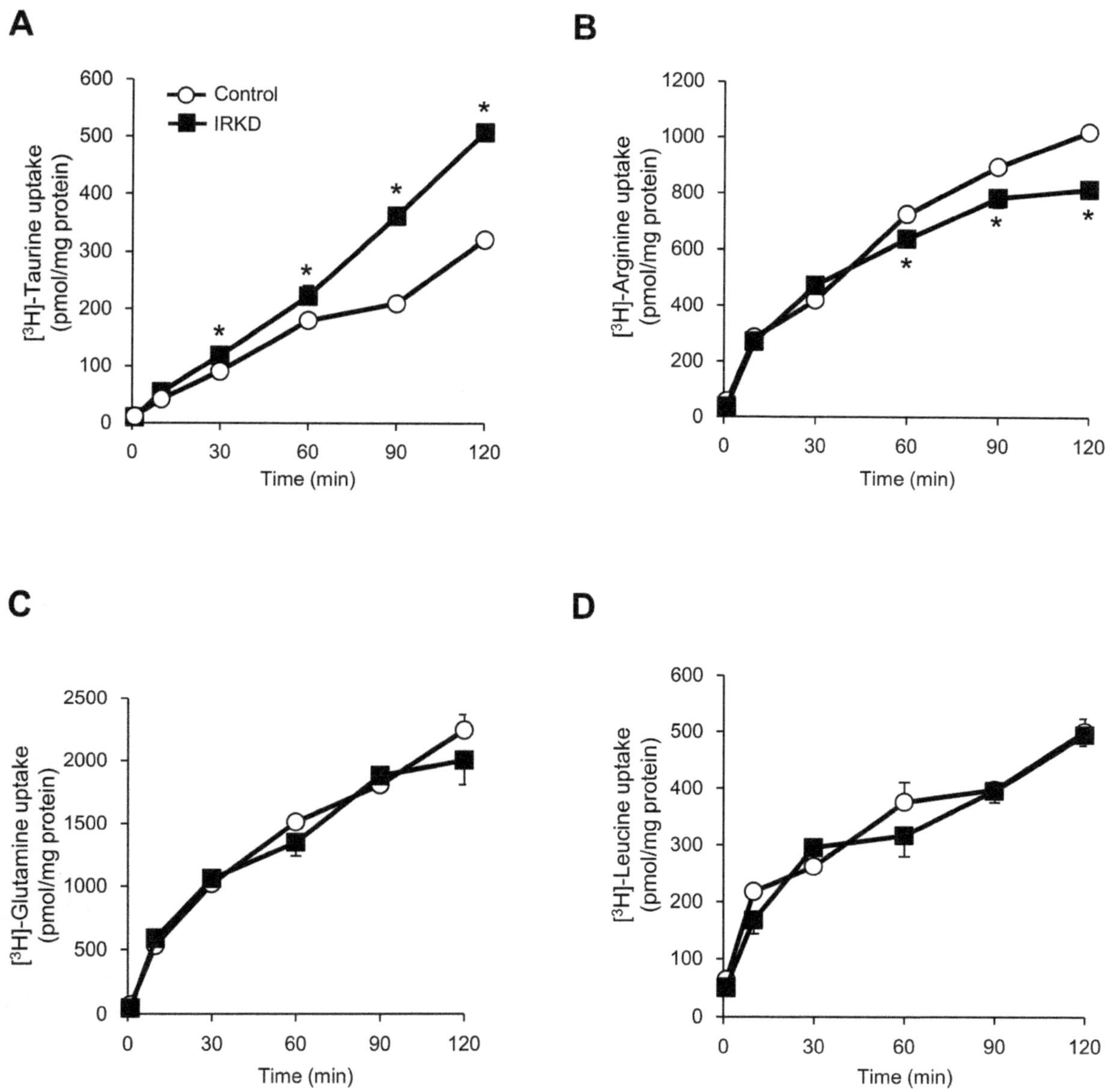

Figure 5. Time course of [^{3}H] taurine and amino acid uptake in control and IRKD αTC1-6 cells. $n = 4$ in each group. The data are expressed as the means ± SEM; $*P<0.05$, control vs. IRKD.

relatively increased in the IRKD cells. Of the various metabolites identified as being significantly altered, taurine, arginine, glutamine and leucine (Fig. 4) were chosen for a further analysis because they could potentially affect the glucagon secretion.

The effects of IR knockdown on the taurine and amino acid uptake and synthesis

We examined whether IR knockdown affected the uptake and synthesis of taurine, arginine, glutamine and leucine in αTC1-6 cells. Figure 5A shows the time-dependent [^{3}H] taurine uptake for 120 min in the control and IRKD cells. The IRKD cells exhibited significantly higher levels of taurine uptake than control cells from 30 to 120 min. On the other hand, the arginine uptake in the IRKD cells was shown to decrease from 60 to 120 min compared with the controls (Fig. 5B). There were no significant differences in the glutamine and leucine uptake between the IRKD and control cells (Figs. 5C and D). It is noteworthy that the uptake of labeled nutrients that are metabolized into CO_2, H_2O and other secreted metabolites would not be included in the measurement, because the assay measures the radioactivity trapped in the cells, so the values obtained in this study may have underestimated the actual values.

Next, we compared the enzymes involved in taurine, arginine and glutamine metabolism in control and IRKD cells (Fig. 6). The gene expression levels of the major synthetic enzymes for taurine (cysteine dioxygenase 1 (*Cdo1*), which converts cysteine to cysteine sulfinic acid, and cysteine sulfinic acid decarboxylase (*Csad*), which converts cysteine sulfinic acid to hypotaurine); arginine (argininosuccinate synthase 1 (*Ass1*), which converts citrulline to argininosuccinate, and argininosuccinate lyase (*Asl*), which converts argininosuccinate to arginine) and glutamine (glutamine synthase (*Glul*)) were examined. As shown in Fig. 6A, the expression of *Csad*, the rate-limiting enzyme required for taurine synthesis, was significantly elevated in IRKD cells compared with the control

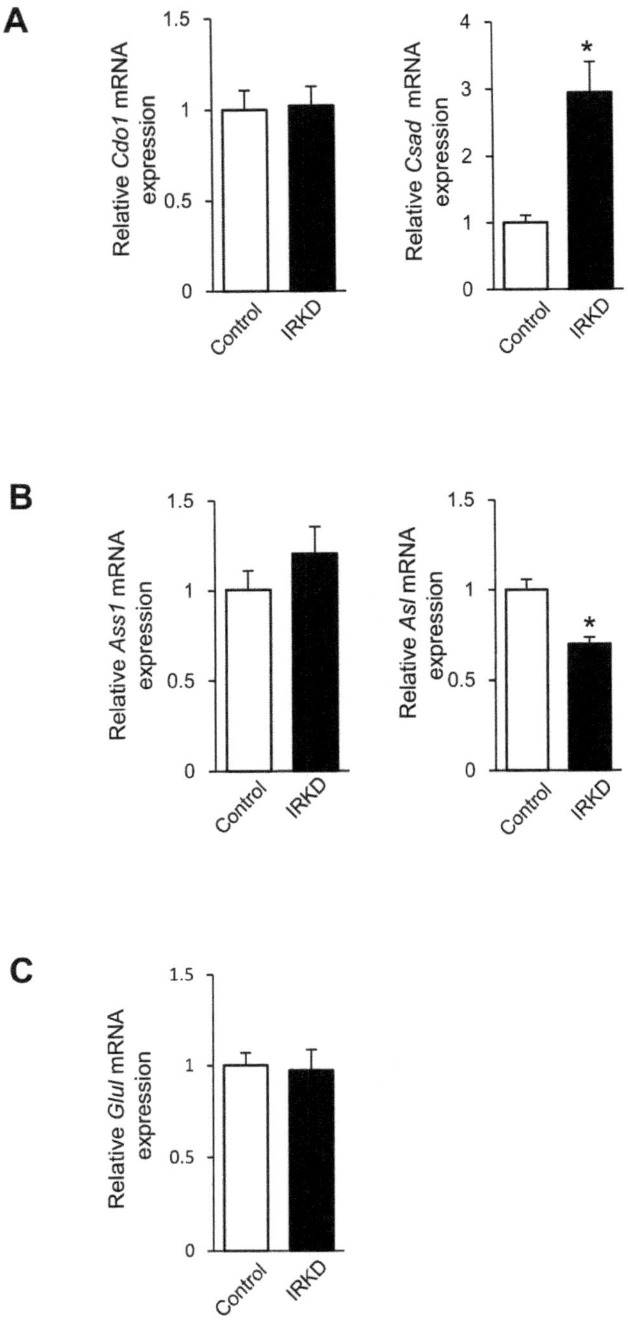

Figure 6. Altered gene expression of the major enzymes required for taurine, arginine and glutamine synthesis in IRKD αTC1-6 cells. The relative expression of *Cdo1*, *Csad*, *Ass1*, *Asl* and *Glul* genes in the control and IRKD αTC1-6 cells incubated for 3 h with KRB containing 5.6 mM glucose was measured by quantitative real-time PCR and normalized to the expression of the reference gene, *Actb*. $n = 4$ in each group. The bars represent the means ± SEM; *$P<0.05$, control vs. IRKD.

cells. In contrast, the mRNA expression of *Asl*, an enzyme that catalyzes the final step of arginine biosynthesis, was decreased in IRKD cells (Fig. 6B). We found no significant difference in the *Glul* expression between IRKD and control cells (Fig. 6C).

Effects of taurine on the glucagon secretion by αTC1-6 cells and islets

Because taurine was considered to be one of the most likely candidate metabolite stimulating glucagon secretion, we determined the effects of taurine supplementation on the glucagon release and synthesis. Consequently, supplementation of taurine enhanced the glucagon secretion in a concentration-dependent manner in the αTC1-6 cells, and this increase in glucagon secretion by taurine was inhibited by adding insulin (Fig. 7A). On the other hand, taurine concentration-dependently reduced the glucagon content in these cells, and the reduction disappeared with the addition of insulin (Fig. 7B). This result suggests that insulin suppresses the stimulatory effect of taurine on glucagon secretion in the αTC1-6 cells.

We also assessed the glucagon secretion in response to three different concentrations of glucose (1.5, 5.6 and 30 mM) with or without 10 mM taurine in control and IRKD cells. Since 10 mM taurine supplementation tended to increase the glucagon release in control αTC1-6 cells (albeit not reaching statistical significance at the 5.6 mM glucose level), and thus could be assumed to enhance glucagon secretion depending upon the glucose concentration, the treatment with a 10 mM concentration of taurine was subsequently examined in IRKD cells and islets. The treatment with 10 mM taurine had no effect on the glucagon released by the control αTC1-6 cells and control islets (Figs. 8A and C); however, when both αTC1-6 cells and islets with knocked down IR were treated with 30 mM glucose plus 10 mM taurine, the glucagon secretion was significantly augmented compared with that in vehicle-treated ones (Figs. 8B and D).

Discussion

This study revealed that there were differential levels of metabolites, together with the abnormal glucagon response to glucose, in an *in vitro* model of intra-islet insulin-deficient α-cells. Notably, taurine was found to be markedly elevated, and was shown to stimulate glucagon secretion in the α-cells, thus suggesting that it might exaggerate the paradoxical secretion of glucagon from α-cells under conditions of insulin deficiency.

We succeeded in generating an αTC1-6 cell line with stable knockdown of the IR. αTC1-6 is a clonal murine α-cell line that specifically produces glucagon but not insulin [17]. This cell line possesses an advantage over primary islets in that it is a homogeneous cellular population and has been used previously to study glucagon secretion and gene expression [15,17–19,27]. IR knockdown in stable α-cell lines could reproduce the circumstances reflecting a chronic deficiency of extracellular insulin, which may reflect the pathophysiology of α-cells in insulin deficiency. Namely, in insulin deficiency, where β-cells are lost, α-cells lack the tonic restraint normally provided by the high concentrations of insulin from juxtaposed β-cells [3]. Clinical studies have shown that in type 1 diabetes, glucose, administered either intravenously or orally, can actually stimulate glucagon secretion [28], while the glucagon response to low glucose is blunted [29,30], indicating that these "opposite" or "paradoxical" changes in the glucagon dynamics may lead to disrupted glucose homeostasis. Thus, exploring the mechanisms responsible for glucose-regulated glucagon dysfunction in an insulin-deficient α-cell model may shed a light on the pathogenesis of glycemic instability in insulin-deficient type 1 diabetes.

In this study, IRKD cells exhibited paradoxical glucagon behavior at different concentrations of glucose. The islets with IRKD also showed a paradoxical pattern, although the statistically different points found in islets and αTC1-6 cells were different; the

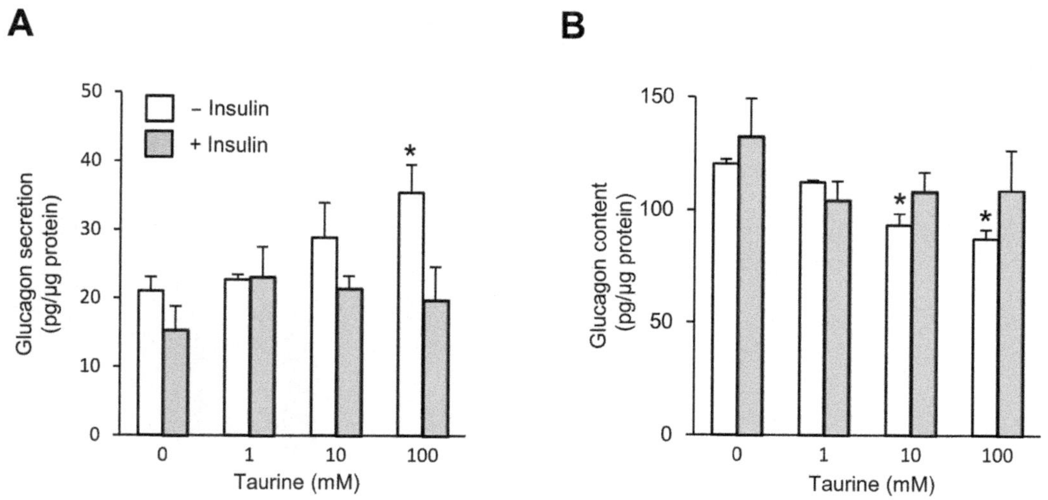

Figure 7. Taurine-stimulated glucagon secretion and cell contents in control αTC1-6 cells with or without insulin. (**A**) Cells were preincubated for 1 h with KRB containing 5.6 mM glucose, and were subsequently stimulated for 2 h with 0, 1, 10 or 100 mM taurine and treated with or without insulin (100 nM). $n = 6$ in each group. (**B**) The total protein content and total glucagon content. $n = 6$ in each group. The bars represent the means ± SEM; *$P<0.05$, vs. vehicle-treated cells.

glucagon secretion in response to low glucose was significantly abolished in islets with IRKD, while that in response to high glucose was significantly exaggerated in the αTC1-6 cells with IRKD. This might have been due to the phenotypic differences between the isolated islets and αTC1-6 cells, or to the differences caused by the transient or stable knock-down of the IR. Diao et al. [15] have previously reported that glucagon secretion is abolished in response to low glucose in isolated islets and in αTC1-6 cells expressing insulin receptor siRNA, whereas glucagon release at the high glucose concentration remained the same as in the control cells. The difference between these two studies may be explained by the different concentrations of glucose used during the preincubation period (5.6 mM in our study and 25 mM in the latter study). Another previous study showed that there was paradoxical glucagon gene expression under both high- and low-glucose conditions in the islets of α-cell specific insulin receptor knockout mice [16]. Furthermore, siRNA-mediated knockdown of the IR in glucagon-secreting InR1G cells promoted enhanced glucagon secretion [16]. Our data are consistent with these findings, and may support the idea that IR expression is essential for glucose-regulated glucagon release.

A novel finding of the present study is the distinct metabolomic patterns between the IRKD and control αTC1-6 cells. The TCA cycle metabolites, such as *cis*-aconitic acid and 2-oxoglutaric acid, the metabolites of the pentose phosphate and nucleotide synthesis pathways and several essential and conditionally essential amino acids were decreased in IRKD cells. These results may reflect the reduced bioenergetic and biosynthetic requirements in IRKD cells due to their decreased viability and proliferation. Regarding the effect of the glucose concentration, no meaningful metabolic differences were seen between IRKD and control cells. The most remarkable difference between the two types of cells was that taurine was abundant in IRKD cells, while it was almost undetectable in control αTC1-6 cells. The quantities of taurine at different glucose concentrations were similar, although the effects of taurine on glucagon secretion were different at the different glucose concentrations in the IRKD cells. This may suggest that intracellular and extracellular taurine have different effects on glucagon secretion at the same glucose concentrations.

Of the various metabolites evaluated, taurine, arginine, glutamine and leucine were considered to potentially exert some effects on the glucagon secretion. Taurine has been reported to inactivate the ATP-sensitive K^+-channels either directly via an interaction with the sulfonylurea receptor (SUR) on the channel, or indirectly via an associated protein that binds to the SUR in skeletal muscle fibers [31]. In neurons and cardiac cells, taurine-modulated calcium flux has been reported [32,33]. Furthermore, it has been proposed that the administration of taurine leads to the opening of voltage-gated calcium channels and a subsequent decrease in the intracellular insulin levels in β-cell lines [34]. Together, these data suggest that taurine enhances glucagon release partly by altering the electrogenic response in α-cells. Our data showing an increase of taurine uptake and synthesis in IRKD cells compared with control cells are consistent with the metabolomic results of the comparatively elevated cellular taurine level in IRKDs, and may account for their exaggerated glucagon response under the high glucose condition.

The intracellular amino acids, arginine, glutamine and leucine, were assumed to play a role in glucagon release, at least in part, through the activation or inactivation of AMPK and mTOR, which are two important energy/nutrient centers [35]. mTOR has been proposed as a downstream component of an energy-sensing pathway, with AMPK as the primary cellular energy sensor [36]. Increases in AMPK activity stimulate glucagon secretion in α-cells [37]. However, both the AMPK and mTOR activity were unchanged after the removal of IR in the present study, which is in accordance with the results of a previous study [15]. Cellular arginine is known to induce glucagon release through a mechanism mediated by nitric oxide [38,39], regardless of the glucose concentration [40]. Thus, the decreased arginine uptake and synthesis observed in IRKD cells may partly contribute to the inhibition of glucagon release at the low glucose concentration in these cells.

Finally, taurine was shown to stimulate glucagon secretion in αTC1-6 cells. Taurine is present in most mammalian tissues, including the pancreatic islets, and regulates the osmolarity, ion channel activity and glucose homeostasis. It has been shown that taurine administration strongly suppresses the glucose-stimulated secretion of insulin from isolated mouse islets [41], and also that

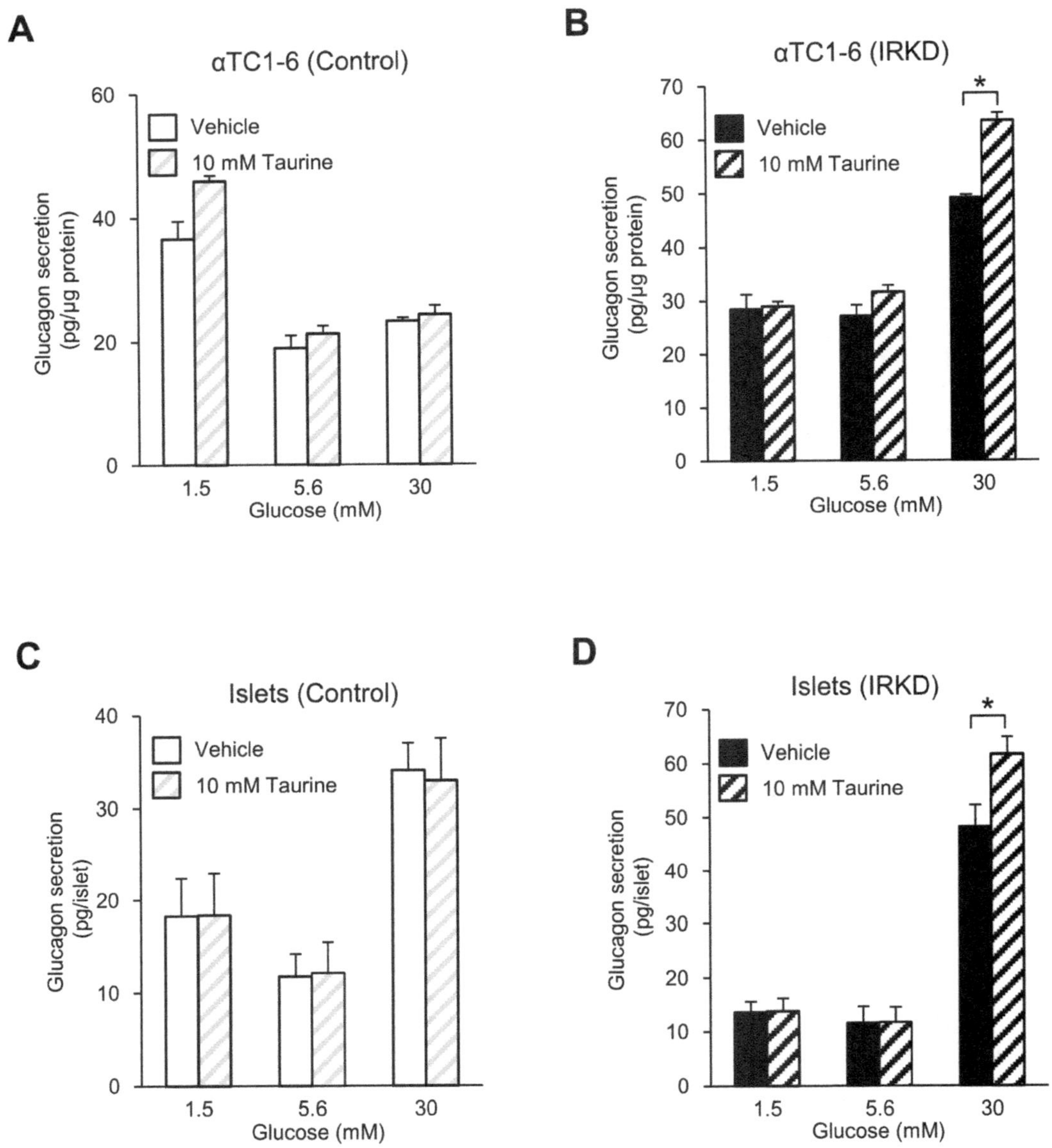

Figure 8. Exaggerated glucose-stimulated glucagon secretion in IRKD αTC1-6 cells and islets in the presence of taurine. αTC1-6 cells (**A, B**) or islets (**C, D**) were preincubated for 1 h with KRB containing 5.6 mM glucose, and were subsequently stimulated for 2 h with 1.5, 5.6 or 30 mM glucose with or without 10 mM taurine. $n=6$ (**A, B**) or 3 (**C, D**) in each group. The bars represent the means ± SEM; *$P<0.05$, taurine-treated vs. vehicle-treated cells or islets.

the intraperitoneal injection of taurine inhibits the increase in serum insulin induced by glucose administration [42]. On the contrary, it has been reported that taurine enhances glucose-stimulated insulin release from cultured rat fetal islets [43]. Another report showed that taurine supplementation to mice improved the insulin secretion and enhanced glucagon secretion from isolated islets [44]. The results showing that the extracellular taurine concentration-dependently reduced the glucagon content in αTC1-6 cells may reflect a relative excess of glucagon exocytosis compared to its biosynthesis. Together, these data indicate a possible glucagonotropic action of taurine in α-cells.

Our results also showed that taurine paradoxically exaggerated the glucagon secretion under the high glucose concentration in both IRKD cells and islets with IRKD, suggesting that it could worsen the aberrant α-cell function under the condition of chronic insulin deficiency. Taurine is known to move passively through the anionic volume regulatory channels [45]. At the 30 mM glucose concentration, the uptake of supplemented taurine into IRKD cells would be higher, because of its high osmolarity, in order to regulate the cell volume compared to that at the 1.5 or 5.6 mM glucose concentration. Therefore, the effects of taurine supplementation on glucagon secretion may be elicited only at 30 mM glucose in IRKD cells and islets. Glucose elevation reduces the activation of both K_{ATP} channels and the P/Q-type Ca^{2+}-current, which accordingly decrease the glucagon secretion at high glucose levels in physiological α-cells [46]. When insulin signaling is impaired, the K_{ATP} and Ca^{2+} channel activity or sensitivity is altered [47]. Taurine might therefore play a role in the glucagon secretion from IRKD cells by affecting the K_{ATP} and Ca^{2+} channels. Conceivably, the combination of a high glucose (30 mM) concentration and 10 mM taurine supplementation can "optimize" the membranous electrical activity for glucagon exocytosis in IRKD cells and islets. However, all of these causal mechanisms are only speculative, and therefore, should be fully evaluated in the future.

It is notable that taurine was accumulated, and may contribute to paradoxical glucagon secretion in this insulin-deficient α-cell model. While some beneficial effects of taurine supplementation for reducing blood glucose and restoring insulin sensitivity have been found in type 2 diabetes, in type 1 diabetes, taurine might exert adverse effects on the glucose stability as a result of α-cell dysfunction.

In conclusion, our study indicates that the metabolic alterations induced by IRKD in α-cells, especially the increase of taurine, may lead to a distorted glucagon response in IRKD αTC1-6 cells, i.e., an *in vitro* model of insulin-deficient α-cells, thus suggesting the importance of taurine in the paradoxical glucagon response and the resultant glucose instability in insulin-deficient type 1 diabetes. Further *in vivo* studies to assess the long-term relevance of taurine to the glucagon secretion and glycemic control in insulin-deficient type 1 diabetes are needed to investigate the clinical implications of our findings.

Supporting Information

Figure S1 Metabolites in the principle metabolic pathways of control and IRKD αTC1-6 cells detected by CE-TOFMS.

Acknowledgments

We thank Dr. Yoshinori Moriyama for providing the kind gift of the αTC1-6 cells and Dr. Hideyuki Hayashi for helpful advice.

Author Contributions

Conceived and designed the experiments: YMM. Performed the experiments: MB YMM. Analyzed the data: MB YMM JT AI TH. Contributed reagents/materials/analysis tools: MB YMM. Wrote the paper: MB YMM. Edited and revised manuscript: AI TH. Approved the final version of the manuscript: TH.

References

1. Reynolds C, Molnar GD, Horwitz DL, Rubenstein AH, Taylor WF, et al. (1997) Abnormalities of endogenous glucagon and insulin in unstable diabetes. Diabetes 26: 36–45.
2. The Diabetes Control and Complications Trial Research Group (1998) Effect of intensive therapy on residual beta-cell function in patients with type 1 diabetes in the diabetes control and complications trial. A randomized, controlled trial. Ann Intern Med 128: 517–523.
3. Unger RH, Orci L (2010) Paracrinology of islets and the paracrinopathy of diabetes. Proc Natl Acad Sci U S A 107: 16009–16012.
4. Siafarikas A, Johnston RJ, Bulsara MK, O'Leary P, Jones TW, et al. (2012) Early loss of the glucagon response to hypoglycemia in adolescents with type 1 diabetes. Diabetes Care 35: 1757–1762.
5. Pörksen S, Nielsen LB, Kaas A, Kocova M, Chiarelli F, et al. (2007) Meal-stimulatd glucagon release is associated with postprandial blood glucose level and does not interfere with glycemic control in children and adolescents with new-onset type 1 diabetes. J Clin Endocrinol Metab 92: 2910–2916.
6. Bessho M, Murase-Mishiba Y, Tsutsumi C, Haseda F, Imagawa A, et al. (2013) Glycaemic instability correlates with a hyperglucagonaemic response in patients with type 1 diabetes without residual beta-cell function. Diabetes Res Clin Pract 102: e38–e40.
7. Taborsky GJ Jr (2010) The physiology of glucagon. J Diabetes Sci Technol 4: 1338–1344.
8. Gaisano HY, Macdonald PE, Vranic M (2012) Glucagon secretion and signaling in the development of diabetes. Front Physiol 3: e349.
9. Gerich JE, Tsalikian E, Lorenzi M, Schneider V, Bohannon NV, et al. (1975) Normalization of fasting hyperglucagonemia and excessive glucagon responses to intravenous arginine in human diabetes mellitus by prolonged infusion of insulin. J Clin Endocrinol Metab 41: 1178–1180.
10. Wendt A, Birnir B, Buschard K, Gromada J, Salehi A, et al.(2004) Glucose inhibition of glucagon secretion from rat alpha-cells is mediated by GABA released from neighboring beta-cells. Diabetes 53: 1038–1045.
11. Rorsman P, Berggren PO, Bokvist K, Ericson H, Möhler H, et al. (1989) Glucose-inhibition of glucagon secretion involves activation of GABAA-receptor chloride channels. Nature 341: 233–236.
12. Ishihara H, Maechler P, Gjinovci A, Herrera PL, Wollheim CB (2003) Islet beta-cell secretion determines glucagon release from neighbouring alpha-cells. Nat Cell Biol 5: 330–335.
13. Kawamori D, Akiyama M, Hu J, Hambro B, Kulkarni RN (2011) Growth factor signaling in the regulation of α-cell fate. Diabetes Obes Metab 13, Suppl 1: 21–30.
14. Bollyky J, Greenbaum CJ (2007) Editorial: The role of glucagon in postprandial hyperglycemia–the jury's still out. J Clin Endocrinol Metab 92: 2879–2881.
15. Diao J, Asghar Z, Chan CB, Wheeler MB (2005) Glucose-regulated glucagon secretion requires insulin receptor expression in pancreatic alpha-cells. J Biol Chem 280: 33487–33496.
16. Kawamori D, Kurpad AJ, Hu J, Liew CW, Shih JL, et al. (2009) Insulin signaling in alpha cells modulates glucagon secretion in vivo. Cell Metab 9: 350–361.
17. Hamaguchi K, Leiter EH (1990) Comparison of cytokine effects on mouse pancreatic alpha-cell and beta-cell lines. Viability, secretory function, and MHC antigen expression. Diabetes 39: 415–425.
18. Hayashi M, Otsuka M, Morimoto R, Hirota S, Yatsushiro S, et al. (2001) Differentiation-associated Na+-dependent inorganic phosphate cotransporter (DNPI) is a vesicular glutamate transporter in endocrine glutamatergic systems. J Biol Chem 276: 43400–43406.
19. Hayashi M, Yamada H, Uehara S, Morimoto R, Muroyama A, et al. (2003) Secretory granule-mediated co-secretion of L-glutamate and glucagon triggers glutamatergic signal transmission in islets of Langerhans. J Biol Chem 278: 1966–1974.
20. Yaekura K, Yada T (1998) [Ca2+]i-reducing action of cAMP in rat pancreatic beta-cells: involvement of thapsigargin-sensitive stores. Am J Physiol 274: C513–C521.
21. Lambert IH (2004) Regulation of the cellular content of the organic osmolyte taurine in mammalian cells. Neurochem Res 29: 27–63.
22. Timbrell JA, Seabra V, Waterfield CJ (1995) The in vivo and in vitro protective properties of taurine. Gen Pharmacol 26: 453–462.
23. Soga T, Heiger DN (2000) Amino acid analysis by capillary electrophoresis electrospray ionization mass spectrometry. Anal Chem 72: 1236–1241.
24. Soga T, Ueno Y, Naraoka H, Ohashi Y, Tomita M, et al. (2002) Simultaneous determination of anionic intermediates for Bacillus subtilis metabolic pathways by capillary electrophoresis electrospray ionization mass spectrometry. Anal Chem 74: 2233–2239.
25. Soga T, Ohashi Y, Ueno Y, Naraoka H, Tomita M, et al. (2003) Quantitative metabolome analysis using capillary electrophoresis mass spectrometry. J Proteome Res 2: 488–494.
26. Chang RC, Stadlin A, Tsang D (2001) Effects of tumor necrosis factor alpha on taurine uptake in cultured rat astrocytes. Neurochem Int 38: 249–254.
27. Paul GL, Waegner A, Gaskins HR, Shay NF (1998) Histidine availability alters glucagon gene expression in murine alphaTC6 cells. J Nutr 128: 973–976.
28. Greenbaum CJ, Prigeon RL, D'Alessio DA (2002) Impaired beta-cell function, incretin effect, and glucagon suppression in patients with type 1 diabetes who have normal fasting glucose. Diabetes 51: 951–957.
29. Gerich JE, Langlois M, Noacco C, Karam JH, Forsham PH (1973) Lack of glucagon response to hypoglycemia in diabetes: evidence for an intrinsic pancreatic alpha cell defect. Science 182: 171–173.
30. Bergenstal RM, Polonsky KS, Pons G, Jaspan JB, Rubenstein AH (1983) Lack of glucagon response to hypoglycemia in type I diabetics after long-term optimal therapy with a continuous subcutaneous insulin infusion pump. Diabetes 32: 398–402.
31. Tricarico D, Barbieri M, Camerino DC (2000) Taurine blocks ATP-sensitive potassium channels of rat skeletal muscle fibres interfering with the sulphonylurea receptor. Br J Pharmacol 130: 827–834.
32. El Idrissi A (2008) Taurine increases mitochondrial buffering of calcium: role in neuroprotection. Amino Acids 34: 321–328.
33. Satoh H, Sperelakis N (1998) Review of some actions of taurine on ion channels of cardiac muscle cells and others. Gen Pharmacol 30: 451–463.
34. L'Amoreaux WJ, Cuttitta C, Santora A, Blaize JF, Tachjadi J, et al. (2010) Taurine regulates insulin release from pancreatic beta cell lines. J Biomed Sci 17, Suppl 1: S1–S11.
35. Newsholme P, Bender K, Kiely A, Brennan L (2007) Amino acid metabolism, insulin secretion and diabetes. Biochem Soc Trans 35: 1180–1186.
36. Gleason CE, Lu D, Witters LA, Newgard CB, Birnbaum MJ (2007) The role of AMPK and mTOR in nutrient sensing in pancreatic beta-cells. J Biol Chem 282: 10341–10351.
37. Leclerc I, Sun G, Morris C, Fernandez-Millan E, Nyirenda M, et al. (2011) AMP-activated protein kinase regulates glucagon secretion from mouse pancreatic alpha cells. Diabetologia 54: 125–134.

38. Henningsson R, Lundquist I (1998) Arginine-induced insulin release is decreased and glucagon increased in parallel with islet NO production. Am J Physiol 275: E500–E506.
39. Henningsson R, Alm P, Lindström E, Lundquist I (2000) Chronic blockade of NO synthase paradoxically increases islet NO production and modulates islet hormone release. Am J Physiol Endocrinol Metab 279: E95–E107.
40. Salehi A, Meidute Abaraviciene S, Jimenez-Feltstrom J, Ostenson CG, Efendic S, et al. (2008) Excessive islet NO generation in type 2 diabetic GK rats coincides with abnormal hormone secretion and is counteracted by GLP-1. PLoS One 3: e2165.
41. Tokunaga H, Yoneda Y, Kuriyama K (1983) Streptozotocin-induced elevation of pancreatic taurine content and suppressive effect of taurine on insulin secretion. Eur J Pharmacol 87: 237–243.
42. Kulakowski EC, Maturo J (1984) Hypoglycemic properties of taurine: not mediated by enhanced insulin release. Biochem Pharmacol 33: 2835–2838.
43. Cherif H, Reusens B, Dahri S, Remacle C, Hoet JJ (1996) Stimulatory effects of taurine on insulin secretion by fetal rat islets cultured in vitro. J Endocrinol 151: 501–506.
44. Ribeiro RA, Bonfleur ML, Amaral AG, Vanzela EC, Rocco SA (2009) Taurine supplementation enhances nutrient-induced insulin secretion in pancreatic mice islets. Diabetes Metab Res Rev 25: 370–379.
45. Brès V, Hurbin A, Duvoid A, Orcel H, Moos FC, et al. (2000) Pharmacological characterization of volume-sensitive, taurine permeable anion channels in rat supraoptic glial cells. Br J Pharmacol 130: 1976–1982.
46. Zhang Q, Ramracheya R, Lahmann C, Tarasov A, Bengtsson M, et al. (2013) Role of KATP channels in glucose-regulated glucagon secretion and impaired counterregulation in type 2 diabetes. Cell Metab 18: 871–882.
47. Leung YM, Ahmed I, Sheu L, Gao X, Hara M, et al. (2006) Insulin regulates islet alpha-cell function by reducing K_{ATP} channel sensitivity to adenosine 5′-triphosphate inhibition. Endocrinology 147: 2155–2162.

Permissions

All chapters in this book were first published in PLOS ONE, by The Public Library of Science; hereby published with permission under the Creative Commons Attribution License or equivalent. Every chapter published in this book has been scrutinized by our experts. Their significance has been extensively debated. The topics covered herein carry significant findings which will fuel the growth of the discipline. They may even be implemented as practical applications or may be referred to as a beginning point for another development.

The contributors of this book come from diverse backgrounds, making this book a truly international effort. This book will bring forth new frontiers with its revolutionizing research information and detailed analysis of the nascent developments around the world.

We would like to thank all the contributing authors for lending their expertise to make the book truly unique. They have played a crucial role in the development of this book. Without their invaluable contributions this book wouldn't have been possible. They have made vital efforts to compile up to date information on the varied aspects of this subject to make this book a valuable addition to the collection of many professionals and students.

This book was conceptualized with the vision of imparting up-to-date information and advanced data in this field. To ensure the same, a matchless editorial board was set up. Every individual on the board went through rigorous rounds of assessment to prove their worth. After which they invested a large part of their time researching and compiling the most relevant data for our readers.

The editorial board has been involved in producing this book since its inception. They have spent rigorous hours researching and exploring the diverse topics which have resulted in the successful publishing of this book. They have passed on their knowledge of decades through this book. To expedite this challenging task, the publisher supported the team at every step. A small team of assistant editors was also appointed to further simplify the editing procedure and attain best results for the readers.

Apart from the editorial board, the designing team has also invested a significant amount of their time in understanding the subject and creating the most relevant covers. They scrutinized every image to scout for the most suitable representation of the subject and create an appropriate cover for the book.

The publishing team has been an ardent support to the editorial, designing and production team. Their endless efforts to recruit the best for this project, has resulted in the accomplishment of this book. They are a veteran in the field of academics and their pool of knowledge is as vast as their experience in printing. Their expertise and guidance has proved useful at every step. Their uncompromising quality standards have made this book an exceptional effort. Their encouragement from time to time has been an inspiration for everyone.

The publisher and the editorial board hope that this book will prove to be a valuable piece of knowledge for researchers, students, practitioners and scholars across the globe.

List of Contributors

Thomas U. Greiner
The Wallenberg Laboratory and Sahlgrenska Center for Cardiovascular and Metabolic Research, Department of Molecular and Clinical Medicine, Institute of Medicine, University of Gothenburg, Gothenburg, Sweden

Tuulia Hyötyläinen and Matej Orešič
VTT Technical Research Centre of Finland, Espoo, Finland
Steno Diabetes Center, Gentofte, Denmark

Mikael Knip
Children's Hospital, University of Helsinki and Helsinki University Central Hospital, Helsinki, Finland
Diabetes and Obesity Research Program, University of Helsinki, Helsinki, Finland
Folkhälsan Research Center, Helsinki, Finland
Department of Pediatrics, Tampere University Hospital, Tampere, Finland

Fredrik Bäckhed
The Wallenberg Laboratory and Sahlgrenska Center for Cardiovascular and Metabolic Research, Department of Molecular and Clinical Medicine, Institute of Medicine, University of Gothenburg, Gothenburg, Sweden
Novo Nordisk Foundation Center for Basic Metabolic Research, Section for Metabolic Receptology and Enteroendocrinology, Faculty of Health Sciences, University of Copenhagen, Copenhagen, Denmark

Sirin A. I. Adham, Hasina Al Rawahi and Sumaya Habib
Department of Biology, College of Science, Sultan Qaboos University, P. O. Box 36, 123 Muscat, Oman

Mansour S. Al Moundhri
Department of Medicine, College of Medicine, Sultan Qaboos University, P.O. Box 35, 123 Muscat, Oman

Alicia Viloria-Petit and Brenda L. Coomber
Department of Biomedical Sciences, Ontario Veterinary College, University of Guelph, Guelph, ON, Canada

Nicole Scheuing, Reinhard W. Holl and Julia M. Hermann
Institute of Epidemiology and Medical Biometry, Central Institute for Biomedical Technology, University of Ulm, Ulm, Germany

Gerd Dockter
Cystic Fibrosis Centre, Saarland University Hospital for Pediatric and Adolescent Medicine, Homburg/Saar, Germany

Sibylle Junge
Clinic for Pediatric Pneumology and Neonatology, Hannover Medical School, Hannover, Germany

Cordula Koerner-Rettberg and Manfred Ballmann
Department of Pediatric Pulmonology, St. Josef Hospital Pediatric Clinic, Ruhr University Bochum, Bochum, Germany

Lutz Naehrlich
Department of Pediatrics, Justus-Liebig University Giessen, Giessen, Germany

Christina Smaczny
Medical Clinic I, Pneumology and Allergology, University Hospital Frankfurt/Main, Goethe University, Frankfurt/Main, Germany

Doris Staab
Division of Pulmonology and Immunology, Department of Pediatrics, Charité Berlin, Berlin, Germany

Gabriela Thalhammer
Department for Pediatric Pulmonology and Allergology, Medical University of Graz, Graz, Austria

Silke van Koningsbruggen-Rietschel
Cystic Fibrosis Centre Cologne, Childrens Hospital, University of Cologne, Cologne, Germany

Ahmadou M. Jingi and Samuel Kingue
Department of Internal Medicine and Specialties, Faculty of Medicine and Biomedical Sciences, University of Yaoundé I, Yaoundé, Cameroon

Jean Jacques N. Noubiap
Internal Medicine Unit, Edéa Regional Hospital, Edéa, Cameroon

Arnold Ewane Onana
National Obesity Center, Yaoundé Central Hospital, Yaoundé, Cameroon

Jobert Richie N. Nansseu
Sickle Cell Unit, Mother and Child Centre, Chantal Biya Foundation, Yaoundé, Cameroon

Binhuan Wang
Department of Population Health, Division of Biostatistics, New York School of Medicine, New York, United States of America

André Pascal Kengne
Non-communicable Disease Research Unit, South African Medical Research Council and University of Cape Town, Cape Town, South Africa

Elena Tynkevich, Marie Metzger, Bénédicte Stengel
CESP, Centre for Epidemiology and Population Health, INSERM Unit 1018, Villejuif, France
University Paris-Sud 11, UMRS 1018, Villejuif, France

Martin Flamant
AP-HP, Hôpital Bichat, Department of Physiology, Paris, France

Jean-Philippe Haymann
AP-HP, Hôpital Tenon, Department of Physiology, Paris, France
INSERM UNIT 702, Paris, France
University Pierre et Marie Curie-Paris 6, UMRS 702, Paris, France

Eric Thervet
AP-HP, Hôpital Européen Georges Pompidou, Department of Nephrology, Paris, France
AP-HP, Hôpital Européen Georges Pompidou, DHU Common and Rare Arterial Diseases, Paris, France

Jean-Jacques Boffa
INSERM UNIT 702, Paris, France, 6 University Pierre et Marie Curie-Paris
University Pierre et Marie Curie-Paris 6, UMRS 702, Paris, France
AP-HP, Hôpital Tenon, Department of Nephrology, Paris, France

François Vrtovsnik
AP-HP, Hôpital Bichat, Department of Nephrology, Paris, France

Pascal Houillier
University Paris Descartes-Paris 5, UMRS 775, Paris, France
AP-HP, Hôpital Européen Georges Pompidou, Department of Physiology, Paris, France

Marc Froissart
CESP, Centre for Epidemiology and Population Health, INSERM Unit 1018, Villejuif, France

Nuha Mahmoud Hamdi
Immunology Department, Riyadh Regional Laboratory, King Saud Medical Complex, Riyadh, Kingdom of Saudi Arabia

Fadel Hassan Al-Hababi
Virology Department, Riyadh Regional Laboratory, King Saud Medical Complex, Riyadh, Kingdom of Saudi Arabia

Amr Ekhlas Eid
Nephrology Department, Riyadh Medical Complex, King Saud Medical Complex, Riyadh, Kingdom of Saudi Arabia

Teresa Tamayo and Wolfgang Rathmann
Institute of Biometrics and Epidemiology, German Diabetes Center, Leibniz Center for Diabetes Research at Heinrich-Heine-University, Düsseldorf, Germany
Competence Network Diabetes mellitus (Federal Ministry of Education
and Research, Germany), Sites Düsseldorf, Munich and Greifswald, Germany

Sabine Schipf
Institute for Community Medicine, University Medicine Greifswald, Greifswald, Germany
Competence Network Diabetes mellitus (Federal Ministry of Education
and Research, Germany), Sites Düsseldorf, Munich and Greifswald, Germany

Christine Meisinger
Helmholtz Zentrum München, German Research Center for Environmental Health, Institute of Epidemiology II, Neuherberg, Germany
Competence Network Diabetes mellitus (Federal Ministry of Education and Research, Germany), Sites Düsseldorf, Munich and Greifswald, Germany

Michaela Schunk and Werner Maier
Helmholtz Zentrum München, German Research Center for Environmental Health, Institute of Health Economics and Health Care Management, Neuherberg, Germany
Competence Network Diabetes mellitus (Federal Ministry of Education and Research, Germany), Sites Düsseldorf, Munich and Greifswald, Germany

Christian Herder
Institute for Clinical Diabetology, German Diabetes Center, Leibniz Center for Diabetes Research at Heinrich-Heine- University, Düsseldorf, Germany
German Center for Diabetes Research (DZD e.V.), Sites Düsseldorf and Munich, Germany

Michael Roden
Institute for Clinical Diabetology, German Diabetes Center, Leibniz Center for Diabetes Research at Heinrich-Heine- University, Düsseldorf, Germany
Department of Endocrinology and Diabetology, University Hospital Düsseldorf, Düsseldorf, Germany
German Center for Diabetes Research (DZD e.V.), Sites Düsseldorf and Munich, Germany

Matthias Nauck,
Institute of Clinical Chemistry and Laboratory Medicine, University Medicine Greifswald, Greifswald, Germany
Competence Network Diabetes mellitus (Federal Ministry of Education and Research, Germany), Sites Düsseldorf, Munich and Greifswald, Germany

Annette Peters
Helmholtz Zentrum München, German Research Center for Environmental Health, Institute of Epidemiology II, Neuherberg, Germany
German Center for Diabetes Research (DZD e.V.), Sites Düsseldorf and Munich, Germany
German Center of Cardiovascular Research (DZHK e.V.), Sites Munich and Greifswald, Germany

Henry Völzke
Institute for Community Medicine, University Medicine Greifswald, Greifswald, Germany
German Center of Cardiovascular Research (DZHK e.V.), Sites Munich and Greifswald, Germany
Competence Network Diabetes mellitus (Federal Ministry of Education and Research, Germany), Sites Düsseldorf, Munich and Greifswald, Germany

Sinna P. Ulrichsen, Anil Mor, Elisabeth Svensson and Reimar W. Thomsen
Department of Clinical Epidemiology, Faculty of Health, Aarhus University Hospital, Aarhus, Denmark

Finn B. Larsen
Centre for Public Health and Quality Improvement, Central Denmark Region, Aarhus, Denmark

Miaoxin Chen
Robinson Research Institute, School of Paediatrics and Reproductive Health, The University of Adelaide, Adelaide, Australia, 5005
Department of Obstetrics and Gynaecology, The Affiliated Hospital of Guiyang Medical College, Guiyang, China, 550004
Discipline of Medicine, The University of Adelaide, Adelaide, Australia, 5005

Linda Wu, Robert J. Norman and Rebecca L. Robker
Robinson Research Institute, School of Paediatrics and Reproductive Health

Fang Wu
Discipline of Medicine, The University of Adelaide, Adelaide, Australia, 5005
Department of Emergency, The Affiliated Hospital of Guiyang Medical College, Guiyang, China, 550004

Gary A. Wittert
Discipline of Medicine, The University of Adelaide, Adelaide, Australia, 5005

Leonie K. Heilbronn
Robinson Research Institute, School of Paediatrics and Reproductive Health
Discipline of Medicine, The University of Adelaide, Adelaide, Australia, 5005

I-Ting Chow, Junbao Yang, Theresa J. Gates, Eddie A. James, Duy T. Mai and Carla Greenbaum
Benaroya Research Institute at Virginia Mason, Seattle, WA, United States of America

William W. Kwok
Benaroya Research Institute at Virginia Mason, Seattle, WA, United States of America
Department of Medicine, University of Washington, Seattle, WA, United States of America

Teresa Oviedo Socarrás
Department of General Pathology, Institute of Biological Sciences, Federal University of Minas Gerais, Belo Horizonte, Minas Gerais, Brazil
Department of Livestock Sciences, University of Córdoba, Montería, Córdoba, Colombia

Anilton C. Vasconcelos, Paula P. Campos, Nubia B. Pereira and Jessica P. C. Souza
Department of General Pathology, Institute of Biological Sciences, Federal University of Minas Gerais, Belo Horizonte, Minas Gerais, Brazil

Silvia P. Andrade
Department of Physiology and Biophysics, Institute of Biological Sciences, Federal University of Minas Gerais, Belo Horizonte, Minas Gerais, Brazil

Yérali Gandica and Orlando Oliveira
Center for Computational Physics, Department of Physics, University of Coimbra, Coimbra, Portugal

Tobias Schwarz
Center for Computational Physics, Department of Physics, University of Coimbra, Coimbra, Portugal
Heinz-Brandt-Schule, Berlin, Germany

Rui D. M. Travasso
Center for Computational Physics, Department of Physics, University of Coimbra, Coimbra, Portugal
Center of Ophthalmology and Vision Sciences(COCV), Institute for Biomedical Imaging and Life Sciences (IBILI), Faculty of Medicine, University of Coimbra, Coimbra, Portugal

Haruka Nagasaki, Tokio Katsumata, Pei-Han Tai, Yukari Sekiguchi,

Ryusuke Koshida, Yunshin Jung and Takashi Kudo
Department of Anatomy and Embryology, Faculty of Medicine, University of Tsukuba, Tsukuba, Ibaraki, Japan

Hisashi Oishi
Department of Anatomy and Embryology, Faculty of Medicine, University of Tsukuba, Tsukuba, Ibaraki, Japan
Life Science Center, Tsukuba Advanced Research Alliance (TARA), University of Tsukuba, Tsukuba, Ibaraki, Japan

Satoru Takahashi
Department of Anatomy and Embryology, Faculty of Medicine, University of Tsukuba, Tsukuba, Ibaraki, Japan
Life Science Center, Tsukuba Advanced Research Alliance (TARA), University of Tsukuba, Tsukuba, Ibaraki, Japan
International Institute for Integrative Sleep Medicine (WPI-IIIS), University of Tsukuba, Tsukuba, Ibaraki, Japan

Antonia Garcia-Martín
Bone Metabolic Unit (RETICEF), Endocrinology Division, Hospital Universitario San Cecilio, Instituto de Investigación Biosanitaria de Granada, Granada, Spain
Endocrinology, Hospital Comarcal del Noroeste, Caravaca de la Cruz, Murcia, Spain

Rebeca Reyes-Garcia
Bone Metabolic Unit (RETICEF), Endocrinology Division, Hospital Universitario San Cecilio, Instituto de Investigacio´n Biosanitaria de Granada, Granada, Spain
Endocrinology Unit, Hospital General Universitario Rafael Mendez, Lorca, Murcia, Spain

Beatriz García-Fontana and Manuel Muñoz-Torres
Bone Metabolic Unit (RETICEF), Endocrinology Division, Hospital Universitario San Cecilio, Instituto de Investigación Biosanitaria de Granada, Granada, Spain

Sonia Morales-Santana
Bone Metabolic Unit (RETICEF), Endocrinology Division, Hospital Universitario San Cecilio, Instituto de Investigacio´n Biosanitaria de Granada, Granada, Spain
Proteomic Research Service, Fundación para la Investigación Biosanitaria de Andalucía Oriental -Alejandro Otero- (FIBAO), Granada, Spain

Ana Coto-Montes
Department of Morphology and Cellular Biology (RETICEF), Faculty of Medicine, University of Oviedo, Oviedo, Spain

Manuel Muñoz-Garach
Critical Care and Emergencies Unit, Hospital Universitario San Cecilio, Granada, Spain

Pedro Rozas-Moreno
Endocrinology Division, Hospital General de Ciudad Real, Ciudad Real, Spain

Sebastian Kummer, Ertan Mayatepek and Thomas Meissner
Department of General Pediatrics, Neonatology and Pediatric Cardiology, University Children's Hospital, Duesseldorf, Germany

Anna Stahl-Pehe, Katty Castillo, Christina Bächle, Klaus Straßburger,

Guido Giani and Joachim Rosenbauer
Institute for Biometrics and Epidemiology, German Diabetes Center (DDZ), Leibniz Institute for Diabetes Research at Heinrich Heine University, Duesseldorf, Germany

Christine Graf
Institute of Movement and Neurosciences, German Sport University, Cologne, Germany

Burak Salgin
Department of Paediatrics, Cambridge University, Addenbrooke's Hospital, Cambridge, United Kingdom

Reinhard W. Holl
Institute for Epidemiology and Medical Biometry, University of Ulm, Ulm, Germany

Ligia Petrica, Gheorghe Gluhovschi, Florica Gadalean, Cristina Gluhovschi, Silvia Velciov and Flaviu Bob
"Victor Babes" University of Medicine and Pharmacy, Dept. of Nephrology, Timisoara, Romania
County Emergency Hospital, Timisoara, Romania

Adrian Vlad
"Victor Babes" University of Medicine and Pharmacy, Dept. of Diabetes and Metabolic Diseases, Timisoara, Romania
County Emergency Hospital, Timisoara, Romania

Victor Dumitrascu and Daliborca Vlad
"Victor Babes" University of Medicine and Pharmacy, Department of Pharmacology, Timisoara, Romania
County Emergency Hospital, Timisoara, Romania

Roxana Popescu
"Victor Babes" University of Medicine and Pharmacy, Dept. of Cellular Biology, Timisoara, Romania
County Emergency Hospital, Timisoara, Romania

Oana Milas
County Emergency Hospital, Timisoara, Romania

Sorin Ursoniu
"Victor Babes" University of Medicine and Pharmacy, Dept. of Public Health Medicine, Timisoara, Romania

Yuzhi Ding, Songtao Yuan, Xiaoyi Liu, Chen Zhao, Yuan Fang, Qinglu Song, Dongqing Yuan, Ping Xie and Qinghuai Liu
Department of Ophthalmology, The First Affiliated Hospital of Nanjing Medical University, Nanjing, China

Pingan Mao
Department of Ophthalmology, No. 2 People's Hospital of Changzhou, Changzhou, China

Qiong Huang, Rihua Zhang and Yun Liu
Department of Endocrinology, The First Affiliated Hospital of Nanjing Medical University, Nanjing, China

Dorit Samocha-Bonet and Donald J. Chisholm
Diabetes and Metabolism Division, Garvan Institute of Medical Research, Sydney, Australia
Faculty of Medicine, UNSW (The University of New South Wales), Sydney, Australia

Fiona M. Gribble
Cambridge Institute of Medical Research and Department of Clinical Biochemistry, University of Cambridge, Cambridge, United Kingdom

Adelle C. F. Coster
School of Mathematics and Statistics, UNSW (The University of New South Wales), Sydney, Australia

Kevin H. Carpenter
Disciplines of Genetic Medicine & Paediatrics and Child Health, University of Sydney, Sydney, Australia

Graham R. D. Jones
Faculty of Medicine, UNSW (The University of New South Wales), Sydney, Australia
Department of Chemical Pathology, St. Vincent's Hospital, Sydney, Australia,

Jens J. Holst
NNF Center for Basic Metabolic Research, Department of Biomedical Sciences, University of Copenhagen, Panum Institute, Copenhagen, Denmark

Jerry R. Greenfield
Diabetes and Metabolism Division, Garvan Institute of Medical Research, Sydney, Australia
Faculty of Medicine, UNSW (The University of New South Wales), Sydney, Australia
Department of Endocrinology and Diabetes Center, St. Vincent's Hospital, Sydney, Australia

Matthias Oelze, Swenja Kröller-Schön, Philipp Welschof, Thomas Jansen, Michael Hausding, Yuliya Mikhed, Paul Stamm, Michael Mader, Elena Zinßius, Saule Agdauletova, Anna Gottschlich, Sebastian Steven, Eberhard Schulz, Thomas Münzel and Andreas Daiber
2nd Medical Clinic, Department of Cardiology, Medical Center of the Johannes Gutenberg University, Mainz, Germany

Serge P. Bottari
Laboratory of Fundamental and Applied, Bioenergetics, INSERM U1055, Grenoble-Alpes Universitéet Pôle de Biologie, CHU, Grenoble, France

Eric Mayoux
Boehringer Ingelheim Pharma GmbH & Co. KG, Ingelheim, Germany

Panchalli Wang
Department of Obstetrics and Gynecology, Ditmanson Medical Foundation Chia-Yi Christian Hospital, Chia-Yi City, Taiwan

Mei-Chun Lu
Department of Obstetrics and Gynecology, Ditmanson Medical Foundation Chia-Yi Christian Hospital, Chia-Yi City, Taiwan
Department of Medical Research, Ditmanson Medical Foundation Chia-Yi Christian Hospital, Chia-Yi City, Taiwan

Cheng-Wei Yu
Department of Nutrition, Ditmanson Medical Foundation Chia-Yi Christian Hospital, Chia- Yi City, Taiwan

Yuan-Horng Yan
Department of Medical Research, Ditmanson Medical Foundation Chia-Yi Christian Hospital, Chia-Yi City, Taiwan
Department of Internal Medicine, Ditmanson Medical Foundation Chia-Yi Christian Hospital, Chia-Yi City, Taiwan
Institute of Occupational Medicine and Industrial Hygiene, College of Public Health, National Taiwan University, Taipei, Taiwan

Peiyao Jin, Jinjuan Peng, XunXu and Xi Zhang
Department of Ophthalmology, Shanghai First People's Hospital, Shanghai Jiao Tong University, Shanghai, 20080, China

Haidong Zou
Department of Ophthalmology, Shanghai First People's Hospital, Shanghai Jiao Tong University, Shanghai, 20080, China
Department of Preventative Ophthalmology, Shanghai Eye Disease Prevention and Treatment Center, Shanghai, 200040, China

Weiwei Wang, Jiong Fu, Binjie Shen and Xuelin Bai
Beixinjing Community Health Service Center, Shanghai, China

Chi-Sheng Hung, Mao-Shin Lin, Shyang-Rong Shih, Jyh-Ming Liou, Lee-Ming Chuang, Ming-Fong Chen and Hung-Yuan Li
Department of Internal Medicine, National Taiwan University Hospital, Taipei, Taiwan

Jen-Kuang Lee
Department of Clinical Pathology, Far Eastern Memorial Hospital, New Taipei City, Taiwan

Chung-Yi Yang
Department of Medical Imaging, National Taiwan University Hospital and National Taiwan University College of Medicine, Taipei, Taiwan

Hung-Ren Hsieh
Department of Radiology, National Taiwan University Hospital Yun-Lin Branch, Yun-Lin, Taiwan

Wen-Ya Ma
Division of Endocrinology, Department of Internal Medicine, Cardinal Tien Hospital, Xindian, Taiwan

Pi-Hua Liu
Clinical Informatics and Medical Statistics Research Center, Chang Gung University, Gueishan, Taiwan

Jou-Wei Lin
Department of Internal Medicine, National Taiwan University Hospital Yun-Lin Branch, Yun-Lin, Taiwan

Jung-Nan Wei
Chia Nan University of Pharmacy and Science, Tainan, Taiwan

Te-Chuan Chen
Division of Nephrology, Kaohsiung Chang Gung Memorial Hospital and Chang Gung University College of Medicine, Kaohsiung, Taiwan

Mao-Ling Sung and Chia-Kuang Yen
Department of Cardiology, St. Martin De Porres Hospital, Chiayi, Taiwan

Hsing-Chun Kuo
Institute of Nursing and Department of Nursing, Chang Gung University of Science and Technology, Chronic Diseases and Health Promotion Research Center, CGUST, Taoyuan, Taiwan
Research Center for Industry of Human Ecology, Chang Gung University of Science and Technology, Taoyuan, Taiwan

Shao-Ju Chien
Division of Pediatric Cardiology, Department of Pediatrics, Kaohsiung Chang Gung Memorial Hospital, Chang Gung University College of Medicine, Kaohsiung, Taiwan

Cheng-Nan Chen
Department of Biochemical Science and Technology, National Chiayi University, Chiayi, Taiwan

Megumi Bessho, Yuko Murase-Mishiba Jungo Terasaki and Toshiaki Hanafusa
Department of Internal Medicine (I), Osaka Medical College, Osaka, Japan

Akihisa Imagawa
Department of Internal Medicine (I), Osaka Medical College, Osaka, Japan
Department of Metabolic Medicine, Graduate School of Medicine, Osaka University, Osaka, Japan

Index

A

Acetylsalicylic Acid, 31-32

Adipose Tissue, 11, 20, 81, 192-193, 196, 198-199

Alcohol Intake, 69-70, 72-77, 125

Aldose Reductase, 150-151, 155-157

Anesthesia, 2, 80, 98, 166

Angiogenesis, 21, 97-98, 102, 104-107, 112-114, 207

Artificial Organs, 97, 103

Atherosclerosis, 45-46, 124-125, 127-130, 173, 176, 200, 203, 206-207

Autoantibodies, 2, 9, 88-89, 95

Autoimmune Diabetes, 1, 5, 7, 9-10

B

Beta Cells, 1, 88, 122

Blastocysts, 80, 83, 86

Blood Glucose, 1-2, 4-5, 7, 11, 22-26, 61, 84, 98, 102, 118, 121, 141, 151-153, 160, 162, 165, 168, 170, 175, 183, 186, 221

Blood Pressure, 37-38, 62-63, 65, 82-83, 86-87, 125-126, 135, 145, 159-161, 185-190, 192-198

Blood Sugar, 28, 30, 32

Blood Vessel, 107, 113

Body Mass Index, 23, 25, 36-38, 42-43, 45, 62-63, 72-76, 126, 128, 132, 145, 178-182, 195-197, 201

Bone Mineral Density, 124, 126-128, 130

Breast Cancer, 11-13, 15-21

C

Cancer Cells, 11-12, 16-21, 205

Carbohydrate, 11, 20, 23, 80, 160

Cardiovascular Disease, 28, 30, 35, 46, 48, 61, 78-79, 83, 124-130, 166, 176, 199, 207

Cell Morphology, 14, 16-17, 19

Cell Proliferation, 18, 20, 155, 158, 200-203, 205-207, 210, 216

Cholesterol, 30, 32, 37-38, 42-43, 61-63, 127, 145, 167-168, 170, 175, 186-187, 192-199, 201

Chronic Infections, 23

Chronic Kidney Disease, 36-37, 39, 41, 43, 45-47, 59, 125-126, 130, 143, 148, 199

Connective Tissue, 97, 102, 105

Coronary Heart Disease, 28, 34, 36, 46, 87, 126-128

Ct Scan, 194

Cystic Fibrosis, 22-23, 25-27, 137, 141

D

Diabetic Nephropathy, 50, 53, 142, 148-149, 156, 176

Diabetic Retinopathy, 107-108, 112-114, 150-151, 153-157, 185, 187-191

Dislipidaemia, 127-128

E

Endocrine Cells, 115, 208

Endothelial Cells, 19, 100, 107, 125, 128, 130, 173, 200, 207

Epithelial Ovarian Cancer, 12

Extracellular Matrix, 11, 102, 104, 113

G

Glomerulonephritis, 48, 50, 59

Glucose Metabolism, 1, 4, 7, 9, 22, 24, 26, 79-81, 83, 85, 87, 183

Glucose Tolerance Test, 2, 9, 22-25, 27, 60-61, 115, 118, 178-179, 183-184, 193, 195, 197

Glucose-lowering Drugs, 69-77

Glucotoxicity, 165-166, 173, 175

Granulation Tissue, 97, 102-103

Gut Microbiota, 1-3, 5, 7, 9-10

H

Haematoxylin, 2, 167

Haptoglobin, 37-38, 41-42, 44

Hemoglobin, 26, 97-98, 100, 104, 108, 126-127, 158-159, 163, 166, 186, 193, 195, 197, 199, 201

Hormonal Therapy, 12, 129

Human Leukocyte Antigen, 1

Hydrochlorothiazide, 31-32

Hypertension, 28-29, 33, 35, 37, 47-48, 50, 68, 79, 86, 106, 125-128, 173, 176, 185-189, 192-199

Hypoglycemia, 11-20, 140, 207-208, 221

I

Insulin Therapy, 24, 134, 188

Intracellular Cytokine, 89, 93, 95

Islet Autoimmunity, 1-2, 5

K

Kidney Transplant, 37, 59

L

Liver Disease, 125

Lung Transplantation, 22-23, 26

M
Mast Cells, 97, 100-105
Metabolic Acidosis, 37, 39, 41, 46
Metabolome, 2, 7, 208-211, 213, 215-217, 219, 221
Mitochondrial Dna, 81-82, 86
Monoclonal Antibodies, 1, 201
Mononuclear Cells, 88-89, 98, 201
Myocardial Infarction, 71, 124-125, 129-130, 200

N
Neovascularization, 98, 112, 190
Normoxia, 12, 20, 109

O
Orosomucoid, 37-38, 41-42, 44
Osteoporosis, 124-130
Ovarian Hyperstimulation, 79, 83, 86
Oxidative Stress, 86, 155-157, 162, 165-167, 170-171, 173, 175-177, 206
Oxphos, 81-82, 85

P
Pancreas, 1-2, 4, 9, 67, 84, 88, 107, 115, 122-123, 131, 193, 209
Physical Exercise, 69-70, 72-77
Plasma Fibrinogen, 37-38, 41-42, 44
Preimplantation Embryo, 79, 82, 87
Proteinuria, 30, 32, 36, 38, 41-45, 143, 148, 188

R
Renal Function, 37, 44, 78, 143-144, 148, 160
Retinal Ganglion Cell, 150, 154, 156

S
Skeletal Muscle, 37, 46, 86, 131, 219, 221
Stem Cell, 1, 116, 205
Streptozotocin, 97-98, 102, 115-116, 121-122, 151, 156, 165-166, 176, 207, 222
Sulfonylureas, 70-77, 186

U
Urinary Creatinine, 36-46

V
Vascular Dysfunction, 86, 165-167, 169, 171, 173, 175-177
Vascular Network, 107-109, 112-113
Virus Infection, 47